Practical Guide to
Chronic Pain
Syndromes

Practical Guide to
Chronic Pain
Syndromes

Edited by
Gary W. Jay
Pfizer, Inc.
New London, Connecticut, USA

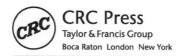

CRC Press
Taylor & Francis Group
Boca Raton London New York

CRC Press is an imprint of the
Taylor & Francis Group, an **informa** business

CRC Press
Taylor & Francis Group
6000 Broken Sound Parkway NW, Suite 300
Boca Raton, FL 33487-2742

First issued in paperback 2017

© 2010 by Taylor & Francis Group, LLC
CRC Press is an imprint of Taylor & Francis Group, an Informa business

No claim to original U.S. Government works

ISBN-13: 978-1-4200-8045-2 (hbk)
ISBN-13: 978-1-138-11214-8 (pbk)

Library of Congress Cataloging-in-Publication Data

Practical guide to chronic pain syndromes / edited by Gary W. Jay.
    p. ; cm.
    Includes bibliographical references and index.
    ISBN-13: 978-1-4200-8045-2 (hardcover : alk. paper)
    ISBN-10: 1-4200-8045-8 (hardcover : alk. paper)   1. Chronic pain. I. Jay,
Gary W.
    [DNLM: 1. Pain. 2. Chronic Disease. 3. Syndrome.
WL 704 P8949 2009]
   RB127 .P725 2009
   616'.0472–dc22

                          2009035194

Visit the Taylor & Francis Web site at
http://www.taylorandfrancis.com

and the CRC Press Web site at
http://www.crcpress.com

Foreword

Pain specialists, noninterventionalists, primary care physicians, medical specialists, fellows, residents, and medical students all want to make clinical decisions about pain efficiently, often with an incomplete knowledge of underlying pathophysiology, while addressing global needs of their patients. Pain management is not part of the routine training for most physicians, yet the majority of patients seek medical attention because they have pain. Pain is typically addressed by primary care practitioners on an acute, time-limited basis, but when first- and second-level strategies fail, patients are referred to pain specialists and/or disease or body system specialists for more thorough evaluation and management. Primary care physicians, typically the first stopping point for patients in pain, as well as specialists from anesthesiology, internal medicine subspecialties, neurology, physical medicine, and psychiatry must be prepared to help people suffering with chronic pain disorders.

Pain and other medical specialists as well as primary care physicians managing patients having chronic pain know that usual acute pain management strategies do not address complex needs of people having many years of continuous pain. Interventionalists focus on performing procedures intended to interrupt pain processing, while medically oriented practitioners skillfully blend multiple medications, many of which primary care physicians are not comfortable prescribing (especially methadone). The field of modern pain management has become highly procedural, often relying upon opioids, involving the use of polypharmacy and the management of patients within multidisciplinary pain clinics.

Dr. Gary Jay and contributors to this book, *Practical Guide to Chronic Pain Syndromes*, have collectively demystified chronic pain, bringing the management of people with persisting pain into the understanding of pain medicine and other specialists. The chapter authors have prepared essential reviews focusing on the information most needed by specialists, fellows, residents, and medical students to confidently and competently manage complex people in pain. In the various pain disorder sections, chapters focus on common, but potentially vexing painful disorders: soft tissue pain syndromes, neuropathic pain, rheumatologic pain, urologic pain, back pain, cancer pain, end-of-life pain, and pain from other causes. In the second section, pharmacologic options are discussed: nonopioid analgesics and adjuvants, opioids, antidepressants, and anticonvulsants, with special attention to the legal aspects for prescribing controlled substances.

Today's specialists evaluating and treating people in pain are medical detectives. They make sense out of painful complaints by following clues, seeing patterns, laying their hands upon their patients, using scientific methods, while balancing clinical suspicion, intuition, and compassion. People living with chronic pain may wish for absolute pain relief, but they are grateful for any pain relief and the opportunity to receive care from clinicians demonstrating concern and ability.

Practical Guide to Chronic Pain Syndromes is a "go to" book when information is needed concisely about some aspect of chronic pain. This book focuses on what matters most for busy clinicians: presentation of chronic pain syndromes, common causes and underlying pathophysiologic mechanisms, differential diagnosis, diagnostic assessment methods (e.g., laboratory studies, imaging, and electrodiagnostic testing), and recommended treatments. While much is said about the importance of evidence-based treatment, for many chronic pain syndromes there are limited well-controlled and randomized studies. The contributors have taken care to keep their messages practical, and readers are sure to find this book one they will keep close at hand.

B. Eliot Cole, MD, MPA
Montclair, New Jersey, U.S.A.

Preface

Chronic pain syndromes (CPS) are complex problems that present a major challenge to health care providers. They are biological, psychological, and sociological in nature, may have an unclear etiology, and, frequently, poor responses to therapy. CPS, if treated in a typical mono- or bimodality manner may not give the patient the best treatment outcome, but as things are now, that may be the best that can be done for these difficult patients. Even the definition of a CPS (of any kind) may be considered unsettled, as some look at it as pain that persists more than three months, while others consider chronic pain to begin after six months. Pain that persists after physiological healing has occurred, typically in three months, posttreatment, for example, tells us nothing new—it becomes an entity in and of itself. The best way to treat it is to understand the complex interactions of the pathophysiology of pain as well as the issues of the psychological and sociological aspects of an individual patient's pain, and deal with it all as best as one can.

The purpose of this book is to give the practitioner the basics and more regarding a number of important, not uncommon, CPS that pain specialists, as well as other medical specialists see. Sometimes the most difficult issue is diagnosis—Clinically speaking, pain is what the patient says it is, and it is up to the clinician to determine what the patient means. Then the treatment phase begins and this may engender the use/need of chronic opioids, physical therapy, and psychological therapy—whatever it may take to help your patient's chronic pain problems.

Chronic pain can be considered to be like diabetes or hypertension—a disease that can be treated and controlled, but not necessarily cured.

Practical Guide to Chronic Pain Syndromes has been written for the noninterventional pain specialist as well as for other physicians who treat chronic pain of one, two, or multiple types. All of the pain syndrome chapters have information on a specific disorder, the pathophysiology, the treatment, any evidence-based medicine issues and, of course, up to date references.

I have elected to place the largest section, "Neuropathic Pain," first. This is followed by a section on probably the most common pain problems: the soft tissue pain syndromes including myofascial pain and fibromyalgia. One of the most frequently missed problems in my longer than a quarter century of patient care is the piriformis syndrome, which is also discussed in detail. Mechanical and neuropathic low back pain are also discussed in detail.

Many times, pain specialists are asked to deal with visceral pain syndromes such as interstitial cystitis and vulvovestibulitis, which are discussed by experts, along with prostatitis.

Cancer pain and palliative care are ever-growing issues and separate chapters dealing with both are included.

The section titled "Other Pain Syndromes" includes chapters on osteoarthritis, electrical injury, and neurogenic thoracic outlet syndrome.

Finally, no book would be complete, practical, and useful if it did not include a medications section.

I want to thank the many erudite, patient focused, and excellent contributors to this textbook. It was an honor and a pleasure to work with you!

It was a long road to get to here, and I believe it has been well worth it for the pain specialists, neurologists, anesthesiologists, physiatrists, urologists, rheumatologists, oncologists, general practitioners, internists, psychologists, nurses, physical therapists, as well as the residents and fellows and others who may benefit from the knowledge contained in these books.

Most of all, our patients should receive the ultimate benefit of this work.

Gary W. Jay, MD

Acknowledgments

First, as always, I want to thank my wonderful wife Suzanne and my incredible daughter Samantha for their love and patience with me during the extended period of time I spent working on this book. Many thanks also go to Byron Scott, R.Ph., my brother by choice, and one of the smartest and best people in the world to talk to; David Longmire, MD, another brother by choice, for his rather droll wit and strange ability to look just like my doppelganger with neither ability getting in the way of his amazing knowledge of neurology (with, of course, special attention to the Autonomic Nervous System); to my new friends at Pfizer (you know who you are) and, of course, to the thousands of patients I had the good fortune to meet, diagnose and treat- you were all my best teachers. After 25 years of clinical practice, when I made the choice to go into Pharma, I knew I would miss you all and I do.

Finally, this book is dedicated to Jim Kapp, who left us all too soon.

Contents

Foreword   *B. Eliot Cole* .... *v*
Preface .... *vii*
Acknowledgments .... *ix*
Contributors .... *xv*

PART I NEUROPATHIC PAIN SYNDROMES

1. **Diabetic Peripheral Neuropathy**   *1*
   Gordon Irving and Richard Irving

2. **HIV/AIDS Neuropathy**   *15*
   Vasanthi Arumugam and Maurice Policar

3. **Central Poststroke Pain**   *23*
   Gary W. Jay

4. **Postherpetic Neuralgia**   *30*
   Rajbala Thakur, Annie G. Philip, and Jonathan C. Weeks

5. **Management of Pain Related to Amputation**   *50*
   Steven Stanos

6. **Pathophysiology of Complex Regional Pain Syndrome**   *62*
   Robert J. Schwartzman

7. **Meralgia Paresthetica**   *81*
   Elizabeth A. Sekul

8. **Compression Neuropathies**   *85*
   Gabriel E. Sella

9. **Quantitative Clinical, Sensory, and Autonomic Testing
   of Chronic Neuropathic Pain**   *102*
   David R. Longmire

PART II SOFT TISSUE PAIN SYNDROMES

10. **The Myofascial Pain Syndrome**   *115*
   Gary W. Jay

11. Piriformis Syndrome   *140*
Gary W. Jay

12. Fibromyalgia   *144*
Gary W. Jay

PART III LOW BACK PAIN

13. Low Back Pain and Sciatica: Pathogenesis, Diagnosis
and Nonoperative Treatment   *181*
Anthony H. Wheeler

14. Neuropathic Low Back Pain   *206*
Joseph F. Audette, Joseph Walker III, and Alec L. Meleger

PART IV GENITOURINARY PAIN SYNDROMES

15. Interstitial Cystitis   *228*
Neel Shah, Hossein Sadeghi-Nejad, and Robert Moldwin

16. Chronic Prostatitis/Chronic Pelvic Pain Syndrome—A Urologist's
Perspective   *242*
Richard A. Watson and Hossein Sadeghi-Nejad

17. Female Chronic Pelvic Pain   *261*
Frank F. Tu, Sangeeta Senapati, Gregory Goldstein, and Alexandra Roybal

PART V CANCER PAIN AND PALLIATIVE CARE

18. Cancer Pain   *271*
Judith A. Paice

19. Palliative Care Pain Management   *285*
Kathleen Broglio

PART VI OTHER CHRONIC PAIN SYNDROMES

20. Chronic Pain Following Electrical Injury   *301*
Elena N. Bodnar

21. Neurogenic Thoracic Outlet Syndrome—A Biopsychosocial Approach
312
Allen J. Togut

22. Osteoarthritis   *318*
Thomas J. Romano

PART VII MEDICATIONS

23. Nonopiate Analgesics and Adjuvants *327*
Gary W. Jay

24. Opioid Medications and Correct Medical Usage—An Update *343*
Gary W. Jay

25. Legal Issues in Pain Management *367*
Jennifer Bolen

26. Antidepressant Medications *391*
Gary W. Jay

27. Anticonvulsant Medications *397*
Gary W. Jay

Index *407*

Contributors

Vasanthi Arumugam   Elmhurst Hospital Center, Mount Sinai School of Medicine, Elmhurst, New York, U.S.A.

Joseph F. Audette   Department of Physical Medicine and Rehabilitation, Spaulding Rehabilitation Hospital, Harvard Medical School, Boston, Massachusetts, U.S.A.

Elena N. Bodnar   Electrical Trauma Program, Department of Surgery, The University of Chicago, Chicago, Illinois, U.S.A.

Jennifer Bolen   The Legal Side of Pain®, The J. Bolen Group, LLC, Knoxville, Tennessee, U.S.A.

Kathleen Broglio   New York University School of Medicine, Bellevue Pain Center, New York, New York, U.S.A.

Gregory Goldstein   Northwestern University, Evanston, Illinois, U.S.A.

Gordon Irving   Swedish Pain and Headache Center and University of Washington Medical School, Seattle, Washington, U.S.A.

Richard Irving   Department of Electrical Engineering, University of Washington, Seattle, Washington, U.S.A.

Gary W. Jay   Clinical Disease Area Expert-Pain, Pfizer, Inc., New London, Connecticut, U.S.A.

David R. Longmire   Department of Internal Medicine, University of Alabama at Birmingham School of Medicine, Huntsville Regional Medical Campus, Huntsville, Alabama, U.S.A.

Robert Moldwin   Pelvic Pain Center, The Arthur Smith Institute for Urology; Long Island Jewish Medical Center, New Hyde Park, New York, U.S.A.

Alec L. Meleger   Department of Physical Medicine and Rehabilitation, Spaulding Rehabilitation Hospital, Harvard Medical School, Boston, Massachusetts, U.S.A.

Judith A. Paice   Cancer Pain Program, Division of Hematology–Oncology, Feinberg School of Medicine, Northwestern University, Chicago, Illinois, U.S.A.

Annie G. Philip   Department of Anesthesiology, University of Rochester School of Medicine and Dentistry, Rochester, New York, U.S.A.

Maurice Policar   Elmhurst Hospital Center, Mount Sinai School of Medicine, Elmhurst, New York, U.S.A.

Thomas J. Romano   Private Practice, Martins Ferry, Ohio, U.S.A.

Alexandra Roybal   Northwestern University, Evanston, Illinois, U.S.A.

Hossein Sadeghi-Nejad   UMDNJ New Jersey Medical School, Newark; Hackensack University Medical Center, Hackensack; and VA NJ Health Care System, East Orange, New Jersey, U.S.A.

Robert J. Schwartzman   Department of Neurology, Drexel University College of Medicine, Philadelphia, Pennsylvania, U.S.A.

Elizabeth A. Sekul   Medical College of Georgia, Augusta, Georgia, U.S.A.

Gabriel E. Sella   Department of Community Medicine, Faculty of Medicine, West Virginia University, Morgantown, West Virginia, U.S.A.

Sangeeta Senapati   NorthShore University HealthSystem, Evanston, and Pritzker School of Medicine, Chicago, Illinois, U.S.A.

Neel Shah   UMDNJ New Jersey Medical School, Newark, New Jersey, U.S.A.

Steven Stanos   Center for Pain Management, Rehabilitation Institute of Chicago, Department of Physical Medicine and Rehabilitation, Northwestern University Medical School, Feinberg School of Medicine, Chicago, Illinois, U.S.A.

Rajbala Thakur   Department of Anesthesiology, University of Rochester School of Medicine and Dentistry, Rochester, New York, U.S.A.

Allen J. Togut   The Commonwealth Medical College of Pennsylvania, Wilkes-Barre, Pennsylvania, U.S.A.

Frank F. Tu   NorthShore University HealthSystem, Evanston, and Pritzker School of Medicine, Chicago, Illinois, U.S.A.

Joseph Walker III   Department of Physical Medicine and Rehabilitation, Spaulding Rehabilitation Hospital, Harvard Medical School, Boston, Massachusetts, U.S.A.

Richard A. Watson   Touro University College of Medicine & Hackensack University Medical Center, Hackensack; and UMDNJ New Jersey Medical School, Newark, New Jersey, U.S.A.

Jonathan C. Weeks   Department of Anesthesiology, University of Rochester School of Medicine and Dentistry, Rochester, New York, U.S.A.

Anthony H. Wheeler   Pain and Orthopedic Neurology, Charlotte, North Carolina, U.S.A.

1   Diabetic Peripheral Neuropathy

Gordon Irving

Swedish Pain and Headache Center and University of Washington Medical School, Seattle, Washington, U.S.A.

Richard Irving

Department of Electrical Engineering, University of Washington, Seattle, Washington, U.S.A.

THE DISORDER

Diabetes is currently on the rise around the globe. In 2007, the estimated total prevalence of diabetes (diagnosed and undiagnosed) in the United States was 7.8%, with the majority of affected individuals being 60 years and older. As the rate of diabetes has increased there has been an associated rise in prevalence of diabetic neuropathy (1).

Diabetic peripheral sensory polyneuropathy is one of the most common ailments associated with diabetes. Although it is possible to reverse the effects if treated early, diabetic neuropathy often results in permanent loss of function and death of the small nerve fibers, most commonly affecting the feet. It affects approximately 50% of the patients who have diabetes mellitus.

Despite its prevalence, the onset of symptoms is often mild and can go unnoticed for long periods of time, with most patients not experiencing any pain. However, approximately 11% experience chronic, painful symptoms (2).

Painful diabetic peripheral neuropathy (DPN) is associated with substantial patient burden due to interference with daily function, especially in those with suboptimal pain management. The severity of neuropathic pain is significantly associated with overall patient burden, employment disruption, and productivity. Not surprisingly, most interference is reported to result from reduced walking ability (3). The medical costs of DPN may account for up to 27% of the direct medical costs of diabetes, although the proportion due to pain is unclear (2).

Neuropathy is present in over 80% of diabetic patients with foot ulcers. Ulcers are more common because of decreased sensation perception of pressure and impairment of the microcirculation and integrity of the skin. Muscle imbalances may lead to anatomic deformities. Once an ulcer has occurred, aggressive therapy and protective measures should be taken to avoid secondary infection. The risk of lower limb amputation is high if there is a history of a previous foot ulcer, neuropathy, peripheral vascular disease, or poor glycemic control (4).

DIAGNOSIS

The diagnosis of DPN is based on the history. The pain may be spontaneous, continuous, or intermittent and is often worse at night. It affects the long nerve fibers of the extremities, so the pain tends to be felt first in the toes and may progress to the hands. The pain is usually described as burning, stabbing, tingling, numb, hot, cold, or itchy.

General Examination of the Feet

Visual inspection may reveal several abnormalities such as claw toes due to atrophy of the small intrinsic muscles, allowing unopposed action of the larger muscles. Charcot arthropathy may be present and is characterized by a collapse of the midfoot arch and bony prominences. Sweating may be diminished or absent resulting in dry, scaly, cracked skin, allowing access to infection.

The feet or hands may reveal sensory abnormalities with diminution or heightened perception to touch, pinprick sensation, or hot and cold. Allodynia (nonpainful stimulation perceived as painful) may be present with patient complaints of being unable to have their feet under the bedclothes at night as the pressure of the sheet irritates them.

Testing Methods

- The Semmes-Weinstein monofilament is a simple calibrated nylon filament. It is inexpensive, easy to use, and rapid and reproducible, with a specificity of 90%. It should be placed at right angles to the skin and the pressure increased until it buckles. This indicates that a 10-g pressure has been applied. Unfortunately, the sensitivity has been reported to be only 44% to 71% depending on how many skin areas are tested, and the prevalence between examiners varied between 3.4% and 29.3% (5).
- Vibration testing is done with a 128-Hz tuning fork placed at the bony prominence at the base of the first toe and is quick and easy to do. The sensitivity and specificity have been reported to be 53% and 99%, respectively (6). If no vibration is felt, the diagnosis is probably DPN. Loss of vibration sense predicts a high probability of foot ulceration and has been suggested as predicting mortality from diabetic complications (7, 8).

Pain Scales

There are several neuropathic pain scales, such as the Leeds Assessment of Neuropathic Symptoms and Signs (LANSS) Pain Scale and the Neuropathic Pain Scale, that have been devised to aid the diagnosis. Young et al. described the simple patient-completed questionnaire below (9).

1. What is the type of sensation felt? (maximum 2 points)
   a. Burning, numbness, or tingling (2 points)
   b. Fatigue, cramping, or aching (1 point)
2. Where is the location of symptoms? (maximum 2 points)
   a. Feet (2 points)
   b. Calves (1point)
   c. Elsewhere (no points)
3. Have the symptoms ever awakened you at night?
   a. Yes (1 point)
4. When is the pain worse? (maximum 2 points)
   a. At night (2 points)
   b. Day and night (1 point)
   c. Present only during the day (0 points)

5. What makes the pain better? (maximum 2 points)
    a. Walking around (2 points)
    b. Standing (1 point)
    c. Sitting or lying or no relief (0 points)

Total score:

0–2: Normal
3–4: Mild
5–6: Moderate
7–9: Severe

Additional Tests

Nerve conduction velocity (NCV) tests may be normal, as they only measure large fiber function and the majority of abnormalities are at the small fiber level.

Thermal thresholds in isolation or as part of quantitative sensory nerve testing may be more appropriate indicators of dysfunction of small-diameter sensory nerve fibers but are not widely available. Nerve or skin biopsies are useful only where the etiology is unclear or for research purposes.

Corneal confocal microscopy is a noninvasive evaluation of the middle layer of the cornea at a depth of 62 μm. Pictures taken of the corneal fiber density in this layer have been reported to closely correlate with the peripheral fiber density as measured by the much more invasive skin biopsy (10).

If the presentation of neuropathy is not symmetrical, another cause should be considered. Other differential peripheral neuropathic pain diagnoses to consider include the following:

*   Entrapment neuropathy
*   Alcoholism
*   HIV infection
*   Paraneoplastic syndrome
*   Monoclonal gammopathy
*   Vitamin deficiencies
*   Amyloidosis
*   Drugs and toxins: vincristine, cisplatin, isoniazid, arsenic, thallium
*   Vasculitic neuropathy
*   Fabry disease

PATHOPHYSIOLOGY

The pathophysiology of DPN is complex and not fully understood. Most theories involve interactions between metabolic and ischemic factors have been shown to create nerve damage. Several studies have begun to uncover the specific pathogenesis of diabetic neuropathy.

Hyperglycemia

By comparing animal axonal models that mimic the human disorders, it has become clear that hyperglycemia, or insulin deficiency, is a major culprit of DPN (11). The resulting damage occurs in DPN for both type 1 and type 2 diabetics. Common metabolic factors include the following:

*   *Advanced glycosylation end products*—Glycosylation of tissue and plasma proteins can result in advanced glycosylation end products, which tend to

increase in concentration in diabetic patients. These end products are thought to play a major role in diabetic microvascular complications.
- *Sorbitol*—Glucose metabolism is more pronounced in patients with hyperglycemia. Accumulation of sorbitol interferes with cell metabolism by raising cell osmolarity and decreasing intracellular myoinsitol.
- *Oxidative stress*—Reduced antioxidants and prolonged exposure to reactive oxygen species lead to peripheral nerve damage and degeneration.

In the more severe type 1 DPN, insulin and C-peptide deficiencies augment the deficits in Na^+/K^+-ATPase and endothelial nitric oxide. These deficiencies result in gene regulatory abnormalities of neurotrophic factors, their receptors, and cell-adhesive proteins (12).

Disease Progression
In both experimental models and human diabetic subjects, there is an initial metabolic phase that is responsive to metabolic corrections. During this initial phase, damage, as caused by the processes described above, can often be reversed (13).

Progression of disease leads to a structural phase that is increasingly nonresponsive to therapeutic interventions. Abnormalities during the structural phase add to the severity of axonal pathology and result in severe consequences with respect to nerve function (14).

Metabolic Changes
One of the earliest metabolic abnormalities is shunting of excessive glucose through the polyol pathway, resulting in intracellular accumulation of sorbitol and fructose with depletion of other osmolytes such as taurin and myoinositol. The latter interferes with phosphoinositide turnover, resulting in insufficient diacylglycerol for activation of Na^+/K^+-ATPase. In type 1 DPN, the more severe effect on Na^+/K^+-ATPase is accounted for by additional insults caused by insulin and C-peptide deficiencies (15).

Unmyelinated fiber abnormalities occur early and are reflected in thermal hyperalgesia and allodynia. Damage to small myelinated Aδ and unmyelinated C-fibers underlies these functional abnormalities, which translate to abnormal pain sensation—a common symptom in diabetic patients with DPN. Damage to the axonal membranes of C-fibers induces increased formation of Na^+ channels and α-adrenergic receptors, facilitating ectopic discharges (16, 17).

The initial damage to small peripheral fibers appears to be coupled with impaired neurotrophic support by nerve growth factor and insulin, itself, both of which are specifically neurotrophic for small nociceptive ganglion cells of the dorsal root ganglia. This may explain the more severe degenerative changes of these fibers in type 1 versus type 2 diabetes (18).

TREATMENT

Prevention of Progression of DPN
Currently, DPN is treated symptomatically, but studies have shown a link between glycemic control and microvascular complications such as neuropathy.

Although there does not appear to be a close link to pain control, getting the HbA1c down to 7or less should be a priority.

Encouraging the patient to develop a list of achievable goals may assist with lifestyle changes. These goals should include, where relevant, smoking cessation, weight loss, and regular exercise. Getting the patient to want to change and to believe he or she can change may require a different type of therapeutic approach such as motivational interviewing (19).

Described in this section are several nonpharmacological and pharmacological treatments that have been shown to be effective in a number of trials. By one estimate, most therapies for DPN result in a 30% to 50% reduction in pain. This level of improvement may be disappointing to patients (20).

Nonpharmacological Treatment
There are several nonpharmacological treatments that have been shown to have some efficacy in small trials. Treatment should also include foot care.

Transcutaneous Electrical Nerve Stimulation
TENS versus sham stimulation had positive results in 31 patients (21). Pain, numbness, and allodynia improved significantly in a small, randomized, double-blind study of 19 patients with mild to moderate DPN in the group treated with TENS (22).

Acupuncture
There have been no large placebo-controlled studies evaluating the efficacy of acupuncture for DPN, but small open-label trials have reported some benefit (23).

Spinal Cord Stimulation
Spinal cord stimulation has been reported to provide long-term relief for some patients with DPN, but there have been no placebo-controlled studies (24).

Transcranial Magnetic Stimulation
TMS is a noninvasive technology whereby an electric current is passed through an insulated circular or figure-eight coil to produce a magnetic pulse. When the coil is applied to the head, the magnetic pulse is capable of passing uninterrupted through the skin, skull, and ultimately to the cortex.

Repetitive transcranial magnetic stimulation (rTMS) has been shown to produce long-lasting effects in some small-scale clinical trials. According to one trial, it might be effective in alleviating DPN (25).

Foot Care Advice
When discussing the care of the DPN foot, advice should include the following:

1. Avoiding walking barefoot.
2. Wearing well-fitted, not tight shoes.
3. Feeling the inside of the shoes before putting them on in case there is a stone or anything that may cause skin damage.
4. Washing feet twice a day to ensure that patients examine their feet at least that often.

5. The importance of careful nail cutting, even having a podiatrist do the cutting to avoid cutting the skin.
6. Treating all blisters and abrasions early.

Pharmacological Treatment

Frequently, patients take more than one drug for their pain. A cross-sectional, community-based survey of 255 patients with DPN found that a majority of patients (79.2%) had taken at least one medication and more than half (52.1%) had taken at least two for DPN during the preceding week (26).

Nonsteroidal anti-inflammatory drugs (NSAIDs) were the most commonly used medications, with 46.7% reporting their use, although there is little evidence to support their efficacy. NSAIDs have a high potential for renal impairment in patients with diabetic neuropathy. Other frequently used medications were short- and long-acting opioids (43.1%), anticonvulsants (27.1%), second-generation antidepressants (18%), and tricyclic antidepressants (TCAs) (11.4%) (26).

Acetyl-L-Carnitine

Acetyl-L-carnitine (ALC) has reported beneficial effects on the metabolic abnormalities underlying the acute nerve conduction velocity slowing in experimental diabetes, such as Na^+/K^+-ATPase activity, endoneurial blood flow, and oxidative stressors (27).

A European and North American multicenter trial of 1346 patients with type 1 and type 2 diabetes and DPN received ALC, either 1500 or 3000 mg/day. None of the NCV or amplitude measures showed any significant improvement, but vibratory perception in the lower and upper extremities showed highly significant improvements. Pain also improved significantly in patients taking ALC 3000 mg/day both at 26 weeks and at the end of the trial at 52 weeks. Sural nerve biopsies also demonstrated increased nerve fiber regeneration (28).

ALC has a good safety profile and should be considered early in the disease, as results appear to be better the earlier the patient is treated (29).

ACE Inhibitors

The ACE inhibitor trandolapril was shown to improve peripheral neuropathy even in normotensive patients with diabetes. In general, the ACE inhibitor class of medications appears to have some protective effect against microvascular complications and organ damage from diabetes (30).

Lipid-Lowering Agents

Hypertriglyceridemia is a risk factor for development of diabetic neuropathy, and there is evidence that lipid-lowering agents may prevent DPN microvascular complications (31).

The lipid-lowering HMG-CoA reductase inhibitors (statins) may also possess neuroprotective properties in their own right (32).

Aldose Reductase Inhibitors

Metabolism of blood glucose via the polyol pathway, where aldose reductase is a key enzyme, may be important in the development of diabetic neuropathy. Therefore, blocking aldose reductase may reduce this risk of diabetic neuropathy.

In a one-year, placebo-controlled study, the aldose reductase fidarestat has been reported to be superior to placebo for reducing pain as well as the progression of peripheral diabetic neuropathy (33).

A postmarketing surveillance of more than 5000 patients on epalrestat, another aldose reductase inhibitor, was reported to show improvement of subjective symptoms, including spontaneous pain, in patients with DPN (34). In a three-year study, epalrestat was effective in slowing down the development of neuropathy as measured by changes in median nerve conduction velocity compared with controls. However, there was no significant difference in pain between the treated and untreated group (35).

α-Lipoic Acid

A meta-analysis of 1258 patients with DPN reported that infusions of α-lipoic acid (600 mg/day intravenously) ameliorated neuropathic symptoms and deficits after three weeks (36).

The ALADIN III (Alpha-Lipoic Acid in Diabetic Neuropathy) study showed that oral treatment with 600 mg three times a day resulted in a favorable effect on neuropathic deficits after six months (37).

The SYDNEY 2 (Symptomatic Diabetic Neuropathy 2) trial suggests that treatment for five weeks using 600 mg of α-lipoic acid orally every day reduces the paresthesias and numbness to a clinically meaningful degree (38).

All studies have reported a highly favorable safety profile. The drug is licensed in Germany, but not in the United Kingdom or the United States, for the treatment of DPN; however, it is sold as a food supplement in the latter two countries.

Tricyclic Antidepressants

Despite their widespread use, none of the TCAs has been approved by the FDA for treatment of DPN or any type of pain. A review found the total number of patients in clinical trials of the various TCAs for treatment of DPN to be less than 200, with no single study having more than 50 patients (39). That review found no difference in efficacy among the various kinds of TCAs, with an number needed to treat (NNT) of 3 (95% CI, 2.4–4.0) for improvement of pain of 50% or more. A 2005 Cochrane Collaborative analysis of five diabetic neuropathic pain trials of antidepressants reported that the NNT for amitriptyline's effectiveness was 1.3 (95% CI, 1.2–1.5; relative risk, 12.4; 95% CI, 5.2–29.2) (40).

Amitriptyline is the best studied TCA in DPN; other agents in this class include imipramine, clomipramine, desipramine, and nortriptyline. Their analgesic effect is independent of their antidepressant effect. Analgesia is thought to be the result of the inhibition of serotonin and norepinephrine reuptake, as well as sodium channel modulation.

The pain-relieving effect of amitriptyline is correlated with the total plasma concentration. If the plasma concentration exceeded 300 nmol/L, 70% of patients were responders on the daily rating of pain and 90% were responders on the global rating. Only 20% were responders at plasma concentrations below 300 nmol/L. This is lower than the reported corresponding level for the treatment of depression, which is 500 nmol/L (41).

Because of variable absorption, blood levels of amitriptyline should be taken. In a randomized controlled trial (RCT) of amitriptyline, it was found that total plasma levels of amitriptyline at a daily dose of 75 mg/day ranged from 56 to 925 nmol/L (42).

TCAs have a considerable adverse event burden. Ray et al. reported a slight increase in sudden cardiac death with TCA doses greater than 100 mg/day. There was no evidence that TCA doses lower than 100 mg increased the risk of sudden cardiac death (43). This is of obvious concern in the patient with diabetes who has a higher risk of heart disease. Some authors recommend baseline and follow-up electrocardiograms (ECGs) throughout treatment with TCAs (44).

Serotonin Norepinephrine Reuptake Inhibitors

There is general agreement that serotonin norepinephrine reuptake inhibitors (SNRIs) such as duloxetine, velafaxine and the newer SNRI's milnacipran, desvenlafaxine and venlafaxine are safer to use than TCAs and are a better option in patients with cardiac disease. However, the risk of hyponatremia due to the syndrome of inappropriate secretion of antidiuretic hormone (SIADH) is thought to be greater in elderly patients using selective serotonin reuptake inhibitors (SSRIs/SNRIs) than in those using TCAs (45). Hyponatremia should be considered in all patients who develop drowsiness, confusion, or convulsions while taking an antidepressant.

Venlafaxine

Results for the primary end point of pain intensity on the VAS showed that the 150 to 225 mg of venlafaxine ER significantly reduced pain intensity compared with placebo at week 6. Results with 75 mg were not different from those with placebo (46).

Another trial compared venlafaxine with imipramine for treatment of painful neuropathies. Treatment with either venlafaxine or imipramine significantly reduced pain compared with placebo; no significant difference was seen between the venlafaxine and imipramine groups (47).

In a multicenter, prospective, open-label study of 97 patients older than 80 years with depressive syndrome, not DPN, extended-release venlafaxine was found to be safe and effective in the elderly. Adverse events were reported by seven patients, but no serious events were reported. The most frequent adverse events were dizziness, gastric pain, and nausea. Treatment with venlafaxine over 24 weeks did not produce any clinically significant changes in blood pressure, heart rate, or other variables. The authors suggest that venlafaxine is particularly useful in the treatment of the elderly due to a low potential for drug–drug interaction (48).

Duloxetine

The efficacy of duloxetine in the treatment of DPN was established in three double-blind, placebo-controlled RCTs that included a total of 1139 patients. Patients with comorbid depression were excluded (49, 50).

The FDA-approved dosage of duloxetine 60 mg daily demonstrated rapid onset of action (within the first week of treatment) and sustained pain relief. All doses of duloxetine were well tolerated, with no significant changes in concentrations of hemoglobin A1C or triglycerides. Adverse events that were reported more often in the duloxetine group than in the placebo group were somnolence and constipation; these were mild to moderate (51).

Milnacipran and Desvenlafaxine

There have been no studies reported as yet on the efficacy of these drugs on DPN.

Antiepileptic Drugs

In the elderly, antiepileptic drugs may cause significant central nervous system side effects, especially dizziness and drowsiness, which not infrequently lead to discontinuation of treatment. Cognitive side effects are common and may go unrecognized in older patients, particularly in patients with communication problems.

Pregabalin

The efficacy of pregabalin in DPN has been established in three double-blind, placebo-controlled RCTs that included a total of 730 patients. It demonstrated early and sustained improvement in pain and a beneficial effect on sleep with dosages ranging from 150 to 600 mg daily. The most common treatment-related adverse events in the 300- and 600-mg/day groups were dizziness (27.2% and 39%, respectively), somnolence (23.5% and 26.8%, respectively), and peripheral edema (7.4% and 13.4%, respectively) (52–54).

Gabapentin

In one randomized trial of DPN, gabapentin was initiated at a dosage of 300 mg, three times daily, and increased during a period of four weeks in increments of 300 mg (from 900 to a maximum of 3600 mg/day). Beginning at week 2 and continuing throughout the trial, patients treated with gabapentin showed statistically significant improvements in pain scores compared with those who received placebo (55).

Sodium Channel Blockers

Sodium channel blockers have not been shown to be effective in patients with painful diabetic neuropathy. Carbamazepine cannot be recommended due to inadequate evidence in painful diabetic neuropathy. The successor drug, oxcarbazepine, has been withdrawn from clinical trials because of lack of efficacy (56). Neither topiramate nor lamotrigine has been shown to be effective (57, 58).

Opioids

The weak opioid, tramadol, is effective in painful DPN, but more severe pain often requires stronger opioids such as oxycodone (59). Two trials over four and six weeks have demonstrated significant pain relief and improvement in quality of life following treatment with controlled-release oxycodone, in a dose range of 10 to 100 mg (mean 40 mg/day). In these trials, antidepressants and anticonvulsants were not discontinued throughout the trial. As expected, adverse events were frequent and typical of opioid-related side effects (60, 61).

Combination therapy is common in treating DPN but has been poorly researched. In a study that titrated the maximum tolerable dose of a combination treatment of gabapentin and morphine compared with monotherapy of each drug, the maximum tolerable dose was significantly lower but efficacy was better, suggesting an additive interaction between the two drugs (62).

Isosorbide Dinitrate Spray

In a study of 22 DPN patients, 11 patients using topical isosorbide dinitrate had benefit and continued with the spray before bedtime compared with only four patients receiving placebo. There were virtually no adverse effects (63).

TABLE 1 Pharmacological Treatment Tier Recommendations

Drug	Dworkin et al. (66)	Attal et al. (67)	Argoff et al. (68)	Moulin et al. (69)
Antidepressants				
TCA	1	1	1	1
Duloxetine	NR	2	1	2
Venlafaxine	2	2	2	2
Bupropion	2	NR	—[a]	NR
Paroxetine	2	NR	NE	NR
Citalopram	2	NR	NE	NR
Antiepileptics				
Gabapentin	1	1	2	1
Pregabalin	1	1	1	1
Lamotrigine	NR	NR	2	NR
Valproate	NR	2	NR	4
Topiramate	NR	NE	NR	4
Phenytoin	NR	NR	—[a]	NR
Opioids				
Tramadol	1	2	2	3
Oxycodone/methadone	1	2	1	3
Topicals				
Lidocaine 5%	1	2	—[b]	2
Capsaicin	3	2	—[b]	3
Others				
Mexilitine	3	NE	NR	4
Clonidine	3	NE	NR	4

1 = first tier, 2 = second tier, 3 = third tier, 4 = fourth tier.
[a]>1 RCT.
[b]Mechanism of action.
Abbreviations: NR, no recommendations; NE, not considered effective.

Local Anesthetics

Lidocaine 5% patches may be effective for treating patients with DPN (64, 65). Some patients find that cutting the patch and wrapping it around their toes and then putting socks on will decrease their nighttime pain and allow a better night's sleep.

Summary of Pharmacological Treatments

There have been three published task force recommendations for pharmacological therapies in neuropathic pain and one consensus guidelines published on DPN. Drugs were evaluated and ranked based on recommendations from tier 1 to 4, with tier 1 drugs being the most recommended, as shown in Table 1.

Comorbidities

When deciding which medication to choose, other factors must play a role.

- Obesity: Avoid or monitor carefully TCAs or a gabapentinoid (gabapentin, pregabalin), all of which have significant risk of weight gain.
- Poor sleep: Consider any of the tier 1 medications in Table 1.
- Smoking: To encourage smoking cessation consider bupropion to assist in decreasing withdrawal symptoms.

- Polypharmacy: Consider a gabapentinoid and/or venlafaxine.
- Depression or anxiety: Consider duloxetine, venlafaxine, or TCAs because of fewer drug to drug interactions.

Surgical Treatment

If the presentation of pain is atypical, with pain felt over individual nerve dermatomes, entrapment neuropathy should be considered. A Tinel sign should be looked for over the deep peroneal or posterior tibial nerve. The superficial peroneal nerve, as it goes around the head of the fibula, may also be tender to touch, leading to a possibility of entrapment at this site. Although there are advocates of decompression in these cases, there is controversy as to whether surgical nerve decompression surgery is effective (70, 71).

REFERENCES

1. Centers for Disease Control and Prevention. Diabetes: disabling, deadly, and on the rise, 2008. Available at: http://www.cdc.gov/features/dsDiabetesTrends/. Accessed October 15, 2009.
2. Gordois A, Scuffhart P, Shearer A, et al. The health care costs of diabetic peripheral neuropathy in the US. Diabetes Care 2003; 26:1790–1795.
3. Tolle T, Xu X, Sadosky AB. Painful diabetic neuropathy: a cross sectional survey of health state impairment and treatment patterns. J Diabetes Complications 2006; 20: 26–33.
4. Litzelman DK, Marriott DJ, Vinicor F. Physiological predictors of foot lesions in patients with NIDDM. Diabetes Care 1997; 20:382.
5. McGill M, Molyneaux L, Spencer R, et al. Possible sources of discrepancies in the use of the Semmes-Weinstein monofilament. Impact on prevalence of insensate foot and workload requirements. Diabetes Care 1999; 22:598–602.
6. Perkins BA, Olaleye D, Zinman B, et al. Simple screening tests for peripheral neuropathy in the diabetes clinic. Diabetes Care 2001; 24:250.
7. Young MJ, Breddy JL, Veves A, et al. The prediction of diabetic neuropathic foot ulceration using vibration perception thresholds. Diabetes Care 1994; 17:557–560.
8. Coppini DV, Bowtell PA, Weng C, et al. Showing neuropathy is related to increased mortality in diabetic patients—a survival analysis using an accelerated failure time model. J Clin Epidemiol 2000; 53:519–523.
9. Young MJ, Boulton AJ, Macleod AF, et al. A multicenter study of the prevalence of diabetic peripheral neuropathy in the United Kingdom hospital clinic population. Diabetologia 1993; 36:150.
10. Quattrini C, Tavakoli M, Jeziorska M, et al. Surrogate markers of small fiber damage in human diabetic neuropathy. Diabetes 2007; 56(8):2148–2154.
11. Vincent, AM, Russell, JW, Low, P, Feldman, EL. Oxidative stress in the pathogenesis of diabetic neuropathy. Endocr Rev 2004;25:612.
12. Pierson CR, Zhang W, Murakawa Y, et al. Early gene responses of trophic factors differ in nerve regeneration in type 1 and type 2 diabetic neuropathy. J Neuropathol Exp Neurol 2002; 61:857–871.
13. Sima AAF. C-peptide and diabetic neuropathy. Expert Opin Investig Drugs 2003; 12:1471–1488.
14. Sima AAF, Zhang W, Li Z-G, et al. Molecular alterations underlie nodal and paranodal degeneration in type 1 diabetic neuropathy and are prevented by C-peptide. Diabetes 2004; 53:1556–1563.
15. Sima AAF. Pathological mechanisms involved in diabetic neuropathy: can we slow the process? Curr Opin Investig Drugs 2006; 7:324–337.
16. Hirade M, Yasuda H, Omatsu-Kaube M, et al. Tetrodotoxin-resistant sodium channels of dorsal root ganglion neurons are readily activated in diabetic rats. Neuroscience 1999; 90(3):933–939.

17. Lee YH, Ryn TG, Park SJ, et al. Alpha-1 adrenoreceptor involvement in painful diabetic neuropathy: a role in allodynia. Neuroreport 2000; 11:1417–1420.
18. Kamiya H, Murakawa Y, Zhang W, et al. Unmyelinated fiber sensory neuropathy differs in type 1 and type 2 diabetes. Diabetes Metab Res Rev 2005; 21:448–458.
19. Diabetes Control and Complications Trial Research Group. Effect of intensive diabetes treatment on nerve conduction in the Diabetes Control and Complications Trial. Ann Neurol 1995; 38(6):869–880.
20. Mendell JR, Sahenk Z. Painful sensory neuropathy. N Engl J Med 2003; 348(13):1243–1255.
21. Kumar D, Marshall HJ. Diabetic peripheral neuropathy: amelioration of pain with transcutaneous electrostimulation. Diabetes Care 1997; 20(11):1702–1705.
22. Forst T, Nguyen M, Forst S, et al. Impact of low frequency transcutaneous electrical nerve stimulation on symptomatic diabetic neuropathy using the new Salutaris device. Diabetes Nutr Metab 2004; 17(3):163–168.
23. Abuaisha BB, Costanzi JB, Boulton AJ. Acupuncture for the treatment of chronic painful peripheral diabetic neuropathy: a long-term study. Diabetes Res Clin Pract 1998; 39:115–121.
24. Daousi C, Benbow SJ, MacFarlane IA. Electrical spinal cord stimulation in the long-term treatment of chronic painful diabetic neuropathy. Diabet Med 2005; 22(4):393–398.
25. Khedr EM, Kotb H, Kamel NF, et al. Longlasting antalgic effects of daily sessions of repetitive transcranial magnetic stimulation in central and peripheral neuropathic pain. J Neurol Neurosurg Psychiatry 2005; 76(6):833–838.
26. Gore M, Brandenburg N, Tai K, et al. A survey of pain medication use among patients with painful diabetic peripheral neuropathy (DPN). Diabetes 2004; 52(suppl 2):A126.
27. Lowitt S, Malone JI, Salem AF, et al. Acetyl-L-carnitine corrects altered peripheral nerve function of experimental diabetes. Metabolism 1995; 44:677–680.
28. Sima AAF, Calvani M, Mehra M, et al. Acetyl-L-carnitine improves pain, vibratory perception and nerve morphology in patients with chronic diabetic peripheral neuropathy: an analysis of two randomized, placebo-controlled trials. Diabetes Care 2005; 28:96–101.
29. Amato A, Sima AAF. The protective effect of acetyl-L-carnitine on symptoms, particularly pain, in diabetic neuropathy. Diabetes Res Clin Pract 2002; 56:173–180.
30. Malik RA, Williamson S, Abbott C, et al. Effect of angiotensin-converting-enzyme (ACE) inhibitor trandolapril on human diabetic neuropathy: randomised double-blind controlled trial. Lancet 1998; 352(9145):1978–1981.
31. Fried LF, Forrest KY, Ellis D, et al. Lipid modulation in insulin dependent diabetes mellitus: effect on microvascular outcomes. J Diabetes Complications 2001; 15(3):113–119.
32. Leiter LA. The prevention of diabetic microvascular complications of diabetes: is there a role for lipid lowering? Diabetes Res Clin Pract 2005; 68(suppl 2):S3–S14.
33. Hotta N, Toyota T, Matsuoka K, et al. Clinical efficacy of fidarestat, a novel aldose reductase inhibitor, for diabetic peripheral neuropathy: a 52-week multicenter placebo-controlled double-blind parallel group study. Diabetes Care 2001; 24(10):1776–1782.
34. Hotta N, Sakamoto N, Shigeta Y, et al. Clinical investigation of epalrestat, an aldose reductase inhibitor, on diabetic neuropathy in Japan: Diabetic Neuropathy Study Group in Japan. J Diabetes Complications 1996; 10(3):168–172.
35. Hotta N, Akanuma Y, Kawamori R, et al. Long-term clinical epalrestat, an aldose reductase inhibitor, on diabetic neuropathy in type 2 diabetic patients: the 3-year, multicenter, comparative Aldose Reductase Inhibitor-Diabetes Complications Trial. Diabetes Care 2006; 29(7):1538–1544.
36. Ziegler D, Nowak H, Kempler P, et al. Treatment of symptomatic diabetic polyneuropathy with the antioxidant α-lipoic acid: a meta-analysis. Diabet Med 2004; 21:114–121.
37. Ziegler D. Thioctic acid for patients with symptomatic diabetic neuropathy. A critical review. Treat Endocrinol 2004; 3:1–17.

38. Ziegler D, Ametov A, Barinov A, et al. Oral treatment with alpha-lipoic acid improves symptomatic diabetic polyneuropathy: the SYDNEY 2 trial. Diabetes Care 2006; 29(11):2365–2370.

39. McQuay HJ, Tramer M, Nye BA, et al. A systematic review of antidepressants in neuropathic pain. Pain 1996; 68:217–227.

40. Saarto T, Wiffen PJ. Antidepressants for neuropathic pain. Cochrane Database Syst Rev 2005; 4:CD005454. Available at: www.cochrane.org/reviews/en/ab005454.html. Accessed October 13, 2009.

41. Leijon G, Boivie J. Central post-stroke pain—a controlled trial of amitriptyline and carbamazepine. Pain 1989; 36:27–36.

42. Sindrup S. Antidepressants and chronic pain. In: Jensen T, Wilson P, Rice A, eds. Clinical Pain Management: Chronic Pain. London, UK: Arnold, 2003:chap 18.

43. Ray W, Meredith S, Thapa P, et al. Cyclic antidepressants and the risk of sudden cardiac death. Clin Pharmacol Ther 2004; 75:234–241.

44. Dworkin R, Backonja M, Rowbotham M. Advances in neuropathic pain: diagnosis, mechanisms and treatment recommendations. Arch Neurol 2003; 60:1524–1534.

45. Antai-Otong D. Antidepressants in late-life depression: prescribing principles. Perspect Psychiatr Care 2006; 42:149–153.

46. Rowbotham MC, Goli V, Kunz NR, et al. Venlafaxine extended release in the treatment of painful diabetic neuropathy: a double-blind, placebo-controlled study. Pain 2004; 110:697–706.

47. Sindrup SH, Bach FW, Madsen C, et al. Venlafaxine versus imipramine in painful polyneuropathy: a randomized, controlled trial. Neurology 2003; 60:1284–1289.

48. Baca E, Roca M, Garcia-Calvo C, et al. Venlafaxine extended-release in patients older than 80 years with depressive syndrome. Int J Geriatr Psychiatry 2006; 21:337–343.

49. Goldstein DJ, Lu Y, Detke MJ, et al. Duloxetine versus placebo in patients with painful diabetic neuropathy. Pain 2005; 116:109–118.

50. Raskin J, Pritchett YL, Wang F, et al. A double-blind, randomized multicenter trial comparing duloxetine with placebo in the management of diabetic peripheral neuropathic pain. Pain Med 2005; 6:348–356.

51. Wernicke J, Lu Y, D'Souza D, et al. Duloxetine at doses of 60 mg QD and 60 mg BID is effective in treatment of diabetic neuropathic pain (DNP). J Pain 2004; 5:48.

52. Lesser H, Sharma U, LaMoreaux L, et al. Pregabalin relieves symptoms of painful diabetic neuropathy: a randomized controlled trial. Neurology 2004; 63:2104–2110.

53. Richter RW, Portenoy R, Sharma U, et al. Relief of painful diabetic peripheral neuropathy with pregabalin: a randomized, placebo-controlled trial. J Pain 2005; 6: 253–260.

54. Rosenstock J, Tuchman M, LaMoreaux L, et al. Pregabalin for the treatment of painful diabetic peripheral neuropathy: a double-blind, placebo-controlled trial. Pain 2004; 110:628–638.

55. Backonja M, Beydoun A, Edwards KR, et al. Gabapentin for the symptomatic treatment of painful neuropathy in patients with diabetes mellitus: a randomized controlled trial. JAMA 1998; 280:1831–1836.

56. Dogra S, Beydoun S, Mazzola J, et al. Oxcarbazepine in painful diabetic neuropathy: a randomized, placebo-controlled study. Eur J Pain 2005; 9:543–554.

57. Thienel U, Neto W, Schwabe SK, et al. Topiramate in painful diabetic polyneuropathy: findings from three double-blind placebo-controlled trials. Acta Neurol Scand 2004; 110:221–231.

58. Vinik AI, Tuchman M, Safirstein B, et al. Lamotrigine for treatment of pain associated with diabetic neuropathy: results of two randomized, double-blind, placebo-controlled studies. Pain 2007; 128:169–179.

59. Harati Y, Gooch C, Swenson M, et al. Double-blind randomized trial of tramadol for the treatment of the pain of diabetic neuropathy. Neurology 1998; 50:1842–1846.

60. Watson CP, Moulin D, Watt-Watson J, et al. Controlled-release oxycodone relieves neuropathic pain: a randomized controlled trial in painful diabetic neuropathy. Pain 2003; 105:71–78.

61. Gimbel JS, Richards P, Portenoy RK. Controlled-release oxycodone for pain in diabetic neuropathy: a randomized controlled trial. Neurology 2003; 60:927–934.
62. Gilron I, Bailey JM, Tu D, et al. Morphine, gabapentin, or their combination for neuropathic pain. N Engl J Med 2005; 352:1324–1334.
63. Yuen KC, Baker NR, Rayman G. Treatment of chronic painful diabetic neuropathy with isosorbide dinitrate spray: a double-blind placebo-controlled cross-over study. Diabetes Care 2002; 25(10):1699–1703.
64. Devers A, Galer BS. Topical lidocaine patch relieves a variety of neuropathic pain conditions: an open-label study. Clin J Pain 2000; 16(3):205–208.
65. Barbano RL, Herrmann DN, Hart-Gouleau S, et al. Effectiveness, tolerability, and impact on quality of life of the 5% lidocaine patch in diabetic polyneuropathy. Arch Neurol 2004; 61(6):914–918.
66. Dworkin R, Backonja M, Rowbotham M. Advances in neuropathic pain: diagnosis, mechanisms and treatment recommendations. Arch Neurol 2003; 60:1524–1534.
67. Attal N, Cruccu G, Haanpaa M, et al. EFNS guidelines on pharmacological treatment of neuropathic pain. Eur J Neurol 2006; 13:1153–1169.
68. Argoff CE, Backonja MM, Belgrade M, et al. Diabetic peripheral neuropathic pain: consensus guidelines for treatment. J Fam Pract 2006; suppl:3–19.
69. Moulin DE, Clark AJ, Gilron I, et al. Pharmacological management of chronic neuropathic pain—consensus statement and guidelines from the Canadian Pain Society. Pain Res Manage 2007; 12:13–21.
70. Dellon AL. How to improve the results of peripheral nerve surgery. Acta Neurochir Suppl 2007;100:149–151.
71. Chaudhry V, Stevens JC, Kincaid J, et al. Practice advisory utility of surgical decompression for treatment of diabetic neuropathy. Report of the therapeutics and Technology Assessment Subcommittee of the American Academy of Neurology. Neurology 2006; 66:1805–1808.

HIV/AIDS Neuropathy

Vasanthi Arumugam and Maurice Policar

Elmhurst Hospital Center, Mount Sinai School of Medicine, Elmhurst, New York, U.S.A.

THE DISORDER

There are several forms of peripheral neuropathy related to HIV/AIDS, but the most common is distal sensory polyneuropathy (DSP). DSP has become the most frequent neurologic syndrome associated with HIV infection, and the pain associated with this condition can be debilitating. Several factors such as age, use of antiretroviral medication (ARV), severity of HIV infection, diabetes, and alcohol abuse have been related to an increased risk of developing DSP (1). However, studies of subgroups who received highly active antiretroviral therapy (HAART) have not shown a relationship between virologic and immunologic status, and the development of symptomatic sensory neuropathies (2). There are two subtypes of DSP: the type solely associated with HIV infection and the type associated with antiretroviral treatments, sometimes referred to as antiretroviral toxic neuropathy (ATN) (3). When caused by ARV, the clinical presentation may be the same except for a temporal relationship with ARV use. Neuropathy in HIV can also result from other causes, such as chronic hepatitis C infection, vitamin deficiency, or chemotherapy.

Occurring in the middle and late stages of HIV infection, DSP commonly presents as painful feet. Neuropathy related to ARV toxicity may occur at any stage of HIV infection. When DSP is caused by medications, the most common culprits are antiretroviral agents, but medications such as dapsone, isoniazid, and chemotherapeutic agents have also been implicated. Nucleoside reverse transcriptase inhibitors (NRTIs) are the class of drugs most frequently associated with peripheral neuropathy.

Prevalence

The prevalence of DSP varies from 9% to 63% in different series (4). Although the incidence has progressively decreased since the introduction of HAART (5), DSP has become more prevalent. This increase in prevalence is most likely due to the increased survival of those infected with HIV, the occurrence of comorbidities with similar complications, and the use of antiretroviral therapy (6).

DIAGNOSIS

The diagnosis of the peripheral neuropathy syndrome in HIV-infected patients is generally based upon the clinical picture.

DSP commonly presents as tingling and numbness in the toes bilaterally, and then gradually spreads proximally from the lower extremities, rarely involving the upper extremities. Early painful dysesthesias of the lower extremities are common, but patients may also complain of numbness. These symptoms are typically most severe on the soles of the feet and are worse at night or after walking (7). There is sensory loss in a stocking distribution, and ankle jerks are decreased or absent. Knee jerks are occasionally decreased and may be absent in severe cases. Vibratory, pain, and temperature sensation is usually decreased, but muscle weakness is not a prominent symptom of DSP and generally occurs only in advanced disease.

Compared with DSP that is related to HIV infection, that related to antiretroviral toxicity is indistinguishable, except for the temporal relationship of ARV use with onset, and eventual resolution with discontinuation. Whereas HIV-related DSP may take weeks to months to develop, ATN generally occurs shortly after exposure and may not be related to cumulative exposure to ARV (8). Specific agents in the NRTI class are most commonly associated with DSP, particularly the so-called "d" drugs: ddI (didanosine), ddC (zalcitabine), and d4T (stavudine). As a result of the frequency of ATN, and other adverse drug reactions, prescribing patterns in the developed world have changed to limit the use of these agents. In developing countries, however, ARV regimens still commonly contain stavudine. Concern about a possible relationship of ATN and the class of ARV known as protease inhibitors led to a recent study by Ellis and colleagues. The investigators concluded that the independent risk of DSP attributable to protease inhibitors, if any, is very small (9).

It can be clinically difficult to distinguish between HIV-associated and drug-induced neuropathy. Numbness, tingling, and pain are common in both types. Both predominantly affect the distal extremities, mostly in the lower limbs. The upper extremities may become involved late in the course and may be more commonly affected with drug toxicity. A beneficial response after withdrawal of the offending agent can help identify ARV as the cause. It has been noted that a transient intensification of symptoms ("coasting") can occur for four to eight weeks after drug withdrawal and before improvement begins (6).

In patients with significant weakness, or an asymmetric presentation, additional diagnoses should be considered. Electrodiagnostic studies including electromyography and nerve conduction studies may be helpful when there is doubt about the diagnosis (4). Nerve biopsy is rarely indicated, and a skin biopsy may be helpful in some cases. A careful history of antiretroviral therapies with a review of other medications should be done to exclude possible iatrogenic causes.

Laboratory evaluation in DSP is relatively unrevealing, but it should exclude other causes of this type of neuropathy. Testing should include the following:

Vitamin B_{12} and folate levels
Thyroid-stimulating hormone assay
Fasting blood sugar
Liver function tests
Blood urea nitrogen and creatinine
Serum protein electrophoresis and immunoelectrophoresis
Screening test for syphilis

Electrophysiologic findings show small or absent sural sensory nerve activation potentials. Nerve conduction studies usually confirm a length-dependent axonal polyneuropathy. Needle electromyography shows acute or chronic partial denervation of distal lower limb muscles.

Nerve biopsy is rarely indicated to exclude other neurologic diagnoses. Features include loss of myelinated and unmyelinated fibers with axonal degeneration and macrophage activation (10).

Skin biopsy may be positive in some patients with negative electrodiagnostic studies (4).

The presence of a low epidermal nerve fiber density (<11 fibers/mm) has been noted in persons with DSP. This finding was associated with an increased likelihood of developing DSP in one study (11).

PATHOPHYSIOLOGY

The pathogenesis of DSP is not well understood and is thought to be multifactorial.

There is little evidence to support direct infection of the neurons by HIV-1, suggesting that this is not likely to be an important mechanism for neuronal injury (12). In vitro studies suggest roles for viral proteins such as gp120 in the indirect stimulation of axonal degeneration and/or cell death (3).

The envelope glycoprotein gp120 may produce neurotoxicity within the dorsal root ganglion, and in vitro studies have suggested that gp120 induces apoptosis in rodent dorsal root ganglion cultures and lowers the threshold for excitation (7).

Neuropathologic changes of the dorsal root ganglia include inflammatory infiltrates of lymphocytes and activated macrophages and low numbers of neurons. The amount of macrophage activation in the dorsal root ganglion relates with symptomatic DSP (7).

The prominent presence of proinflammatory cytokines including TNF-alpha, interferon alpha, interleukin 6, and other inflammatory mediators including nitric oxide has been shown in dorsal root ganglia in AIDS. This may lead to neuronal hyperexcitability as has been seen in animal models (7).

In patients receiving NRTIs, therapy interferes with DNA synthesis and causes mitochondrial abnormalities (13). These abnormalities are thought to underlie the pathogenesis of antiretroviral-related DSP. This view is supported by the evidence showing increased serum lactate concentrations and decreased serum concentrations of acetylcarnitine in patients with this condition (7). Elevated blood lactate levels occurred in 90% of those with DSP who were using stavudine (14).

A prospective study of 509 patients again identified older age and receipt of stavudine and didanosine as being more frequent in those developing DSP, but the mitochondrial haplogroup T was also more frequent in this group (15).

TREATMENT

Distal Sensory Polyneuropathy

Management of DSP is largely symptomatic and usually aimed at ameliorating the painful dysesthesias. Correcting nutritional and metabolic abnormalities when present may be helpful. Various classes of medication have been used in the treatment of DSP.

Tylenol/NSAIDs
Acetaminophen or nonsteroidals (NSAIDs) are the initial treatment for mild pain. If this is inadequate, other treatment should be considered.

Tricyclic Antidepressants
Tricyclic antidepressants are still used for the treatment of HIV-associated neuropathies, despite the absence of efficacy noted in two small studies (16, 17). Either nortriptyline or amitriptyline may be used. In patients who experience nighttime pain primarily, amitriptyline is a sound alternative. Treatment may be initiated with lower doses to reduce possible side effects such as sedation, urinary retention, dry mouth, and orthostatic hypotension. A starting dose of 25 mg at night is gradually increased to 75 mg or as high as 100 to 150 mg if needed. For patients with daytime pain, oral nortriptyline is often used, since it has a less sedative effect. A starting dose of 10 mg/day is gradually increased to 30 mg three times a day.

Anticonvulsants

Gabapentin
Gabapentin has been widely used in the treatment of DSP. The use of gabapentin for the treatment of painful HIV-related neuropathy was found to reduce pain better than placebo in small groups of patients in two studies (18, 19). Beneficial effects begin with higher doses. The usual starting daily dose is 300 mg/day in three divided doses, but doses can be increased to a maximum of 3600 mg/day. Slow escalation of doses should allow for tolerance to side effects such as somnolence and dizziness.

Pregabalin
Pregabalin is an anticonvulsant designed as a more potent successor to gabapentin. Although pregabalin may be used for the treatment of patients with HIV-associated painful peripheral neuropathy, a randomized, double-blind, placebo-controlled study (20) showed no long-term difference in end point mean pain score between pregabalin and placebo groups. Important to note is that there was a larger-than-usual placebo effect in this study compared with similar studies, possibly negating the effect of pregabalin.

Lamotrigine
Lamotrigine has also been studied in HIV-DSP. In a randomized, placebo-controlled trial (21), lamotrigine alone showed improved pain control over placebo, but only in patients receiving neurotoxic antiretroviral therapy. There was a seven-week dose escalation phase, followed by a maintenance phase. In a different double-blind, placebo-controlled trial (22), lamotrigine, 200 to 400 mg daily, when used in combination with other medications for neuropathic pain, did not demonstrate medication efficacy better than placebo.

Other Agents

Memantine
The use of memantine for the treatment of HIV-associated peripheral neuropathy was evaluated in a placebo-controlled study enrolling 45 subjects. This

N-methyl-d-aspartate (NMDA) receptor antagonist used in the treatment of Alzheimer's disease was not effective at reducing HIV-associated peripheral neuropathy (23).

Prosaptide
A randomized trial evaluating the polypeptide prosaptide for HIV-associated sensory neuropathies (24) showed that, although prosaptide was safe, it is not an effective agent in the treatment of HIV-associated peripheral neuropathy.

Tramadol
Tramadol 50 mg po bid or narcotics are reserved for those with breakthrough pain, as part of a broader treatment regimen. In refractory cases of peripheral neuropathy, the patient may respond to combinations of medications.

Topical

Lidocaine gel
In a double-blind, placebo-controlled multicenter study, lidocaine 5% gel was a safe but ineffective agent in the treatment of pain in HIV-associated DSP (25). The gel was applied once daily to skin over the area of pain.

Capsaicin patch
A double-blind multicenter study randomized 307 subjects with HIV-related peripheral neuropathy to compare high-concentration capsaicin patch versus a low-concentration capsaicin patch. The high-concentration patch had a greater reduction of pain intensity over a 12-week period, 23% versus 11% (26), when applied for 30 to 90 minutes once daily.

Cannabis
Cannabis may be useful in the management of painful HIV-associated sensory neuropathy. A prospective, randomized, placebo-controlled trial of 50 patients with painful HIV-associated sensory neuropathy (27) showed that smoked cannabis reduced daily pain better than placebo (34% vs. 17%). Fifty-two percent of the group treated with cannabis reported a reduction in pain greater than 30% as opposed to the placebo group who experienced a 24% reduction in pain. The first cannabis cigarette reduced chronic pain by a median of 72% vs. 15% with placebo ($p < 0.001$). The patients smoked up to one cigarette three times a day, containing approximately 1 g of cannabis with 3.56% tetrahydrocannabinol (THC).

Acupuncture
In a case series, 21 subjects with HIV-related neuropathy received acupuncture treatment, which demonstrated that subjective pain and symptoms of neuropathy were reduced during the period of acupuncture. The total subjective peripheral neuropathy summary score was reduced by approximately 50% (28).

Healing Touch
A review of anecdotal reports of healing touch (29) found that there are many positive outcomes, but none of the findings were conclusive.

Plasmapheresis/Intravenous Gamma Globulin
Kiprov et al. (30) treated HIV neuropathy with plasmapheresis and intravenous gamma globulin. It appears that the combination of plasmapheresis and intravenous gamma globulin was a potent immunomodulatory therapy for patients with HIV-related neuropathy.

It has been recognized that unhealthy behaviors may be employed by HIV-positive patients suffering from DSP. As part of a larger study on self-care and HIV (31), investigators identified specific unhealthy self-care behaviors such as cigarette smoking, alcohol consumption, and illicit drug use which were employed to alleviate pain. It was concluded that the clinician must partner with the patient to address any unhealthy behavior that may exacerbate DSP.

Antiretroviral Toxic Neuropathy
Treatment of ATN should include the discontinuation of drugs that cause peripheral neuropathy. About two-thirds of these patients will eventually respond to the NRTI discontinuation.

Two large studies (32, 33) demonstrated the beneficial effect of using lamotrigine in patients with ATN rather than DSP. Dose escalation occurred over seven weeks to reach a maximum of 400 to 600 mg/day in two divided doses.

Acetyl-L-carnitine has been used as treatment for painful ATN in HIV patients. In an open-label study (34), acetyl-L-carnitine was found to be effective in symptomatic treatment of painful neuropathy but had no observable effect on neurophysiologic parameters. In another double-blind, placebo-controlled, multicenter study (35), investigators looked at acetyl-L-carnitine in the symptomatic treatment of ATN. Using the Visual Analog Scale, acetyl-L-carnitine was found to significantly reduce the subject's pain rating in comparison to placebo.

Amitriptyline, mexiletine, topical capsaicin, 5% lidocaine, and gabapentin may also be useful therapeutic modalities for treating ATN.

In a prospective study (36), 11 HIV/AIDS patients with a drug-induced neuropathy were enrolled. Noninvasive skin electrodes were placed on the leg, and low-voltage current was passed for 20 minutes every day for 30 days. Although only seven individuals completed the study, the results support the notion that low-voltage electroacupuncture improves the condition of the neuropathic HIV/AIDS patient.

General Measures
Podiatrist evaluation (to develop plan of care, including exercise, care of feet, etc.)
> Loose shoes or no shoes
> Soak feet
> Short walks
> Blanket bridge to protect feet while sleeping

Initiation of HAART may help in DSP
Vitamin supplements may be considered—mainly B_1, B_{12}, and folate
Other supplements including magnesium, α-lipoic acid, γ-linolenic acid
Avoidance of alcohol
Control blood sugar if applicable
Alternative therapy: massage, yoga, hypnosis, and meditation

REFERENCES

1. de Freitas MRG. Infectious neuropathy. Curr Opin Neurol 2007; 20(5:)548–552.
2. Morgello S, Estanislao L, Simpson D, et al. HIV-associated distal sensory polyneuropathy in the era of highly active antiretroviral therapy: the Manhattan HIV Brain Bank. Arch Neurol 2004; 61:546–551.
3. Cornblath DR, Hoke A. Recent advance in HIV neuropathy. Curr Opin Neurol 2006; 19(5:)446–450.
4. Nardin RA, Freeman R. Clinical manifestations, diagnosis, and treatment of HIV-associated peripheral neuropathy. UpToDate Online version 16.2, 2008. Accessed July 2008.
5. Lichteinstein KA, Arnon C, Baron A, et al. Modification of drug-associated symmetrical peripheral neuropathy by host and disease factors in the HIV outpatient study cohort. Clin Infect Dis 2005; 40:148–157.
6. Nicholas PK, Mauceri L, Slate Ciampa A, et al. Distal sensory polyneuropathy in the context of HIV/AIDS. J Assoc Nurses AIDS Care 2007; 18(4:)32–40.
7. McArthur JC, Brew BJ, Nath A. Neurological complications of HIV infection. Lancet Neurol 2005; 4(9:)543–555.
8. Arenas-Pinto A, Bhaskaran K, Dunn D, et al. The risk of developing peripheral neuropathy induced by nucleoside reverse transcriptase inhibitors decreases over time: evidence from the Delta trial. Antiviral Ther 2008; 13(2:)289–295.
9. Letendre S, McCutchan JA, Ellis RJ. Neurologic complications of HIV disease and their treatment. Top HIV Med 2008; 16(1:)15–22.
10. Ferrari S, Vento S, Monaco S, et al. Human immunodeficiency virus-associated peripheral neuropathies. Mayo Clin Proc 2006; 81(2:)213–219.
11. Hermann DN, McDermott MP, Sowden JE, et al. Is skin biopsy a predictor of transition to symptomatic HIV neuropathy? A longitudinal study. Neurology 2006; 66:857–861.
12. Pardo CA, McArthur JC, Griffin JW. HIV neuropathy: insights in the pathology of HIV peripheral nerve disease. J Peripher Nerv Syst 2001; 6:21–27.
13. Lewis W, Dalakas MC. Mitochondrial toxicity of antiviral drugs. Nat Med 1995; 1:417–422.
14. Brew BJ, Tisch S, Law M. Lactate concentrations distinguish between nucleoside neuropathy and HIV neuropathy. AIDS 2003; 17:1094–1096.
15. Hulgan T, Haas DW, Haines JL, et al. Mitochondrial haplogroups and peripheral neuropathy during antiretroviral therapy: an adult AIDS clinical trials group study. AIDS 2005; 19:1341–1349.
16. Kieburtz K, Simpson D, Yiannoutsos C, et al. A randomized trial of amitriptyline and mexiletine for painful neuropathy in HIV infection. AIDS Clinical Trial Group 242 Protocol Team. Neurology 1998; 51(6:)1682–1688.
17. Shlay JC, Chaloner K, Max MB, et al. Acupuncture and amitriptyline for pain due to HIV-related peripheral neuropathy: a randomized controlled trial. Terry Bearn Community Programs for Clinical Research on AIDS. JAMA 1998; 280(18:)1590–1595.
18. Hahn K, Arendt G, Braun JS, et al. A placebo-controlled trial of gabapentin for painful HIV-associated sensory neuropathies. J Neurol 2004; 251(10:)1260–1266.
19. La Spina I, Porazzi D, Maggiolo F, et al. Gabapentin in painful HIV-related neuropathy: a report of 19 patients, preliminary observations. Eur J Neurol 2001; 8(1:)71–75.
20. Simpson DM, Murphy TK, Durso-De Cruz E, et al. A randomized, double-blind, placebo-controlled, multicenter trial of pregabalin vs. placebo in the treatment of neuropathic pain associated with HIV neuropathy. XVII International AIDS Conference, Mexico City, Mexico, August 3–8, 2008. Abstract THAB0301.
21. Simpson DM, McArthur JC, Olney R, et al. Lamotrigine for HIV-associated painful sensory neuropathies: a placebo-controlled trial. Neurology 2003; 60(9:)1508–1514.
22. Silver M, Blum D, Grainger J, et al. Double-blind, placebo-controlled trial of lamotrigine in combination with other medications for neuropathic pain. J Pain Symptom Manag 2007; 34(4:)446–454. Epub July 26, 2007.

23. Schifitto G, Yiannoutsos CT, Simpson DM, et al. A placebo-controlled study of memantine for the treatment of human immunodeficiency virus-associated sensory neuropathy. J Neurovirol 2006; 12(4:)328–331.

24. Evans SR, Simpson DM, Kitch DW, et al. A randomized trial evaluating Prosaptide™ for HIV-associated sensory neuropathies: use of an electronic diary to record neuropathic pain. PLoS ONE 2007; 2(6:) e551. Available at: http://www.plosone.org/article/citationList.action?articleURI=info%3Adoi%2F10. 1371%2Fjournal.pone.0000551. Accessed July 2008.

25. Estanislao L, Carter K, McArthur J, et al. A randomized controlled trial of 5% lidocaine gel for HIV-associated distal symmetric polyneuropathy. J Acquir Immune Defic Syndr 2004; 37(5:)1584–1586.

26. Simpson DM, Brown S, Tobias J, et al. Controlled trial of high-concentration capsaicin patch for treatment of painful HIV neuropathy. Neurology 2008; 70(24:)2305–2313.

27. Abrams DI, Jay CA, Shade SB, et al. Cannabis in painful HIV-associated sensory neuropathy: a randomized placebo-controlled trial. Neurology 2007; 68(7:)515–521.

28. Phillips KD, Skelton WD, Hand GA. Effect of acupuncture administered in a group setting on pain and subjective peripheral neuropathy in persons with human immunodeficiency virus disease. J Altern Complement Med 2004; 10(3:)449–455.

29. Wardell DW, Weymouth KF. Review of studies of healing touch. J Nurs Scholarsh 2004; 36(2:)147–154.

30. Kiprov DD, Stricker RB, Miller RG. Treatment of HIV neuropathy with plasmapheresis and intravenous gamma globulin: an update. VIII International AIDS Conference, Amsterdam, The Netherlands, July 19–24, 1992. Abstract PuB 7281.

31. Nicholas PK, Voss JG, Corless IB. Unhealthy behaviours for self-management of HIV-related peripheral neuropathy. AIDS Care 2007; 19(10:)1266–1273.

32. Simpson DM, Olney R, McArthur JC, et al. A placebo-controlled trial of lamotrigine for painful HIV-associated neuropathy. Neurology 2000; 54(11:)2115–2119.

33. Simpson DM, McArthur JC, Olney R, et al. Lamotrigine for HIV-associated painful sensory neuropathies: a placebo-controlled trial. Neurology 2003; 60(9:)1508–1514.

34. Osio M, Muscia F, Zampini L, et al. Acetyl-L-carnitine in the treatment of painful antiretroviral toxic neuropathy in human immunodeficiency virus patients: an open label study. J Peripher Nerv Syst 2006; 11(1:)72–76.

35. Youle M, Osio M; ALCAR Study Group. A double-blind, parallel-group, placebo-controlled, multicentre study of acetyl-L-carnitine in the symptomatic treatment of antiretroviral toxic neuropathy in patients with HIV-1 infection. HIV Med 2007; 8(4:)241–250.

36. Galantino ML, Eke-Okoro ST, Findley TW, et al. Use of noninvasive electroacupuncture for the treatment of HIV-related peripheral neuropathy: a pilot study. J Altern Complement Med 1999; 5(2:)135–142.

3 | Central Poststroke Pain

Gary W. Jay

Clinical Disease Area Expert-Pain, Pfizer, Inc., New London, Connecticut, U.S.A.

THE DISORDER

Central poststroke pain (CPSP) was originally thought to be "thalamic" pain, as described by Dejerine and Roussy (1), although it was described even earlier in 1883 (2). Dejerine and Roussy (1) characterized their eponymous thalamic pain syndrome as including hemiplegia, hemiataxia and hemiastereognosis, difficulties with both superficial and deep sensation; persistent, paroxysmal, typically intolerable pain; and choreoathetoid movements. This syndrome is now known as central poststroke pain syndrome.

DIAGNOSIS

The reported incidence of CPSP varies widely from 2% (3) to 8% (4) in stroke patients and to 25% (5) in patients with lateral medullary infarctions (Wallenberg's syndrome).

CPSP is broadly defined as central neuropathic pain, secondary to lesions or dysfunction in the central nervous system. It is typically characterized by constant or intermittent pain and sensory abnormalities, most commonly of thermal sensation (6).

The pain is typically described as burning, scalding, or freezing and burning. Early diagnosis can be difficult, as the patients who develop CPSP may develop the problem long after their cerebral vascular accident (CVA), causing misdiagnosis or significant delay prior to treatment. Also, as these patients may have cognitive or speech difficulties, as well as depression, anxiety, and sleep problems, diagnosis may be further complicated. They may also develop spontaneous dysesthesias and stimulus-evoked sensory disturbances including dysesthesia, hyperalgesia, and allodynia (6, 7).

The onset of the pain may be immediate or be delayed for months to years (7–9). In 40% to 60% of CPSP patients, the onset of their centrally related pain post stroke may occur more than one month after the CVA (10). The pain may encompass a large part of the contralateral body, but it may also involve only a small area.

Sensory abnormalities are also associated with CPSP. These may include altered sensory processing: warm and cold stimulation applied to the skin may be perceived as paresthesias or dysesthesias rather than cold or warm (4,7). Allodynia is found in 55% to 70% of patients (11, 12). Hyperalgesia and dysesthesia are also frequently seen (13).

Evaluation of the CPSP patient may be more complex than that of the typical pain patient, at least in part for reasons noted above. The pain history must be accompanied by a pain-specific sensory examination, musculoskeletal and

23

myofascial evaluation, and basic psychological evaluation. Specialized sensory testing may also be needed, something that a neurologist can easily learn but may need specialized tools (14).

PATHOPHYSIOLOGY

Locations of the lesions inducing the CPSP have been demonstrated to be referable to the spinothalamocortical tract/pathway, typically associated with abnormal evoked sensations in the peripherally affected area (10,15,16). While at least three thalamic regions, which directly or indirectly receive spinothalamic projections, appear to be involved in the development of CPSP—the ventroposterior thalamus including the posteriorly and inferiorly located nuclei bordering on that region, the reticular nucleus, and the medial intralaminar region—it is the ventroposterior thalamic region that is proposed to be most significantly involved in central pain (17–19). It should also be noted that cerebrovascular lesions located above the diencephalon, that is, in the parietal lobe, may also induce CPSP (11,17,20).

While damage to the spinothalamocortical pathway appears to be a necessary condition in CPSP, it is thought that the spontaneous pain linked to CPSP is secondary to hyperexcitability or spontaneous discharges in thalamic or cortical neurons that have lost part of their normal input (21).

CPSP is most typically associated with a single lesion, associated with either a focal gray or white matter lesion; the lesion may be at the spinal, brain stem, or cerebral level, but it is always contralateral to the pain of CPSP; CPSP is associated with abnormal somatic senses, particularly thermal and/or pain sensations—most commonly, a loss of sensation is seen, but one may also see an exaggerated sensation of pain or temperature. The pain of CPSP may unilaterally involve the contralateral (to the lesion) face, body, and extremities, or it may be focal, involving only a limb, part of a limb, or the face; it is almost always within the region of somatic motor or sensory impairment; it may begin at the time of the CVA or be delayed for months (22).

Studies using magnetic resonance imaging and positron emission tomography (PET) scan have demonstrated anatomical lesions and associated information. One study using functional magnetic resonance imaging and diffusion tensor imaging found that in CPSP, there is an important role of damage of lateral nociceptive thalamoparietal fibers, along with release of activity of anterior cingulate and posterior parietal regions (23). An older study using single-photon emission computerized tomography found a contralateral relative hyperactivity in a central region corresponding with the thalamic region in patients with CPSP (24).

The "disinhibition hypothesis" of CPSP suggests that there is an excessive response (including dysesthesias/hyperalgesia/allodynia) associated with a loss of sensation secondary to a lesion of a "lateral nucleus" of the thalamic or "corticothalamic pathways." It was also thought that injury to a cool-signaling lateral thalamic pathway disinhibits a nociceptive medial thalamic pathway, producing both burning, cold, ongoing pain and cold allodynia. Using quantitatively evaluated sensory testing, it was found that, in CPSP, tactile allodynia occurs in disturbances of thermal/pain pathways that can spare the tactile signaling pathways, and that cold hypoesthesia itself is not necessary or sufficient for cold allodynia (25).

Another way of evaluating CPSP using PET scan technology revealed a striking loss of opioid receptor availability widely distributed throughout a great deal of the hemisphere contralateral to the pain (especially in the thalamus, anterior and posterior cingulate cortex, insula, S2, and lateral prefrontal cortex) (26).

It has previously been pointed out that decreased opioid receptor binding can also indicate the release of endogenous opioids during pain (27). The authors of the previous study (26) found that the location and distribution of the diminished receptor binding was more extensive and showed little overlap as compared to the other group (27). It is thought possible that the loss of opioid receptor availability in CPSP may be secondary to a reduction or downregulation of opioid receptors, resulting in a reduction of effectiveness of endogenous, opioid-mediated, analgesic mechanisms (26).

A later study looked at peripheral versus central neuropathic pain (28). The authors used PET scans to evaluate patients with peripheral ($n = 7$) and CPSP ($n = 8$) neuropathic pain patients. They found that in CPSP patients, interhemispheric comparison indicated a significant decrease in opioid binding in posterior midbrain, medial thalamus, and the insular, temporal, and prefrontal cortices contralateral to the painful side. The patients with peripheral neuropathic pain did not show any lateralized decrease in opioid binding. The authors concluded that decreases in opioid binding were much more extensive than anatomical cortical lesions and were not colocalized with the lesions: metabolic depression (diaschisis) and/or degeneration of opioid receptor–bearing neurons secondary to central lesions appears to be a likely mechanism (28).

Sympathetic dysfunction has also been felt to play a role in central pain secondary to signs of abnormal sympathetic activity: edema, hypohidrosis, trophic skin changes, changes in skin color, and decreased skin temperature (12,29). It is also noted that some or many of these changes may be secondary to "movement allodynia," which makes the patient keep the affected limb motionless (9).

Reports of CPSP associated with abnormal "epileptiform" activities in thalamic cells may be involved with central pain (30, 31). This would also indicate that some aspects of the problem may be secondary to cortical involvement, as epileptiform discharges are associated with that region, typically. Another group also noted that central pain may be a manifestation of partial epileptic seizures (32).

TREATMENT
Treatment of the CPSP is difficult and options are limited.

The most common first-line drug is amitriptyline, with other drugs including opiates treated as second line (10). Amitriptyline is thought to be helpful, secondary to its reuptake inhibition of serotonin and norepinephrine (33). In a controlled trial of amitriptyline and carbamazepine, only patients on amitriptyline reached a statistically significant reduction in pain compared to placebo. Patients on carbamazepine did not but had "some pain relief" and more side effects (34).

Aside from amitriptyline, anticonvulsants including lamotrigine and gabapentin have been reported to provide pain relief with better safety than carbamazepine and phenytoin (35–39). In spite of the articles suggesting lamotrigine provided good relief of CPSP, a Cochrane review found that lamotrigine had only limited evidence that it would be useful, and it was, in fact, unlikely to be of benefit for the treatment of neuropathic pain (40).

Other antidepressants and anticonvulsants have also been tried in the treatment of CPSP, but none has become a primary or gold-standard treatment (41–46).

Intravenous lidocaine appeared to be helpful in patients with CPSP (47, 48). Intravenous naloxone was not helpful in CPSP (49), while intrathecal baclofen, an agonist of GABA-B receptors, did provide relief for CPSP patients (50).

Stimulation of the primary motor cortex for intractable deafferentation pain, as well as central stroke pain, has been used successfully. The mechanism of pain relief by this form of electrical stimulation of MI is uncertain (51, 52). However, motor cortex stimulation is felt to be the treatment of choice in poststroke pain, thalamic pain, or anesthesia dolorosa of the face (53).

One group looked at the effectiveness of chronic subthreshold stimulation of the contralateral precentral gyrus in patients with intractable neuropathic pain for more than 15 years. They found that patients with trigeminal neuralgia had a greater positive effect than those with CPSP. They note that positive effects can last for 10 years in long-term follow-up (54).

Repetitive transcranial magnetic stimulation of the primary motor cortex has also been used successfully, as long as the postcentral gyrus (M1) is stimulated (55). Another group found this modality to give good but transient relief (56).

Transcutaneous electrical nerve stimulation (TENS), both high and low frequency, was tested on patients with CPSP ($n = 15$). Four patients obtained pain relief. Three patients continued to use TENS ipsilaterally with good effect at 23 to 30 months, while in one-third of the patients, TENS temporarily increased their pain (57).

One undesirable effect of repetitive deep brain stimulation (DBS) is the reduction of the seizure threshold, known as kindling (58–62). An associate of the author (personal communication) described a patient whose pain was only partially reduced with the original stimulus parameters of DBS. In an attempt to improve pain control, that individual used the external controller to increase the amount of stimulation above the amount used by the attending neurosurgeon. After several days of this maneuver, the patient suffered a first-ever focal onset, secondarily generalized seizure. To the author's knowledge, this patient may represent the first case of self-induced kindling of seizures in a human patient using DBS for pain control. Other treatments include sympathetic blockade, as well as surgical interventions including cordotomy, dorsal root entry zone lesions, thalamotomy, or cortical and subcortical ablation (63–69).

REFERENCES

1. Dejerine J, Roussy G. Le syndrome thalamique. Rev Neurol 1906; 14:521–532.
2. Greiff N. Zur localization der hemichorea. Arch Psychol Nervenkrankheiten 1883; 14:598.
3. Bowsher D. Sensory consequences of stroke (Letter). Lancet 1993; 341:156.
4. Andersen G, Vestergaard K, Ingeman-Neilsen M, et al. The incidence of central poststroke pain. Pain 1995; 61:187–193.
5. MacGowan DJ, Janal MN, Clark WC, et al. Central poststroke pain and Wallenberg's lateral medullary infarction: frequency, character and determinants in 63 patients. Neurology 1997; 49:120–125.

6. Henry JL, Lalloo C, Yashpal K. Central poststroke pain: an abstruse outcome. Pain Res Manag 2008; 13(1):41–49.
7. Leijon G, Boivie J, Johansson I. Central post-stroke pain—neurological symptoms and pain characteristics. Pain 1989; 36:13–25.
8. Holmgren H, Leijon G, Boivie J, et al. Central post-stroke pain—somatosensory evoked potentials in relation to location of the lesion and sensory signs. Pain 1990; 40:43–52.
9. Bowsher D. The management of central post-stroke pain (Review). Postgrad Med J 1995; 71:598–604.
10. Hansson P. Post-stroke pain case study: clinical characteristics, therapeutic options and long-term follow-up. Eur J Neurol 2004; 11(suppl 1):22–30.
11. Wessel K, Vieregge P, Kessler C, et al. Thalamic stroke: correlation of clinical symptoms, somatosensory evoked potentials and CT findings. Acta Neurol Scand 1994; 90:167–173.
12. Bowsher D. Central pain: clinical and physiological characteristics. J Neurol Neurosurg Psychiatry 1996; 61:62–69.
13. Mersky HH, Lindblom U, Mumford JM, et al. Pain terms: a current note with definitions and notes on usage. Pain Suppl 1986; 3:216–221.
14. Backonja MM, Galer BS. Pain assessment and evaluation of patients who have neuropathic pain. Neurol Clin 1998; 16(4):775–789.
15. Boivie J. Central pain. In: Wall PD, Melzack R, eds. Textbook of Pain. 3rd ed. New York: Churchill Livingstone, 1994:3;902.
16. Jensen TS, Lenz FA. Central post-stroke pain: a challenge for the scientist and the clinician (Editorial). Pain 1995; 61:62–69.
17. Lenz FA. Ascending modulation of thalamic function and pain: experimental and clinical data. In: Sicuteri F, ed. Advances in Pain Research and Therapy. New York: Raven, 1992:177–196.
18. Jones EG. Thalamus and pain. APS J 1992:1:58–61.
19. Boivie J. Hyperalgesia and allodynia in patients with CNS lesions. In: Willis WDJ, ed. Hyperalgesia and Allodynia. New York: Raven, 1992:363–373.
20. Sandy R. Spontaneous pain, hyperpathia and wasting of the hand due to parietal lobe haemorrhage. Eur Neurol 1985; 24:1–3.
21. Vestergaard K, Nielsen J, Andersen G, et al. Sensory abnormalities in consecutive, unselected patients with central post-stroke pain. Pain 1995; 61:177–186.
22. Casey K. Central pain: distributed effects of focal lesions (Editorial). Pain 2004; 108:205–206.
23. Seghier ML, Lazeyras F, Vuilleumier P, et al. Functional magnetic resonance imaging and diffusion tensor imaging in a case of central poststroke pain. J Pain 2005; 6(3):208–212.
24. Cesaro P, Mann MW, Moretti JL, et al. Central pain and thalamic hyperactivity: a single photon emission computerized tomographic study. Pain 1991; 47(3):329–336.
25. Greenspan JD, Ohara S, Sarlani E, et al. Allodynia in patients with post-stroke central pain (SPSP) studied by statistical quantitative sensory testing within individuals. Pain 2004; 109:357–366.
26. Willoch F, Schindler F, Wester HJ, et al. Central poststroke pain and reduced opioid receptor binding within pain processing circuitries: a [^{11}C]diprenorphine PET study. Pain 2004; 108:213–220.
27. Zubieta JK, Smith YR, Bueller JA, et al. Regional mu opioid receptor regulation of sensory and affective dimensions of pain. Science 2001; 293:311–315.
28. Maarrawi J, Peyron R, Mertens P, et al. Differential brain opioid receptor availability in central and peripheral neuropathic pain. Pain 2007; 127:183–194.
29. Riddoch G. The clinical features of central pain. Lancet 1938; 234:1093–1098, 1150–1056, 1205–1209.
30. Gorecki J, Hirayama T, Dostrovsky JO, et al. Thalamic stimulation and recording in patients with deafferentation and central pain. Stereotact Funct Neurosurg 1989; 52:120–126.

31. Yamashiro K, Iwayama K, Kurihara M, et al. Neurones with epileptiform discharge in the central nervous system and chronic pain: experimental and clinical investigations. Acta Neurochir Suppl (Wien) 1991; 52:130–132.

32. Scholz J, Vieregge P, Moster A. Central pain as a manifestation of partial epileptic seizures. Pain 1999; 80:445–450.

33. Jensen TS, Lenz FA. Central post-stroke pain: a challenge for the scientist and the clinician. Pain 1995; 61:161–164.

34. Leijon G, Boivie J. Central Post-stoke pain—a controlled trial of amitriptyline and carbamazepine. Pain 1989; 36(1):27–36.

35. Frese A, Husstedt IW, Ringelstein EB, et al. Pharmacologic treatment of central post-stroke pain. Clin J Pain 2006; 22(3):252–260.

36. Chen B, Stitik TP, Foye PM, et al. Central post-stroke pain syndrome: yet another use for gabapentin? Am J Phys Med Rehabil 2002; 81(9):718–720.

37. Nicholson BD. Evaluation and treatment of central pain syndromes. Neurology 2004; 62(5 suppl 2):S30–S36.

38. Backonja MM. Use of anticonvulsants for treatment of neuropathic pain. Neurology 2002; 59(5 suppl 2):S14–S17.

39. Jensen TS. Anticonvulsants in neuropathic pain: rationale and clinical evidence. Eur J Pain 2002; 6 suppl A:61–68.

40. Wiffen PJ, Rees J. Lamotrigine for acute and chronic pain. Cochrane Database Syst Rev 2007; 18(2):CD006044.

41. Davidoff G, Guarrachini M, Roth E, et al. Trazodone hydrochloride in the treatment of dysesthetic pain in traumatic myelopathy: a randomized, double blind, placebo-controlled study. Pain 1987; 29:151–161.

42. Ekbom K. Tegretol, a new therapy of tabetic lightning pains. Acta Med Scand 1966; 179:251–252.

43. Swerdlow M. Anticonvulsants in the therapy of neuralgic pain. Pain Clin 1986; 1:9–19.

44. Awerbuch A. Treatment of thalamic pain syndrome with Mexilitene. Ann Neurol 1990; 28:233.

45. Leijon G, Boivie J. Treatment of neurogenic pain with antidepressants. Nordisk Psykiatrisk Tidsskrift 1989b; 43(suppl 20):83–87.

46. Portenoy RK, Foley KM, Inturrisi CE. The nature of opioid responsiveness and its implications for neuropathic pain: new hypotheses derived from studies of opioid infusions. Pain 1990; 43:272–286.

47. Kastrup J, Petersen P, Dejgard A, et al. Intravenous lidocaine infusion—a new treatment of chronic painful diabetic neuropathy? Pain 1987; 28:69–75.

48. Backonja MM, Gombar KA. Response of central pain syndromes to intravenous lidocaine. J Pain Symptom Manage 1992; 7(3):172–178.

49. Bainton T, Fox M, Bowsher D, et al. A double-blind trial of naloxone in central post-stroke pain. Pain 1992; 48(2):159–162.

50. Taira T, Hori T. Intrathecal baclofen in the treatment of post-stroke central pain, dystonia and persistent vegetative state. Acta Neurochir Suppl 2007; 97(pt 1):227–229.

51. Saitoh Y, Yoshimine T. Stimulation of primary motor cortex for intractable deafferentation pain. Acta Neurochir Suppl 2007; 97(pt 2):51–56.

52. Cioni B, Meglio M. Motor cortex stimulation for chronic non-malignant pain: current state and future prospects. Acta Neurochir Suppl 2007; 97(pt 2):45–49.

53. Lazorthes Y, Sol JC, Fowo S, et al. Motor cortex stimulation for neuropathic pain. Acta Neurochir Suppl 2007; 97(pt 2):37–44.

54. Rasche D, Ruppolt M, Stippich C, et al. Motor cortex stimulation for long-term relief of chronic neuropathic pain: a 10 year experience. Pain 2006; 121(1–2):43–52.

55. Hirayama A, Saitoh Y, Kishima H, et al. Reduction of intractable deafferentation pain by navigation-guided repetitive transcranial magnetic stimulation of the primary motor cortex. Pain 2006; 122(1/2):22–27.

56. Lefaucheur JP, Drouot X, Menard-Lefaucheur I, et al. Neurogenic pain relief by repetitive transcranial magnetic cortical stimulation depends on the origin and the site of pain. J Neurol Neurosurg Psychiatry 2004; 75(4):612–616.

57. Leijon G, Boivie J. Central post-stroke pain—the effect of high and low frequency TENS. Pain 1989; 38(2):187–191.
58. Hirato M, Watanabe K, Takahashi A, et al. Pathophysiology of central (thalamic) pain: combined change of sensory thalamus with cerebral cortex around central sulcus. Stereotact Funct Neurosurg 1994; 62:300–303.
59. Douglas RM, Goddard G. Long-term potentiation of the perforant path–granule cell synapse in the rat hippocampus. Brain Res 1975; 86:205–215.
60. Goddard GV, Douglas RM. Does the engram of kindling model the engram of normal long-term memory? Can J Neurol Sci 1975; 2(4):385–394.
61. Racine RJ, Gartner JG, Burnham WM. Epileptiform activity and neural plasticity in limbic structures. Brain Res 1972; 47(1):262–268.
62. Racine RJ, Tuff L, Zaide J. Kindling, unit discharge patterns and neural plasticity. Can J Neurol Sci 1975; 2(4):395–405.
63. Siegfried J. Long term results of electrical stimulation in the treatment of pain my means of implanted electrodes. In: Rizzi C, Visentin TA, eds. Pain Therapy. Amsterdam, The Netherlands: Elsevier, 1983:463–475.
64. Tasker R, de Carvalho G, Dostrovsky JO. The history of central pain syndromes, with observations concerning pathophysiology and treatment. In: Casey KL, ed. Pain and Central Nervous Disease: The Central Pain Syndromes. New York: Raven, 1991:31–58.
65. Siegfried J, Demierre B. Thalamic electrostimulation in the treatment of thalamic pain syndrome. Pain 1984 (suppl 2):116.
66. Tasker R. Pain resulting from central nervous system pathology (central pain). In: Bonica JJ, ed. The Management of Pain. Philadelphia: Lea and Febiger, 1990:264–280.
67. Edgar RE, Best LG, Quail PA, et al. Computer-assisted DREZ microcoagulation: post-traumatic spinal deafferentation pain. J Spinal Dis 1993; 6:48–56.
68. Nashold BS, Bullitt E. Dorsal root entry zone lesions to control central pain in paraplegics. J Neurosurg 1981; 55:414–419.
69. Loh L, Nathan PW, Schott GD. Pain due to lesions of central nervous system removed by sympathetic block. Br Med J 1981; 282:1026–1028.

4   Postherpetic Neuralgia

Rajbala Thakur, Annie G. Philip, and Jonathan C. Weeks

Department of Anesthesiology, University of Rochester School of Medicine and Dentistry, Rochester, New York, U.S.A.

Postherpetic neuralgia (PHN) is a chronic neuropathic condition that may be associated with severe, intractable pain that can last for years and cause significant suffering. Its exact incidence and prevalence is unknown, but it is estimated to affect about 500,000 to 1 million Americans (1, 2). It is the most common complication following an episode of acute herpes zoster. Herpes zoster is caused due to reactivation of varicella zoster virus that has lain dormant in a sensory ganglion following a chicken pox causing primary varicella infection. This reactivation is due to an age-, disease-, or drug-related decline in cellular immunity. The most important risk factors for PHN are age 60 years or older, and severe acute pain and rash during acute herpes zoster. There is a relative paucity of data on its natural history due to the lack of population-based studies of zoster-related pain. Multiple studies consistently indicate that the majority of patients experience resolution of pain over weeks to months following rash onset (3–6). Persistent pain one year after the initial diagnosis of PHN has been described to be present in 20% of patients over the age of 60 (7–9). The exact number of patients who enjoy a complete resolution of PHN is unknown.

Prevention strategies for PHN include administration of zoster vaccine, treatment with antiviral therapy within 72 hours of rash onset, and aggressive pain control. Treatment of PHN includes medications such as gabapentin, pregabalin, topical lidocaine, tricyclic antidepressants, tramadol, opioids, and capsaicin cream. There may be a small but potentially significant role of invasive interventions in the treatment of PHN.

THE DISORDER

Definition
The term PHN is used to describe persistent, unilateral, dermatomal pain following the appearance and healing of a zoster rash. Historically, time points used to describe PHN have ranged from one to six months after a zoster episode (10). Recent research supports defining PHN as pain that persists for more than 120 days after the onset of the rash (11). Clinical presentation includes a constellation of characteristics, but heterogeneous symptoms and signs, none of which, by itself, is pathognomonic of the disease state. Pain may be continuous or episodic, spontaneous or evoked, and may or may not be accompanied by itching.

Symptoms

- *Stimulus-independent pain*: Intermittent sharp, stabbing, electrical shock-like lancinating pain and/or continuous throbbing and burning dysesthetic pain is common.
- *Stimulus-evoked pain*: Allodynia, an excessively painful response to an innocuous stimulus, is a common symptom of PHN and may be the most debilitating symptom associated with this disorder. Tactile allodynia can be so severe that patients with truncal PHN may not be able to tolerate the sensation of clothing against their skin at the affected site. A cool breeze or air-conditioning may evoke pain in patients with craniofacial involvement; shaving and wearing hats or glasses may become problematic.
- *Pruritus*: Chronic itching with or without comorbid pain may be present and can become problematic for some patients with PHN. Serious, self-inflicted injury may result secondary to scratching, especially if the affected body part is insensate.
- *Psychosocial symptoms*: The presence of persistent, unremitting pain can result in psychosocial sequelae including anxiety, depression, and social isolation (2–15). The patient's ability to perform job-related and household tasks may be affected, causing significant reduction in global quality-of-life indicators (14,16).
- *Nonspecific symptoms*: Chronic fatigue, anorexia, weight loss, and insomnia (12) are frequently associated with PHN resulting in significant disability.

Signs

- *Skin discoloration*: Skin can be normal in appearance or exhibit areas of hyperpigmentation, hypopigmentation, or scarring in the affected dermatomes. Affected areas may also exhibit a persistent reddish or brownish hue.
- *Sensory abnormalities*: Involved areas may be hypesthetic. This can be found even in regions that exhibit tactile allodynia. Hyperalgesia (abnormally increased pain perception to a noxious stimulus) or dysesthesia (uncomfortable but not painful sensation to touch) are also common findings in PHN. The areas of altered tactile sensitivity may grow wider than the sites originally affected by the zoster rash. Alterations in temperature sensation have also been demonstrated.
- *Motor abnormalities*: In select cases, residual motor weakness may be present due to the involvement of motor neurons as a bystander effect, in addition to the more typically involved sensory ganglion (17). Evidence of facial paralysis in the form of ptosis or loss of the nasolabial fold in cases of facial nerve involvement, and a truncal bulge, resulting from intercostal muscle weakness may be present. Myofascial trigger points and reduced joint range of motion may be seen in severe cases when pain has resulted in excessive guarding.

DIAGNOSIS

A diagnosis of PHN is made primarily on the basis of clinical findings. A history of a unilateral dermatomal rash, followed by persistent pain in the same distribution, usually establishes the diagnosis. Occasionally, patients report having a pain-free hiatus that has been observed to last for a period of weeks to as long as 12 months. In a study of 156 patients with PHN, Watson et al. (5) noted that 25% of patients with a poor outcome said that they could recall a time after the rash when they had little or no pain. The recurrence of dermatomal pain is not associated with a recurrent episode of herpes zoster but may coincide with a period of increased emotional or physical stress. In cases where a definitive history of rash is not available, a definitive diagnosis of varicella zoster virus (VZV)-related pain would require serial serologic assessments that are unlikely to be obtained in most clinical settings.

PHN can cause a significant deleterious effect on health-related quality of life (4,18–20). In addition, it can result in fatigue, insomnia, anxiety, depression, and suicidal ideation. Hence, in addition to a thorough history and physical examination, assessment should include screening for any psychological comorbidities and the overall impact the pain has had on the patient.

Laboratory Diagnosis
Diagnostic tests have a limited role in clinical practice and are predominantly used in a clinical research setting. Standardized Quantitative Sensory testing can distinguish between phenotypic subtypes of PHN patients that could potentially be correlated to different pathogenic mechanisms. This is a potentially fruitful area of future research, especially if these insights help to identify therapeutic targets. Skin biopsy studies and nerve conduction studies can help confirm the diagnoses and potentially provide uniformity for clinical analgesic trials.

PATHOPHYSIOLOGY
A variety of pathophysiological mechanisms are postulated in an attempt to explain the heterogeneity of signs and symptoms seen in patients with PHN. Viral reactivation followed by replication causes neural and inflammatory damage in the involved sensory ganglion and peripheral nerve, inducing a cycle of peripheral as well as central sensitization that result in ongoing chronic pain. Severity of neural damage correlates with the severity of the acute syndrome and subsequent PHN (21). Our existing knowledge of the pathophysiological mechanisms of PHN is limited. Multiple studies (22–28) including neuroanatomical autopsy studies, skin biopsy studies, and studies of sensory dysfunction and pharmacological responses have led to the impression that two distinct pathophysiological mechanisms contribute substantially to the development of PHN: sensitization and deafferentation.

Sensitization
1. Peripheral sensitization of intact C-nociceptor fibers is depicted by minimal sensory loss in areas of marked allodynia and reduced thermal sensory threshold (23, 24, 27, 29, 30), resulting in heat hyperalgesia (29). This results in the spontaneous burning pain that is commonly seen in these patients.
2. Central sensitization may result from sprouting of A-beta fibers, centrally, in response to partial loss of C-fiber input. Regenerating A-beta fibers make contact with those central receptors that previously received input from the C-fibers, resulting in the development of tactile allodynia and hyperalgesia (24, 27). These observations support the hypothesis that in a subset of PHN patients, allodynia may be maintained by input from partially intact, but sensitized, nociceptors resulting in central sensitization (24, 31). Glutamate, an N-methyl D-aspartate (NMDA) receptor agonist, is the major neurotransmitter involved in this process.

TABLE 1 Risk Factors in PHN

Well replicated

- Age >60 yr
- Severity of rash
- Severity of acute pain
- Painful prodrome

Less well replicated

- Female gender
- Polyneuropathy
- Physical and emotional stress
- Craniofacial distribution

Deafferentation

In a subset of PHN patients, there is a complete loss of both large- and small-diameter sensory afferent fibers. This loss of peripheral input results in the development of spontaneous discharges in the deafferentated central neurons, leading to intrinsic changes in the central nervous system. This produces constant pain in addition to severe mechanical allodynia in the area of sensory loss (24, 31, 32).

The above data suggests that there may be different underlying mechanisms in the generation and maintenance of this chronic pain state that are responsible for the varied presentations of pain in patients with PHN. A mechanistic approach for selecting specific pharmacological treatment options is an extremely desirable goal that has not yet been achieved. Any factors that can increase the extent of neural damage caused by the viral load, or accentuate the effect of the damage, lead to an increase in the incidence, severity, and duration of the PHN pain (see Table 1 for a list of risk factors). Increasing age is the strongest risk factor in both immunocompetent and immunocompromised individuals (4,33–35). In one study, the overall prevalence of PHN was 15 and 27 times as high at 30 and 60 days, respectively, in persons older than 50 years of age compared to younger patients. Each one-year increment in age was associated with 9% and 12% increases in the prevalence of PHN at 30 and 60 days, respectively (36). In addition to the waning immunity and neurological comorbidities, presence of subclinical polyneuropathy is more likely in the elderly; hence, even a smaller viral load can lead to increased damage (37, 38). Other powerful risk factors include the presence of a painful prodrome, increased severity of acute pain, and severity of rash (39–41). All of these factors seem to correspond with the degree of neural damage and are independent risk factors contributing to the incidence and severity of PHN. Each one of these may independently explain the postulated pathophysiological mechanisms for this disease state.

TREATMENT

Management includes strategies for prevention as well as treatment of PHN. The main therapies for PHN prevention include primary varicella vaccine, zoster vaccine, and antiviral medications. There is some data to suggest a beneficial effect of amitriptyline in PHN prevention.

Prevention Strategies

Varicella Vaccine
Childhood varicella vaccination reduces the incidence of chicken pox and subsequent herpes zoster and PHN. A live, attenuated Oka varicella vaccine entered into widespread use in 1995 and has led to a marked decrease in the incidence of chicken pox (42). The vaccine virus establishes latency in sensory ganglia, like wild-type VZV, but appears to cause herpes zoster much less frequently. Hence, childhood varicella vaccination should eventually result in an overall decrease in the incidence of herpes zoster and PHN (43).

Some experts speculate that the incidence of herpes zoster could increase in younger adults in the near future because a decline in the incidence of varicella may reduce the population's exposure to VZV, prevent opportunities for subclinical immune boosting to VZV, and increase the risk for VZV reactivation (44, 45).

Zoster Vaccine
This live, attenuated varicella vaccine was developed with the goal of conferring an immunologic boost to the age-related waning immunity of older adults. This is especially important in light of the fact that natural immune boosting opportunities will eventually decline as mentioned above. The Shingles Prevention Study—a large, multicenter, randomized, placebo-controlled trial—was conducted to evaluate the efficacy and safety of herpes zoster vaccination (46). The results of the trial indicated that the herpes zoster vaccine reduces the likelihood of developing herpes zoster in immunocompetent individuals 60 years of age or older. Important results of this study included a decrease in the incidence of herpes zoster by 51.3%, a reduction in the overall burden of illness by 61.1%, and a decrease in the incidence of PHN by 66.5% (47). The effect on decreasing the incidence of herpes zoster was less in older subjects, but the effect on reducing the severity of illness was greater in older subjects. Therefore, the overall reduction in burden of illness, the primary end point of the study, was maintained across all age groups. On the basis of these data, the FDA approved the use of the herpes zoster vaccine in individuals 60 years and older. This live, attenuated vaccine is contraindicated in children, pregnant women, and immunocompromised individuals.

Antiviral Agents
Three oral antiviral medications, including acyclovir, famciclovir, and valacyclovir, have been assessed in patients with herpes zoster for their role in the prevention of PHN or lessening its severity. Results of clinical trials indicate that all three agents mentioned decrease both zoster pain and the risk of developing PHN to some degree. The results of the individual trials could be questioned for consistency of evidence, but taken together, a strong case can be made for the use of antiviral therapy in treatment for herpes zoster–associated pain and in decreasing the incidence and chronicity of PHN pain (4,9,48–55). Early antiviral therapy is recommended to reduce viral replication and resultant neural damage and, thus, decrease the incidence and severity of PHN. A meta-analysis of the trials involving the use of acyclovir showed that in patients who were at least 50 years of age, the proportion with persistent pain at six months was 15%, as

compared with 35% in the placebo group (4). In comparing famciclovir (500 mg every eight hours) to placebo in a subgroup of subjects who were at least 50 years of age and who had persistent pain after skin healing, the median duration of PHN was 163 days in the placebo group and 63 days in the famciclovir group ($P = 0.004$) (53). In a randomized trial of patients who were at least 50 years of age, comparison of valacyclovir (1000 mg every eight hours) and acyclovir resulted in equivalent rates of cutaneous healing (54). Valacyclovir significantly shortened the median time to resolution of zoster-associated pain (38 days vs. 51 days, $P = 0.001$). The proportion of patients experiencing pain at six months was 25.7% in the acyclovir group and 19.3% in the valacyclovir group ($P = 0.02$). Famciclovir and valacyclovir were compared (55) and showed similar effect on rash healing, acute pain resolution, and the percentage of patients with persistent pain at six months. All three drugs are comparable in their efficacy and safety profile. Valacyclovir and famciclovir enjoy a more favorable dosing regimen (three times per day) compared to acyclovir (five times per day) and are thus easier to use. On the other hand, acyclovir is the least expensive of the three. Other antiviral agents include brivudine and foscarnet. Brivudine with once-a-day dosing is not available in the United States. Foscarnet is only available in intravenous formulation and has not been studied in PHN prevention.

Amitriptyline

A small, placebo-controlled, randomized trial evaluated the effect of a 25-mg daily dose of amitriptyline in patients older than 60 years of age. In this protocol, the amitriptyline was initiated within 48 hours of rash onset (56). The amitriptyline group showed a 50% decrease in pain prevalence at six months with an number needed to treat (NNT) of 5. Treatment with amitriptyline may have a beneficial effect on the incidence of PHN, but its use should be weighed carefully against potential serious side effects in elderly or otherwise frail patients. In clinical practice, nortriptyline is used more commonly because of its better safety and tolerability profile.

Gabapentin and Pregabalin

Use of neuromodulating medications like gabapentin and pregabalin may also decrease the severity of pain in acute herpes zoster and reduce the incidence of PHN beyond what can be achieved by antiviral therapy alone. In clinical practice, these medications are started early on, but there is no evidence in human studies to support its efficacy as a preventive strategy. There is promising data in acute postoperative pain in humans (57) but only animal data is available in PHN pain (58).

Corticosteroids

Two double-blind randomized controlled trials of corticosteroids given for a duration of 21 days did not show any effect on the incidence or duration of PHN (59, 60). The available evidence does not support the routine use of corticosteroids as a strategy to prevent PHN.

Invasive Interventions

There is no compelling evidence to support the use of invasive interventions for the prevention of PHN pain. Interventions such as epidural steroid injections, epidural local anesthetic infusions, sympathetic blocks, perilesional infiltration of local anesthetics, and steroids are used for pain management in patients who are refractory to conservative therapy. The hypothesis behind the interventional approach is that aggressive management of acute pain, itself, may prevent, or at least decrease, the severity and duration of chronic PHN pain. Uncontrolled clinical trials involving the use of sympathetic blocks in herpes zoster have claimed a reduction in the development of PHN (61, 62). Other studies, however, failed to replicate this effect (63). Thus, currently available evidence is inadequate to definitively support the routine use of sympathetic blocks or epidural blocks as a strategy for preventing PHN.

Key Points in Prevention of PHN

---

1. Zoster vaccination is recommended for older immunocompetent adults with the aim of decreasing the incidence of herpes zoster, the incidence and severity of PHN, and the overall burden of illness.
2. Early antiviral therapy within 72 hr of rash onset is recommended to hasten the rate of healing, minimize neural damage, and decrease pain caused by the acute illness. In addition, this may decrease the incidence and duration of postherpetic neuralgia.
3. Amitriptyline in acute herpes zoster can be used to decrease the risk of PHN.
4. No evidence exists to support the use of corticosteroids in PHN prevention.
5. Poor evidence regarding the role of invasive interventions in reducing the risk of PHN.

Clinical Treatments

In clinical practice, gabapentin, pregabalin, topical lidocaine patches, and tramadol are used as first-line medications followed by opioids and tricyclic antidepressants. This is largely based on the better tolerability of the first-line medications. Gabapentin, pregabalin, and lidoderm patch are FDA approved for PHN pain, although tricyclic antidepressants (TCAs) and opioids also have a well-established efficacy record (Table 2). Capsaicin cream is not commonly used, although it has been shown to be efficacious in two small randomized trials. There is a limited role for invasive interventions and alternative modalities, but these are utilized for patients who are refractory to conservative modalities. Recent studies have evaluated the relative efficacy of these treatments (64, 65). Additionally, consensus recommendation and guidelines for the pharmacotherapeutic management of neuropathic pain, including PHN, have been published and serve as useful guides in selecting treatment options (66–68) for an individual patient.

Gabapentinoids

Gabapentin and pregabalin have greater evidence of efficacy, are well tolerated, and are much safer compared to antiepileptics previously used to treat neuropathic pain conditions. Although the precise mechanism of action is not well understood, data derived from rodent models suggests that it acts at the alpha-2 delta-1 subunit of voltage-dependent calcium channels to decrease calcium influx, which, in turn, decreases the release of glutamate, norepinephrine, and substance P. These neurotransmitters are thought to be involved in maintaining central sensitization in chronic neuropathic pain states.

TABLE 2 Pharmacological Options for the Management of PHN (65, 72, 77, 87, 90, 94)

Medication	Starting dose	Dose titration	Common side effects	Caution/comments	Pooled NNT[a]
Gabapentin	100–300 mg	Start qhs and increase to tid dosing; increase by 100–300 mg every 3 days to total dose of 1800–2400 mg/day in three divided doses	Somnolence, dizziness, fatigue, ataxia, peripheral edema, and weight gain	Decrease dose in patients with renal impairment. QOD dosing in dialysis patients. Avoid sudden discontinuation.	4.4
Pregabalin	50 mg tid or 75 mg bid	300–600 mg/day in 7–10 days in two divided doses	Somnolence, fatigue, dizziness, peripheral edema and weight gain, blurred vision, and euphoria	Decrease dose in patients with renal impairment.	4.9
Topical Lidocaine	5% patch	Can use up to 3 patches 12 hr/day	Local erythema, rash, blisters	Known hypersensitivity to amide local anesthetics. Do not use on skin with open lesions.	2.0
Tramadol	50 mg every 6 hr prn	Can titrate up to 100 mg q 6 hr. Maximum daily dose: 400 mg. Extended-release dosing once a day	Nausea/vomiting, constipation, drowsiness, and dizziness	Be careful in patients with seizure disorder and concomitant use of SSRI, SSNRI, and TCAs. Decrease dose in patients with hepatic or renal disease.	4.8
[b] TCAs Nortriptyline Desipramine Amitriptyline	10–25 mg qhs. Start at a lower dose in elderly	Increase by 10–25 mg weekly with a target dose of 75–150 mg; once-in-24 hr dose	Sedation, dry mouth, blurred vision, weight gain, urinary retention, constipation, sexual cysfunction	Cardiac arrhythmic disease, glaucoma, suicide risk, seizure disorder. Risk of serotonin syndrome with concomitant use of tramadol, SSRI, or SNRIs. Amitriptyline has the most anticholinergic effects.	2.6
Opioids Morphine Oxycodone [c] Methadone [d] Fentanyl patch	15 mg q 6 hr prn 5 mg q 6 hr prn 2.5 mg tid 12 mcg/hr	Titrate at weekly intervals balancing analgesia and side effects. If patient tolerating, the medications can titrate faster.	Nausea/vomiting, constipation, drowsiness, and itching	Driving impairment and cognitive dysfunction during treatment initiation. Be careful in patients with sleep apnea. Additive effects of sedation with neuromodulating medications.	2.7
Topical Capsaicin	0.025–0.075% Cream	Apply 3–4 times a day over affected region	No systemic side-effects. Burning and stinging sensation at the application site.	Avoid contact with eyes, nose, and mouth. Application of lidocaine gel locally may be helpful prior to capsaicin cream application.	3.3

[a]NNT: Number of pain patients that need to be treated to achieve a 50% reduction in pain intensity in one patient.
[b]Obtain baseline EKG in patients with history of cardiac disease.
[c]Has a long and unpredictable half-life, hence need for extra caution in elderly patients.
[d]May need to start a patient on short-acting opioid medications before changing over to a Fentanyl patch.

Gabapentin

The optimal dosing schedule for gabapentin has not been well characterized. A recent review suggested that dosing should be initiated at 300 mg on the first day, followed by 300 mg twice daily on the second day, and then increased to 300 mg three times daily on the third day (69). At that point, gabapentin should be more slowly titrated with a goal of reaching 600 mg three times daily over the ensuing two weeks. A more gradual titration may be better tolerated in elderly frail individuals. As the drug is excreted renally, patients on dialysis should be started on a single dose of 100 mg given one hour after dialysis treatment on alternate days. This dose can be titrated up slowly and cautiously. There is good evidence to support the use of gabapentin in PHN pain. In two large clinical trials, its use was shown to be associated with a statistically significant reduction in daily pain ratings as well as improvements in sleep, mood, and quality of life at daily dosages of 1800 to 3600 mg (70, 71). A meta-analyses of two randomized controlled trials revealed that the pooled NNT for gabapentin in the treatment of PHN is approximately 4.4 (95% CI, 3.3–6.1) (72) (Table 2).

Common side effects include somnolence, gait or balance problems, dizziness, and mild peripheral edema. In general, these side effects are short lived but do require monitoring and, occasionally, dosage adjustment.

Pregabalin

Pregabalin is one of the newer anticonvulsants approved by FDA for use in PHN pain and fibromyalgia. Pregabalin also has a demonstrated anxiolytic effect in patients with generalized anxiety disorder (73, 74). This anxiolytic effect may complement its analgesic effect and provide additional benefit in PHN patients. Its mechanism of action is thought to be the same as gabapentin.

No optimal dosing schedule has been studied, and both fixed as well as flexible dosing schedules seem to be efficacious (75, 76). Three double-blind randomized controlled trials comprising a total of 776 patients with PHN showed superior pain relief and improved pain-related sleep interference compared to placebo. Doses in these studies ranged between 150 and 600 mg/day (77). In a meta-analysis, NNT for pregabalin was found to be 4.9 (3.66–7.58) (72) (Table 2).

There does not seem to be any difference in efficacy between gabapentin and pregabalin. Pregabalin does have a perceived advantage secondary to the ease of twice-daily dosing and a simpler titration process, which may result in a more rapid response to treatment.

Clearance of the drug is directly proportional to creatinine clearance; the dosage needs to be adjusted when creatinine clearance is less than 60 mL/min.

Frequently reported side effects are somnolence, balance problems, peripheral edema, and dizziness.

Tricyclic Antidepressants

Amitriptyline is the most widely studied antidepressant for PHN pain and, in fact, for many neuropathic pain conditions. The available evidence suggests that nortriptyline and desipramine (78) are equally effective (72, 79) and are better tolerated compared to amitriptyline; these agents may be preferred in frail patients. Both amitriptyline and nortriptyline are often helpful in patients with associated insomnia. Desipramine causes significantly less sedation and should be preferred in patients who may be either intolerant to the aforementioned agents or are taking other analgesics with sedating properties. A number of proposed mechanisms may explain the analgesic efficacy of these medications in neuropathic pain. These include inhibition of reuptake of norepinephrine and serotonin, glutamatergic transmission, and sodium channel blockade (80–82). These medications should be started at a low dose, typically 25 mg at night, and titrated up slowly to a target dose of 75 to 100 mg/day. Elderly frail individuals can be started at an even lower dose of 10 mg at night. Concomitant use with selective serotonin reuptake inhibitors (SSRI) antidepressants should be monitored carefully as there is a risk of developing toxic serum levels of TCAs with this combination. A number of randomized controlled trials and meta-analyses of these agents show good evidence of efficacy in the treatment of pain associated with PHN. Pooled data in these meta-analyses have shown an NNT of 2.1 to 2.6 (72, 83, 84) (Table 2). Major side effects include tachyarrhythmia, prolongation of the QT interval with the potential of life-threatening arrhythmias, and worsening of acute angle glaucoma. It is prudent to review a baseline EKG before starting these medications in elderly patients or those who possess other cardiac risk factors (85, 86). Minor side effects include dryness of mouth, dizziness, weight gain, sedation, constipation, urinary retention, and orthostatic hypotension.

Selective Dual Reuptake Inhibitors
The selective dual reuptake inhibitor duloxetine is FDA approved for use in diabetic polyneuropathic pain and fibromyalgia. Its efficacy in PHN has not been studied. Clinically, this medication seems to be better tolerated than TCAs and, hence, is used in clinical practice for PHN pain.

Opioids
Opioids are used in the treatment of PHN pain, and their use is supported by the results of well-designed clinical trials as well as years of clinical experience. These medications are recommended as second- or third-line analgesics (66–68) based upon concerns for their side effects, potential development of tolerance, and misuse and abuse. Available evidence suggests that the efficacy of opioids is comparable to TCAs and better than that of anticonvulsant agents. The analgesic efficacy of oral oxycodone was evaluated in a double-blind crossover trial (87). Treatment with oxycodone resulted in a significant reduction in allodynia, steady pain, and spontaneous paroxysmal pain. This treatment also resulted in superior scores for global effectiveness, disability reduction, and patient preference compared to placebo. In another randomized crossover study comparing opioids (morphine or methadone), tricyclic antidepressants (nortriptyline or desipramine), and placebo, morphine (mean dose 91 mg/day) or methadone (mean dose 15 mg/day) used as a rescue analgesic was associated with superior pain relief as compared to placebo. This study also made a direct comparison of opioids and TCAs. The NNT for opioids was 2.79 (2.01–4.6) compared to 3.73 (2.43–7.99) for the antidepressants (88).

Common opioid-related side effects such as nausea, sedation, urinary retention, pruritis, and constipation should be anticipated and managed proactively. Counseling and appropriate monitoring for tolerance, physical dependence, opioid-induced hyperalgesia, immune suppression, and hypogonadism is needed in chronic opioid therapy. Misuse and drug addiction are less of a concern in elderly patients, but drug diversion by family members is a possibility and should be considered and appropriately monitored.

Tramadol

Tramadol is a unique analgesic medication with a dual mechanism of action. It has a weak mu agonist effect, like opioids, and an inhibitory effect on the reuptake of serotonin and norepinephrine, like TCAs. Tramadol can be dosed 50 to 100 mg every six hours on an as-needed basis. The daily dose should not exceed 400 mg. Lower doses should be used in the elderly and in patients with impaired renal function. It is available as an extended release preparation and, also, as a combination product with acetaminophen.

A randomized controlled trial involving 127 patients compared the use of sustained release tramadol to placebo. Superior pain relief and improved quality of life was seen with the use of tramadol (89). The NNT was 4.8 (95% CI, 3.5–6.0) (Table 2).

Side effects include nausea, vomiting, dizziness, constipation, urinary retention, somnolence, and headache. Concomitant use with medications that are inhibitors of CYP2D6, such as SSRIs, SNRIs, and TCAs, can lead to serotonin syndrome. Abuse of tramadol is thought to be rare but has been observed. There is an increased risk of seizures in patients treated with tramadol who have a history of seizures or are also receiving drugs that can reduce the seizure threshold.

Lidoderm Patch

A 5% Lidoderm patch provides a local analgesic effect and is FDA approved for use in PHN. The mechanism of action of lidocaine in the treatment of neuropathic pain is thought to be due to inhibition of ionic fluxes necessary for the conduction of ectopic action potentials generated by damaged nociceptors. Efficacy can be ascertained within two weeks of initiation of treatment. An inherent advantage of topical therapies is that they are associated with few systemic effects due to minimal systemic absorption of the medication. Lidoderm 5% patch should be used only on intact skin, can be cut to fit the affected area, and should be left on for 12 hours in a 24-hour period. In select circumstances, use can be extended to 18 hours, if need be. A randomized controlled trial showed greater efficacy associated with the use of Lidoderm patches as compared to vehicle-controlled patches in PHN patients presenting with allodynia (90, 91). Side effects were similar in both groups and the suggested NNT for Lidoderm patch was 2.0 (90) (Table 2). In another placebo-controlled crossover trial that analyzed efficacy of Lidoderm 5% patch in 40 patients with chronic neuropathic pain including 22 with PHN, the NNT was found to be 4.4 (92). Lidocaine gel can be used in place of Lidoderm 5% patch, as it has also shown efficacy in PHN patients with allodynia (93). It is interesting to note that patients may respond well to topical lidocaine even if the skin at the targeted site is completely devoid of nociceptors (34).

Topical Capsaicin

Capsaicin (trans-8-methyl-N-vanillyl-6-nonenamide) is a drug that depletes substance P and may be effective in inhibiting pain. It is an agonist of the vanilloid receptor (TRPV1) present on afferent nociceptor terminals. There are no systemic effects with local application. It is commercially available in two concentrations: 0.025% and 0.075%. Pooled data from two placebo-controlled studies demonstrated superior pain relief following three to four times daily application of 0.075% capsaicin to the painful area with an NNT of 3.3 (94, 95) (Table 2). Blinding in these studies is challenging given that the medication produces a distinct burning sensation on initial application. In clinical practice, it is difficult to use, especially in patients who already have significant allodynia—the very patients most likely to benefit from this therapy. In clinical practice, a patient can be advised to apply a local anesthetic cream such as EMLA followed by capsaicin application for better tolerability. Recent pilot studies have evaluated a single application of a high concentration (8%) of capsaicin following a local anesthetic application. The results of these initial studies suggest this approach may produce prolonged relief of pain in some PHN patients (96).

Other Topical Treatments
Topical anti-inflammatory preparations such as aspirin/diethyl ether, indomethacin, and diclofenac/diethyl ether mixtures have been studied in a randomized, placebo-controlled trial with aspirin and indomethacin showing superior pain relief but not diclofenac (97). No definitive conclusions can be drawn about efficacy of these preparations, as significant heterogeneity was detected in this and other studies. The evidence for use of other compounded topical agents, including ketamine, TCAs, and vincristine, is weak, and these are not used in mainstream clinical practice.

Combination Therapy
Use of combination therapy is common in clinical practice despite paucity of convincing evidence advocating this approach. One recent study did demonstrate that the combination of gabapentin and morphine was superior to either of these medications used alone in relieving pain in patients with either painful diabetic neuropathy or PHN (98).

In clinical practice, a combination of gabapentin, tramadol, and lidoderm patch is used commonly as an initial analgesic regimen for PHN. The goal of combination therapy is to have a synergistic, or at least additive, effect in terms of improved pain relief. Disadvantages of combination therapy may include an increased risk of side effects, as the number of medications is increased so is the difficulty in determining which medication is useful and/or which one is responsible for the side effects. Conversely, adverse effects may potentially be minimized as lower doses of each medicine may be used. Ideally, medications that can cause similar side effects, for example, sedation, should not be started simultaneously. There should be a judicious interval of at least a week or more before a new medication is introduced to the regimen.

Miscellaneous
A variety of other agents have been evaluated in the treatment of PHN or other neuropathic pain conditions. Other antiepileptic or antidepressants, besides those mentioned previously, may have potential efficacy but have not been shown to have convincing benefit as yet. NMDA antagonists, including ketamine, dextromethorphan, and memantine, have been studied but no conclusive evidence of their efficacy has been shown. Similarly, the sodium channel blocker mexiletine has not demonstrated convincing benefit. Furthermore, this particular agent is usually avoided given its high-toxicity profile. The use of these

medications can be considered in select circumstances, when more conventional treatments have failed.

Invasive Interventional Strategies

A number of interventional strategies, including local anesthetic infiltration, peripheral nerve blocks, dorsal root ganglion blocks, sympathetic nerve blocks, epidural local anesthetics with or without steroids, and intrathecal steroids, have been tried in the prevention and treatment of PHN. In clinical practice, invasive treatments are considered for patients with pain refractory to conventional treatment. At present, there is no conclusive evidence available for the efficacy of these interventions. This points more toward the lack of adequate research as opposed to the conclusion that these interventions are inherently ineffective.

Sympathetic Nerve Blocks

Sympathetic nerve blocks are utilized in clinical practice for the treatment of both acute pain associated with herpes zoster and chronic pain of PHN. These include stellate ganglion blocks for craniofacial involvement and thoraco-lumbar sympathetic blocks for truncal involvement. Unfortunately, there is no quality evidence supporting the use of this treatment modality. A review by Kumar et al. (99) details multiple case studies, four retrospective studies, and one randomized controlled study showing that sympathetic blocks provided short-term pain relief. These studies reported that 41% to 50% of patients presenting with long-standing PHN noted short-term relief following the blocks, but the efficacy waned over time based on the long-term follow-up (99). In clinical practice, sympathetic blocks are reserved as a treatment option for cases in which more conservative treatments have failed to provide adequate pain relief.

Neuraxial Blocks

The authors occasionally use continuous epidural local anesthetic infusions (e.g., 0.0625% bupivacaine) for a period of one to two weeks in outpatients with intractable PHN pain. We have found this to be beneficial for severe cases, but literary evidence for this therapy is lacking. Furthermore, it requires home nursing services and significant coordination of care by the treating physician. In general, it is reserved for the most severe cases. In conventional practice, single-shot epidural injections of both local anesthetic and steroids are more often used in patients with pain refractory to conservative treatment.

A few randomized, placebo-controlled trials have shown promising results with the use of subarachnoid methyl prednisone plus 90 mg of lidocaine in providing good to excellent analgesia in patients with PHN. It has been shown that interleukin-8, an inflammatory mediator, is associated with pain in inflammatory reactions; and there is high concentration of interleukin-8 in the CSF of patients with intractable PHN. Thus, theoretically, intrathecal steroid injections may potentially be beneficial. These results did show a decrease in CSF interleukin-8 concentration by 50% in patients who received intrathecal methyl prednisone and that correlated with 70% pain relief (100). Safety concerns regarding the use of such high dosages of intrathecal lidocaine in elderly patients and production of adhesive arachnoiditis with intrathecal methyl prednisone have precluded its routine use. In any case, these results have not been confirmed by independent investigators.

In conclusion, currently available evidence does not lend convincing support to the routine use of neuraxial blocks in the treatment of PHN.

Peripheral Nerve and Dorsal Root Ganglion Blocks

As is the case for interventions described above, there is limited evidence available (101) for the use of intercostal nerve blocks in providing long-term relief in truncal PHN. Occasionally, we have performed dorsal root ganglion blocks with steroids in patients with intractable PHN and found them to be helpful. Hypothetically, if an inflammatory process at the level of the dorsal root ganglion is considered to play a role in the persistence of PHN pain, this treatment approach may seem rational. There is, however, no convincing evidence to support the routine use of this treatment.

Spinal Cord Stimulation

Spinal cord stimulation and other neuromodulatory devices are playing an increasing role in the management of chronic neuropathic pain states. The mechanism of action is thought to be at the level of the dorsal horn causing inhibition or reversal of central sensitization by suppressing the excessive firing of hyperexcitable, wide dynamic range neurons. It may also result in increased levels of the inhibitory neurotransmitters GABA and serotonin and decreased levels of excitatory neurotransmitters glutamate and aspartate that, in turn, leads to decreased central hypersensitization. The effects of spinal cord stimulation were studied prospectively in a case series of 28 patients (4 patients with herpes zoster and 24 patients with PHN). Long-term relief was obtained in 82% of the patients with PHN (102). Patients served as their own controls by intermittently switching their spinal cord stimulator (SCS) off and then monitoring for the reappearance of their pain symptoms. This is an interesting case series, but the lack of a formal control group diminishes the quality of the evidence, although it would be difficult to have a purely control group with such a therapy.

Surgical Approaches

Surgical approaches described in the literature for the treatment of PHN are peripheral neurectomies, nerve avulsion, dorsal root entry zone lesioning, cordotomy, rhizotomy, and surgical sympathectomy. In general, these are quite drastic procedures with no proven, long-term benefit. Surgical treatments are largely avoided given the limited body of literature to support their use, the potential for serious sequelae, and the expanding list of safer and more efficacious options.

Key Points in the Pharmacological Management of PHN

---

1. Gabapentin, pregabalin, tricyclic antidepressants, tramadol, Lidoderm patch, and opioids have convincing evidential support in the treatment of PHN.
2. The use of spinal cord stimulation is promising but studies with a formal control group are needed before a recommendation can be made for its widespread use.
3. The use of intrathecal steroids with lidocaine in the treatment of PHN has moderately good evidence, but this evidence has not been reproduced by independent investigators and there is a significant risk of neurological sequelae. This treatment cannot be recommended in clinical practice.

Psychological Interventions

The efficacy of cognitive behavioral therapy and other psychological therapies has not been studied specifically in patients with PHN. There is ample data to support the use of these therapies in other chronic pain states. Arguably this data can be extrapolated to apply to PHN patients as well. PHN has been demonstrated to adversely affect the quality of life, mood, physical and social functioning in afflicted patients. It follows that the use of relaxation therapy, diversion techniques and imagery, may potentially be of benefit (103).

Transcutaneous Electrical Nerve Stimulation

There have been variable responses reported to transcutaneous electrical nerve stimulation (TENS) therapy in patients with PHN. TENS is still offered clinically to many patients on a trial basis given its excellent safety profile. Those patients who have a favorable response to the trial therapy can procure a TENS device for more long-term use. There are a few small group series (104) that showed efficacy with use of this modality. However, other similar reports failed to demonstrate any benefit. It is postulated that the antinociceptive effect of TENS is due to an increase in levels of endorphins and enkephalins in response to a low-level electrical stimulation. In presence of allodynia, it should be tried on a mirror image region for about 10 minutes before applying to the affected area. TENS may be especially useful in patients with associated myofascial pain that may result secondary to excessive guarding.

Acupuncture

The routine use of acupuncture cannot be recommended as there is insufficient clinical experience or evidence available to advocate its efficacy. A possible mechanism of pain relief is due to release of endorphins secondary to stimulation of peripheral nerves. Case studies and anecdotal evidence suggest that acupuncture may be of benefit in relieving PHN pain.

CONCLUSION

PHN is the most common complication of herpes zoster in the elderly. Recent advances in the understanding, prevention, and treatment of PHN include the development and implementation of zoster vaccine, knowledge of the role of antiviral therapy and aggressive pain management in PHN prevention, identification of effective pharmacological treatments, and acceptance of PHN as a study model of neuropathic pain. Despite all these advances, we must recognize the limitations of available treatment modalities in addressing the tremendous health and economic burden related to acute and chronic zoster disease. The epidemiology of this illness is expected to change in a dramatic and potentially unpredictable way secondary to the implementation of VZV and zoster vaccination programs. Therefore, prevention of herpes zoster and PHN should be the critical focus in an attempt to decrease the substantial burden of this illness. After the widespread application of primary varicella vaccination, the universal administration of zoster vaccination to the target population should follow. Future areas of research should include the development of effective vaccination protocols for special needs populations and identifying the therapeutic targets in the early course of disease. At present, there is sound evidence for the efficacy of certain pharmacological therapies including amitriptyline, other

TCAs, gabapentin, pregabalin, lidoderm patches, tramadol and opioids. Therapy should be individualized with consideration given to sequential trials of these medications alone or in combination. Referral to a specialist should be made early in the course of the disease if pain control is inadequate despite institution of these measures. Interventional modalities such as spinal cord stimulation may play an important role, especially in patients with intractable pain; further studies will be needed before this can be recommended for widespread use. Optimization of physical and emotional well-being is the overall goal; hence, education of the patient and caregivers, along with psychosocial support, cannot be overemphasized.

REFERENCES

1. Bennett GJ. Neuropathic pain: an overview. In: Borsook D, ed. Molecular Neurobiology of Pain. Seattle, Washington: IASP Press, 1997:109–113.
2. Bowsher D. The lifetime occurrence of herpes zoster and prevalence of post-herpetic neuralgia: a retrospective survey in an elderly population. Eur J Pain 1999; 3(4):335–342.
3. Wood MJ, Kay R, Dworkin RH, et al. Oral acyclovir therapy accelerates pain resolution in patients with herpes zoster: a meta-analysis of placebo-controlled trials. Clin Infect Dis 1996; 22(2):341–347.
4. Dworkin RH, Schmader KE. The epidemiology and natural history of herpes zoster and postherpetic neuralgia. In: Watson CPN, Gershon AA, eds. Herpes Zoster and Postherpetic Neuralgia. 2nd revised and enlarged edition. New York: Elsevier, 2001:39–64.
5. Watson CPN, Watt VR, Chipman M, et al. The prognosis with postherpetic neuralgia. Pain 1991; 46(2):195–199.
6. Helgason S, Petursson G, Gudmundsson S, et al. Prevalence of postherpetic neuralgia after a first episode of herpes zoster: prospective study with long term follow up. BMJ 2000; 321(7264):794–796.
7. Donahue JG, Choo PW, Manson JE, et al. The incidence of herpes-zoster. Arch Intern Med 1995; 155(15):1605–1609.
8. De Moragas M, Kierland RR. The outcome of patients with herpes zoster. Arch Dermatol 1957; 75:193–196.
9. Kost RG, Straus SE. Postherpetic neuralgia: pathogenesis, treatment, and prevention. N Eng J Med 1996; 335(1):32–42.
10. Dworkin RH, Portenoy RK. Proposed classification of herpes-zoster pain. Lancet 1994; 343(8913):1648.
11. Arani RB, Soong SJ, Weiss HL, et al. Phase specific analysis of herpes zoster associated pain data: a new statistical approach. Stat Med 2001; 20(16):2429–2439.
12. Schmader KE. Epidemiology and impact on quality of life of postherpetic neuralgia and painful diabetic neuropathy. Clin J Pain 2002; 18(6):350–354.
13. Arvin AM. Varicella-zoster virus. Clin Microbiol Rev 1996; 9(3):361–381.
14. Mauskopf J, Austin R, Dix L, et al. The Nottingham health profile as a measure of quality-of-life in zoster patients—convergent and discriminant validity. Qual Life Res 1994; 3(6):431–435.
15. Shaikh S, Ta CN. Evaluation and management of herpes zoster ophthalmicus. Am Fam Physician 2002; 66(9):1723–1730.
16. Oster G, Harding G, Dukes E, et al. Pain, medication use, and health-related quality of life in older persons with postherpetic neuralgia: results from a population-based survey. J Pain 2005; 6(6):356–363.
17. Haanpää M, Hakkinen V, Nurmikko T. Motor involvement in acute herpes zoster. Muscle Nerve 1997; 20(11):1433–1438.

18. Dworkin RH, Portenoy RK. Pain and its persistence in herpes zoster. Pain 1996; 67 (2–3):241–251.
19. Schmader K. Postherpetic neuralgia in immunocompetent elderly people. Vaccine 1998; 16(18):1768–1770.
20. Schmader K. Herpes zoster in older adults. Clin Infect Dis 2001; 32(10):1481–1486.
21. Bennett GJ. Hypotheses on the pathogenesis of herpes zoster-associated pain. Ann Neurol 1994; 35:S38–S41.
22. Watson CPN, Deck JH, Morshead C, et al. Postherpetic neuralgia: further post-mortem studies of cases with and without pain. Pain 1991; 44(2):105–117.
23. Oaklander AL. The density of remaining nerve endings in human skin with and without postherpetic neuralgia after shingles. Pain 2001; 92(1–2):139–145.
24. Fields HL, Rowbotham M, Baron R. Postherpetic neuralgia: irritable nociceptors and deafferentation. Neurobiol Dis 1998; 5(4):209–227.
25. Rowbotham MC, Petersen KL, Fields HL. Is postherpetic neuralgia more than one disorder? Pain Forum 1998; 7(4):231–237.
26. Bowsher D. Sensory change in postherpetic neuralgia. In: Watson CPN, ed. Herpes Zoster and Postherpetic Neuralgia. Amsterdam, The Netherlands: Elsevier, 1993: 97–101.
27. Baron R, Saguer M. Postherpetic neuralgia: are C-nociceptors involved in signaling and maintenance of tactile allodynia? Brain 1993; 116:1477–1496.
28. Baron R, Saguer M. Mechanical allodynia in postherpetic neuralgia: evidence for central mechanisms depending on nociceptive C-fiber degeneration. Neurology 1995; 45(12):S63–S65.
29. Rowbotham MC, Yosipovitch G, Connolly MK, et al. Cutaneous innervation density in the allodynic form of postherpetic neuralgia. Neurobiol Dis 1996; 3(3): 205–214.
30. Pappagallo M, Oaklander AL, Quatrano-Piacentini AL, et al. Heterogenous patterns of sensory dysfunction in postherpetic neuralgia suggest multiple pathophysiologic mechanisms. Anesthesiology 2000; 92(3):691–698.
31. Petersen KL, Fields HL, Brennum J, et al. Capsaicin evoked pain and allodynia in post-herpetic neuralgia. Pain 2000; 88(2):125–133.
32. Wasner G, Kleinert A, Binder A, et al. Postherpetic neuralgia: topical lidocaine is effective in nociceptor-deprived skin. J Neurol 2005; 252(6):677–686.
33. Jung BF, Johnson RW, Griffin DRJ, et al. Risk factors for postherpetic neuralgia in patients with herpes zoster. Neurology 2004; 62(9):1545–1551.
34. Ragozzino MW, Melton LJ, Kurland LT, et al. Population-based study of herpes-zoster and its sequelae. Medicine 1982; 61(5):310–316.
35. Opstelten W, Mauritz JW, de Wit NJ, et al. Herpes zoster and postherpetic neuralgia: incidence and risk indicators using a general practice research database. Fam Pract 2002; 19(5):471–475.
36. Choo PW, Galil K, Donahue JG, et al. Risk factors for postherpetic neuralgia. Arch Intern Med 1997; 157(11):1217–1224.
37. Baron R, Haendler G, Schulte H. Afferent large fiber polyneuropathy predicts the development of postherpetic neuralgia. Pain 1997; 73(2):231–238.
38. Mcculloch DK, Fraser DM, Duncan LPJ. Shingles in diabetes-mellitus. Practitioner 1982; 226(1365):531–532.
39. Higa K. Acute herpetic pain and post herpetic neuralgia. Eur J Pain 1993; 14(4):79–90.
40. Nagasako EM, Johnson RW, Griffin DRJ, et al. Rash severity in herpes zoster: correlates and relationship to postherpetic neuralgia. J Am Acad Dermatol 2002; 46(6):834–839.
41. Dworkin RH, Boon RJ, Griffin DRG, et al. Postherpetic neuralgia: impact of famci-clovir, age, rash severity, and acute pain in herpes zoster patients. J Infect Dis 1998; 178:S76–S80.
42. Seward JF, Watson BM, Peterson CL, et al. Varicella disease after introduction of varicella vaccine in the United States, 1995–2000. JAMA 2002; 287(5):606–611.
43. Goldman GS. Universal varicella vaccination: efficacy trends and effect on herpes zoster. Int J Toxicol 2005; 24(4):205–213.

44. Thomas SL, Wheeler JG, Hall AJ. Contacts with varicella or with children and protection against herpes zoster in adults: a case–control study. Lancet 2002; 360(9334):678–682.
45. Brisson M, Gay NJ, Edmunds WJ, et al. Exposure to varicella boosts immunity to herpes-zoster: implications for mass vaccination against chickenpox. Vaccine 2002; 20(19–20):2500–2507.
46. Oxman MN, Levin MJ, Johnson GR, et al. A vaccine to prevent herpes zoster and postherpetic neuralgia in older adults. N Engl J Med 2005; 352(22):2271–2284.
47. Gnann JW. Vaccination to prevent herpes zoster in older adults. J Pain 2008; 9(1):S31–S36.
48. Dworkin RH, Johnson RW, Breuer J, et al. Recommendations for the management of herpes zoster. Clin Infect Dis 2007; 44:S1–S26.
49. Jackson JL, Gibbons R, Meyer G, et al. The effect of treating herpes zoster with oral acyclovir in preventing postherpetic neuralgia—a meta-analysis. Arch Intern Med 1997; 157(8):909–912.
50. Crooks RJ, Jones DA, Fiddian AP. Zoster-associated chronic pain: an overview of clinical-trials with acyclovir. Scand J Infect Dis 1991; 80:62–68.
51. Decroix J, Partsch H, Gonzalez R, et al. Factors influencing pain outcome in herpes zoster: an observational study with valaciclovir. J Eur Acad Dermatol Venereol 2000; 14(1):23–33.
52. Degreef H, Andrejevic L, Aoki F, et al. Famciclovir, a new oral antiherpes drug: results of the first controlled clinical-study demonstrating its efficacy and safety in the treatment of uncomplicated herpes-zoster in immunocompetent patients. Int J Antimicrob Agents 1994; 4(4):241–246.
53. Tyring S, Barbarash RA, Nahlik JE, et al. Famciclovir for the treatment of acute herpes-zoster: effects on acute disease and postherpetic neuralgia: a randomized, double-blind, placebo-controlled trial. Ann Intern Med 1995; 123(2):89–96.
54. Beutner KR, Friedman DJ, Forszpaniak C, et al. Valaciclovir compared with acyclovir for improved therapy for herpes-zoster in immunocompetent adults. Antimicrob Agents Chemother 1995; 39(7):1546–1553.
55. Tyring SK, Beutner KR, Tucker BA, et al. Antiviral therapy for herpes zoster: randomized, controlled clinical trial of valacyclovir and famciclovir therapy in immunocompetent patients 50 years and older. Arch Fam Med 2000; 9(9):863–869.
56. Bowsher D. The effects of pre-emptive treatment of postherpetic neuralgia with amitriptyline: a randomized, double-blind, placebo-controlled trial. J Pain Symptom Manage 1997; 13(6):327–331.
57. Dahl JB, Mathiesen O, Moiniche S. 'Protective premedication': an option with gabapentin and related drugs? A review of gabapentin and pregabalin in the treatment of post-operative pain. Acta Anaesthesiol Scand 2004; 48(9):1130–1136.
58. Kuraishi Y, Takasaki I, Nojima H, et al. Effects of the suppression of acute herpetic pain by gabapentin and amitriptyline on the incidence of delayed postherpetic pain in mice. Life Sci 2004; 74(21):2619–2626.
59. Wood MJ, Johnson RW, McKendrick MW, et al. A randomized trial of acyclovir for 7 days or 21 days with and without prednisolone for treatment of acute herpes zoster. N Engl J Med 1996; 22:341–347.
60. Whitley RJ, Weiss H, Gnann JW, et al. Acyclovir with and without prednisone for the treatment of herpes zoster: a randomized, placebo-controlled trial. Ann Intern Med 1996; 125(5):376–383.
61. Colding A. The effect of sympathetic blocks on herpes zoster. Acta Anaesthesiol Scand 1969; 13:113–141.
62. Dan K, Higa K, Noda B. Nerve block for herpetic pain. Adv Pain Res Ther 1985; 9:831–838.
63. Yanagida H, Suwa K, Corssen G. No prophylactic effect of early sympathetic blockade on postherpetic neuralgia. Anesthesiology 1987; 66(1):73–76.
64. Dworkin RH, Schmader KE. Treatment and prevention of postherpetic neuralgia. Clin Infect Dis 2003; 36(7):877–882.

65. Dworkin RH, Backonja M, Rowbotham MC, et al. Advances in neuropathic pain: diagnosis, mechanisms, and treatment recommendations. Arch Neurol 2003; 60(11):1524–1534.

66. Attal N, Cruccu G, Haanpää M, et al. EFNS guidelines on pharmacological treatment of neuropathic pain. Eur J Neurology 2006; 13(11):1153–1169.

67. Dworkin RH, O'Connor AB, Backonja M, et al. Pharmacologic management of neuropathic pain: evidence-based recommendations. Pain 2007; 132(3):237–251.

68. Moulin DE, Clark AJ, Gilron I, et al. Pharmacological management of chronic neuropathic pain: consensus statement and guidelines from the Canadian Pain Society. Pain Res Manage 2007; 12:13–21.

69. Backonja M, Glanzman RL. Gabapentin dosing for neuropathic pain: evidence from randomized, placebo-controlled clinical trials. Clin Ther 2003; 25(1):81–104.

70. Rowbotham M, Harden N, Stacey B, et al. Gabapentin for the treatment of postherpetic neuralgia: a randomized controlled trial. JAMA 1998; 280(21):1837–1842.

71. Rice ASC, Maton S. Gabapentin in postherpetic neuralgia: a randomized, double-blind, placebo-controlled study. Pain 2001; 94(2):215–224.

72. Hempenstall K, Nurmikko TJ, Johnson RW, et al. Analgesic therapy in postherpetic neuralgia: a quantitative systematic review. PloS Med 2005; 2(7):628–644.

73. Montgomery SA, Tobias K, Zornberg GL, et al. Efficacy and safety of pregabalin in the treatment of generalized anxiety disorder: a 6-week, multicenter, randomized, double-blind, placebo-controlled comparison of pregabalin and venlafaxine. J Clin Psychiatry 2006; 67(5):771–782.

74. Rickels K, Pollack MH, Feltner DE, et al. Pregabalin for treatment of generalized anxiety disorder: a 4-week, multicenter, double-blind, placebo-controlled trial of pregabalin and alprazolam. Arch Gen Psychiatry 2005; 62(9):1022–1030.

75. Dworkin RH, Corbin AE, Young JP, et al. Pregabalin for the treatment of postherpetic neuralgia: a randomized, placebo-controlled trial. Neurology 2003; 60(8):1274–1283.

76. Freynhagen R, Strojek K, Griesing T, et al. Efficacy of pregabalin in neuropathic pain evaluated in a 12-week, randomized, double-blind, multicentre, placebo-controlled trial of flexible- and fixed-dose regimens. Pain 2005; 115(3):254–263.

77. Frampton JE, Foster RH. Pregabalin in the treatment of postherpetic neuralgia. Drugs 2005; 65(1):111–118.

78. Rowbotham MC, Reisner LA, Davies PS, et al. Treatment response in antidepressant-naive postherpetic neuralgia patients: double-blind, randomized trial. J Pain 2005; 6(11):741–746.

79. Watson CPN, Vernich L, Chipman M, et al. Nortriptyline versus amitriptyline in postherpetic neuralgia: a randomized trial. Neurology 1998; 51(4):1166–1171.

80. Dick IE, Brochu RM, Purohit Y, et al. Sodium channel blockade may contribute to the analgesic efficacy of antidepressants. J Pain 2007; 8(4):315–324.

81. Offenbaecher M, Ackenheil M. Current trends in neuropathic pain treatments with special reference to fibromyalgia. CNS Spectr 2005; 10(4):285–297.

82. Guay DRR. Adjunctive agents in the management of chronic pain. Pharmacotherapy 2001; 21(9):1070–1081.

83. Collins SL, Moore RA, Mcquay HJ, et al. Antidepressants and anticonvulsants for diabetic neuropathy and postherpetic neuralgia: a quantitative systematic review. J Pain Symptom Manage 2000; 20(6):449–458.

84. Sindrup SH, Jensen TS. Efficacy of pharmacological treatments of neuropathic pain: an update and effect related to mechanism of drug action. Pain 1999; 83(3):389–400.

85. Sansone RA, Todd T, Meier BP. Pretreatment ECGs and the prescription of amitriptyline in an internal medicine clinic. Psychosomatics 2002; 43(3):250–251.

86. Vieweg WVR, Wood MA. Tricyclic antidepressants, QT interval prolongation, and torsade de pointes. Psychosomatics 2004; 45(5):371–377.

87. Watson CPN, Babul N. Efficacy of oxycodone in neuropathic pain: a randomized trial in postherpetic neuralgia. Neurology 1998; 50(6):1837–1841.

88. Raja SN, Haythornthwaite JA, Pappagallo M, et al. Opioids versus antidepressants in postherpetic neuralgia: a randomized, placebo-controlled trial. Neurology 2002; 59(7):1015–1021.

89. Boureau F, Legallicier P, Kabir-Ahmadi M. Tramadol in post-herpetic neuralgia: a randomized, double-blind, placebo-controlled trial. Pain 2003; 104(1–2):323–331.
90. Galer BS, Rowbotham MC, Perander J, et al. Topical lidocaine patch relieves postherpetic neuralgia more effectively than a vehicle topical patch: results of an enriched enrollment study. Pain 1999; 80(3):533–538.
91. Rowbotham MC, Davies PS, Verkempinck C, et al. Lidocaine patch: double-blind controlled study of a new treatment method for post-herpetic neuralgia. Pain 1996; 65(1):39–44.
92. Meier T, Wasner G, Faust M, et al. Efficacy of lidocaine patch 5% in the treatment of focal peripheral neuropathic pain syndromes: a randomized, double-blind, placebo-controlled study. Pain 2003; 106(1–2):151–158.
93. Rowbotham MC, Davies PS, Fields HL. Topical lidocaine gel relieves postherpetic neuralgia. Ann Neurol 1995; 37(2):246–253.
94. Bernstein JE, Korman NJ, Bickers DR, et al. Topical capsaicin treatment of chronic postherpetic neuralgia. J Am Acad Dermatol 1989; 21(2):265–270.
95. Watson CPN, Tyler KL, Bickers DR, et al. A randomized vehicle-controlled trial of topical capsaicin in the treatment of postherpetic neuralgia. Clin Ther 1993; 15(3):510–526.
96. Backonja M. High-concentration capsaicin for treatment of PHN and HIV neuropathy pain. Eur J Pain 2007; 11(1):S40.
97. DeBenedittis G, Lorenzetti A. Topical aspirin/diethyl ether mixture versus indomethacin and diclofenac/diethyl ether mixtures for acute herpetic neuralgia and postherpetic neuralgia: a double-blind crossover placebo-controlled study. Pain 1996; 65(1):45–51.
98. Gilron I, Bailey JM, Tu DS, et al. Morphine, gabapentin, or their combination for neuropathic pain. N Engl J Med 2005; 352(13):1324–1334.
99. Kumar V, Krone K, Mathieu A. Neuraxial and sympathetic blocks in herpes zoster and postherpetic neuralgia: an appraisal of current evidence. Reg Anesth Pain Med 2004; 29(5):454–461.
100. Kotani N, Kushikata T, Hashimoto H, et al. Intrathecal methylprednisolone for intractable postherpetic neuralgia. N Engl J Med 2000; 343(21):1514–1519.
101. Doi K, Nikai T, Sakura S, et al. Intercostal nerve block with 5% tetracaine for chronic pain syndromes. J Clin Anesth 2002; 14(1):39–41.
102. Harke H, Gretenkort P, Ladleif HU, et al. Spinal cord stimulation in postherpetic neuralgia and in acute herpes zoster pain. Anesth Analg 2002; 94(3):694–700.
103. Haythornthwaite JA, Clark MR, Pappagallo M, et al. Pain coping strategies play a role in the persistence of pain in post-herpetic neuralgia. Pain 2003; 106(3):453–460.
104. Nathan PW, Wall PD. Treatment of post-herpetic neuralgia by prolonged electric-stimulation. Br Med J 1974; 3(5932):645–647.

5 Management of Pain Related to Amputation

Steven Stanos

Center for Pain Management, Rehabilitation Institute of Chicago, Department of Physical Medicine and Rehabilitation, Northwestern University Medical School, Feinberg School of Medicine, Chicago, Illinois, U.S.A.

> Verily, it is a thing wondrous strange and prodigious and which scarce can be credited, unless by such as have seen with their eyes and heard with their ears, the patients who many months after the cutting away of the leg, grievously complained that they felt exceeding great pain of that leg so cut off.
>
> —Pare, Ambroise*

THE DISORDER

Approximately 150,000 persons undergo an amputation in the United States each year (1). Amputations are commonly the result of trauma (i.e., military injury, work-related or motor vehicle accidents) or diabetes-related peripheral vascular disease. Pain after amputation remains an enigma. Phantom limb pain (PLP) typically is associated with amputation of a limb but has also been reported with other surgical procedures including removal of organs (i.e., tongue, breast, teeth, genitals, and the bladder). Sensations related to amputation or loss of limb can be divided into three separate types: (*i*) PLP, (*ii*) residual limb (stump) pain (RLP), and (*iii*) phantom limb sensations (PLS). Compensatory pain related to phantom sensations has been recognized more recently as an important additional condition and is usually due to musculoskeletal pain secondary to changes in body or limb movement (i.e., neck, low back, and/or joint pain proximal to the affected residual limb).

Various survey reports have shown PLP to have a significant negative impact on function and quality of life. Sherman et al. found that 51% of patients with PLP reported lifestyle limitations on more than six days per month, approximately one-third for more than 15 hr/day (2). A systematic review of acute and chronic PLP management found that although up to 70% of patients report pain, there is little evidence-based medicine to guide treatment (3). This chapter will review epidemiology, pathophysiology, treatment options (pharmacologic and nonpharmacologic), and novel approaches to managing acute and chronic pain related to amputation.

---

* Pare A. Les aeuvres d'Ambroise Pare. Paris: Gabriel Buon, 1598 (Histoire du defunct Roy Charles IX, 10 Book, Chap 41, p. 401). Quoted in Livingston WK. Pain Mechanisms. New York: Macmillan, 1943.

DIAGNOSIS

Epidemiology
The reported incidence of PLP varies widely between 2% and 98% (4). A greater number of patients (80–100%) experience phantom sensations (5). The recent review of posttraumatic amputation pain by Schley et al. reported 53.8% of patients with phantom sensations, a greater prevalence of RLP (61.5%) and residual sensations (78.5%). Continuous sensations or pain were rare immediately after surgery (PLP 6.9%, PLS 14.3%, RLP 12.5%). Twenty-eight percent reported PLP immediately after amputation and 41% with the onset of phantom phenomena one year after surgery. In most patients, pain was stable or decreased in severity over a six-month to 12-month period (6). More recent epidemiological studies show that up to one-fourth of amputees report severe chronic pain (7, 8).

History
PLP has been reported as early as the 1560s by Ambroise Pare, a French surgeon (Pare, 1598). Pare described a number of surgical procedures to help limit infection and improve survival after surgical trauma (9). Dualism theory in the 1600s struggled in understanding the basic causes of phantom pain. Rene Descartes (1596–1650) described the mind to be "deceived" by "signals from the body" (10). Silas Weir Mitchell coined the term "phantom limb pain" 300 years after Pare in descriptions of PLP by soldiers he treated as a union physician in the American Civil War. Mitchell classically described PLP, in addition to posttraumatic neuralgias, and causalgias. His eloquent descriptions of wounded soldiers' PLP in the *Atlantic Monthly* brought the condition to the focus of the American public (11).

Modern brain imaging has led to a greater understanding of potential causes of phantom pain initiated by deafferentation of neural pathways after limb loss, facilitating cortical reorganization of somatotopic maps (12). In the last 10 years, Ramachandran and others have introduced a novel understanding and treatment approach based on the interaction of vision with the PLS, using mirror reflection visual feedback to create the illusion of a normal limb (from the contralateral extremity) superimposed on the phantom. This approach is based on the theory that with an amputation, motor commands are sent from the cortex to the affected extremity and lose the normally dampened feedback created by proprioception. The amputated limb and loss of proprioceptive feedback lead to amplified motor output and sensations of pain or spasm (13).

Definitions
Phantom phenomenon has been classified as it relates to three general presentations following amputation (14):

1. Phantom pain: painful sensations referred to the phantom limb.
2. Phantom sensation: any sensation, other than pain, in the phantom limb.
3. Stump or "residual" pain: pain localized to the residual limb or extremity proximal to the amputation.

Phantom pain is described by a number of descriptors such as burning, tingling, cramping, shocking, and paresthesia-like (i.e., "pins and needles"). Amputees may experience an unpleasant itch to more severe clenching and squeezing sensations. Phantom sensation can be classified as exteroceptive

TABLE 1 Factors That May Modulate the Experience of
Phantom Pain

Internal factors	External factors
Genetic predisposition	Weather change
Anxiety/emotional distress	Touching the stump
Attention/distraction	Use of prosthesis
Urination/defecation	Spinal anesthesia
Other disease (cerebral hemorrhage,	Rehabilitation
Prolapsed intervertebral disk)	

and/or proprioceptive (i.e., tingling, itching, pressure, movement, warmth or cold). Others may describe the phantom as a general awareness of the limb (15). Some phantom pain may closely reflect pain experienced during the preamputation state in the affected extremity. In a study of lower limb amputations, Hanley et al. found acute RLP to be the best overall predictor of chronic PLP at 24 months. Higher levels of pain before or soon after amputation may predict those at risk for chronic pain (16).

Other Common Phantom Phenomena

Besides phantom pain, individuals may report a habitual posture of the phantom (i.e., flexed at the elbow, hand clenched, hand twisted) as well as telescoping sensations. These postures may spontaneously change, remain fixed in awkward or painful positions, or be activated by rubbing or touching the residual limb or more proximal structures. Telescoping of phantom pain and sensations includes the shrinking or fading of the sensation over time (14). More common in upper limb amputations, telescoping involves shortening or shrinking back of sensations from the distal part of the phantom proximally toward the residual limb. Shukla et al. described telescoping in two-thirds of patients (17). Telescoping may be related to cortical distortion of primary somatosensory maps (S1) (15).

Internal and external factors may help to modulate phantom pain and sensations including genetic, affective, attention, organ function, and other disease states. External factors commonly reported include weather change, touch or pressure to the residual limb, prosthesis use, and spinal anesthesia (Table 1) (14).

Residual Limb Pain

RLP is commonly described as aching, burning, or throbbing. Ehde et al. reported RLP to be as common as PLP in lower limb amputees and more distressing (18). RLP may be related to nerve transection and spontaneous neural activity (i.e., neuroma), scar, soft tissue changes, and central sensitization. Neuroma formation may be idiopathic or related to suboptimal surgical technique, where the goal is to bury the severed nerve or neuroma under large soft tissue masses serving to limit and protect the neural tissue from pressure and irritation. Many times, limited soft tissue coverage, increased adhesion of tissues, or surgical complications may lead to persistent pain in the perioperative and long-term follow-up period. Neuromas, many times palpable under the skin, cause focal pain or pain that radiates distally to the end of the residual limb. Neuroma pain has been reported to aggravate PLP. Good postoperative management which may limit neuroma formation includes edema control and early desensitization of the affected skin area (19)

TABLE 2 Differential Diagnosis of Residual Limb Pain

Neuroma
Infection of soft tissue
Prosthesis use, malalignment
Contact dermatitis
Epidermoid cysts
Joint contracture
Vascular disease
Central sensitization

RLP has been suggested to be related to allodynia or hyperpathia, or spontaneous pain of peripheral and central origin. A differential diagnosis of RLP includes neuroma, infection, skin breakdown, dermatitis, joint contracture, and vascular disease (Table 2) (20).

PATHOPHYSIOLOGY
A number of theories proposed to explain phantom pain can be classified as either peripheral or central causes.

Peripheral and Central Changes
Animal models have demonstrated that after injury to a nerve, primary afferent axons regenerate or sprout acquiring abnormal properties including spontaneous discharge and abnormal sensitivity to noradrenaline. Sympathetic efferent fibers may interact with sensory afferents modulating afferent activity such as spontaneous pain. Similar changes in neural processing are noted proximally at the dorsal root ganglion and dorsal horn of the spinal cord. Furthermore, second-order neurons that primarily respond to noxious stimuli start responding to inputs from low-threshold, mechanosensitive A-beta fibers that normally carry nonnoxious stimuli, leading to exaggerated pain and allodynia (21). This central sensitization may lead to spontaneous PLP, touch-evoked PLP, and mechanical residual limb allodynia (22). Chabal et al. injected a potassium channel blocker into neuromas in residual limbs of amputees leading to analgesia, suggesting that ion channel excitability contributes to phantom pain (23). Unfortunately, peripheral blocking of neuromas may lead to transient or lack of analgesic response in clinical practice. Ongoing input from sensitized tissue, including neuromas, is critical, but not the sole component to PLP and may be an important first step in alterations in central somatosensory processing (central sensitization), including changes more proximally in the central nervous system.

Supraspinal Plasticity: Cortical Reorganization
More recent evidence suggests cortical reorganization is an additional component to supraspinal changes responsible for phantom phenomena (24). Long-lasting input from the limb and cortical pain memory enhanced excitability and reorganization of the somatosensory zone correlating to the area of pain. Lotze et al. reported that use of a myoelectric prosthesis in upper extremity amputees was associated with reduced cortical reorganization and decreased PLP over time (25). A number of rehabilitation approaches have more recently been developed theoretically focusing on reversing cortical reorganization, or

TABLE 3 Phantom Limb Pain Therapies

Nonpharmacologic
  Sensory discrimination training
  Mirror therapy
  Relaxation therapy
  Aerobic exercise
  Desensitization techniques
  TENS
Pharmacologic
  Epidural anesthesia
  Regional anesthesia
  Oral medications
  Tricyclic antidepressants
  Selective serotonin norepinephrine reuptake inhibitors
  Opioids
  Anticonvulsants
  Antiarrhythmics
  GABAergic medications (benzodiazepines)
  Topical analgesics and counter-irritants (capsaicin)
  NMDA receptor antagonists (ketamine, dextromethorphan, memantine, and amantadine)
  Alpha-adrenoceptor agonist (clonidine)

Abbreviations: NMDA, *N*-methyl-D-aspartate; TENS, transcutaneous electrical nerve stimulation.

reversing maladaptive plasticity within the sensorimotor cortex with the clinical goal of potentially decreasing PLP and PLS. Techniques developed include the use of virtual techniques such as imagining the phantom in various positions, mirror or mirror box therapy, and computer-based virtual therapies (i.e., virtual limb and distraction-based techniques).

TREATMENT
A number of pharmacologic and nonpharmacologic approaches may be useful in decreasing pain and potentially improving quality of life in patients with PLP (Tables 3 and 4).

TABLE 4 Treatment for Phantom Pain

Medical	Nonmedical	Surgical
Antidepressants	TENS	Neurectomy
Anticonvulsants	Acupuncture	Stump revision
Lidocaine/mexiletine	Biofeedback	Rhizotomy
Opioids/tramadol	Intrathecal drug delivery system	Cordotomy
NMDA receptor antagonist	Stump massage/ electromagnetically shielding stump liner	Tractotomy
Mirtazapine	Stump ultrasound	DREX lesion
IV salmon calcitonin	Electroconvulsive therapy	Lobectomy
Clonazepam	Nerve blocks/perineural infusion	Sympathectomy
Baclofen	Psychological therapy/CBT	Spinal cord and peripheral nerve stimulation
Clonidine/tizanidine	Immersive virtual reality	Deep brain stimulator

Abbreviations: NMDA, *N*-methyl-D-aspartate; TENS, transcutaneous electrical nerve stimulation; CBT, cognitive behavioral therapy; DREZ, dorsal root entry zone.

Pharmacologic Update

A number of pharmacologic approaches are used in the treatment of pain despite the paucity of randomized, placebo-controlled studies. Common intraoperative and perioperative techniques include regional nerve blocks (i.e., posterior tibial or sciatic), epidural infusions including various medications (meperidine, paracetamol, clonidine, bupivacaine, morphine, and ketamine), and transcutaneous electrical nerve stimulation. A systematic review found poor quality of studies and contradictory results, which failed to provide evidence to support any specific intervention (3).

Evidence for pharmacotherapy in PLP and RLP is based primarily on more indirect evidence for neuropathic pain conditions (22). Treatment for neuropathic pain and PLP, in general, includes the use of opioids, anticonvulsants, antidepressants, systemic and spinal opioids, local anesthetics, and regional anesthesia. This section will briefly review oral medications commonly used in the outpatient management of PLP and PLS, reviewing recent literature and novel approaches to therapy.

Tricyclic Antidepressants

Tricyclic antidepressants including reuptake inhibitors of monoamines (serotonin and norepinephrine) may potentiate endogenous inhibitory descending spinal pathways. Amitriptyline has the most evidence across neuropathic pain states, with mean dosage of 75 to 150 mg/day (26). Few studies have directly examined tricyclic agents in PLP. Wilder-Smith et al. examined amitriptyline, titrated from 25 mg to a maximum of 75 mg/day over one month, in patients with chronic PLP and RLP due to trauma. After one month, pain was "almost completely inhibited" in 67% of patients (average dose 56 mg/day) (27). Quantitative sensory testing in patients demonstrated significantly enhanced antinociception on the residual limb in treatment responders. Kuiken et al. studied the use of mirtazapine, serotonin/norepinephrine modulator (α_2-antagonist and serotonergic agonist), in a three-month case study of PLP with doses ranging between 7.5 and 30 mg/day showing improved sleep and analgesia (28).

Opioids

A recent trial of opioids in a cohort of cancer patients undergoing amputation demonstrated analgesic efficacy upon application of the WHO analgesic ladder. Patients complaining of PLS, PLP, and RLP decreased from 69%, 60%, and 31%, respectively, at one month to 32%, 32%, and 5%, at the end of two years, most of which used mild- and moderate-strength opioids included in steps II and III of the WHO ladder, respectively (29). A study of amitriptyline in PLP conducted by Wilder-Smith et al. also demonstrated efficacy of tramadol dosed twice a day, with an average dose of 523 mg/day. Tramadol, a nonscheduled, weak mu agonist, has an additional proposed mechanism of action blocking reuptake of serotonin and norepinephrine. Tramadol's dual mechanism of action may be a critical reason why studies have suggested efficacy in other neuropathic pain conditions, some of which included patients with phantom pain.

Methadone, a mu opioid receptor agonist with N-methyl-D-aspartate (NMDA) receptor antagonist effects, has demonstrated clinical efficacy in neuropathic pain (30). The clinical significance of methadone's NMDA receptor antagonist effects remains unclear (31). A case series including four patients with severe PLP demonstrated efficacy of methadone, started at 5 mg twice per day and titrated to effect in patients who had failed opioids (32). Average dose in this small series at two to four months of therapy was 25.5 mg/day.

Anticonvulsants

More recently, gabapentin, an anticonvulsant and Ca channel modulator, has been the most popular medication used in a wide variety of neuropathic pain conditions and off-label for PLP despite limited evidence-based support. Bone et al. examined gabapentin in PLP patients in a randomized, double-blind, placebo-controlled study with daily doses titrated to 2400 mg/day. The study found significantly greater pain intensity differences in treatment versus placebo (33). However, Nikolajsen et al. found no difference between gabapentin and placebo in reducing postamputation RLP and PLP with treatment during the first 30 days after surgery (34).

Pharmacologic Approaches of Decreasing Cortical Excitability

Taken from a greater understanding of neuroplasticity as identified on modern neuroimaging of PLP, medications involved in decreasing cortical plasticity have become ideal candidates for drug study and development. The NMDA receptor is thought to be a key receptor involved in synaptic plasticity and central sensitization in animal models of chronic pain. In animal models of neuropathic pain, NMDA receptor antagonists decrease spontaneous pain and pain-related behavior in evoked pain (35). Blocking the NMDA receptor could serve to block or limit central sensitization and, hence, phantom phenomena (36).

Common NMDA receptor antagonists include methadone, ketamine, memantine, and dextromethorphan. Ketamine, a highly competitive NMDA antagonist usually given by parenteral route, is limited clinically secondary to the compound's psychomimetic and dissociative side effects. Wilson et al. assessed the effect of preemptive epidural ketamine in combination with bupivacaine in patients undergoing lower limb amputation and found improved analgesia in the ketamine group versus saline in the immediate postoperative period but failed to show benefit between the groups at one year (37). Focus has shifted to identifying or developing less competitive NMDA antagonists with potentially improved tolerability. Recent literature has examined memantine and dextromethorphan. Memantine, a derivative of amantadine, is a noncompetitive NMDA receptor blocker (38) that is used for the treatment of Parkinson's disease, dementia, and spasticity. A recent case report of two patients with severe lower limb PLP refractory to high-dose opioids and adjunctive medications reported profound analgesic response to memantine titrated to 10 mg bid (39). A five-week, randomized, placebo-controlled study of memantine (5–20 mg/day) failed to demonstrate efficacy of memantine compared to placebo in evoked or spontaneous pain in a study of patients with traumatic nerve injuries (mostly due to amputation and nerve resection) (40). Wiech et al. investigated the effect of memantine (30 mg/day) on intensity of chronic PLP and cortical reorganization, measured by assessing functional organization of the primary somatosensory cortex with neuromagnetic source imaging. The four-week crossover trial found no difference at baseline compared to placebo on the intensity of chronic PLP and changes in functional organization (41). Dextromethorphan, a noncompetitive NMDA receptor antagonist, was reported to be successful in a case series of PLP (42). All patients reported a 50% decrease in pain intensity, improved mood, and lower sedation in the three-month study. Doses of dextromethorphan ranged from 120 to 270 mg/day. Previous studies using dextromethorphan in neuropathic and cancer-related pain conditions failed to show benefit at lower doses (range, 40–90 mg/day) (43, 44).

Nonpharmacologic Approaches

Common physical modalities for PLP treatment include acupuncture, residual limb vibration (45), desensitization techniques (i.e., contrast baths, scrub and carry treatments), ultrasound, and massage. More recent research and clinical practice has included sensory training techniques. Sensory training for PLP includes two basic approaches: (*i*) sensory discrimination training and (*ii*) mirror therapy (virtual visual feedback). Sensory stimulation applied to the limb has been shown to lead to significant improvement in PLP and reversal of cortical sensory reorganization (46).

Mirror Therapy

Virtual visual feedback has become a growing area of research and an active area of therapy for treatment of PLP. The amputee places the contralateral limb in view of a mirror usually placed at the patient's midline or in a box and, while moving the intact limb, imagines moving the phantom hand while continuing to view the intact limb in its reflection. This visual "illusion" was first described by Ramachandran and Rogers-Ramachandran (47). Persons with the amputated limb use a mirror or mirror box to reflect an image of the intact limb, providing the patient with the visual illusion that two "intact" limbs exist. Mercier and Sirigu studied eight patients with upper limb phantom pain who underwent training two times per week for eight weeks, where a virtual image of a missing limb was created while performing different movements following the movement with the phantom limb. Patients showed a 38% decrease in "background pain," with five of eight reporting greater than 30% reduction in pain. Predictors of effectiveness were related more by susceptibility to the virtual visual feedback than lesion type and duration of deafferentation (48). A recent case report described a "home-based" patient-delivered mirror therapy program for a lower limb amputee as an efficacious, low-cost treatment delivered primarily independently by the patients with minimal health care resources and without the guidance of a structured supervised exercise program (49) (Fig. 1). The patient's self-designed protocol included the use of a discount store bought mirror placed on its edge on the floor. Exercises included 20 to 30 minute sessions two to three times per week, exercising the "intact" foot in front of the mirror in a number of movements while incorporating deep breathing and other relaxation techniques learned as part of a structured multidisciplinary program. The patient reported decreased pain, increased control of his phantom, enjoyment from practice, and decreased use of opioid and anticonvulsant medications.

Relaxation-Assisted Biofeedback Training for PLP

Biofeedback-assisted relaxation training has been shown to be effective in classic studies and case reports of PLP (50, 51). Combined EMG-assisted thermal biofeedback resulted in complete elimination of PLP after treatment and maintained at 3- and 12-month follow-up in a patient with extreme PLP of the right

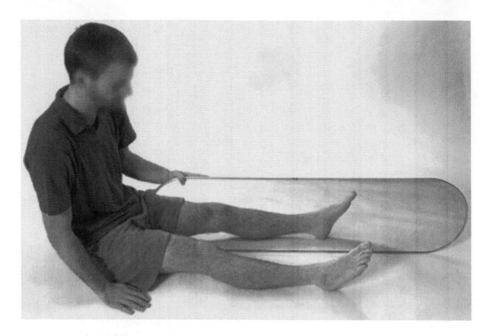

FIGURE 1 Home-Based Mirror therapy. From Ref. 49.

upper limb (52). Electrodes were placed at the bicep muscle above the residual limb and on the contralateral limb. The two-phase training (six sessions each) consisted of training the patient to increase perceptual awareness of the residual limb sensations and muscular tension, with exercises aimed at increasing and decreasing tension in the residual limb. The second phase included instruction on training to increase skin temperature in the affected limb by decreasing burning pain of the phantom. Harden et al. examined the effectiveness of biofeedback in the treatment of nine PLP patients who received up to seven thermal and autogenic biofeedback sessions over a four- to six-week period pilot study. At the conclusion of the study, patients reported an average of 39% decrease in daily pain, with three reporting greater than 50% reduction (53).

SUMMARY

PLS, PLP, and RLP continue to be a challenge to clinicians and a source of potentially severe and disabling pain to patients. Pharmacologic therapy may include the use of antidepressants, anticonvulsants, opioids, and NMDA receptor antagonists. Modern brain imaging has offered additional evidence to the underlying cortical changes related to loss of a limb, which may lead to central sensitization and plasticity, and serve as the final pathway in understanding the complex pathophysiology of PLS, pain, and residual limb symptoms. A greater appreciation of central changes in neural processing may also serve as a clinical target for treatment including mind–body treatments such as biofeedback-assisted relaxation training and mirror therapy. A multimodal approach based on pharmacologic and nonpharmacologic approaches is the cornerstone of effective management.

REFERENCES

1. Dillingham TR, Pezzin LE, MacKenzie EJ. Limb amputation and limb deficiency: epidemiology and recent trends in the United States. South Med J 2002; 95:875–883.
2. Sherman RA, Sherman CJ, Parker L. Chronic phantom and stump pain among American veterans: results of a survey. Pain 1984; 18:83–95.
3. Halbert J, Crotty M, Cameron I. Evidence for the optimal management of acute and chronic phantom pain: a systematic review. Clin J Pain 2002; 18:84–92.
4. Jensen TS, Nikolajsen L. Phantom pain and other phenomena after amputation. In: Wall PD, Melzack R, eds. Textbook of Pain. 4th ed. New York: Churchill Livingstone, 1999:799–814.
5. Jensen TS, Krebs B, Nielsen J, et al. Phantom limb, phantom pain and stump pain in amputees during the first 6 months following limb amputation. Pain 1983; 17:243–256.
6. Schley MT, Wilms P, Toepfner S, et al. Painful and nonpainful phantom and stump sensations in acute traumatic amputees. J Trauma 2008; 65:858–864.
7. Desmond DM, Maclachlan M. Affective distress and amputation-related pain among older men with long-term traumatic limb amputations. J Pain Symptom Manage 2006; 31:362–368.
8. Ephraim PL, Wegener ST, MacKenzie EJ, et al. Phantom pain, residual limb pain, and bck pain in amputees: results of a national survey. Arch Phys Med Rehabil 2005; 86:1910–1919.
9. Zimmermann M. The history of pain concepts and treatment before IASP. In: Merskey H, Loeser J, Dubner R, eds. The Paths of Pain 1975–2005. Seattle: IASP Press, 2005.
10. Wall PP. Pain: The Science of Suffering. New York: Columbia University Press, 2000: 20–21.
11. Woodhouse A. Phantom limb sensation. Clin Exp Pharmacol Physiol 2005; 32:132–134.
12. Ramachandran VS. Plasticity and functional recovery in neurology. Clin Med 2005;5:368–373.
13. Ramachandram VS, Rogers-Ramachandran D, Cobb S. Touching the phantom limb. Nature 1995; 377:489–490.
14. Nikolajsen L, Jensen TS. Phantom limb pain. Br J Anaesth 2001; 87:107–116.
15. Ramachandran VS, Hirstein W. The perception of phantom limbs. The D.O. Hebb lecture. Brain 1998; 121:1603–1630.
16. Hanley M, Jensen MP, Smith DG, et al. Preamptation pain and acute pain predict chronic pain after lower extremity amputation. J Pain 2007; 8(2):102–109.
17. Shukla GD, Sahu SC, Tripathi RP, et al. A psychiatric study of amputees. Br J Psychiatry 1982; 141:50–53.
18. Ehde DM, Czerniecki JM, Smith DG, et al. Chronic phantom sensations, phantom pain, residual lib pain, and other regional pain after lower limb amputation. Arch Phys Med Rehabil 2000; 81:1039–1044.
19. Esquenazi A. Upper limb amputee rehabilitation and prosthetic restoration. In: Braddom RL, ed. Physical Medicine and Rehabilitation. 3rd ed. Philadelphia: Saunders, 2007:267–282.
20. Kuiken TA, Miller L, Lipschutz R, et al. Rehabilitation of people with lower limb amputation. In: Braddom RL, ed. Physical Medicine & Rehabilitation. 3rd ed. Philadelphia: Saunders Elsevier, 2007:283–323.
21. Woolf CJ. Evidence for a central component of post-injury pain hypersensitivity. Nature 1983; 306(5944):686–688.
22. Baron R, Wasner G, Lindner V. Optimal treatment of phantom limb pain in the elderly. Drugs Aging 1998; 12:361–376.
23. Chabal C, Jacobson L, Russell LC, et al. Pain responses to perineuronal injection of normal saline, gallamine, and lidocaine in humans. Pain 1989; 36:321–325.
24. Flor H. Cortical reorganization and chronic pain: implications for rehabilitation. J Rehabil Med 2003; 41(suppl):66–72.

25. Lotze M, Grodd W, Birbaumer N, et al. Dose use of a myoelectric prosthesis prevent cortical reorganization and phantom limb pain? Nat Neurosci 1999; 2:501–502.
26. Max MB, Cunane M, Schafer SC, et al. Amitriptyline relieves diabetic neuropathy pain in patients with normal or depressed mood. Neurology 1987; 37:589–596.
27. Wilder-Smith C, Hill L, Laurent S. Postamputation pain and sensory changes in treatment-naïve patients: characteristics and responses to treatment with tramadol, amitriptyline, and placebo. Anesthesiology 2005; 103:619–628.
28. Kuiken T, Schechtman L, Harden RN. Phantom limb pain treatment with mirtazapine: c case series. Pain Pract 2005; 5:356–360.
29. Mishra S, Bhatnager S, Gupta D, et al. Incidence and management of phantom limb pain according to the World health Organization analgesic ladder in amputees of malignant origin. Am J Hosp Palliat Care 2008; 24:455–462.
30. Gorman A, Elliott K, Inturrisi C. The D- and L-isomer of methadone bind to the non-competitive site on the N-methyl-D-aspartate (NMDA) receptor in rat forebrain and spinal cord. Neurosci Lett 1997; 223:5–8.
31. Carpenter K, Chapman V, Dickenson A. Neuronal inhibitory effects of methadone are predominantly opioid receptor mediated in the rat spinal cord in vivo. Eur J Pain 2000; 4:19–26.
32. Bergmans S, Snijdelaar D, Katz, et al. Methadone for phantom limb pain. Clin J Pain 2002; 18:203–205.
33. Bone M, Crithchley P, Buggy D. Gabapentin in postamputation phantom limb pain: a randomized, double-blind, placebo-controlled, cross-over study. Reg Anesth Pain Med 2002; 27:481–486.
34. Nikolajsen L, Finnerup NB, Kramp S, et al. A randomized study of the effects of gabapentin on postamputation pain. Anesthesiology 2006; 105:1008–1015.
35. Mao J, Price DD, Haes R, et al. Intrathecal treatment with dextrorphan or ketamine reduces pain-related behavior in a rat model of peripheral mononeuropathy. Brain Res 1993; 605:164–168.
36. Warncke T, Stubhaung A, Jorum E. Preinjury treatment with morphine or ketamine inhibits the development of experimentally induced secondary hyperalgesia in man. Pain 2000; 86:293–303.
37. Wilson J, Nimmo A, Fleetwood-Walker S, et al. A randomized double blind trial of the effect of pre-emptive epidural ketamine on persistent pain after lower limb amputation. Pain 2008; 135:108–118.
38. Borman J. Memantine is a potent blocker of N-methyl-D-aspartate (NMDA) receptor channels. Eur J Pharmacol 1989; 166:591–592.
39. Hackworth R, Tokarz K, Fowler I, et al. Profound pain reduction after induction of memantine treatment in two patients with severe phantom limb pain. Anesth Analg 2008; 107:1377–1379.
40. Nikolajsen L, Gottrup H, Kristensen A, et al. Memantine (a N-methyl-D-aspartate receptor antagonist) in the treatment of neuropathic pain after amputation or surgery: a randomized, double-blinded, cross-over study. Anesth Analg 2000; 91:960–966.
41. Wiech K, Kiefer T, Topfner S, et al. A placebo-controlled randomized crossover trial of the N-methyl-D-aspartic acid receptor antagonist, memantine, in patients with chronic phantom limb pain. Anesth Analg 2004; 98:408–413.
42. Abraham R, Marouani N, Weinbroum A. Dextromethorphan mitigates phantom pain in cancer amputees. Ann Surg Oncol 2003; 10:268–274.
43. McQuay H, Carroll D, Jadad A, et al. Dextromethorphan for the treatment of neuropathic pain: a double-blind randomized controlled crossover trial with integral n-of-1 design. Pain 1994; 59:127–133.
44. Mercadante S, Casuccio A, Genovese G. Ineffectiveness of dextromethorphan in cancer pain. J Pain Symptom Manage 1998; 16:317–322.
45. Lundeberg T. relief of pain from a phantom limb by peripheral stimulation. J Neurol 1985; 232:79–82.
46. Flor H, Denke C, Schaefer M, et al. Effect of sensory discrimination training on cortical reorganization and phantom limb pain. Lancet 2001; 357:1763–1764.

47. Ramachandran VS, Rogers-Ramachandran D. Synaesthesia in phantom limbs induced with mirrors. Proc Biol Sci 1996; 263:377–386.
48. Mercier C, Sirigu A. Training with virtual visual feedback to alleviate phantom limb pain. Neurorehabil Neural Repair. 2009; 23:587–594.
49. Darnall BD. Self-delivered home-based mirror therapy for lower limb phantom pain. Am J Phys Med Rehabil 2009; 88:78–81.
50. Arena JG, Sherman RA, Bruno GM, et al. The relationship between situational stress and phantom limb pain: cross-lagged correlational data from six month pain logs. J Psychosom Res 1990; 34:71–77.
51. Doughery J. Relief of phantom limb pain after EMG biofeedback-assisted relaxation: a case report. Behav Res Ther 1980; 18:355–357.
52. Belleggia G, Birbaumer N. Treatment of phantom limb pain with combined EMG and thermal biofeedback: a case report. Appl Psychophysiol Biofeedback 2001; 26:141–146.
53. Harden R, Houle T, Green S, et al. Biofeedback in the treatment of phantom limb pain: a time-series analysis. Appl Pscyhophysiol Biofeedback 2005; 30:83–93.

6 Pathophysiology of Complex Regional Pain Syndrome

Robert J. Schwartzman

Department of Neurology, Drexel University College of Medicine, Philadelphia, Pennsylvania, U.S.A.

INTRODUCTION

The application of recent statistical methods and internal and external validation techniques has recently redefined complex regional pain syndrome (CRPS) I and II (1–3). These criteria were designed to provide an objective evaluation of CRPS I and II and to distinguish it from neuropathic conditions in which significant autonomic symptoms are present.

The signs and symptoms of CRPS cluster into four statically distinct subgroups (factors) that have been derived by internal validation from a series of 123 patients that met earlier IASP criteria of CRPS (4, 5). These are (*i*) pain, allodynia, hyperalgesia, and hyperpathia and the signs and symptoms of (*ii*) temperature asymmetry and color change; (*iii*) edema and sweating asymmetry; and (*iv*) motor dysfunction with atrophy and dystrophy. Factor analysis is a statistical technique that identifies signs and symptoms (factors) that are collated statistically such that if one sign or symptom in a given factor is present, other signs or symptoms in the factor will also be present (6). If four sign categories and three of four symptom categories are present in a possible CRPS patient, the sensitivity of these criteria for the diagnosis of CRPS is 0.85 with a specificity of 0.69.

Cluster analysis, the overall pattern of CRPS signs and symptoms that are present in individual patients, does not reveal distinct subgroups in CRPS (6) but does suggest three statistically distinct CRPS subtypes: (*i*) a mild predominant vasomotor syndrome; (*ii*) a limited neuropathic pain and sensory syndrome; and (*iii*) severe syndrome with all classic features (6).

There is now general agreement that the pain of CRPS is usually disproportionate to the primary injury and is regional in that it does not respect a nerve or root distribution. It is severe, unrelenting, burning, and deep in muscle and joint and is most often associated with mechano and thermal allodynia, hyperalgesia, and hyperpathia in later stages. Neurogenic edema, autonomic dysregulation, a profound movement disorder, atrophy, and dystrophy are associated (7, 8). The process often spreads to contiguous areas of the body, spreads in a mirror distribution, and may become generalized (9). Over time the process becomes centralized with dysfunction of the CNS control of autonomic, somatosensory, and motor systems (10). However, even in its most severe form, patients may achieve a profound remission, the longest of which is now nine years (11, 12).

The reported incidence of CRPS after injuries is variable due to the fact that in some studies, patients were evaluated weeks to months after symptom onset while other series studied more chronic patients (13–18). There is also variability in the incidence and severity of CRPS in population-based studies (19, 20). The most recent population-based study from the Netherlands (most patients are seen at regional centers) documents an incidence of 40.4 for females and 11.9 for males per 100,000 person-years at risk (20). The Olmsted County, Minnesota, study reported a much lower incidence of 8.57 for females and 2.16 for males per 100,000 per year at risk (19). However, this population-based study most likely is not representative of an urban community and was done retrospectively and by less skilled generalists. This study also reported that the majority of CRPS patients underwent spontaneous resolution of symptoms. This clearly is not the case in the over 5000 patients seen by the author. Our own (Department of Neurology, Drexel University College of Medicine) database of 1900 CRPS patients is in agreement with the demographics reported from other studies. There is an approximate 4:1 female preponderance whose average age at onset varies from 37 to 60 years of age (21–23). In this database, bone fractures, sprains, and trauma were the overwhelming majority of initiating events and the upper body was slightly more involved than the lower. As previously noted (7), more than half of the patients had the affected extremity immobilized following injury. After one year, most of the signs and symptoms were present and demonstrated increases in severity with disease duration.

LABORATORY TESTS FOR CRPS
The gold standard to diagnose CRPS is the clinical examination based on factor analysis as noted earlier. However, laboratory tests can help to confirm the clinical impression.

Skin Temperature
Differences of skin temperature between the affected and normal side are a measure of sympathetic vasoconstrictor activity. A difference of 1.5°C between sides has been suggested as diagnostic (23). In general, in acute CRPS the extremity is warm but with time becomes cold, although in a subgroup of patients the affected extremity is initially cold. Whole body warming and cooling have demonstrated a marked difference in temperature between affected and normal sides with controlled thermoregulations (body suit) (24).

Peripheral Vasoconstrictor Reflex
The peripheral vasoconstrictor reflex measured by laser Doppler fluxmetry is mediated by α-adrenergic sympathetic fibers. Rhymic cycling of cutaneous skin blood flow occurs in healthy controls but is lost in CRPS patients (25). Several authors have demonstrated an absent vasoconstrictor response to arousal maneuvers, deep inspiration, or the cold pressor test in CRPS patients that is normally evoked in healthy individuals (26–28). Importantly, the vasoconstrictor response is normal in posttraumatic patients without clinical evidence of CRPS, which is often a difficult diagnostic problem (29, 30).

Radiography
The major radiographic manifestations of CRPS are (*i*) diffuse osteoporosis with patchy demineralization of periarticular areas; (*ii*) subperiosteal bone resorption; and (*iii*) increased endosteal resorption of cortical bone. Most often these radiographic features are late manifestations of the illness (31).

Triple-Phase Bone Scan

The characteristic scintigraphic findings in CRPS I, particularly in early stages are (*i*) accelerated blood flow into the affected area; (*ii*) increased diffuse activity during the blood pool phase; and (*iii*) increased periarticular uptake in the delayed static phase (32–35). Unfortunately, the diagnostic sensitivity of the triple-phase bone scan technique is usually less than 50% and decreases with disease duration (36–38).

Sudomotor function tests, sympathetic skin responses, EMG, somatosensory evoked potentials, psychological assessment, and MRI often help in ruling out other disorders, but in general are nonspecific, time consuming, difficult to perform, and not helpful (38).

PATHOPHYSIOLOGY

CRPS most often follows peripheral trauma, a surgical procedure, or soft-tissue injury. However, approximately 10% of patients have a CNS injury of pain pathways (39, 40). At the site of injury in which nerve trunks (CRPS II) or C and A-delta fibers are damaged (CRPS I), an "inflammatory soup" develops composed of substances that originate from blood, inflammatory cells, or are upregulated and released by resident immune cells. This mixture of sensitizing and depolarizing compounds consists of cytokines interleukin-1 (IL-1), IL-6, tumor necrosis factor α (TNF-α), prostaglandin E2, serotonin (5-hydroxytryptamine), lipoxygenase, epinephrine, protons, adenosine, nerve growth factor, brain-derived neurotrophic factor, and neurotrophin-3 (8,41). There is a rapid and active interaction from the site of injury to the large (touch), small (nociceptive), and satellite cells (microglia-like) of the dorsal root ganglia (DRG) maintained by orthograde and retrograde transport. A breakdown of the peripheral nerve–blood barrier occurs at the affected dermatomal levels (42). Fibroblasts, macrophages, and lymphocytes produce and secrete growth factors that are transported to the DRG and neurons of the dorsal horn (DH), which alter G-protein-coupled receptors, transmitters, and synaptic modulators that enhance depolarization of pain transmission neurons (PTNs) (43). Profound changes occur within the affected C and A-delta fibers of the involved areas that induce peripheral nociceptive terminal membrane sensitization and subsequent depolarization. These include (*i*) activation of intracellular phosphokinase A and phosphokinase C (43) and (*ii*) increased phosphorylation, density, and location of tetrodotoxin-resistant sodium channels on PTNs of the DH (44). It has recently been shown in nerve-injured mice that blood-borne macrophages (presumably from the site of injury) may actually infiltrate the spinal cord and differentiate into fully functioning microglia that may also secrete inflammatory cytokines that in turn may alter the function of PTNs (45).

The afferent barrage from the site of injury may be a critical feature in initiating CRPS. In general, C-fibers fire at 1 Hz frequency in nonpainful conditions, which is subthreshold for pain perception (43). The high-frequency injury barrage (50–200 Hz) that occurs at the site of injury, particularly that from mechanoinsensitive C-fibers, may be critical for central sensitization of PTNs of the DH (46). Its clinical manifestations are (*i*) a lower threshold to fire DH neurons; (*ii*) spread of pain extraterritorially; (*iii*) mechano and thermal allodynia; (*iv*) increased receptive field size of affected DH neurons; and (*v*) central pain processing dysregulation manifested by hyperpathia (47–49). The basis of this physiological state is a high-frequency-sustained nociceptive barrage that releases glutamate and the neuromodulators substance P (SP) and calcitonin gene–related protein (CGRP) on PTNs. This causes slow excitatory postsynaptic potentials, which last for seconds and are the basis for temporal summation that releases the Mg^{2+} block of the glutamatergic NMDA receptor. This leads to an influx of Ca^{2+}, which initiates transcription of immediate early response genes (c-Fos and c-Jun) and the activation of enzymes as well as the transcription of new proteins, channels, and receptors (43,50).

Experimental evidence suggests that central sensitization is similar to long-term potentiation (LTP) that occurs in the CA1 region of the hippocampus that is induced by enhanced synaptic currents. Long-term depression (LTD) is the opposite in which synaptic currents are diminished (50). A perceptual correlate of LTP and LTD has been shown in patients (51). A sustained nociceptive barrage in PTNs activates voltage-gated calcium and nonspecific ion channels. This is correlated with the "wind-up" phenomenon in which nociceptive input causes repetitive firing of PTNs and enhances pain (48). Partial nerve or distal axonal injury is clearly present in CRPS type II, and Oaklander's recent studies suggest that CRPS I may be secondary to small-fiber degeneration associated with minimal nerve injury to terminal twigs of C and A-delta fibers (52) in soft tissue. The mechanisms that cause damage to axonal pain afferents in soft tissue are not clear but (*i*) crossed after-discharge in which potassium from actively conducting fibers diffuses and depolarizes contiguous axons and (*ii*) abnormalities from the "inflammatory soup" (such as reactive oxygen species or products of Wallerian degeneration) have been suggested (53, 54). Another important physiological correlate of nerve injury is instability of the axon membrane that causes potential oscillations that initiate ectopic firing near the DRG (55, 56).

Partial nerve injury induces a number of molecular biological and physiological changes in the DH that include (*i*) induction of cyclooxygenase, (*ii*) down-regulation of the μ opioid receptor, and (*iii*) a phenotypic switch of touch to pain fibers (expression of SP and brain-derived neurotrophic factor on touch fibers). This expression of novel genes may allow low-threshold mechanoreceptors to induce central sensitization (57).

In both experimental pain models and as now demonstrated in patients, blockade of the NMDA receptor reduces the pain of CRPS, which supports a critical role for this receptor in the maintenance of chronic pain in this syndrome (12,58–60).

Patients with CRPS suffer mechanical and thermal allodynia, hyperalgesia, deep muscle pain, hyperpathia, and often hypoesthesia in affected areas. These sensations may be the clinical correlates of LTP or LTD, and their physiological correlates have also been demonstrated in nociceptive neurons (47,61,62).

Glutamatergic AMPA receptors (GluR2/3 subunits) mediate fast pain (A-delta fiber) that is experienced after acute injury (63). A major component of synaptic plasticity of PTNs is due to the number and conductance of AMPA receptors in the postsynaptic membrane, which is dependent on synaptic NMDA modulation (64). A critical process in the induction and maintenance of LTP and LTD of PTNs is dependent upon the concentration and spatial and temporal influx of calcium through the NMDA receptor. These factors determine either the aggregation (LTP) or dispersal (LTD) of AMPA receptors at the postsynaptic membrane (65). Intracellular calcium-calmodulin–dependent protein kinase II is critical for LTP by providing anchoring sites for AMPA receptors and increasing their conductance (66). Regulatory and enhancing proteins located in the postsynaptic density control other important signaling cascades such as Ras-mitogen-activated protein kinase and inositide 3-kinase during calcium influx (59,67,68). Ras-mitogen-activated protein kinase expression regulates transcription factors such as cyclic adenosine 5′ monophosphate response element binding protein, which is one pathway for gene expression initiated by Ca^{2+} influx through NMPA receptors (50,69). Central (DH) and peripheral (C and A-delta fiber) sensitization is enhanced by the products of novel gene expression which lower the firing threshold of damaged C and A-delta fiber terminals at the site of injury and increase the sensitivity of PTNs in the DRG and DH. Failure of inhibitory circuitry in the DH may also contribute to central sensitization (62).

LTD, the possible basis of clinical hypoesthesia often noted in the injured area, requires NMDA receptor activation, a rise in intracellular Ca^{2+} in PTNs, and is spike timing regulated (70, 71). NMDA activation may also induce internalization of AMPA receptors, dephosphorylation of their GluR1 subunits, and increased AMPA receptor degradation after endocytosis (72). LTD is also enhanced by upregulation of gamma-aminobutyric acid (GABA) and glycinergic-mediated inhibition (73). These mechanisms of LTP and LTD are clearly present in experimental models of neuropathic pain but have not been proven in CRPS patients.

THE SICKNESS RESPONSE

Pain facilitation from immune to brain communication is known as the sickness response. This is the body's initial nonspecific immune response to infection or injury and occurs within hours of the inciting event. It is caused by immune to brain interaction that initiates nervous system–mediated processes that include pain facilitation (74). Mast cells, macrophages, monocytes, and leukocytes are activated and recruited to the site of infection or injury (42). These immune cells secrete proinflammatory cytokines that include IL-1, IL-6, and TNF-α that activate paraganglia which synapse on vagal sensory fibers which project to the brainstem via the vagus and glossopharyngeal nerves (75, 76). Sickness-induced pain facilitation can be induced by intraperitoneal injection of lipopolysaccharide from the cell walls of Gram-negative bacteria or by infusion of proinflammatory cytokines (77, 78). In experimental pain models, it can be blocked by IL-1 antagonists, TNF-α-binding proteins, or subdiaphragmatic vagotomy (78–80).

On a molecular level, the immune system is pivotal for both the induction and maintenance of central sensitization (8). Experimental animal models have demonstrated that following injury or inflammation, there is activation of glial cells at the appropriate spinal level (42,81,82). Pretreatment with compounds that block microglial and astrocytic activation blocks neuropathic pain (83–85). Microglial activation is important in the induction of neuropathic pain, while astrocytes appear important in its maintenance (86–88). As noted earlier, immune cells activated at the site of injury may invade the DH and become functionally active (45) and thus contribute to the maintenance of neuropathic pain.

Recent clinical data suggest that proinflammatory cytokines may not be critical to pain maintenance, as improvement of signs and symptoms of the syndrome was noted in the face of increased levels of IL-6 and TNF-α (89). However, specific aspects of pain such as hyperalgesia may be related to specific proinflammatory cytokines (TNF-α) (90). Most studies suggest, however, that the differential expression patterns of cytokines with a shift toward proinflammatory profiles and downregulation of inhibitory profiles (decreased IL-4 and IL-10) occur in the syndrome (91–94).

Complicating the issues of the role of cytokines in the pathogenesis of CRPS is the interaction between pain, stress, and innate immunity. Quantitative analysis of lymphocytic subsets in CRPS patients versus controls shows a decrease of $CD8^+$ lymphocytes and a lower percentage of IL-2-producing T-cell subpopulations with no change of the TH2 response (95). Neutrophils of CRPS patients who had high stress scores and stress hormone concentrations demonstrated decreased expression of CD62L and CD11b/CD18 markers and had impaired ability to phagocytize zymosan particles as compared to controls. In vitro incubation of neutrophils with catecholamine from highly stressed CRPS patients demonstrated impaired neutrophil function (95). Thus, it is possible that CRPS patients may be expressing the immune-suppressive effects of the neuroendocrine stress response rather than differential cytokine expression specific to this syndrome.

THE ROLE OF THE SYMPATHETIC NERVOUS SYSTEM IN THE PAIN OF CRPS

Experimental and clinical evidence documents the importance of the sympathetic nervous system in the pain of CRPS (8,96). Stressors such as physical and mental activity and emotional upset activate the sympathetic nervous system and increase pain in CRPS patients (97). There is a subset of CRPS patients (usually early in the course of the illness) that has sympathetically maintained pain (98). Patients who have had relief of CRPS pain by sympathectomy may have a return of pain if norepinephrine is injected into the formerly affected area (99). Modification of sympathetic outflow by total body cooling reproduces mechanical hyperalgesia in those areas that demonstrated (SMP) earlier and not in those painful areas that were sympathetically independent (SIP) (100). Complete pain relief has been accomplished by sympatholysis in some CRPS patients and in those that are sympathetically maintained lasts longer than the induced conduction blockade. This suggests that sympathetically maintained pain may be important for the maintenance of central sensitization of PTNs in some patients (10).

Anatomical connections of the sympathetic nervous system to peripheral nociceptive afferents at the site of injury and within the DRG have been demonstrated following axotomy in experimental pain models (8,100,101). In the DRG, sympathetic fibers form basket terminals around large mechanoreceptor neurons and innervate thinly myelinated A-delta afferents. They are induced to sprout by lymphocyte inhibitory factor and are guided by upregulation of p75 on these target neurons (101). Epinephrine from the adrenal gland sensitizes mechanoreceptors, and there are interactions of sympathetic fibers, bradykinin, neurotrophic factors, and prostanoids on nociceptive afferents (8). Other potential mechanisms of coupling of sympathetic and sensory systems occur due to the expression of adrenoreceptors on mechanosensitive sensory afferents after nerve injury as well as the upregulation of α-1 adrenoreceptors in hyperalgesic skin shown in CRPS patients (97,102). Prolonged hindlimb ischemia followed by reperfusion in an experimental rat pain model produces (*i*) a hyperemic warm extremity that lasts for four hours and then demonstrates dystrophic signs within 24 hours, (*ii*) changes in the contralateral extremity, and (*iii*) long-lasting pinprick, hyperalgesia, and thermal mechanoallodynia. The model suggests that ischemia may sensitize and activate deep nociceptors of muscle ligaments and joints which characterize clinical CRPS (103).

AUTONOMIC DYSREGULATION AND EDEMA

In patients with acute CRPS, the extremity is warm and vasodilated (104). Sympathetic preganglionic neurons of the intermediolateral column of the spinal cord project to sympathetic ganglia that in turn innervate the effector cells of various tissues. These neurons are under differential control from brainstem and hypothalamic centers and have characteristic tonic and reflex discharge patterns depending on the tissues innervated (thermoregulatory, nutritive, sudomotor, and muscle) (105, 106). Controlled thermoregulation (cooling and heating the body while measuring distal extremity blood flow and temperature) has demonstrated diminished vasoconstrictor responses, increased cutaneous perfusion, and decreased phasic sympathetic vasoconstrictor reflexes in CRPS patients (29,107,108). Further support for decreased sympathetic outflow and transmitter release in acute CRPS is (*i*) reduced levels of norepinephrine, (*ii*) its metabolite 3,4-dihydroxyphenylethyleneglycol, and (*iii*) the associated vasoconstrictive neuropeptide which colocalizes with norepinephrine in terminal sympathetic varicosities in the venous effluent from the affected extremity (109, 110).

Central inhibition and a functional loss of cutaneous sympathetic vasoconstriction and associated wave-like fluctuations (vasomotion) are primary manifestations of sympathetic paralysis in acute CRPS (25). A spinal contribution to this deficit is suggested by its pattern of bilateral sympathetic dysfunction in these patients (25–27).

NEUROGENIC EDEMA

Localized neurogenic inflammation occurs in acute CRPS. CGRP levels are increased in the acute but not the chronic stage of the illness and may also cause increased axon reflex sweating by their action on peripheral sweat glands (30). Acute CRPS patients demonstrate increased axon reflex vasodilatation, and transcutaneous electrical nerve stimulation elicits protein extravasation in patients but not controls. Intradermal infusion of SP in the affected arm caused axon reflex vasodilation in the unaffected arm of CRPS patients but not in the contralateral side of controls (111, 112). Continuous intra-arterial infusion of SP induces edema, inflammation and mechanical but not thermal pain (113). Enhanced leukocytoendothelial cell interaction in CRPS patients is demonstrated by an increase in leukocyte rolling and their firm adherence to the walls of postcapillary venules (113). Bone scintigraphy, analysis of joint fluid, synovial biopsy, and MRI all demonstrate plasma extravasation in early acute CRPS (114–117).

Endothelial function may be impaired in early CRPS as assessed by waveforms and the increase in diameter and blood flow of the brachial artery in CRPS patients (118). Plasma endothelin levels were found to be normal in severe CRPS patients versus healthy controls and other painful conditions (119). In the intermediate stage of illness, ET-1, IL-6, and TNF-α were found to be elevated in blister fluid of the affected extremity of CRPS patients, whereas nitrate/nitrite was decreased (120). The exact role of nitric oxide, prostacyclin, and endothelin in the vasodilation noted in early CRPS is not clear (118). At the present time, it appears that sympathetic dysfunction and neurogenic inflammation are the major causes of the warm affected extremity in early CRPS. The return of normal sympathetic-induced vasoconstrictor function may coincide with recovery from acute CRPS I (121).

Supersensitivity to circulating catecholamines is the dominant mechanism for the vasoconstriction (cold CRPS) noted in chronic CRPS patients. Many mechanisms for the phenomenon may contribute such as an increased density of adrenoreceptors in affected blood vessels, increased affinity of ligands for these receptors, decrease in neurotransmitter uptake, or an upregulation of second messenger systems (104,122). There is a negative correlation between the duration of CRPS (intermediate to later stages) and temperature asymmetry (108,110), and it is generally accepted that a 2°C difference between sides strongly suggests CRPS rather than a posttraumatic or other pain syndrome (24). Temperature and blood flow changes are dynamic through the course of the disease and are most evident during median to high levels of sympathetic tone but may be equal at baseline (104). Thermography during static and controlled thermoregulation (whole body cooling and warming) increases temperature differences significantly (123).

SYMPATHETICALLY MAINTAINED PAIN

Differential sympathetic efferent output affects both cutaneous and deep somatic pain. A recent study has demonstrated that all components of sympathetically maintained pain are dynamic and decrease with illness duration. The sympathetically maintained component of deep somatic pain (bones, joints, tendons) was more affected by sympathetic blockade in acute patients than cutaneous pain (124). The chronic ischemia reperfusion model of CRPS I pain supports the role of enhanced sympathetically mediated vasoconstriction in the pain of CRPS, as it could be relieved by decreasing vasoconstriction or enhancing vasodilatation (125, 126). A prospective study in patients who were to undergo repeat carpal tunnel surgery demonstrated that those patients with abnormal preoperative sympathetic function had recurrent CRPS I (127).

A recent pathologic study of the amputated limbs of two CRPS I patients demonstrates some of the pathologic changes that may underlie the physiological sympathetic modulated phenomena seen in patients. These findings include (*i*) loss of vascular endothelial integrity, (*ii*) inappropriate expression of NPY (a vasoconstriction modulatory protein expressed with norepinephrine in the innervation to superficial arterioles), (*iii*) loss of calcitonin gene–related peptide (neuropeptide that modulates vasodilatation) expression on cutaneous vasculature, and (*iv*) vascular hypertrophy (128).

Sudomotor dysfunction is prevalent at some point of the illness in a majority of CRPS patients. Eccrine sweat glands are located in hairy skin and are innervated by sympathetic postganglionic cholinergic fibers as opposed to epinephrine at all other sympathetic effector sites (129). Sweat glands are also innervated by fibers that stain for vasoactive intestinal peptide, CGRP, SP, and tyrosine hydroxylase that also are thought to modulate sweat production (130). Most studies demonstrate increased resting sweat production of the affected extremities (131). An adrenergic sweat response in CRPS-affected limbs, by ionophoresis, provides evidence for adrenergic activation of a system that is physiologically not under adrenergic control (132).

The sympathetic nervous system may also play a role in edema formation by stimulation of lymphatics and increase of capillary filtration capacity (a measure of microvascular permeability), although the major mechanism is neurogenic inflammation mediated by vasoactive neuropeptides (111,133–135).

THE MOVEMENT DISORDER OF CRPS

The movement disorder of CRPS consists of (*i*) difficulty initiating, maintaining, and loss of precision of distal movement, (*ii*) weakness, (*iii*) decrease of active and passive range of movement, (*iv*) tremor, (*v*) spasms and myoclonus, (*vi*) neglect of affected parts, and (*vii*) kinematically demonstrated abnormalities of grip and target reaching (96,136,137).

This aspect of CRPS was not recognized earlier, as it was thought to be either psychogenic or related to patient splinting due to pain. It may be seen prior to or concomitant with autonomic system dysfunction. It occurs to some degree (at least one component) in approximately 70% of patients, may appear suddenly, or gradually spread to all extremities (138). The sympathetic nervous system has profound effects upon skeletal muscle contraction, neuromuscular transmission, anterior horn cell function, and spinal cord reflexes. Intrafusal fibers of the muscle spindle are sympathetically innervated as are anterior horn cells (8). The movement disorder of CRPS has been dramatically improved by sympathetic blockade (139). In the spinal cord, SP and CGRP are found in the dorsal, ventral, and intermediolateral columns. In tissue culture, these neuropeptides have been shown to induce prolonged depolarization of anterior horn cells, which is blocked by GABA$_b$ agonists (baclofen). The release of these neuropeptides from nociceptive afferents modulates the gain and persistence of nociceptive flexor withdrawal reflexes (140). The clinical expression of disordered nocifensor reflex function may be the flexed protective posture of the affected extremity. In general, nerve conduction velocity, needle EMG, and somatosensory evoked potentials are negative in CRPS patients (141).

Patients with CRPS that suffer dystonia have impaired reciprocal inhibition between flexor and extensor muscles, a decreased threshold of the tonic and phasic components of the stretch reflex, as well as impaired H reflex inhibition by vibration (141). Dorsal horn interneuronal circuits that mediate presynaptic inhibition are also impaired, as these patients are unable to dampen reflex activity by proximal muscle proprioceptive input. GABAergic mechanisms are involved, as intrathecal baclofen is often effective in decreasing dystonia and spasms (142).

The pivotal role of GABAergic interneurons in dystonia is suggested by their supraspinal descending projections from the brainstem, motor cortex, and the descending nociceptive inhibitory complex as well as their direct and collateral nociceptive afferent input. The clinical manifestation of this disordered circuitry is a decreased reciprocal inhibition threshold of the stretch reflex (141). Further clinical manifestations of this disordered inhibitory circuitry are the increased dystonia and nociceptive flexor withdrawal that occurs with emotional stress, movement, and cold and tactile stimulation (143).

Relative sparing of the first two digits is frequently seen in upper extremity dystonia (143). A possible explanation is that polysynaptic interneuronal circuits for flexor reflexes are distributed equally to all digits but there is a larger direct cortical motor projection to digits I and II which are thus less reliant on interneurons (143). A recent functional MRI study of dystonia in CRPS patients versus 17 controls in which patients imagined movement of their dystonic arm demonstrated reduced activation of the ipsilateral premotor and prefrontal cortex, frontal operculum, anterior insular cortex, and superior temporal gyrus. Contralaterally reduced activation was seen in the inferior parietal and primary sensory cortex. No difference between controls and patients was noted during executed movements or imagined movement of the unaffected arm. This altered activation pattern was interpreted as demonstrating an interface between pain associated distributed loops and higher motor control (144). A recent epidemiologic study that evaluated factors that influence the onset of these movement disorders concluded that dystonia in CRPS has a highly variable onset latency, is associated with an increased risk of spread to other extremities, and may be associated with maladaptive neuroplasticity (145). It was also noted that hyperacusis is common in severely affected CRPS-related dystonia patients and suggested that central involvement spreads beyond sensorimotor processing areas (146).

The tremor of CRPS is associated with the other movement disorders of CRPS but occasionally appears alone (16,23,143,147–149). Its characteristics are (*i*) a frequency of 3 to 7 Hz; (*ii*) it is most often intentional but may be postural kinetic; (*iii*) it is rarely seen as the only motor feature; and (*iv*) most likely it is an enhancement of an intentional tremor.

Myoclonus is frequently seen in severe CRPS patients (16,23,150, 151). Clinically, myoclonic jerks can be seen at rest, are aggravated by movement, and are associated with spasms and dystonia. A recent study utilizing intermuscular and corticomuscular coherence analysis demonstrated increased intermuscular coherence in the 6- to 12-Hz band similar to that seen in physiological tremor. Side-to-side coherence was seen in two patients, which is suggestive of a central oscillatory drive (152).

A neglect-like syndrome (both cognitive and motor) has been clearly documented in CRPS patients (136). PET and SPECT studies of chronic CRPS patients have demonstrated decreased activity of the thalamus contralateral to the affected limb (153–155). However, one study suggested that these findings may be time dependent, as an earlier SPECT evaluation demonstrated hyperfusion (155). CRPS patients and others with chronic pain demonstrate neglect-like symptoms and have metabolic changes in the frontal cortex and thalamus during neglect. Sympathetically maintained pain and chronic pain patients are anatomically similar by functional studies (156). Clinically, CRPS patients demonstrated more involuntary leg movements than other chronic pain patients by functional MRI (157). Abnormalities of target reaching and grip as well as a mismatch between sensory input and motor output have also been described as components of the motor syndrome seen in CRPS patients (158, 159).

CORTICAL REORGANIZATION DURING CRPS

The recent application of functional MRI, PET, magnetoencephalography, and SPECT correlate sensory parameters and changes in distributed anatomical loops with disease progression (160–165). Transcranial stimulation studies in CRPS patients versus controls have demonstrated (*i*) a smaller cortical motor representation opposite an affected extremity, (*ii*) reduction of intracortical inhibition and an increase in I-wave facilitation contralateral to the affected extremity (sensory motor hyperexcitability), and (*iii*) that the disease process affects the indirect neural circuits that effect sensory input and motor output from the cortex (166–168).

PET analysis utilizing F18–2DG of the CNS in 18 CRPS patients versus controls revealed a bilateral increase in glucose metabolism of SII and contralateral increases in midanterior and posterior cingulate cortex, anterior and posterior parietal cortex, posterior insula, thalamus, and cerebellum. Glucose metabolism was decreased contralateral to the affected extremity in the prefrontal and motor cortex. The bilateral glucose metabolism increase in the midanterior and posterior cingulate cortex was correlated with disease duration. SPECT studies, utilizing statistical subtraction analysis pre- and posttreatment, revealed a correlation of rCBF in the thalamus, frontal, and parietal lobe to pain relief (163).

Functional imaging of allodynia in CRPS demonstrates widespread activations in the contralateral (side opposite the affected hand) SI, bilateral insular, parietal association cortices, as well as the anterior and posterior cingulate cortices and the motor cortex. The demonstrated nociceptive as well as cognitive and motor area metabolic increases support a shift from tonically active sensory systems (visual and vestibular cortices) to somatosensory processing areas (164). Functional imaging in CRPS patients with pinprick hyperalgesia also demonstrated a widespread neuronal matrix that includes cognitive and motor areas (90). Functional MRI studies have also demonstrated that patterns of cortical reorganization, a reduction of SI and SII signals, paralleled impaired tactile discrimination that also correlated with mean sustained pain levels (169). Clinical correlations of these pain-driven cortical metabolic changes are mislocalization of tactile stimuli in CRPS patients and a return to normal of tactile discrimination with pain reduction (160,164).

TREATMENT OF CRPS

Present therapy for many CRPS patients, particularly long-standing patients (>2 years), is unsuccessful. The usual or standard treatments with nonsteroidal anti-inflammatory, agents, anticonvulsants, narcotics, and sympatholytic agents have recently been reviewed and will not be covered here (170).

The use of multiday ketamine infusions and five-day subanesthetic infusions has been a significant advance in moderately severe patients. Ketamine coma has been dramatically effective in approximately 50% of severe intractable patients who have suffered longer than five years (12, 58, 60, 171).

Therapy with drugs that block inflammatory cytokines particularly TNF-α and IL-1 and IL-6 has proven to be efficacious both in their own right and in maintaining effects achieved with ketamine (172, 173).

Present gene array techniques suggest that the function and significance of a vast array of genes turned on by specific forms of nociceptive pain will be discovered and will direct future therapy for this crippling syndrome.

REFERENCES

1. Harden RN, Bruehl S, Galer BS, et al. Complex regional pain syndrome: are the IASP diagnostic criteria valid and sufficiently comprehensive? Pain 1999; 83(2):211–219.
2. Bruehl S, Harden RN, Galer BS, et al. External validation of IASP diagnostic criteria for complex regional pain syndrome and proposed research diagnostic criteria. International Association for the Study of Pain. Pain 1999; 81(1/2):147–154.

3. Bruehl S, Lofland KR, Semenchuk EM, et al. Use of cluster analysis to validate IHS diagnostic criteria for migraine and tension-type headache. Headache 1999; 39(3):181–189.
4. Merskey H, Bogduk N. Classification of Chronic Pain: Description of Chronic Pain Syndrome and Definition of Pain Terms. 2nd ed. Seattle, WA: IASP Press, 1994.
5. Bruehl S, Harden RN, Galer BS, et al. Complex regional pain syndrome: are there distinct subtypes and sequential stages of the syndrome? Pain 2002; 95(1/2): 119–124.
6. Harden RN, Bruehl SP. Diagnostic criteria; the statistical derivation of the four criterion factors. In: Wilson PR, Stanton-Hicks M, Harden RN, eds. CRPS: Current Diagnosis and Therapy; Progress in Pain Research and Management. Vol 32. Seattle, WA: IASP Press, 2005:45–58.
7. Schwartzman RJ, McLellan TL. Reflex sympathetic dystrophy. Arch Neurol 1987; 44(5):555–561.
8. Schwartzman RJ, Alexander GM, Grothusen J. Pathophysiology of complex regional pain syndrome. Expert Rev Neurother 2006; 6(5):669–681.
9. Maleki J. "Sensitization": is there a cure? Pain Med 2002; 3(4):294–297.
10. Jänig W, Baron R. Complex regional pain syndrome: mystery explained? Lancet Neurol 2003; 2(11):687–697.
11. Kiefer RT, Rohr P, Ploppa A, et al. Complete recovery from intractable complex regional pain syndrome, CRPS-type I, following anesthetic ketamine and midazolam. Pain Pract 2007; 7(2):147–150.
12. Kiefer RT, Rohr P, Ploppa A, et al. Efficacy of ketamine in anesthetic dosage for the treatment of refractory complex regional pain syndrome: an open-label phase II study [published online ahead of print February 5, 2008]. Pain Med.
13. Omer G, Thomas S. Treatment of causalgia. Review of cases at Brooke General Hospital. Tex Med 1971; 67(1):93–96.
14. Bohm E. Das suddeutsche syndrome. Hefte Zur Unfallheilkunde 1985; 174:241–250.
15. Atkins RM, Duckworth T, Kanis JA. Features of algodystrophy after Colles' fracture. J Bone Joint Surg Br 1990; 72(1):105–110.
16. Veldman PH, Reynen HM, Arntz IE, et al. Signs and symptoms of reflex sympathetic dystrophy: prospective study of 829 patients. Lancet 1993; 342(8878):1012–1016.
17. Bickerstaff DR, Kanis JA. Algodystrophy: an under-recognized complication of minor trauma. Br J Rheumatol 1994; 33(3):240–248.
18. Dijkstra PU, Groothoff JW, ten Duis HJ, et al. Incidence of complex regional pain syndrome type I after fractures of the distal radius. Eur J Pain 2003; 7(5):457–462.
19. Sandroni P, Benrud-Larson LM, McClelland RL, et al. Complex regional pain syndrome type I: incidence and prevalence in Olmsted county, a population-based study. Pain 2003; 103(1/2):199–207.
20. de Mos M, de Bruijn AG, Huygen FJ, et al. The incidence of complex regional pain syndrome: a population-based study. Pain 2007; 129(1/2):12–20.
21. Zyluk A. The natural history of post-traumatic reflex sympathetic dystrophy. J Hand Surg Br 1998; 23(1):20–23.
22. Allen G, Galer BS, Schwartz L. Epidemiology of complex regional pain syndrome: a retrospective chart review of 134 patients. Pain 1999; 80(3):539–544.
23. Birklein F, Riedl B, Sieweke N, et al. Neurological findings in complex regional pain syndromes—analysis of 145 cases. Acta Neurol Scand 2000; 101(4):262–269.
24. Wasner G, Schattschneider J, Baron R. Skin temperature side differences—a diagnostic tool for CRPS? Pain 2002; 98(1/2):19–26.
25. Bej MD, Schwartzman RJ. Abnormalities of cutaneous blood flow regulation in patients with reflex sympathetic dystrophy as measured by laser Doppler fluxmetry. Arch Neurol 1991; 48(9):912–915.
26. Rosén L, Ostergren J, Fagrell B, et al. Skin microvascular circulation in the sympathetic dystrophies evaluated by videophotometric capillaroscopy and laser Doppler fluxmetry. Eur J Clin Invest 1988; 18(3):305–308.

27. Kurvers HA, Jacobs MJ, Beuk RJ, et al. The spinal component to skin blood flow abnormalities in reflex sympathetic dystrophy. Arch Neurol 1996; 53(1):58–65.
28. Schürmann M, Gradl G, Fürst H. A standardized bedside test for assessment of peripheral sympathetic nervous function using laser Doppler flowmetry. Microvasc Res 1996; 52(2):157–170.
29. Schürmann M, Gradl G, Andress HJ, et al. Assessment of peripheral sympathetic nervous function for diagnosing early post-traumatic complex regional pain syndrome type I. Pain 1999; 80(1/2):149–159.
30. Birklein F, Schmelz M, Schifter S, et al. The important role of neuropeptides in complex regional pain syndrome. Neurology 2001; 57(12):2179–2184.
31. Gradl G, Steinborn M, Wizgall I, et al. Acute CRPS I (morbus sudeck) following distal radial fractures—methods for early diagnosis. Zentralbl Chir 2003; 128(12):1020–1026.
32. Genant HK, Kozin F, Bekerman C, et al. The reflex sympathetic dystrophy syndrome. A comprehensive analysis using fine-detail radiography, photon absorptiometry, and bone and joint scintigraphy. Radiology 1975; 117(1):21–32.
33. Kozin F, Genant HK, Bekerman C, et al. The reflex sympathetic dystrophy syndrome. II. Roentgenographic and scintigraphic evidence of bilaterality and of periarticular accentuation. Am J Med 1976; 60(3):332–338.
34. Intenzo C, Kim S, Millin J, et al. Scintigraphic patterns of the reflex sympathetic dystrophy syndrome of the lower extremities. Clin Nucl Med 1989; 14(9):657–661.
35. Kozin F, Soin JS, Ryan LM, et al. Bone scintigraphy in the reflex sympathetic dystrophy syndrome. Radiology 1981; 138(2):437–443.
36. Werner R, Davidoff G, Jackson MD, et al. Factors affecting the sensitivity and specificity of the three-phase technetium bone scan in the diagnosis of reflex sympathetic dystrophy syndrome in the upper extremity. J Hand Surg Am. 1989; 14(3):520–523.
37. Lee GW, Weeks PM. The role of bone scintigraphy in diagnosing reflex sympathetic dystrophy. J Hand Surg Am 1995; 20(3):458–463.
38. Rommel O, Häbler HJ, Schürmann M. Laboratory tests for complex regional pain syndrome. In: Wilson PR, Stanton-Hicks M, Harden RN, eds. CRPS: Current Diagnosis and Therapy. Vol 32. Seattle, WA: IASP Press, 2005:chap 26.
39. Gellman H, Keenan MA, Stone L, et al. Reflex sympathetic dystrophy in brain-injured patients. Pain 1992; 51(3):307–311.
40. Schwartzman RJ, Gurusinghe C, Gracely E. Prevalence of complex regional pain syndrome in a cohort of multiple sclerosis patients. Pain Physician 2008; 11(2):133–136.
41. Shu X, Mendell LM. Nerve growth factor acutely sensitizes the response of adult rat sensory neurons to capsaicin. Neurosci Lett 1999; 274(3):159–162.
42. Marchand F, Perretti M, McMahon SB. Role of the immune system in chronic pain. Nat Rev Neurosci 2005; 6(7):521–532.
43. Woolf CJ, Salter MW. Neuronal plasticity: increasing the gain in pain. Science 2000; 288(5472):1765–1769.
44. England S, Bevan S, Docherty RJ. PGE2 modulates the tetrodotoxin-resistant sodium current in neonatal rat dorsal root ganglion neurons via the cyclic AMP-protein kinase A cascade. J Physiol 1996; 495(pt 2):429–440.
45. Zhang J, Shi XQ, Echeverry S, et al. Expression of CCR2 in both resident and bone marrow-derived microglia plays a critical role in neuropathic pain. J Neurosci 2007; 27(45):12396–12406.
46. Weidner C, Schmelz M, Schmidt R, et al. Functional attributes discriminating mechano-insensitive and mechano-responsive C nociceptors in human skin. Neuroscience 1999; 19(22):10184–10190.
47. Davies SN, Lodge D. Evidence for involvement of N-methylaspartate receptors in 'wind-up' of class 2 neurons in the dorsal horn of the rat. Brain Res 1987; 424(2):402–406.
48. Dickenson AH, Sullivan AF. Evidence for a role of the NMDA receptor in the frequency dependent potentiation of deep rat dorsal horn nociceptive neurons following C fibre stimulation. Neuropharmacology 1987; 26(8):1235–1238.

49. Kilo S, Schmelz M, Koltzenburg M, et al. Different patterns of hyperalgesia induced by experimental inflammation in human skin. Brain 1994; 117(pt 2):385–396.
50. Sheng M, Kim MJ. Postsynaptic signaling and plasticity mechanisms. Science 2002; 298(5594):776–780.
51. Klein T, Magerl W, Hopf HC, et al. Perceptual correlates of nociceptive long-term potentiation and long-term depression in humans. J Neurosci 2004; 24(4):964–971.
52. Oaklander AL, Rissmiller JG, Gelman LB, et al. Evidence of focal small-fiber axonal degeneration in complex regional pain syndrome-I (reflex sympathetic dystrophy). Pain 2006; 120(3):235–243.
53. van der Laan L, Kapitein PJ, Oyen WJ, et al. A novel animal model to evaluate oxygen derived free radical damage in soft tissue. Free Radical Res 1997; 26(4): 363–372.
54. Amir R, Devor M. Functional cross-excitation between afferent A- and C-neurons in dorsal root ganglia. Neuroscience 2000; 95(1):189–195.
55. Cummins TR, Dib-Hajj SD, Black JA, et al. Sodium channels and the molecular pathophysiology of pain. In: Sandkühler J, Bromm B, Gebhart GF, eds. Nervous System Plasticity and Chronic Pain. Amsterdam, The Netherlands: Elsevier Press, 2000:13–19.
56. Lyu YS, Park SK, Chung K, et al. Low dose of tetrodotoxin reduces neuropathic pain behaviors in an animal model. Brain Res 2000; 871(1):98–103.
57. Zhou XF, Chie ET, Deng YS, et al. Injured primary sensory neurons switch phenotype for brain-derived neurotrophic factor in the rat. Neuroscience 1999; 92(3):841–853.
58. Harbut RE, Correll GE. Successful treatment of a nine-year case of complex regional pain syndrome type-I reflex sympathetic dystrophy with intravenous ketamine-infusion therapy in a warfarin-anticoagulated adult female patient. Pain Med 2002; 3(2):147–155.
59. Petrenko AB, Yamakura T, Baba H, et al. The role of N-methyl-D-aspartate (NMDA) receptors in pain: a review. Anesth Analg 2003; 97(4):1108–1116.
60. Goldberg ME, Domsky R, Scaringe D, et al. Multi-day low dose ketamine infusion for the treatment of complex regional pain syndrome. Pain Physician 2005; 8(2):175–179.
61. Thompson SW, King AE, Woolf CJ. Activity-dependent changes in rat ventral horn neurons in vitro; summation of prolonged afferent evoked postsynaptic depolarizations produce a d-2-amino-5-phosphonovaleric acid sensitive windup. Eur J Neurosci 1990; 2(7):638–649.
62. Sandkühler J, Chen JG, Cheng G, et al. Low-frequency stimulation of afferent Adelta-fibers induces long-term depression at primary afferent synapses with substantia gelatinosa neurons in the rat. J Neurosci 1997; 17(16):6483–6491.
63. Hollmann M, Heinemann S. Cloned glutamate receptors. Annu Rev Neurosci 1994; 17:31–108.
64. Kim MJ, Dunah AW, Wang YT, et al. Differential roles of NR2A- and NR2B-containing NMDA receptors in Ras-ERK signaling and AMPA receptor trafficking. Neuron 2005; 46(5):745–760.
65. Song I, Huganir RL. Regulation of AMPA receptors during synaptic plasticity. Trends Neurosci 2002; 25(11):578–588.
66. Carroll RC, Beattie EC, von Zastrow M, et al. Role of AMPA receptor endocytosis in synaptic plasticity. Nat Rev Neurosci 2001; 2(5):315–324.
67. Popescu G, Auerbach A. Modal gating of NMDA receptors and the shape of their synaptic response. Nat Neurosci 2003; 6(5):476–483.
68. Pérez-Otaño I, Ehlers MD. Homeostatic plasticity and NMDA receptor trafficking. Trends Neurosci 2005; 28(5):229–238.
69. Hoeger-Bement MK, Sluka KA. Phosphorylation of CREB and mechanical hyperalgesia is reversed by blockade of the cAMP pathway in a time-dependent manner after repeated intramuscular acid injections. J Neurosci 2003; 23(13):5437–5445.
70. Bi GQ, Rubin J. Timing in synaptic plasticity: from detection to integration. Trends Neurosci 2005; 28(5):222–228.

71. Morishita W, Marie H, Malenka RC. Distinct triggering and expression mechanisms underlie LTD of AMPA and NMDA synaptic responses. Nat Neurosci 2005; 8(8):1043–1050.
72. Liang F, Huganir RL. Coupling of agonist-induced AMPA receptor internalization with receptor recycling. J Neurochem 2001; 77(6):1626–1631.
73. Gaiarsa JL, Caillard O, Ben-Ari Y. Long-term plasticity at GABAergic and glycinergic synapses: mechanisms and functional significance. Trends Neurosci 2002; 25(11):564–570.
74. Watkins LR, Maier SF. The pain of being sick: implications of immune-to-brain communication for understanding pain. Annu Rev Psychol 2000; 51:29–57.
75. Layé S, Bluthé RM, Kent S, et al. Subdiaphragmatic vagotomy blocks induction of IL-1 beta mRNA in mice brain in response to peripheral LPS. Am J Physiol 1995; 268(5 pt 2):R1327–R1331.
76. Bernard J, Gauriau F. Brainstem and pain: a complementary role with regard to the thalamus. In: Wilson PR, Stanton-Hicks M, Harden NR, eds. Current Diagnosis and Therapy. Seattle, WA: IASP Press, 2005:139–154.
77. Mason P. Lipopolysaccharide induces fever and decreases tail flick latency in awake rats. Neurosci Lett 1993; 154(1/2):134–136.
78. Watkins LR, Goehler LE, Relton J, et al. Mechanisms of tumor necrosis factor-alpha (TNF-alpha) hyperalgesia. Brain Res 1995; 692(1/2):244–250.
79. Maier SF, Wiertelak EP, Martin D, et al. Interleukin-1 mediates the behavioral hyperalgesia produced by lithium chloride and endotoxin. Brain Res 1993; 623(2):321–324.
80. Watkins LR. Thermal hyperalgesia and mechanical allodynia produced by intrathecal administration of the human immunodeficiency virus-1 (HIV-1) envelope glycoprotein, gp120. Brain Res 2000; 861(1):105–116.
81. DeLeo JA, Yezierski RP. The role of neuroinflammation and neuroimmune activation in persistent pain. Pain 2001; 90(1/2):1–6.
82. Tsuda M, Inoue K, Salter MW. Neuropathic pain and spinal microglia: a big problem from molecules in "small" glia. Trends Neurosci 2005; 28(2):101–107.
83. Milligan ED, Mehmert KK, Hinde JL, et al. Thermal hyperalgesia and mechanical allodynia produced by intrathecal administration of the human immunodeficiency virus-1 (HIV-1) envelope glycoprotein, gp120. Brain Res 2000; 861(1):105–116.
84. Milligan ED, Twining C, Chacur M, et al. Spinal glia and proinflammatory cytokines mediate mirror-image neuropathic pain in rats. J Neurosci 2003; 23(3):1026–1040.
85. Aumeerally N, Allen G, Sawynok J. Glutamate-evoked release of adenosine and regulation of peripheral nociception. Neuroscience 2004; 127(1):1–11.
86. Kreutzberg GW. Microglia: a sensor for pathological events in the CNS. Trends Neurosci 1996; 19(8):312–318.
87. Raghavendra V, Tanga F, DeLeo JA. Inhibition of microglial activation attenuates the development but not existing hypersensitivity in a rat model of neuropathy. J Pharmacol Exp Ther 2003; 306(2):624–630.
88. Watkins LR, Maier SF. Immune regulation of central nervous system functions: from sickness responses to pathological pain. J Intern Med 2005; 257(2):139–155.
89. Munnikes RJ, Muis C, Boersma M, et al. Intermediate stage complex regional pain syndrome type 1 is unrelated to proinflammatory cytokines. Mediators Inflamm 2005; 6:366–372.
90. Maihöfner C, Handwerker HO, Neundörfer B, et al. Mechanical hyperalgesia in complex regional pain syndrome: a role for TNF-alpha? Neurology 2005; 65(2):311–313.
91. Alexander GM, van Rijn MA, van Hilten JJ, et al. Changes in cerebrospinal fluid levels of pro-inflammatory cytokines in CRPS. Pain 2005; 116(3):213–219.
92. Schinkel C, Gaertner A, Zaspel J, et al. Inflammatory mediators are altered in the acute phase of posttraumatic complex regional pain syndrome. Clin J Pain 2006; 22(3):235–239.
93. Uçeyler N, Eberle T, Rolke R, et al. Differential expression patterns of cytokines in complex regional pain syndrome. Pain 2007; 132(1/2):195–205.

94. Sabsovich I, Guo TZ, Wei T, et al. TNF signaling contributes to the development of nociceptive sensitization in a tibia fracture model of complex regional pain syndrome type I [published online ahead of print November 20, 2007]. Pain.
95. Kaufmann I, Eisner C, Richter P, et al. Lymphocyte subsets and the role of TH1/TH2 balance in stressed chronic pain patients. Neuroimmunomodulation 2007; 14(5):272–280.
96. Schwartzman RJ. Autonomic system and pain. In: Appenzeller O, ed. Handbook of Clinical Neurology. Amsterdam, The Netherlands: Elsevier, 2000:307–347.
97. Drummond PD, Finch PM, Skipworth S, et al. Pain increases during sympathetic arousal in patients with complex regional pain syndrome. Neurology 2001; 57(7):1296–1303.
98. Raja SN, Treede RD, Davis KD, et al. Systemic alpha-adrenergic blockade with phentolamine: a diagnostic test for sympathetically maintained pain. Anesthesiology 1991; 74(4):691–698.
99. Torebjörk E, Wahren L, Wallin G, et al. Noradrenaline-evoked pain in neuralgia. Pain 1995; 63(1):11–20.
100. Baron R, Schattschneider J, Binder A, et al. Relation between sympathetic vasoconstrictor activity and pain and hyperalgesia in complex regional pain syndromes: a case–control study. Lancet 2002; 359(9318):1655–1660.
101. McLachlan EM, Jänig W, Devor M, et al. Peripheral nerve injury triggers noradrenergic sprouting within dorsal root ganglia. Nature 1993; 363(6429):543–546.
102. Drummond PD, Skipworth S, Finch PM. Alpha 1-adrenoceptors in normal and hyperalgesic human skin. Clin Sci (Lond) 1996; 91(1):73–77.
103. Coderre TJ, Xanthos DN, Francis L, et al. Chronic post-ischemia pain (CPIP): a novel animal model of complex regional pain syndrome-type I (CRPS-I; reflex sympathetic dystrophy) produced by prolonged hindpaw ischemia and reperfusion in the rat. Pain 2004; 112(1/2):94–105.
104. Wasner G, Baron R. Factor II: vasomotor changes—pathophysiology and measurement. CRPS: current diagnosis and therapy. In: Wilson P, Stanton-Hicks M, Norman Harden R, eds. Progress in Pain Research and Management. Vol 32. Seattle, WA: IASP Press, 2005:81–106.
105. Jänig W, Häbler HJ. Organization of the autonomic nervous system: structure and function. In: Vinken PJ, Bruyn GW, eds. The Autonomic Nervous System, Part I: Normal Functions. Handbook of Clinical Neurology. Vol 74. Amsterdam, The Netherlands: Elsevier Science, 1999:1–52.
106. Jänig W, McLachlan EM. Neurobiology of the autonomic nervous system. In: Mathias CJ, Bannister R, eds. Autonomic Failure—A Textbook of Clinical Disorders of the Autonomic Nervous System. Oxford, UK: Oxford University Press, 1999:3–15.
107. Kurvers HA, Jacobs MJ, Beuk RJ, et al. Reflex sympathetic dystrophy: evolution of microcirculatory disturbances in time. Pain 1995; 60(3):333–340.
108. Birklein F, Riedl B, Neundörfer B, et al. Sympathetic vasoconstrictor reflex pattern in patients with complex regional pain syndrome. Pain 1998; 75(1):93–100.
109. Harden RN, Duc TA, Williams TR, et al. Norepinephrine and epinephrine levels in affected versus unaffected limbs in sympathetically maintained pain. Clin J Pain 1994; 10(4):324–330.
110. Wasner G, Schattschneider J, Heckmann K, et al. Vascular abnormalities in reflex sympathetic dystrophy (CRPS I): mechanisms and diagnostic value. Brain 2001; 124(pt 3):587–599.
111. Leis S, Weber M, Isselmann A, et al. Substance-P-induced protein extravasation is bilaterally increased in complex regional pain syndrome. Exp Neurol 2003; 183(1):197–204.
112. Leis S, Weber M, Schmelz M, et al. Facilitated neurogenic inflammation in unaffected limbs of patients with complex regional pain syndrome. Neurosci Lett 2004; 359(3):163–166.
113. Gradl G, Finke B, Schattner S, et al. Continuous intra-arterial application of substance P induces signs and symptoms of experimental complex regional pain

syndrome (CRPS) such as edema, inflammation and mechanical pain but no thermal pain. Neuroscience 2007; 148(3):757–765.

114. Renier JC, Arlet J, Bregeon C, et al. The joint in algodystrophy. Joint fluid, synovium, cartilage. Rev Rhum Mal Osteoartic 1983; 50(4):255–260.

115. Oyen WJ, Arntz IE, Claessens RM, et al. Reflex sympathetic dystrophy of the hand: an excessive inflammatory response? Pain 1993; 55(2):151–157.

116. Leitha T, Korpan M, Staudenherz A, et al. Five phase bone scintigraphy supports the pathophysiological concept of a subclinical inflammatory process in reflex sympathetic dystrophy. Q J Nucl Med 1996; 40(2):188–193.

117. Graif M, Schweitzer ME, Marks B, et al. Synovial effusion in reflex sympathetic dystrophy: an additional sign for diagnosis and staging. Skeletal Radiol 1998; 27(5):262–265.

118. Duman I, Sanal HT, Dincer K, et al. Assessment of endothelial function in complex regional pain syndrome type I. Rheumatol Int 2008; 28(4):329–333.

119. Eisenberg E, Erlich T, Zinder O, et al. Plasma endothelin-1 levels in patients with complex regional pain syndrome. Eur J Pain 2004; 8(6):533–538.

120. Groeneweg JG, Huygen FJ, Heijmans-Antonissen C, et al. Increased endothelin-1 and diminished nitric oxide levels in blister fluids of patients with intermediate cold type complex regional pain syndrome type 1. BMC Musculoskelet Disord 2006; 7:91.

121. Wasner G, Heckmann K, Maier C, et al. Vascular abnormalities in acute reflex sympathetic dystrophy (CRPS I): complete inhibition of sympathetic nerve activity with recovery. Arch Neurol 1999; 56(5):613–620.

122. Fleming WW, Westfäll DP. Adaptive supersensitivity. In: Trendelenburg U, Weiner N, eds. Catecholamines I, Handbook of Experimental Pharmacology. Springer-Verlag, 1988:509–559.

123. Niehof SP, Huygen FJ, van der Weerd RW, et al. Thermography imaging during static and controlled thermoregulation in complex regional pain syndrome type 1: diagnostic value and involvement of the central sympathetic system. *Biomed Eng Online* 2006; **5:**30. doi:10.1186/1475-925X-5-30.

124. Schattschneider J, Binder A, Siebrecht D, et al. Complex regional pain syndromes: the influence of cutaneous and deep somatic sympathetic innervation on pain. Clin J Pain 2006; 22(3):240–244.

125. Xanthos DN, Bennett GJ, Coderre TJ. Norepinephrine-induced nociception and vasoconstrictor hypersensitivity in rats with chronic post-ischemia pain [published online ahead of print December 11, 2007]. Pain.

126. Xanthos DN, Coderre TJ. Sympathetic vasoconstrictor antagonism and vasodilatation relieve mechanical allodynia in rats with chronic postischemia pain. J Pain 2008.

127. Ackerman WE III, Ahmad M. Recurrent postoperative CRPS I in patients with abnormal preoperative sympathetic function. J Hand Surg Am 2008; 33(2):217–222.

128. Albrecht PJ, Hines S, Eisenberg E, et al. Pathologic alterations of cutaneous innervation and vasculature in affected limbs from patients with complex regional pain syndrome. Pain 2006; 120(3):244–266.

129. Low PA, Opfer-Gehrking TL, Kihara M. In vivo studies on receptor pharmacology of the human eccrine sweat gland. Clin Auton Res 1992; 2(1):29–34.

130. Low PA, Kennedy WR. Cutaneous effectors as indicators of abnormal sympathetic function. In: Morris JL, ed. Autonomic Innervation of the Skin. Amsterdam, The Netherlands: Harwood Academic, 1997:165–212.

131. Chelimsky TC, Low PA, Naessens JM, et al. Value of autonomic testing in reflex sympathetic dystrophy. Mayo Clin Proc 1995; 70(11):1029–1040.

132. Chémali KR, Gorodeski R, Chelimsky TC. Alpha-adrenergic supersensitivity of the sudomotor nerve in complex regional pain syndrome. Ann Neurol 2001; 49(4):453–459.

133. Howarth D, Burstal R, Hayes C, et al. Autonomic regulation of lymphatic flow in the lower extremity demonstrated on lymphoscintigraphy in patients with reflex sympathetic dystrophy. Clin Nucl Med 1999; 24(6):383–387.

134. Schürmann M, Zaspel J, Gradl G, et al. Assessment of the peripheral microcirculation using computer-assisted venous congestion plethysmography in post-traumatic complex regional pain syndrome type I. J Vasc Res 2001; 38(5):453–461.
135. Weber M, Birklein F, Neundörfer B, et al. Facilitated neurogenic inflammation in complex regional pain syndrome. Pain 2001; 91(3):251–257.
136. Galer BS, Jensen M. Neglect-like symptoms in complex regional pain syndrome: results of a self-administered survey. J Pain Symptom Manage 1999; 18(3):213–217.
137. van Hilten JJ, Blumberg H, Schwartzman RJ. Factor IV: movement disorders and dystrophy—pathophysiology and measurement. In: Wilson P, Stanton-Hicks M, Harden RN, eds. CRPS: Current Diagnosis and Therapy, Progress in Pain Research and Management. Seattle, WA: IASP Press, 2005:119–137.
138. van de Beek WJ, Vein A, Hilgevoord AA, et al. Neurophysiologic aspects of patients with generalized or multifocal tonic dystonia of reflex sympathetic dystrophy. J Clin Neurophysiol 2002; 19(1):77–83.
139. Price DD, Long S, Wilsey B, et al. Analysis of peak magnitude and duration of analgesia produced by local anesthetics injected into sympathetic ganglia of complex regional pain syndrome patients. Clin J Pain 1998; 14(3):216–226.
140. Woolf C, Wiesenfeld-Hallin Z. Substance P and calcitonin gene-related peptide synergistically modulate the gain of the nociceptive flexor withdrawal reflex in the rat. Neurosci Lett 1986; 66(2):226–230.
141. van de Beek WJ, Schwartzman RJ, van Nes SI, et al. Diagnostic criteria used in studies of reflex sympathetic dystrophy. Neurology 2002; 58(4):522–526.
142. van Hilten JJ, van de Beek WJ, Roep BO. Multifocal or generalized tonic dystonia of complex regional pain syndrome: a distinct clinical entity associated with HLA-DR13. Ann Neurol 2000; 48(1):113–116.
143. van Hilten JJ, van de Beek WJ, Vein AA, et al. Clinical aspects of multifocal or generalized tonic dystonia in reflex sympathetic dystrophy. Neurology 2001; 56(12):1762–1765.
144. Gieteling EW, van Rijn MA, de Jong BM, et al. Cerebral activation during motor imagery in complex regional pain syndrome type 1 with dystonia. Pain 2008; 134(3):302–309.
145. van Rijn MA, Marinus J, Putter H, et al. Onset and progression of dystonia in complex regional pain syndrome. Pain 2007; 130(3):287–293.
146. de Klaver MJ, van Rijn MA, Marinus J, et al. Hyperacusis in patients with complex regional pain syndrome related dystonia. J Neurol Neurosurg Psychiatry 2007; 78(12):1310–1313.
147. Schwartzman RJ, Kerrigan J. The movement disorder of reflex sympathetic dystrophy. Neurology 1990; 40(1):57–61.
148. Deuschl G, Blumberg H, Lücking CH. Tremor in reflex sympathetic dystrophy. Arch Neurol 1991; 48(12):1247–1252.
149. Navani A, Rusy LM, Jacobson RD, et al. Treatment of tremors in complex regional pain syndrome. J Pain Symptom Manage 2003; 25(4):386–390.
150. Marsden CD, Obeso JA, Traub MM, et al. Muscle spasms associated with Sudeck's atrophy after injury. Br Med J (Clin Res Ed) 1984; 288(6412):173–176.
151. van der Laan L, Veldman PH, Goris RJ. Severe complications of reflex sympathetic dystrophy: infection, ulcers, chronic edema, dystonia, and myoclonus. Arch Phys Med Rehabil 1998; 79(4):424–429.
152. Munts AG, Van Rootselaar AF, Van Der Meer JN, et al. Clinical and neurophysiological characterization of myoclonus in complex regional pain syndrome. Mov Disord 2008; 23(4):581–587.
153. Iadarola MJ, Max MB, Berman KF, et al. Unilateral decrease in thalamic activity observed with positron emission tomography in patients with chronic neuropathic pain. Pain 1995; 63(1):55–64.
154. Fukumoto M, Ushida T, Zinchuk VS, et al. Contralateral thalamic perfusion in patients with reflex sympathetic dystrophy syndrome. Lancet 1999; 354(9192):1790–1791.

155. Fukui S, Shigemori S, Nosaka S. Changes in regional cerebral blood flow in the thalamus after electroconvulsive therapy for patients with complex regional pain syndrome type 1 (preliminary case series). Reg Anesth Pain Med 2002; 27(5):529–532.

156. Apkarian AV, Thomas PS, Krauss BR, et al. Prefrontal cortical hyperactivity in patients with sympathetically mediated chronic pain. Neurosci Lett 2001; 311(3):193–197.

157. Frettlöh J, Hüppe M, Maier C. Severity and specificity of neglect-like symptoms in patients with complex regional pain syndrome (CRPS) compared to chronic limb pain of other origins. Pain 2006; 124(1/2):184–189.

158. Schattschneider J, Wenzelburger R, Deusch G, et al. Kinematic analysis of the upper extremity in CRPS. In: Harden RN, Baron R, Janig W, eds. Progress in Pain Research and Management. Vol 22. Seattle, WA: IASP Press, 2001:119–128.

159. McCabe CS, Haigh RC, Ring EF, et al. A controlled pilot study of the utility of mirror visual feedback in the treatment of complex regional pain syndrome (type 1). Rheumatology (Oxford) 2003; 42(1):97–101.

160. Pleger B, Tegenthoff M, Ragert P, et al. Sensorimotor retuning [corrected] in complex regional pain syndrome parallels pain reduction. Ann Neurol 2005; 57(3):425–429.

161. Vaneker M, Wilder-Smith OH, Schrombges P, et al. Patients initially diagnosed as 'warm' or 'cold' CRPS 1 show differences in central sensory processing some eight years after diagnosis: a quantitative sensory testing study. Pain 2005; 115(1/2):204–211.

162. Shiraishi S, Kobayashi H, Nihashi T, et al. Cerebral glucose metabolism change in patients with complex regional pain syndrome: a PET study. Radiat Med 2006; 24(5):335–344.

163. Wu CT, Fan YM, Sun CM, et al. Correlation between changes in regional cerebral blood flow and pain relief in complex regional pain syndrome type 1. Clin Nucl Med 2006; 31(6):317–320.

164. Maihöfner C, Neundörfer B, Birklein F, et al. Mislocalization of tactile stimulation in patients with complex regional pain syndrome. J Neurol 2006; 253(6):772–779.

165. Maihöfner C, Baron R, DeCol R, et al. The motor system shows adaptive changes in complex regional pain syndrome. Brain 2007; 130(pt 10):2671–2687.

166. Eisenberg E, Chistyakov AV, Yudashkin M, et al. Evidence for cortical hyperexcitability of the affected limb representation area in CRPS: a psychophysical and transcranial magnetic stimulation study. Pain 2005; 113(1/2):99–105.

167. Krause P, Förderreuther S, Straube A. TMS motor cortical brain mapping in patients with complex regional pain syndrome type I. Clin Neurophysiol 2006; 117(1):169–176.

168. Turton AJ, McCabe CS, Harris N, et al. Sensorimotor integration in complex regional pain syndrome: a transcranial magnetic stimulation study. Pain 2007; 127(3):270–275.

169. Pleger B, Ragert P, Schwenkreis P, et al. Patterns of cortical reorganization parallel impaired tactile discrimination and pain intensity in complex regional pain syndrome. Neuroimage 2006; 32(2):503–510.

170. Stengel M, Binder A, Baron R. Update on the diagnosis and management of complex regional pain syndromes. Adv Pain Manag 2007; 1(3):96–104.

171. Correll GE, Maleki J, Gracely EJ, et al. Subanesthetic ketamine infusion therapy: a retrospective analysis of a novel therapeutic approach to complex regional pain syndrome. Pain Med 2004; 5(3):263–275.

172. Schwartzman RJ, Chevlen E, Bengtson K. Thalidomide has activity in treating complex regional pain syndrome. Arch Intern Med 2003; 163(12):1487–1488.

173. Irving G, Schwartzman R, Dogra S, et al. A multicenter, open-label study to evaluate the safety and efficacy of lenalidomide (CC-5013) in the treatment of type-1 complex regional pain syndrome (CRPS). In: Conference on the Mechanisms and Treatment of Neuropathic Pain. 7th International Conference; November 4–6, 2004; Bermuda.

7 Meralgia Paresthetica

Elizabeth A. Sekul

Medical College of Georgia, Augusta, Georgia, U.S.A.

THE DISORDER

Meralgia paresthetica is a painful mononeuropathy of the lateral femoral cutaneous nerve (LFCN). The diagnosis is readily made clinically; however, nerve conductions may aid in verification. The incidence in the general population is 4.3 per 10,000 person-years (1). Etiology can be spontaneous or iatrogenic. Meralgia paresthetica has been reported in all ages but most commonly occurs in middle age. It typically occurs in isolation; however, in 20% of cases, symptoms can be bilateral (2). Although not life threatening, it can be a source of severe discomfort and disability.

Anatomy

The LFCN is a pure sensory nerve with no motor component. Regional variation in the anatomy is common, occurring in up to 30% of cases (3). The most common course of the nerve is as follows: The LFCN arises from the lumbar plexus at the L2-3 level. It transverses through the psoas muscle and exits laterally. It then travels across the anterior iliacus muscle underneath the fascia. Transversing retroperitoneally, it approaches the anterior superior iliac spine. It then crosses or pierces the ilioinguinal ligament to enter into the thigh. The most common site of crossing of the ilioinguinal ligament is 1 cm medial to the anterior superior iliac spine (4); however, it has been noted as far as 6.5 cm medially (5). In 4% of patients, the nerve is on top of the iliac crest (6). Branching of the nerve into an anterior and posterior division typically occurs after the ilioinguinal ligament but may occur at or before the ligament. These divisions then penetrate the fascia lata to supply sensation to the skin over the anterior and lateral thigh, respectively. The cutaneous area of innervation by this nerve is only the anterior–lateral thigh. Its distribution does not extend below the knee (Fig. 1).

DIAGNOSIS

Symptoms of meralgia paresthetica include constant or intermittent numbness, burning, or tingling in the lateral thigh. Symptoms may be exacerbated by prolonged walking or standing. As LFCN is a pure sensory nerve, there is no associated weakness. Back pain is also not a part of the syndrome. If either is present, further evaluation of the L2-3 nerve roots and/or lumbar plexus should be done. When examining a patient with suspected LFCN injury, particular attention should be paid to the strength of the muscles innervated by the L2-3 roots, such as the iliopsoas and hip adductors. Weakness in these muscles points to a radicular or plexus etiology for the numbness and pain. On sensory exam, decreased sensation to pinprick and touch should be present over the anterior and/or lateral thigh area, depending upon whether divisions are involved. The area of altered

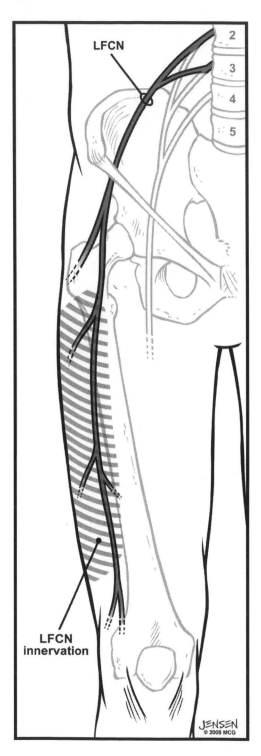

FIGURE 1 Area of innervation of the lateral femoral cutaneous nerve.

sensitivity does not extend below the knee (Fig. 1). Cutaneous hypersensitivity over the area of the LFCN may be present. A Tinel sign, reproduction of the symptoms by tapping on the nerve, may be elicited by tapping on the anterior superior iliac spine or just medial to it. Stretching the nerve by extending the leg backwards may also reproduce symptoms. A newer clinical test of pelvic compression may be useful, but it has not been fully validated as of yet. This test is done by having the patient lay on his side with the affected side up. Then, downward pressure is applied to the anterior iliac spine for 45 seconds. Theoretically, this relieves pressure on the ilioinguinal ligament and, thus, relieves the symptoms (7).

Electrophysiological studies can aid in the diagnosis. Significant differences in side-to-side recordings of conventional LFCN studies are the most reliable parameters for verification of the clinical diagnosis (8). In an obese person, it may be difficult to localize or properly simulate the nerve; therefore, side-to-side comparisons are mandatory to rule out technical difficulties. Some authors advocate the use of somatosensory evoked potentials as a more sensitive measure for diagnosis, particularly in obese individuals. However, studies on this are conflicting.

PATHOPHYSIOLOGY

The most common site of injury to the LFCN is where it crosses the ilioinguinal ligament. There it is subject to compression or injury during surgery or trauma. Injury to the nerve more proximal can also occur. Proximal to this point, pelvic tumors, abscesses, endometriosis, and pelvic inflammatory disease can compromise the nerve. In the psoas muscle, the nerve is particularly vulnerable to compression due to retroperitoneal hemorrhage in patients on anticoagulants. The nerve may also be involved in lumbar plexitis, but other nerve distributions should also be affected. Ischemic nerve injury, such as can occur with diabetes, can also affect this nerve in isolation and the site of injury may occur anywhere along its course.

Compression of the LFCN at the ilioinguinal ligament is more common in overweight individuals or in those who wear tight clothing or large tool belts. Pregnancy or a rapidly expanding lower abdomen due to ascites can also cause compression. Seat belt injury in a motor vehicle accident can trigger this disorder. Injury to the LFCN can occur during surgery via compression if the person is positioned prone or due to direct trauma when operating in the area of the nerve. Patients undergoing hip and lumbar surgeries as well as bone marrow harvesting from the anterior iliac spine are particularly at risk for LFCN injury. Of the patients undergoing total hip replacement and posterior spine surgery, up to 25% will have injury to the LFCN (9, 10). If it was due to positioning during surgery then, typically, symptoms resolve spontaneously within two months (10). Lithotomy position during surgery and delivery has also been implicated in LFCN injuries.

TREATMENT

Conservative treatment is warranted in the majority of patients. Nonsteroidal medications, weight loss when indicated, and avoidance of tight compressive clothing or belts are the first line of treatment. Physical therapy may be helpful. Blockade of the LFCN with regional anesthetic provides complete and immediate relief and is diagnostic, but symptoms will most likely return once the block is worn off. If there is no improvement in symptoms when local anesthetic is injected, then evaluation for a more proximal site of injury should be done. Injecting with a combination of a local anesthetic agent and a corticosteroid can result in a more prolonged or even permanent relief in some patients. Repeat injections at four- to six-week intervals may be necessary. If long-term relief is not achieved after three injections and there was a positive response to blockade, then surgery should be considered (11). The most common site for injection is at the level of the ilioinguinal ligament 1 cm medial to the anterior iliac spine. Because of variation in the nerve, ultrasound guidance may provide a more precise localization for injection and allow for avoidance of direct nerve injection (12). Stimulation and injection via a needle electrode may also aid in localization. Medications for treatment of chronic neuropathic pain such as tricylic antidepressants, gabapentin, or topiramate can also be effective. Topical capsaicin or a lidocaine patch applied to the affected area may be helpful to decrease the surface sensitivity. If the lidocaine patch is used, then contact should be limited to less than 12 hr/day.

If intractable pain continues despite conservative measures, surgical intervention with neurolysis with or without transposition of the LFCN or transection of the nerve may be indicated (13). Transection results in permanent loss of sensation over the anterior–lateral thigh. The exact procedure that best addresses persistent meralgia paresthetica surgically is still controversial.

REFERENCES

1. Van Slobbe AM, Bohnen AM, Bernsen RM, et al. Incidence rates and determinants in meralgia paresthetica in general practice. J Neurol 2004; 251(3):294–297.
2. Eker AD, Woltman HW. Meralgia paresthetica: a report of one hundred and fifty cases. JAMA 1938; 110:1650–1652.
3. Keegan JJ, Holyoke EA. Meralgia paresthetica. An anatomical and surgical study. J Neurosurg 1962; 19:341–345.
4. Williams PH, Trzil KP. Management of meralgia paresthetica. J Neurosurg 1991; 74:76–80.
5. Bjurlin MA, Davis KE, Allin EF, et al. Anatomic variations in the lateral femoral cutaneous nerve with respect to pediatric hip surgery. Am J Orthop 2007; 36(3):143–146.
6. Azmann OC, Dellon ES, Dellon AL. Anatomical course of the lateral femoral cutaneous nerve and its susceptibility to compression and injury. Plast Reconstr Surg 1997; 100:600–604.
7. Nouraei SA, Anand B, Spink G, et al. A novel approach to the diagnosis and management of meralgia paresthetica. Neurosurgery 2007; 60(4):696–700.
8. Seror P. Lateral femoral cutaneous nerve conduction v somatosensory evoked potentials for electrodiagnosis of meralgia paresthetica. Am J Phys Med Rehabil 1999; 78(4):313–316.
9. Bal BS, Haltom D, Aleto T, et al. Early complications of primary total hip replacement performed with a two-incision minimally invasive technique. Surgical technique. J Bone Joint Surg Am 2006; 88(suppl 1)(pt 2):221–233.
10. Yang SH, Wu CC, Chen PQ. Postoperative meralgia paresthetica after posterior spine surgery: incidence, risk factors, and clinical outcomes. Spine 2005; 30(18):E547–E550.
11. Haim A, Pritsch T, Ben-Galim P, et al. Meralgia paresthetica: a retrospective analysis of 79 patients evaluated and treated according to a standard algorithm. Acta Orthop 2006; 77(3):482–486.
12. Hurdle MF, Weingarten TN, Crisostomo RA, et al. Ultrasound-guided blockade of the lateral femoral cutaneous nerve: technical description and review of 10 cases. Arch Phys Med Rehabil 2007; 88(10):1362–1364.
13. Grossman MG, Ducey SA, Nadler SS, et al. Meralgia paresthetica: diagnosis and treatment. J Am Acad Orthop Surg 2001; 9(5):336–344.

8 Compression Neuropathies

Gabriel E. Sella

Department of Community Medicine, Faculty of Medicine, West Virginia University, Morgantown, West Virginia, U.S.A.

THE DISORDER

Compression neuropathies are a diverse group of neural conditions. They share a commonality: a reduction of the perineural space necessary for normal function.

The tissue pressure generally increases on the affected nerve. Vascularity is variably compromised resulting in neural ischemia. If the situation does not resolve in a very timely fashion, that is, if the anatomic structures are not released, the compression and its effects may become chronic with a guarded prognosis for full recovery. Common compression neuropathies result from crush or stretch injuries, ischemia (focal), or lacerations. Clinically, they may be evidenced by loss of strength (LOS), pain, and variable paresthesia (1).

Common symptoms reflect the presence of various types of axonal damage. Thus, ischemic neuropathies tend to show more pain. Small-fiber neuropathies tend to show pain qualities such as "burning" or "lancinating." They may also present with paresthesia, hyperesthesia, dysesthesia, and allodynia. When the neuropathy is symmetrical and distal axonal (i.e., dying back), the neuropathies progress (e.g., from the toes) upward and reflect a "stocking–glove" distribution. Mononeuritis multiplex, for example, in diabetes, shows a specific sensory pathology in the specific root or nerve affected by the condition. Motor symptoms include LOS of various degrees and locations, commonly related to "dying back" nerve involvement. In addition to the weakness, one may present with cramps, fasciculations, and restless leg syndrome. As the disease progresses proximally, one may present with dysarthria and dysphagia (2).

In terms of pattern of involvement, nerve entrapments may occur at common sites of compression or may be secondary to systemic diseases such as diabetes mellitus, myxedema, rheumatoid arthritis, amyloidosis, acromegaly, sarcoidosis, leprosy, AIDS, alcoholism, etc. (3).

Epidemiology

A large British study on the incidence of new compressive neuropathies found in primary care clinics in the year 2000 revealed that the standardized rate per 100,000 was about 491 cases. The study excluded the people presenting with compatible symptoms at specialized clinics. Of interest were the statistics of gender difference. Thus, the overall age-adjusted male to female ratio was 56%. Different compressive neuropathies presented with a variety of gender ratios. The male-to-female patient ratios were 45% for the carpal tunnel syndrome (CTS), 57% for Morton neuroma, 130% for ulnar neuropathy, 80% for meralgia paresthetica, and 209% for radial neuropathy.

In terms of the age range at the first presentation, most neuropathies appeared at 55 to 64 years of age. There were two notable exceptions: CTS was an "early" presentation, at 45 to 54 years of age, and radial nerve palsy appeared "late," at 75 to 84 years of age (4).

The CTS is the most common compressive neuropathy. It may be present in 3% to 9% of people and has a female predilection, with a gender ratio of 3:1 (5, 6).

Entrapment neuropathies account for up to 10% to 20% of neurosurgical practices.

Perioperative neuropathies are found mainly in relation to positioning of the surgical patients during prolonged anesthesia. The most common compressive neuropathies are peripheral. They may affect the median nerve, the ulnar nerve, or the brachial plexus. They may also affect the lumbosacral plexus, the sciatic, the femoral, and the common peroneal nerve. A number of factors contribute to the etiology of these conditions, including the (obese) body habitus, prolonged surgeries, and prolonged bed rest in the immediate postsurgical period (7, 8).

Etiology

Hereditary

HNPP (hereditary neuropathy with liability to pressure palsies) is a condition in which the peripheral nerves show an abnormal sensitivity to external pressure. It is an autosomal dominant genetic trait. Structurally, the condition is evidenced by very thick myelin sheath around the peripheral nerves.

Normal anatomy shows a certain predilection to nerve passage through restricted areas, and a number of natural motions require stretching of the nerves. Normal individuals may get symptoms related to pressure or stretch, such as tingling or numbness or even temporary LOS. Such symptoms are usually self-limiting and may last only a number of seconds or minutes after the nerve relief. Commonly, the affected nerves are the radial, ulnar, and median nerves in the upper limb and the peroneal nerve in the lower limb.

Individuals affected by HNPP may suffer from such symptoms for a number of weeks or months. The symptoms may not be self-limiting and may become permanent.

The management of HNPP may occasionally be surgical. More commonly, it involves occupational therapy and special care for improvement of the ergonomic conditions affecting those individuals (9).

Traumatic

Sports injuries

Flexion activities of the hip may induce urogenital pain and chronic pelvic pain. This occurs more commonly in men who participated in heavy sports such as wrestling, weight lifting, football, and heavy bicycling as teenagers. In many cases, reactive hypertrophy of the pyriformis muscle may cause pudendal and sciatic nerve compression and neuropathy (10, 11).

Thoracic outlet syndrome

Thoracic outlet syndrome (TOS) is related to lower trunk brachial plexus compression neuropathy and may be due to cervical rib in athletes (12). See later in the chapter for a more complete description of TOS.

Nerve entrapment of the lower calf, ankle, and foot in athletes

Muscle compartment syndromes, popliteal artery entrapment, and nerve entrapment syndromes are common clinical considerations in differential diagnosis of lower limb pain, paresthesia, dysesthesia, and weakness. While the etiologies may vary, they have the participation of the individual in consistent athletic activities in common (13).

Bicycle-related injuries

They are common especially in young men. Aside from injuries related to falls, fractures, hematomas, etc., the compressive neuropathies are mainly related to overuse and poor ergonomics. They include the handlebar neuropathies, mainly median and ulnar injuries; saddle-related pudendal nerve compression neuropathy; and hip, knee, and ankle/foot injuries, including symptoms of paresthesia, tendonitis, and metatarsalgia. Treatment is usually symptomatic and relates to physical therapy and improved ergonomics of bicycle use (14).

Tennis-related injuries

This is a sport that requires asymmetrical motions and effort of the upper extremities. Tennis players have been found to have greater strength and range of motion (ROM) of the dominant (used in tennis playing) upper limb compared to the nondominant limb. Nerve conduction studies (NCS) (motor and sensory) of the radial nerve and the ulnar sensory conduction were found to be delayed in the dominant arm of the 21 tennis players studied. The authors concluded that the significant differences may indicate a preclinical state of radial and ulnar nerve compressive neuropathy (15).

Metabolic

Paget's disease is a disease of old age with the predominant feature of bone remodeling resulting in softened bone and structural deformity. The hypertrophic bone may compress adjacent structures such as nerves (e.g., in reduced space foramina) and cause compressive neuropathy.

Infectious disease

Infectious processes may affect the anterior horn cells, resulting in progressive weakness. Such examples include the post-polio syndrome, the Guillain–Barré syndrome, and Lyme disease.

DIAGNOSIS

Clinical Aspects

History

The past medical history needs to include several lines of inquiry: (a) the presence of systemic disease, for example, diabetes or hypothyroidism; (b) medications taken prior to the appearance of symptoms; (c) alcohol use; (d) toxic exposure, such as heavy metals or solvents; (e) infection exposure, for example, HIV, Lyme (tics), leprosy; (f) nutrition habits and possible vitamin deficiency; (g) locomotor difficulties such as gait disturbance, suggestive of hereditary disorders (16).

Physical Examination
A complete physical examination is useful in order to exclude other systemic conditions that may contribute to the compressive neuropathy. Findings such as orthostatic hypotension without compensatory tachycardia may be a sign of autonomic nerve involvement. Respiratory rhythm and volume is needed to rule out respiratory compromise. Systemic disease may show as hepatomegaly, splenomegaly, or lymphadenopathy. Toxic factors such as arsenic poisoning should be considered in the presence of Mees' nail lines and fatigue. A systematic approach is recommended in order to rule out proximal versus distal nerve involvement.

Cervical and Spinal Roots
Testing for vibration sense loss is very important. The sense of vibration may be reduced in cervical root compression, in CTS, and in ulnar neuropathies. In the early presentations, the vibration sense may be normal at 125 and 250 Hz, while it may be reduced at 500 Hz. This pathology usually antedates that of abnormal findings in sensory conduction velocity.

Neuroanatomic Aspects

Cranial Nerves
Testing should include the following: (a) cranial nerve involvement: funduscopic study to rule out vitamin B deficiency and optic pallor; (b) bilateral testing to evaluate the cranial nerves V, VII, IX/X, XI, and XII for LOS, fasciculations, hypotrophy, hypertonus, or atrophy; and (c) sensory testing to light touch, temperature, and sharpness (pinprick) to rule out symmetrical or asymmetrical compressive neuropathies (17).

Compression of the optic nerves by tumors, especially in the region of the optic chiasm and the sphenoid wing, for example, meningioma can cause loss of visual acuity. Surgical decompression may enable recovery of function (18).

Cervical Roots

Long thoracic nerve entrapment
This nerve forms from the cervical roots V–VI–VII. It courses under the large subscapularis muscle and innervates the serratus anterior. Acute injury may be caused by acute compression, such as a direct blow to the area or carrying heavy backpacks, for example, soldiers, campers, etc. Injury may be insidious such as in persons carrying large and heavy purses across the shoulder daily. Injury to the serratus anterior muscle may cause winging of the scapula. The presence of winging may be used as a clinical test for this syndrome. Management consists of reducing the shoulder loads, rest, light shoulder exercise, and, as a last resort, decompressive surgery (19).

Suprascapular nerve entrapment
The suprascapular nerve may be entrapped under the suprascapular ligament, in the presence of a tight, bony notch. The entrapment is followed by a dull pain of uncertain onset. The pain is located in the periscapular region of the shoulder. Motor symptoms include supraspinatus and infraspinatus weakness and eventual hypotrophy. The syndrome mainly affects athletes involved in

repetitive, upper limb sports such as weight lifting, basketball, or volleyball. The clinical diagnosis is aided by the observation of hypotrophy of the supraspinatus and infraspinatus muscles and limited scapulothoracic motion. Electromyography (EMG) studies may show slowing of nerve conduction velocity and signs of denervation. MRI of the shoulder may be useful. Medical management including progressive resistive exercise may be useful. Injections with anesthetics/steroids may relieve any pain symptoms. Surgery should only be contemplated in cases of severe early muscular atrophy (20, 21).

Brachial plexus compressive neuropathies
The brachial plexus may be affected by trauma in any region distal to the root exits from the cervical canal. Its variable course in relation to the scalene muscles exposes it to various compression injuries to those muscles spanning the neck and shoulder. While it is possible to note trauma to the whole plexus, such as in iatrogenic arm traction injuries during neck surgery, most brachial plexopathies show a more regional involvement. Symptoms may be motor, sensory, or mixed. An upper trunk (lateral cord) injury usually involves the shoulder and arm C5 and C6 innervated muscles. Those muscles tend to be weak, and motion of the shoulder and arm may be limited. Sensation will be affected in the lateral forearm area.

A lower trunk (medial cord) injury will affect the C8–T1 innervated muscles. Sensation will be reduced in the medial forearm. Posterior cord injuries may affect the muscles innervated by the axillary and radial nerves. Brachial plexopathy may result from a variety of injuries. These may encompass compressive tumors, for example, Pancoast tumor, compressive lymphadenopathy, radiation therapy–induced scarring, direct surgical trauma, and various motor vehicle accidents.

Treatment of the brachial plexopathies varies with the etiology of each condition. Protection of the nerves and muscles from further damage is paramount. Passive and active exercises need to be judiciously prescribed to guide the muscles toward more normal action and avoid shortening and contracture. Nerve avulsion injuries may take several months or years to repair, and the repair may be incomplete. Surgery with nerve transposition may be contemplated in a few centers specialized in the technique (22, 23).

Thoracic Outlet Syndrome
This condition is usually of vascular etiology. Infrequently, it may be neurogenic. The vascular component expresses itself symptomatically with pulsation loss at the wrist when the arm is abducted as well as nonspecific pain. The neurogenic component involves the lower brachial plexus trunk, primarily, affecting mainly the T1 (sometimes C8) component. There may be sensory loss in the medial forearm and hand. LOS in the abductor pollicis brevis (APB) of the fifth digit is paradigmatic. The usual cause is compression under a fibrous band connecting the transverse process to a cervical rib. EMG studies of the ulnar and medial nerves may show abnormalities consistent with the symptoms. MRI may be useful to identify the vascular or neurogenic compression. Surgery may be necessary for decompression (24).

Median Nerve Entrapment Syndromes

Carpal tunnel syndrome

This is probably the most common example of upper limb compressive neuropathy. It may be present in 3% to 9% of people and has a female predilection. The compression is frequently the result of repetitive motion or excessive use or of physical compression, for example, from ganglion cysts. In this condition, the median nerve is variably compressed in one or more segments of the canal between the metacarpal bones and the overlying flexor retinaculum. The affected individual complains of numbness in the thumb, the forefinger, and the middle finger. Nocturnal pain may ensue in time and may be strong enough to wake up the sufferer. LOS eventually occurs, and the symptoms include easy dropping of objects from the hand (25).

There are two other known syndromes of entrapment of the median nerve that result from proximal nerve compression: (a) the pronator syndrome and (b) the anterior interosseous nerve (AIN) syndrome. The syndromes are generally caused by crushing injuries, lesions compressive lesion, vasculopathies, including A-V fistulas from hemodialysis sites (26).

The pronator syndrome

This is related to entrapment of the median nerve in one of four locations around the pronator muscle. The clinical presentation usually shows an insidious onset that may last up to two years. The main complaint is that of pain in the proximal palmar aspect of the distal arm and in the forearm. Repeated pronation/supination movements tend to enhance the pain. Paresthesia may occur in the radial three and a half digits, same pattern as in CTS. However, the pronator syndrome pain is usually not nocturnal. LOS may be present, but muscular atrophy has not been noted. Provocative clinical tests may be useful, such as resisted pronation. A positive response may reproduce pain, paresthesia, and LOS. Needle EMG may be useful to rule out denervation potentials. Management may be medical or surgical. The medical management is preventive in terms of avoidance of aggravating activities, splints to limit motion and pain, and eventually injections with anesthetics/steroids. Surgical treatment may be attempted if there is poor response to the medical management. It involves finding the area of median compression and decompressing the nerve tissue (27).

The anterior interosseous nerve syndrome

This is an infrequent neuropathy; however, it is relevant to consider it in the differential diagnosis of the painful hand. The neuropathy may be caused, generally, by compression of the AIN from extrinsic causes, for example, trauma or from inflammation. It is a purely motor syndrome, and it presents with variable LOS of the pronator quadratus, flexor pollicis longus, or flexor digitorum profundus. Forearm pain and/or wrist pain may be present. Pain generally precedes the LOS. Pain may exacerbate with activity, especially with repetitive motion. The patient may complain, especially, with difficulty in writing or in picking up small objects. Diagnostic workup aims at the differential diagnosis from other median nerve syndromes. EMG studies are generally useful to localize the muscles affected by this syndrome. Management is aimed at reducing pain and improving muscle strength, first. Avoidance of aggravating factors, splinting, and injections with anesthetics/corticosteroids may be tried for three to four months. Surgical exploration and decompression are other methods of choice (28, 29).

Ulnar Nerve Entrapment Syndromes

Nerve compression may occur (a) at the elbow level or (b) in the canal of Guyon. Sensory dysfunction such as tingling or paresthesia occurs in the fourth and fifth digits of the affected hand. Since the ulnar nerve innervates the small muscles of the hand, weakness may involve the whole hand.

Ulnar neuropathy at the elbow is second only to CTS in the incidence of compressive neuropathies of the upper extremity. There are two common locations of compression: (a) the epicondylar groove and (b) entrapment of the ulnar nerve at the entrance in the cubital tunnel.

The most common complaints are elbow region pain or discomfort, and weakness of grip, wrist, and finger flexion. The Tinel sign, that is, pain elicited by ulnar nerve tapping at the elbow, is usually positive. EMG testing may show slowing of conduction velocity. High-resolution ultrasound may be useful to determine ulnar nerve thickening at the elbow (30, 31). Medical management of the elbow ulnar compressive neuropathy consists of soft splinting for the elbow area. Surgical management is reserved for the chronic cases. It consists of decompression of the ulnar nerve in the location of compression (32).

Ulnar nerve entrapment at the wrist usually occurs in the canal of Guyon; however, it may occur also in the hand, distal to the canal. The symptoms refer to paresthesia of the ulnar two and a half digits and to LOS in the interossei muscles. The finger flexors are normally not affected. Management of the ulnar compressive neuropathy at the wrist consists of splinting, avoidance of repetitive motions of wrist and fingers, and in chronic cases, decompressive surgery of the canal, or compressed distal area of the hand (33).

Radial Nerve Entrapment Syndromes

The radial nerve may be entrapped in several locations. The most common are (a) the axilla and (b) posterior interosseous nerve syndrome.

Axillary radial nerve palsy

This is usually a compressive neuropathy related to prolonged arm positioning over a chair, etc. It is expressed mainly as motor loss of the triceps, ECR, and other radially innervated muscles. The elbow extension, the wrist extension, and the fifth digit extension may be limited. The only sensory deficit occurs in the first dorsal web space.

If the condition is not self-limited, surgical exploration and decompression in the axilla or other locations may be necessary (34).

Posterior interosseous nerve syndrome

This motor syndrome is variably the result of tendinous hypertrophy of the arcade of Frohse and the thickening of the radiocapitellar joint capsule. Vascular compression of the artery of Henry (from the recurrent radial artery) has been described. Repetitive supination motion injury from work activities or from crutches pressing on the supinator muscle may contribute to the condition. The symptoms include a progression of paresis of the extensors of the MCP joints, resulting variably in LOS of the finger extensors and of the thumb abductors. Pain may radiate to the neck and shoulder. Clinical testing for this syndrome may proceed as follows: (a) palpation over the PIN under the supinator muscle may elicit pain; (b) the Tinnel sign, tapping over the radial head immediately distal to the lateral epicondyle, may produce tingling along the radial nerve; (c) passive stretching of the third digit may reproduce pain. EMG studies did not show consistent results. Management of the condition is mainly protective and preventive. Rest and gentle exercise may speed recovery. Anesthetic/steroid injections may offer symptomatic relief. Surgery has been successful in fewer than 50% of cases (35–39).

Lumbosacral Plexus Compressive Neuropathies

Sciatic neuropathy

Sciatic neuropathy or sciatica is a symptom most usually referred to herniation of one to four discs. Depending on the disc that is herniated, the pain of the "sciatica" may be localized to the back or referred to the buttock or the leg. In addition to LS disc herniation, there may be other reasons for the entrapment of the roots that form the sciatic nerve. Stenosis, spondylolisthesis, trauma, spinal tumors, or other injuries may contribute to the condition. The piriformis syndrome is a singular etiology of sciatic pain since the sciatic nerve courses variably through the pirifomis muscle and/or under it. If and when this muscle becomes tight (or in spasm), such as in myofascitis, it may compress and entrap various components of the sciatic nerve.

Prolonged sitting and crossing the legs frequently may contribute to sciatic entrapment in relation to the piriformis muscle.

In terms of management, the sufferer is well advised to change positions often and avoid prolonged sitting and crossing the legs. Sciatica may disappear within six weeks of preventive regimen. If the symptoms of muscle weakness, paresthesia, and tingling do not disappear within six weeks, MRI and EMG studies may contribute to the diagnostic process. The worst case scenario is the sudden or insidious appearance of bladder or bowel control loss, that is, signs of cauda equina. Surgery may be necessary to relieve the sciatic roots entrapment (40).

Cauda equina

Cauda equina syndrome is related to compression or entrapment of the nerve roots in the area of the filum terminale, the bundle of nerve roots distal to the conus medullaris. Compression or inflammation of those terminal nerve roots may cause loss of bladder or bowel control in addition to hyporeflexia pain and occasional LOS in the pelvic area. These are severe symptoms that require appropriate attention in terms of MRI studies and immediate surgery. Lack of immediate attention may cause lower limb paralysis and chronic loss of bowel and bladder control (40).

Lateral femoral cutaneous nerve (meralgia paresthetica)

There is a strong predisposition for this condition during advanced pregnancy and in morbid obesity, where the lateral femoral cutaneous nerve may be compressed in the inguinal ligament before its exit into the sartorius fascia and muscle. The symptoms are exclusively sensory since this is a sensory nerve. They may comprise variably hypoesthesia, paresthesia, hyperesthesia, or dysesthesia in the anterior–lateral aspect of the thigh, sometimes down to the knee region. The symptoms may increase during prolonged standing, walking down steps, and prolonged bed rest. Relief in bed may be obtained by placing a pillow between the thighs (41).

Peroneal neuropathy
The peroneal nerve is more commonly compressed at the level of the fibular head, where it is quite superficially located. Common history includes prolonged squatting or sitting with the legs crossed as well as a history of prolonged bed rest or casting of the calf for fractures, etc. Foot drop is the most common symptom, followed by loss of extension control of the toes. Management may include preventive measures, splints, and gradual physical therapy exercises.

When medical management fails, surgical exploration and removal of the compression may be necessary (40,42).

Tarsal tunnel syndrome
Tarsal tunnel syndrome is usually the result of tibial nerve compression at the ankle. Common causes include trauma, tenosynovitis, and ganglion cysts. Sensory symptoms usually include paresthesia or pain in the sole and/or toes. Motor symptoms include LOS of the intrinsic muscles of the foot. Eventually, one can find lateral clawing of the toes and severe atrophy of the intrinsic flexors of the great toe (42).

Sural nerve entrapment
This nerve entrapment is frequently caused by local ankle trauma, surgical injury, and Achilles tendonitis. The symptoms are usually located at the site of the compression and the lateral course of the nerve in its path to the fifth toe. Treatment is usually conservative and aims at protection of the nerve. If the response is poor, surgery may need to be performed. The usual surgery involves sectioning and excision of the nerve (43).

Dorsal forefoot nerve entrapment
Compression of this nerve can occur as a result of traction injuries, for example, ankle sprains, entrapment at the exit from the fibular neck, or compression from ganglion cysts or midfoot exostoses. It may also be secondary to surgery of the dorsal foot, resulting in painful neuroma. Pain is the major symptom of this nerve entrapment. The therapy may be preventive in terms of wearing appropriate shoes; via injections with anesthetics and steroids; or surgical, such as neurolysis (44).

Deep peroneal nerve entrapment (anterior tibial nerve)
This entrapment has also been described as "the anterior tarsal tunnel syndrome." It may be caused by shoe pressure, compression at the inferior extensor retinaculum, traction, edema, exostoses, or trauma. The main symptoms comprise paresthesia or dysesthesia of the web space between the first and second toe. EMG studies may reveal signs of denervation of the extensor digitorum

brevis muscle. The treatment may be conservative and preventive, such as wearing appropriate shoes to relieve the pressure. It may also consist of anesthetic/steroid injections. If those measures fail, surgical release from the compressive pressure may be necessary (45).

Morton's neuroma

This syndrome is a mechanical entrapment neuropathy. The neuroma occurs most commonly in the intermetatarsal area between the third and fourth toe representing a benign enlargement of the third common branch of the medial plantar nerve. Of interest, inflammation is not a necessary component. Compressive forces and stretch forces on the forefoot, such as in wearing high-heeled shoes may offer a partial explanation for the symptom of pain. There is a female gender prevalence for the condition. The most usual description of the pain is that of "walking on a hot pebble."

Just as the pain may be aggravated by walking in high-heeled shoes, squatting, or working a pedal, it may be relieved by rest. However, any pressure on the sole metatarsal area may enhance the pain.

The clinical diagnosis may be enhanced with EMG studies and with MRI or high-resolution ultrasound studies.

The medical management consists of reducing the pressure and preventing further irritation. Different types of footpads and low-heeled shoes may be useful in reducing the pressure and pain.

Pelvic pain syndrome

The pelvic pain syndrome involves ischial spine and pudendal nerve entrapment. This is a condition found more prevalently in people with a history of major athletic activities before ossification of the spinous process of the ischial bone. The pain occurs in the perineal structures of both genders when the perineum is in positional compression such as in the sitting position. It may be relieved by standing or the supine or prone positions.

Chronic constipation may stretch the pudendal nerve and cause compression (46). Vaginal delivery has been associated with pudendal neuropathy, which may last up to three months (47).

Injections of anesthetics/steroids may be the first step before surgery. When necessary, surgical resection of the neuroma may be an option (48, 49).

Post-polio syndrome

This condition is included with the lumbosacral neuropathies since polio affects the lower limb more than the upper limb. It may also occur in the upper limb, if it was affected by the poliovirus.

This is a condition of distal axonal degeneration and enlarged motor units. The presentation is usually 15 years or longer after the condition of poliomyelitis. The symptoms include increased muscle fatigue, LOS, variable muscle atrophy, and muscle and joint pain. EMG testing shows signs of reinnervation and denervation. Muscular biopsy may show type grouping of reinnervated muscles and compensatory hypertrophy of muscle fibers. Management is nonsurgical and aims at reducing overuse and improving muscular ergonomics (50).

Radiculopathy

Cervical or lumbosacral radiculopathies may result from neural compression at the spinal levels. Arthropathies, disc bulges and herniations, tumors or traumatic cord avulsions are the most common causes. The symptoms usually include pain radiating from the focal spinal region and paresthesia/dysesthesia in a dermatomal pattern. Since the radiculopathies affect the muscles through the different nerves, the subject is discussed in a more focused manner under the topic of the different brachial and lumbosacral nerves, respectively.

Polyneuropathy

Most compressive polyneuropathies are acquired peripheral disorders. They may be secondary to alcoholism, nutritional deficiencies, poisoning, diabetes, renal disease, or compressive tumors. Symptoms may be of sensory, motor, or mixed types. Typical sensory symptoms are "glove or stocking" paresthesias. Motor symptoms include distal LOS. Hyporeflexia is also common.

Electrodiagnosis

NCS and needle EMG are classically utilized in the diagnostic process, including differential diagnosis of compressive neuropathies. They are essential in diagnosing neuropraxia (conduction block) from axonal degeneration.

Motor unit conduction may be measured routinely with NCS. Normal myelinated axonal conduction varies between 40 and 70 m/sec. Sensory unmyelinated axon conduction varies between 0.5 and 2.0 m/sec. It may be measured with neurometry.

A description of the methodology of electromyography is beyond the scope of this text. It is relevant to point out that EMG can be used in serial fashion to evaluate the presence and degree of axonal damage followed in time by the presence of muscular reinnervation.

The testing may be useful within one week of the clinical injury to establish a comparison baseline, within the following three weeks to document axonal functional loss, and after 3 to 12 months to document regeneration. It can also be used intraoperatively to help determine the appropriateness of nerve grafting (51, 52).

The nerve conduction latency is relevant in the evaluation of plexopathies, radiculopathies, polyneuropathies, and mononeuropathies. Latency of response may be indicative of the presence of such neuropathies. The H-reflex, usually performed bilaterally (for symmetry of response) on the gastrocnemius muscle, is used to rule out the early presence of spinal stenosis or bilateral S1 radiculopathies.

Autonomic Studies

Cardiovascular testing: Heart rate variability, blood pressure testing in the standing and tilted positions as well as the response to sustained handgrip may help to rule out the presence of autonomic involvement and small-fiber dysfunction.

Laboratory Studies

The studies may include CSF (cerebrospinal fluid) studies to rule out polyradiculopathies and myelinopathies. Cytological studies may be necessary to rule out lymphoma, Lyme disease, or mononeuritis multiplex.

Nerve Biopsy
Biopsies, more commonly performed on the sural nerve, may serve to rule out leprosy, amyloidosis, vasculitis, sarcoidosis, and other systemic disease (53).

Thermology
Thermography has been useful in identifying asymmetric temperature findings in body regions affected by compressive neuropathy, especially in CTS (54, 55).

Radiologic Studies
MRI is a technique that may use short inversion imaging recovery to display high signal intensity in the affected compressed nerve site. This may be due to the presence of edema in the myelin sheath and the perineurium. Future enhancements of the technique may be necessary to identify reliably compressive neuropathy in smaller nerves.

X-rays may show bone hypotrophy or pathologic fractures or neuropathic arthropathy (54). DEXA scanning may show bone density loss in longstanding neuropathy.

PATHOPHYSIOLOGY
The reduction in structural space results variably in an increase in the tissue pressure. This may bring about a compromise of vascularity. Reduced arteriolar pressure may result in a compromise of the oxygenation and nutrition of the neural tissue. Increased tissue pressure of at least 30 mm Hg may result in venous occlusion and congestion. The process may continue resulting in tissue hypoxia and accumulation of catabolic products and, eventually, in tissue homeostatic compromise (56).

The peripheral nerve has a limited ability to withstand prolonged compression. A mildly compressed segment results in injury to the Schwann cells in myelinated axons. A more severe compression results in axonal compromise. Eventually, the axonal segment peripheral to the injured area may degenerate within 5 to 12 days (Wallerian degeneration) (57).

Classically, Seddon classified the axonal degeneration in order of structural compromise in three categories: neuropraxia, axonotmesis, and neurotmesis. The first category refers to focal demyelination and nerve conduction block in the absence of axonal degeneration. The second category encompasses a continuum of axonal degeneration with intact endoneurium, followed by endoneurial disruption, and finally, by perineurial disruption.

The last category refers to a complete axonal degeneration, including that of the connective tissue components (58).

Also classically, the Seddon classification has been further modified by Sunderland in terms of subdividing the axonotmesis component into three different categories based on the increasing gravity of endoneurial and perineurial compromise (59).

Compression neuropathies encompass an array that can be classified in a variety of forms that may be acute or chronic. The acute forms may be easily reversible and result in no long-term neuronal compromise. The chronic forms result, generally, from longstanding compression and ensue in axonal transport compromise and, in the long term, in fibroblastic scarring of the axon and even of the cell body.

An anatomic classification of compressive neuropathies is presented below.

Spinal Nerve Entrapment/Compressive Disorders

When the spinal nerves are compressed beyond physiologic endurance, a compressive neuropathy may ensue. This may occur in posttraumatic conditions and in spinal foraminal stenosis. The latter is, more commonly, a disease of advancing age. The nerves exiting the affected stenotic spinal canal appear compressed and edematous. Clinically, the affected individual suffers from severe pain and related disability. The etiology is usually related to herniated discs and even to bulging discs. Osteophytes may compress the spinal nerves as well, and the compression level may increase with the growth of the osteophytes.

Depending on the location of the affected nerve, the pain may be found only in the posterior trunk area, the buttock area or may be referred to the lower limb, variably down to the knee and even to the ankle. In addition to the pain, symptoms may include LOS and paresthesia.

The symptomatic cluster caused by variable compression of the lumbosacral roots that form the sciatic nerve is commonly known as *sciatica*.

Nerve Recovery

The healing process from peripheral nerve trauma associated with compression may occur in a number of ways. Classically, three mechanisms are described:

a. *Remyelination*: This may occur within 12 weeks of the clinical onset of the compression injury.
b. *Collateral axonal sprouting*: This originates from the intact axons and may provide new innervation to the lesioned axon. Depending on the length of the compromised axon, this may take a number of months.
c. *Axonal regeneration from the (proximal) site of the original compression injury*: This process may take more than 12 months depending on the length of the compromised axon and on its structural integrity (60).

TREATMENT

Nonsurgical Treatment

The therapy may differ depending on the etiology. Thus, diabetic neuropathy is partly managed by controlling the hyperglycemia and secondary effects thereof. Compressive neuropathy, secondary to tumor impingement, may be treated secondarily to tumor treatment with radiation, chemotherapy, or surgery. Disc disease and radicular impingement may need treatment with neurosurgery.

Various peripheral entrapments may respond to splinting before decompressive surgery is performed. Physical therapy is usually very useful in preventing muscular shortening and contracture. Recovery from compressive neuropathy is usually a slow process, frequently incomplete. Meralgia paresthetica related to obesity or pregnant abdomen pressure may be relieved by weight loss or after delivery, respectively. Periodic nerve area injections with dexamethasone and bupivacaine may provide temporary pain relief.

Most medical management revolves around the control of the pain. A variety of agents may be employed with various degrees in time. The events of tolerance, habituation, and addiction have to be considered by the clinician in addition to the consideration of organ and tissue damage from prolonged use of any agent or combination of agents.

Compression neuropathies are natural sources of neuropathic pain. Such pain, especially the chronic type, responds incompletely to most analgesic regimens available at present. In theory, the tricyclic antidepressants and anticonvulsive medications should be quite useful to reduce the pain frequency and intensity. The first group acts by increasing the available inhibitory neurotransmitters such as serotonin and noradrenaline, for example, amitriptyline. The second group acts by reducing or dampening the abnormal neuronal activity that conducts the pain stimulus in the peripheral and central nervous system, for example, gabapentin, carbamazepine.

Nonopioid agents may be used initially in the course of the treatment. They may include acetaminophen, tramadol, and NSAIDs.

Chronic neuropathic pain sufferers respond poorly to these medications and tend to lead the clinician often to the use of the opiate class. Whereas patients with acute neuropathic pain may be treated symptomatically and successfully with short-acting opioids (e.g., Vicodin, Percocet), the same is not true for sufferers of chronic pain. Long-acting opioids are frequently useful for various periods of time, for example, fentanyl patches, until tolerance and habituation occur.

Other agents that are useful in the treatment of chronic neuropathic pain are local anesthetic patches, for example, Lidoderm.

In chronic conditions, the clinician may have to resort to the concomitant use of a combination of analgesics, where the use of one in a larger dose has outrun its effectiveness.

More invasive treatment of chronic pain may involve electric stimulators or intrathecal morphine implantable pumps (61).

Physical/Occupational Therapy

A variety of physical modalities have been found useful in the treatment of compressive neuropathies, especially in terms of increasing the ability to sustain activities of daily living or even work-related functions. The motivation of the affected person in improving his or her abilities to function is paramount in the success of such therapies, no less than in that of pain control with medication.

Appropriate physical exercise needs to gradually increase the level of function without exhausting the individual or creating more pain. Aquatic therapy (in warm water only) may be particularly useful in increasing the cardiorespiratory and muscular tonus abilities without undue fatigue.

Ergonomics of body position and postural re-education are paramount in redressing postural damage related to muscular hypotrophy, spasm, and sedentariness, for example, partial wheelchair placement.

Psychological and social support are very important adjuvants for the symptomatic improvement of many pain sufferers. The general aim is the reintegration of the suffering person within the family support system and in the social and economic context (62).

Massage Therapy

Massage therapy may be useful in the hands of an experienced practitioner to relieve areas of soft tissue restriction (63).

Acupuncture

One case of acupuncture in radial nerve recovery reported rapid recovery, including wrist ROM, strength, and finger extension. The state of recovery was reviewed four months and one year post injury and was found to be complete (64).

REFERENCES

1. Miller RJ. Acute versus chronic compressive neuropathy. Muscle Nerve 1987; 7:427.
2. Ashbury AK, Gilliat RW, eds. The clinical approach to neuropathy. In: Peripheral Nerve Disorders: A Practical Approach. London, UK: Butterworth, 1984:1–20.
3. Poncelet AN. An algorithm for the evaluation of peripheral neuropathies. Am J Fam Phys 1998; 57(4).
4. Latinovic R, Gulliford MC, Hughes RAC. Incidence of common compressive neuropathies in primary care. J Neurol Neurosurg Psychiatry 2006; 77:263–265.
5. de Krom MC, Knipschild PG, Kester AD, et al. Carpal tunnel syndrome: prevalence in the general population. J Clin Epidemiol 1992; 45:373.
6. Stevens JC, Sun S, Beard CM, et al. Carpal tunnel syndrome in Rochester, Minnesota, 1961 to 1980. Neurology 1988; 38:134.
7. Kroll DA, Caplain RA, Posner K, et al. Nerve injury associated with anesthesia. Anesthesiology 1990; 73:202–207.
8. Warner MA. Perioperative neuropathies. Mayo Clin Proc 1996; 73:567–574.
9. Liebelt J, Parry G. Conservative Management of Hereditary Neuropathy (HNPP). HNPP 2008:1–7.
10. Elftman HO. The evolution of the pelvic floor in primates. Am J Anat 1932; 51:307–346.
11. Abitbol MM. Evolution of the ischial spine and the pelvic floor in the Hominoidea. Am J Phys Anthropol 1988; 75:53–67.
12. Rayan GM. Lower trunk brachial plexus compression neuropathy in young athletes. Am J Sports Med 1988; 16:77–79.
13. McCrory P, Bell S, Bradshaw C. Nerve entrapment of the lower leg, ankle and foot in sport. Sports Med 2002; 32(6):371–391.
14. Thompson MJ, Rivara FP. Bicycle injuries. Am Fam Physician 63:2007–2014, 2017–2018.
15. Colac T, Bamac B, Ozbek A, et al. Nerve conduction studies of upper extremities in tennis players. Br J Sports Med 2004; 38:632–635.
16. McLeod JG. Investigation of peripheral neuropathy. J Neurol Neurosurg Psychiatry 1995; 58:274–283.
17. Thrush D. Investigation of peripheral neuropathies. Br J Hosp Med 1993; 48:13–22.
18. Kayan A, Earl CJ. Compressive lesions of the optic nerves and chiasm pattern of recovery of vision following surgical treatment. Brain 1975; 98:13–28.
19. Novak CB, Mackinnon SE. Surgical treatment of a long thoracic nerve palsy. Ann Thorac Surg 2002; 73:1643.
20. Rengachary SS, Neff JP, Singer PA, et al. Suprascapular entrapment neuropathy: a clinical, anatomical and comparative study. Part 1: Clinical study. Neurosurgery 1979; 5(4):441–446.
21. Torres-Ramos FM, Biundo JJ. Suprascapular neuropathy during progressive resistance exercises in a cardiac rehabilitation program. Arch Phys Med Rehabil 1992; 73:1107.
22. Ferrante MA. Brachial plexopathy: classification, causes and consequences. Muscle Nerve 2004; 30:547.
23. Killer HE, Hess K. Natural history of radiation-induced brachial plexopathy compared with surgically treated patients. J Neurol 1990; 237:247.
24. Levin KH, Wilbourn AJ, Maggiano HJ. Cervical rib and median sternotomy-related brachial plexopathies: a reassessment. Neurology 1998; 50:1407.

25. Dellon AL. Patient evaluation and management considerations in nerve compressions. Hand Clin 1992; 8:229–239.
26. Eversmann WW. Proximal median nerve compression. Hand Clin 1992; 8:307–315.
27. Hartz CR, Linscheid RL, Gramse RR, et al. The pronator teres syndrome: compressive neuropathy of the median nerve. J Bone Joint Surg Am 1981; 63A:885–890.
28. Nakano KK, Lundergan C, Ohihiro MM. Anterior interosseous nerve syndromes: diagnostic methods and alternative treatments. Arch Neurol 1977; 34: 477–480.
29. Schantz K, Riegels-Nielsen P. The anterior interosseous nerve syndrome. J Hand Surg 1992; 17B:510–512.
30. Landau ME, Diaz MI, Barner KC, et al. Changes in nerve conduction velocity across the elbow due to experimental error. Muscle Nerve 2002; 26:838.
31. Beekman R, Shoemaker MC, Van Der A,et al. Diagnostic value of high resolution sonography at the elbow. Neurology 2004; 62:757.
32. Bimmler D, Meyer VE. Surgical treatment of the ulnar nerve entrapment neuropathy: submuscular anterior transposition or simple decompression of the ulnar nerve? Long term results in 79 cases. Ann Chir Main Memb Super 1996; 15:148.
33. Lee CT, Espley AJ. Perioperative ulnar neuropathy in orthopedics: association with tilting the patient. Clin Orthop 2002:106.
34. Nakamichi K, Tachibana S. Radial nerve entrapment by the lateral head of the triceps. J Hand Surg 1991; 16A:748.
35. Cravens G, Kline DG. Posterior interosseous nerve palsies. Neurosurgery 1990; 27(3):397–402.
36. Rinker B, Effron CR, Beasley RW. Proximal radial compression neuropathy. Ann Plast Surg 2004; 52:174.
37. Verhaar J, Spaans F. Radial tunnel syndrome. J Bone Joint Surg 2002; 73A:539.
38. Dickerman RD, Stevens QE, Cohen AJ, et al. Radial tunnel syndrome in an elite power athlete: a case of direct compressive neuropathy. J Periph Nerv Syst 2002; 7:229.
39. Feldman RG, Goldman R, Keyserling WM. Peripheral nerve entrapment syndromes and ergonomic factors. Am J Ind Med 1983; 3:661.
40. Kline DJ, Hudson AR. Lower extremity nerves. In: Nerve Injuries: Operative Results for Major Nerve Injuries, Entrapments and Tumors. Philadelphia: WB Saunders, 1995:389–394.
41. McGillicuddy JE, Harrigan MR. Meralgia paresthetica. Tech Neurosurg 2000; 6(1):50–56.
42. Cimino WR. Tarsal tunnel syndrome: review of the literature. Foot Ankle 1990; 11(1):47–52.
43. Malay DS, McGlamry ED, Nava CA Jr. Entrapment neuropathies of the lower extremities. In: Textbook on Foot Surgery, Vol II, Baltimore, MD: Williams & Wilkins, 1987:668.
44. Meals RA. Peroneal nerve palsy complicating ankle sprain. J Bone Joint Surg Am 1977; 59:966.
45. Dellon AL. Deep peroneal nerve entrapment on the dorsum of the foot. Foot Ankle 1990; 11:73.
46. Amarenco G, Lanoe Y, Perrigot M, et al. A new canal syndrome compression of the pudendal nerve in Alcock's canal or perineal paralysis of cyclists. Presse Med 1987; 16:399.
47. Tetzschner T, Sorensen M, Lose G, et al. Pudendal nerve function during pregnancy and after delivery. Int Urogynecol J Pelvic Floor Dysfunct 1997; 8:66–68.
48. Burns AE, Stewart WP. Morton's neuroma. J Am Podiatry Assoc 1982; 72:135.
49. Sartoris DJ, Brozinsky S, Resnick D. Magnetic resonance images. J Foot Surg 1989; 28:78.
50. Nollet F. Post polio syndrome. Orphanet Encyclopedia 2004:1–8.
51. Parry GJ. Electrodiagnostic studies in the evaluation of peripheral nerve and brachial plexus injuries. Neurol Clin 1992; 10:921.
52. Happel LT, Kline DG, Gelberman RH, eds. Nerve Lesions in Continuity. In: Operative Nerve Repair and Reconstruction. Philadelphia, PA: J.B. Lippincott, 1991:601.

53. Sabin TD, Swift TR, Jacobson RR, Dick PJ, Thomas PK, eds. Leprosy. Peripheral Neuropathy. Philadelphia, PA: Saunders, 1993:1354–1379.
54. Sharma SD, Smith EM, Hazleman BL. Thermographic changes in keyboard operators with chronic forearm pain. BMJ 1997; 314:118.
55. Herrick RT, Herrick SK. Thermography in the detection of carpal tunnel syndrome and other compressive neuropathies. Hand Surg Am 1987; 12(5 pt 2):943–949.
56. Lundborg G, Dahlin L. The pathophysiology of nerve compression. 1992; 4:215.
57. Chaudhry V, Cornblath DR. Wallerian degeneration in human nerves: serial electrophysiological studies. Muscle Nerve 1992; 15:687.
58. Seddon HJ. Three types of nerve injury. Brain 1943; 66.
59. Sunderland S. A classification of peripheral nerves injured producing loss of function. Brain 1951; 74.
60. Seltzer ME. Regeneration of peripheral nerve. In: Sumner AJ, ed. The Physiology of Peripheral Nerve Disease. Philadelphia, PA: Saunders, 1980:358.
61. Siddal PJ, Taylor DA, McClelland JM, et al. Pain report and the relationship of pain to physical factors in the first six months following spinal cord injury. Pain 1991; 81:187–197.
62. Summers JD, Rapoff MA, Varghese G, et al. Psychological factors in chronic spinal cord injury pain. Pain 1991; 47:183,189.
63. Lowe W. Nerve compression and tension. Massage Today 2001; 01(05).
64. Millea PJ, Gelberman RH, eds. Citation: acupuncture treatment of compressive neuropathy of the radial nerve: a single case report of "Saturday Night Palsy". J Altern Complement Med 2005; 11(1):167–169.

9 Quantitative Clinical, Sensory, and Autonomic Testing of Chronic Neuropathic Pain

David R. Longmire

Department of Internal Medicine, University of Alabama at Birmingham School of Medicine, Huntsville Regional Medical Campus, Huntsville, Alabama, U.S.A.

With rare exceptions (1, 2), clinical pain (regardless of its underlying cause) is a neurological phenomenon known universally to human patients. Pain becomes *chronic* only when this unpleasant sensory and emotional experience persists for much longer than expected relative to the severity or duration of the initial noxious stimulus (3, 4). When chronic symptoms are accompanied by other disturbances of vital function, for example, autonomic activity, sleep, and somatic movement, the experience is no longer simply pain, but may be more accurately classified as a chronic pain *syndrome*.

When any irritative pathophysiological process (5) occurs within one or more portions of the central or peripheral nervous system, the resulting unpleasant symptoms may be classified as *neuropathic* in origin (6–9). Of all the known chronic pain syndromes, neuropathic pain is often perceived to be the most likely to be intractable and least likely to be caused by a single etiologic mechanism. This suggests that successful management of any aspect of chronic neuropathic pain can only be attained when established treatments are applied to *all* components of the specific syndrome. The primary purpose of this chapter is to review specific quantitative methods that have been used to assess individual physical or physiological changes that occur in patients with chronic neuropathic pain. The secondary purpose is to differentiate the mechanisms and goals of subjective (clinical, sensory) techniques from those that form the basis of objective (autonomic, sympathetic sudomotor) quantitative testing.

CLINICAL ASSESSMENT OF NEUROPATHIC PAIN

The first step in reaching the correct etiologic diagnosis and classification of each type of pain is the performance of a detailed clinical evaluation (10). For example, the medical *pain* history (11) usually begins with a more detailed documentation of symptom characteristics than might otherwise be expected of a general or acute health problem.

Recording of the spatial characteristics of the pain, whether chronic or acute (12), should be done early in the pain history. The *regions* of symptom onset, patterns of *radiation* or *referral* to other body sites, and any association with loss or excess of somatic sensation within the symptomatic regions have major relevance in the diagnosis of neuropathic pain. In patients who suffer from multiple pain types or regions, or in whom there coexists abnormal perception of different modes of sensory stimulation, documenting clinical data using only verbal descriptors can be overwhelming. Therefore, it is common practice for physicians to have patients draw or shade their pain symptoms on preprinted outlines of the human body, known either as the pain drawing instrument or more simply as the pain drawing. There are many versions or styles of the pain drawing, the most common of which consists of either (a) an anterior and posterior view of the body similar to that found in the McGill Pain Questionnaire (13), or (b) these two views plus two combined lateral and medial views, known as the "walking man" (14). Regardless of which form of pain drawing is selected, it is essential to use a type that does not include lines indicating sensory dermatomes of the type originally reported by Foerster (15, 16). Avoidance of this latter type is important since patients who are naïve to the pain drawing method often seem compelled to indicate their pains by shading only between the lines, the results of which may not reflect the true distribution of their personal symptoms.

In decades past, clinicians who wished to quantify the extent of pain were limited to recording the number of symptomatic zones marked on the pain drawing, or adding the expected surface areas for major body regions (17). At present, the outline of each pain region can be traced using a computer-assisted drafting technique that allows automatic calculation of the area within the perimeter. This has been found to be useful in monitoring decreases or increases of pain extent as a measure of treatment outcome (18, 19).

Specifically, reduction in the number of pain areas *and* the area within each zone over time, or with dose-related changes in treatment, can provide numeric data which have been shown to indicate the relative success of pain symptom management.

In addition, the pain drawing can be used as a convenient place in the medical record to note the severity or *intensity* of every symptomatic area. There are several types of numeric pain scales that can be used for this purpose (20, 21), but the 11-point pain scale (22) seems to be preferred by many patients (23) and is readily applicable to the pain drawing. The anchors or end points of this scale use "0" as indicating no pain at all, and "10" to represent the worst pain imaginable. Unfortunately, there exists a population of physicians who persist in erroneously describing any *verbal* reporting technique as the *Visual* Analog Scale.

A simple but clinically informative quantitative variation on the 11-point verbal pain scale is applied by asking each patient to indicate pain intensity as a fraction. The patient is first asked to give the maximum pain intensity *ever experienced* within a particular pain region, the result of which serves as the denominator. After all values are recorded, the patient is asked to provide the *present* pain intensity score for each region as it is perceived on the day and time of the current clinic visit, which is then recorded as the numerator of the fraction. These simple results provide immediate feedback to the physician as to the success or failure of symptom management. Nevertheless, it must be remembered that, despite the *appearance* of quantifying the patient's pain using any of the methods just described, these values are still purely subjective.

The speed of onset, the intermittent or continuous presentation of pain, responses to palliative or provocative measures, and interference with activities of daily living serve as the next level of important characteristics. Recording the patient's own words to describe the quality of pain is essential in reaching an etiologic diagnosis, particularly for neuropathic pain. Pain *quality* descriptors can also be documented more formally by using the McGill Pain Questionnaire, which has been validated in many studies and translated into multiple languages.

Next, the physical examination (24) is performed with a primary view of determining if there are any structural abnormalities that can explain the source of the pain. In addition to the global physical assessment, standard techniques of a detailed neurological examination are applied with particular detail directed to documentation of any sensory dysfunction. This includes the mapping of reduction or loss of the expected responses to standard stimuli, such as light touch, pressure, pin/point, cold, warm, vibration, and position. Each hypoesthetic or anesthetic region can be shaded on a separate body map of the same design as the pain drawing. Using a similar method, abnormalities of *excessive* sensation (hyperesthesia or allodynia) can be shaded on individual body maps or pain drawing forms. Together these data sheets provide a base upon which anatomic diagnoses can be established, before any laboratory tests are instituted. Sensory abnormalities, while admittedly subjective, can still be quantified using the computer-assisted drafting system noted previously.

It is generally accepted that patients with regional neuropathy often report the coexistence of local sensory loss or distortion of expected sensation within the same territories as their pain. These individuals frequently cite confusion to their physicians by asking how it is possible for a part of the body to have lost normal feeling, and yet have severe pain within the same region. While both sets of positive (hyperesthesia, allodynia) and negative (hypoesthesia, anesthesia) symptoms are sufficiently important to deserve documentation on separate pain drawing forms, they are still personal and subjective and must not be considered to represent any form of purely objective data.

QUANTITATIVE SENSORY TESTING

A method has been developed by which a patient's response to cutaneous thermal stimulation can be evaluated in health and disease in a quantifiable manner. The main purpose of this technique (quantitative sensory testing, QST) (25) is to identify abnormal thresholds of sensation, which are subserved mainly by small-diameter, unmyelinated afferent nerve fibers. The importance of these neural pathways to the maintenance of neuropathic pain cannot be overstated, since there exists an extraordinarily close relationship between thermal and nociceptive fiber systems.

The stimuli used for QST are provided by an extremely well-controlled set of thermal changes that are ordinarily applied to the skin at eight sites over the upper and lower extremities (26). These sites are divided into four homologous pairs, with relative representation over the distal proximal zones over each upper and lower extremity. The physical properties of each set of stimuli are controlled electrically by activating thermal transducers (thermodes) in a manner that can produce temperatures from of 0°C to >50°C. Each temperature stimulus can be varied at a fixed rate, for example, 1.5°C/sec, in a sequence that can evoke identifiable differences in sensation when the appropriate amount of heat or cold stimulation has been changed. Patients and control subjects undergoing QST are asked to provide a verbal response as soon as they perceive a difference in heat or cold sensation while the stimuli are varied. The purpose of this procedure is to measure each patient's threshold of perception for warmth, coolness, heat pain, and cold pain. Pain intensity levels are reported using the 0 to 10 verbal scale described in earlier sections.

One of the major values of QST is the measurable identification of abnormalities of *pure thresholds* of thermal sensation and thermal pain over the chosen test sites. QST also reduces some of the contaminating factors that accompany tests of thermal pain *tolerance*, such as the cold pressor test of single digits (27) or entire distal segments of a limb. The primary importance of QST in clinical practice is based upon the fact that several types of hypoesthesia or analgesia which occur in regional neuropathy are associated with elevated thermal sensory thresholds. In addition, when such thresholds are *reduced*, phenomena such as hyperesthesia, hyperalgesia, or allodynia can be suspected.

Thus far in the development of QST, there are some limitations regarding its potential application to clinical studies of sensory abnormalities and neuropathic pain. Some examples include the subjective nature of the measured verbal response, bias on the part of the patient toward a negative test result (28), and the restricted number and locations of standardized test sites. Earlier concerns regarding the paucity of comprehensive normative data are being addressed as studies performed on healthy control subjects are introduced into the scientific literature.

AUTONOMIC DYSFUNCTION IN NEUROPATHIC PAIN

Historically, large portions of the autonomic nervous system (ANS) have been thought of as only being responsible for the creation of involuntary physiological responses to acute, stressful or noxious stimuli (29, 30). However, it is now accepted that clinical laboratory tests of parasympathetic and sympathetic pathways can be used to detect and quantify many forms of autonomic dysfunction that can occur in systemic illnesses (31). In considering the clinical use of *any* tests of ANS function, it is still essential to remember that such procedures are clearly separate in mechanism and purpose from tests of subjective response to external stimulation, regardless of stimulus modality (32). Since most ANS tests do not directly reflect any aspect of *afferent* function in the processing of clinical pain, they do not suffer the methodological limitations of procedures that require patients' subjective response to stimulation.

For more than half a century, clinical and basic scientists have contributed to current understanding that subsystems within the ANS can play an important role in the modulation and maintenance of certain forms of neuropathic pain (33). Research encouraged by subcommittees of the International Association for the Study of Pain (34) has helped to elucidate the mechanisms and clinical features of certain chronic neuropathic pain syndromes, such as complex regional pain syndrome types I (reflex sympathetic dystrophy) (35) and II (causalgia) (36), and sympathetically maintained pain (37). These efforts have finally led to an acceptance that many forms of pain that occur in individuals whose systemic illnesses have progressed to create abnormalities in sensory *and* autonomic pathways are often maintained through abnormal neural communication within sympathetic fibers.

ANATOMIC AND PHYSIOLOGICAL BASIS OF REGIONAL SYMPATHETIC SUDOMOTOR TESTING

Of the many techniques that have been developed to monitor sympathetic effector subsystems in laboratory settings (38), tests of the *sudomotor* pathways have shown greatest promise in clinical diagnosis. Procedures such as the quantitative sudomotor axon reflex test (39), the Silastic sweat imprint method (40), and sympathetic skin response (41, 42) all provide numeric data which can be compared to results obtained from normal subjects, or from patients with autonomic dysfunction. Unfortunately, all of these methods are limited by the small number of test sites, e.g. 2–8, an effect that reduces the ability to perform accurate assessment of the spatial distribution of sudomotor dysfunction. A separate procedure, the thermoregulatory sweat test (43), can provide a great deal of clinically relevant information about regional loss of sweating, but is time consuming, requires an external thermal challenge and, relative to this chapter, is not readily quantifiable. In the following sections, descriptions of the use of noninvasive tests of sympathetic sudomotor reflexes, using 40 measurements of the passive electrical characteristics of the skin, will be provided. Since this type of procedure does provide sufficient spatial information for clinical diagnosis of regional hyperhidrosis and hypohidrosis, the following description of the functional anatomy of the autonomic pathways that serve as the basis of such testing is relevant.

There is clinical and experimental evidence for input from various portions of the cortex and limbic system into the hypothalamus (44). These findings notwithstanding, it is known that it is really in the preoptic nucleus where thermoregulatory control begins. From there, efferent nerve fibers descend ipsilaterally and remain uncrossed within the brain stem, terminating in the intermediolateral fasciculus of the spinal cord. Within the intermediolateral horn of the spinal cord gray matter, a separate neuronal population, known as sympathetic preganglionic neurons, exists. The axons of these form preganglionic fibers, which travel uninterrupted through the anterior horn from where they eventually leave the spinal cord along with the motor nerve roots.

Shortly thereafter, these fibers separate from the roots and proceed toward the paravertebral sympathetic chain. Their myelination gives rise to their color and thus the segments of these pathways between the root and the chain ganglia are known as the white rami communicantes. After synapsing with neurons in the respective ganglia that are destined to become part of the final common sudomotor path, the postganglionic fibers exit and, due to their unmyelinated state, become identifiable as the *gray* rami communicantes. They return to join the main (mixed) nerve roots which pass through the neural foramina of the spinal column, proceeding to individual territories of skin where clinical and subclinical (electrophysiological) functions are controlled locally. Pathological processes affecting these pathways either (a) create regional hypohidrosis by interrupting normal sweating locally, or (b) irritate such fibers in a manner that forces them to drive the effectors excessively, creating local increases in sweating (hyperhidrosis).

SELECTIVE TISSUE CONDUCTANCE TECHNOLOGY

Selective tissue conductance (STC) technology consists of a painless, noninvasive, quantitative neurophysiological method that has been used clinically for more than a quarter century (45–48) to assess regional dysfunction in the sympathetic sudomotor nerve supply to glabrous skin. In an attempt to provide a safe (49) and objective test that was unrelated to sensory stimulation, Longmire and Woodley based STC technology on the quantitative assessment of *conductance*, as the measure of choice, since this measure of skin is *directly* proportional to the activity of sympathetic sudomotor efferent fibers. In order to ensure that any direct current used to measure conductance would be so low that it could not produce any sensation, or pain, or any other discomfort to the patient or subject, test signals were kept well below sensory threshold. Next, any transcorporeal currents that had been used in monopolar measurement were eliminated by using a bipolar concentric electrode. Its design consisted of a central disk separated from an outer ring by an insulator. This allowed a safe and restricted passage of subthreshold test current between the center contact and the outer ring electrode through very superficial layers of the skin by volume conduction, with no possibility of electrical risk to the function of essential tissues. This aspect of STC technology became known as *spatial selectivity*. The next step in the development of STC technology was the introduction of a procedure that could be used for the avoidance of an iontophoretic effect. This electrochemical phenomenon can contaminate any measurement of DC conductance in biological tissue because of progressively increasing values based upon the duration of application of subsensory current. By making conductance measurements early in the application of the test current, using a method known as *temporal selectivity*, it was possible to eliminate the iontophoretic effect.

By combining the elements of conductance, spatial selectivity, and temporal selectivity, STC was established as "... the relative ability of biological tissue to conduct a weak (DC) electrical signal, which is applied for a selected period of time to a selected, limited and restricted surface area of that tissue ...." Since the conductivity of skin is expressed as a function of the surface area of the electrodes, the international unit of measurement for STC is nanosiemens per square centimeter (nS/cm^2).

QUANTITATIVE STC METHODS APPLIED TO THE MODEL OF PERIPHERAL DIABETIC AUTONOMIC NEUROPATHY

One of the most direct applications of peripheral quantitative STC measurement is in the clinical assessment of patients with painful diabetic autonomic neuropathy (50–52). In these patients, the most common sudomotor abnormalities are distributed in the feet and lower legs along a predominantly *longitudinal* line. Therefore, the most useful montage consists of 20 measurements made over each lower extremity, beginning at the most distal interspace of the third metatarsal and ending just below the inferior margin of the patella. These individual measurements are made sequentially along a generally rectilinear path, the axis of which is located just lateral to the tibia. In order to compensate for differences in leg size, the placement of electrode sites are made in proportion to the length of each limb.

Upon successful completion of all 40 measurements, computerized STC systems automatically display all quantitative results in table form, with columns arranged with the most distal measurements assigned the lower numbers, and progressively more proximal sites matched to the higher columns. Upper and lower rows are arranged to match homologous sites on right and left sides, respectively. During the initial analysis, numeric data which have been presented in table form are inspected independently for the right and left lower limbs *without reference to the opposite limb*. This is followed by a review of the same data presented in a standardized graphic format; STC values obtained using the linear gradient method are plotted on the vertical (y) axis, against distance along the horizontal (x) axis, expressed more commonly as the location of each STC measurement (site number). Values obtained from the most distal sites are plotted to the extreme left of the graph, while those from progressively more proximal sites are plotted along the x-axis from left to right.

STAGING SYSTEM FOR STC RESULTS

The value of systematically repeating laboratory tests of autonomic function on a regular basis is recognized as a way of monitoring the progression of pathophysiological processes that occur in patients with diabetic peripheral neuropathy. Changes that reflect different stages of the disease can thus be documented in a way that will allow the physician to modify treatment. The present system for STC staging is composed of results which can be interpreted in six categories: normal, transitional, and four levels of abnormality. The abnormal results are further divided into categories representing irritative (distal and diffuse hyperhidrosis) or destructive (distal and diffuse hypohidrosis/anhidrosis) stages of peripheral diabetic autonomic neuropathy, which are presented graphically in the following sections.

Normal (STC Stage N)

The determination of a normal result (stage N) is based upon (a) the presence of a distal reference peak (DRP) over the dorsum of the foot, and (b) normal return toward a much lower level over the proximal portions of the anterior tibial aspect of the lower leg. A typical example of this stage is presented in the lowermost graph (A) of Figure 1, measured over the nondominant lower extremity of a nondiabetic, normal control subject.

Transitional (STC Stage T)

The middle graph (B) of Figure 1 displays a classical example of transitional (STC stage T) results. In this graph, there is a second elevation of STC proximal to the DRP value. This stage is thus named to indicate the transition between normal physiological patterns of stage N and any latent or early irritative process developing locally as a potential harbinger of progressive hyperhidrosis that accompanies peripheral diabetic autonomic neuropathy.

Distal Hyperhidrosis (STC Stage I)

Repeated monitoring during the development of peripheral diabetic autonomic neuropathy (PDAN) has revealed that the trough STC values that occur at sites between the dorsum of the feet and proximal transitional peaks will gradually become higher with disease progression. As these values rise, they coalesce graphically to create a relative plateau of selective tissue conductivity over the foot and lower leg. A typical example of the most mild form of sudomotor abnormality (known as *distal hyperhidrosis* or STC stage I) is shown in the uppermost graph (C) of Figure 1. This type of pattern often occurs in individuals with mild diabetes mellitus.

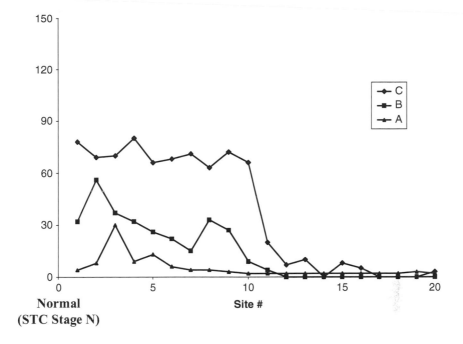

FIGURE 1

Diffuse Hyperhidrosis (STC Stage II)

A more severe form of the sudomotor component of peripheral diabetic autonomic neuropathy often includes a *diffuse hyperhidrosis* (STC stage
II), which is not just the result of poor glycemic control. Indeed, there
are several factors that contribute to the proximal spread of sympathetic
sudomotor excitability from stage I to a more diffuse pattern involving the entire
lower leg. These include the patient's age at onset of diabetes mellitus, the duration of the illness, clinical response to simple dietary restrictions, or to oral antidi-
abetes agents or to insulin, as well as adherence to the treatment plan. Figure 2
includes typical graphic examples of STC results, which represent mild (A),
moderate (B), and severe (C) diffuse hyperhidrosis in the nondominant lower
extremity.

    Another characteristic of advancing autonomic neuropathy is that the spa-
tial distribution of relative *distal* hyperhidrosis spreads proximally until nearly
all values obtained from the feet and the distal, middle, and proximal thirds of
the anterior tibial aspects have become worse, resulting in a more generalized
hyperhidrosis. This increase represents a more severe or chronic pattern of relative hyperhidrosis which correlates with chronicity of painful neuropathy or the
diabetes itself, rather than the severity of loss of glycemic control.

Distal Hypohidrosis (STC Stage III)

Unfortunately, the progression of the neuropathic processes associated with
uncontrolled or chronic diabetes mellitus does not end there. Over time, the
degeneration of nerve fibers eventually proceeds toward the *loss* of sudomotor

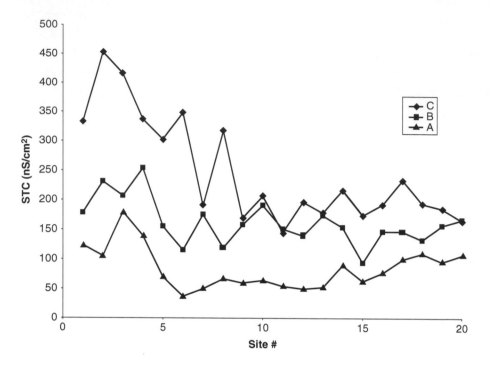

FIGURE 2

fibers in a distal-to-proximal direction (53). In terms of the sympathetic sudomotor nerve supply to the skin, this effect causes changes in numeric STC values, which reflect the development of a *distal hypohidrosis* (STC stage III), with more proximal portions of the leg remaining as hyperhidrotic as they were in STC stage II. Three typical examples of STC stage III are shown in Figure 3, each of which has been obtained from the nondominant lower extremity, with graphs A, B, and C presented in increasing order of severity.

An early indication of relative distal hypohidrosis is that the DRP is absent over the dorsal aspect of the affected foot. This is followed by the reduction of STC levels over the distal third of the anterior tibial aspect of the leg. In more severe or chronic circumstances, the middle third is also reduced or absent, but the values over the proximal third of the anterior tibial region are elevated when compared to the expected euhidrotic or physiologically hypohidrotic state.

Diffuse Hypohidrosis (STC Stage IV)

Finally, the dying back phenomenon continues until progressively greater numbers of sympathetic fibers lose the ability to drive perspiration, and larger areas of the skin become dry and poorly conductive. This results in a *diffuse hypohidrosis* (STC stage IV) over the lower limbs. This term is specifically applied when STC values are extremely low over *all* sites in the linear gradient montage of the feet and lower legs. Figure 4 reveals the graphic presentation of STC data obtained from left and right lower extremities at normal room temperature from a patient with findings that are typical for this STC stage.

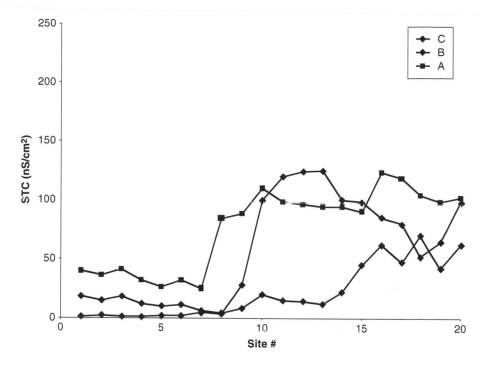

FIGURE 3

It should be noted that there exists a single focus of increased cutaneous irritation at site number 11 on the right lower extremity. Such minor findings can often be seen in patients with severe peripheral neuropathy; their presence does not change the overall classification from STC stage IV (diffuse hypohidrosis).

SUMMARY

The medical management of chronic neuropathic pain can only be accomplished if specific diagnostic tests reveal all of the pathological processes that subserve each syndrome. The initial *qualitative* assessment of any patient suspected of having chronic neuropathic pain is based upon data obtained through the medical history and general physical and neurological examinations. During these two physical assessment portions of the initial examination, emphasis must be placed on evaluating, in detail, both sensory and autonomic (sympathetic) functions. In patients who demonstrate abnormalities of either type, quantitative testing should be performed to ensure (a) confirmation of the anatomic diagnosis, (b) staging of the severity of the illness progression, and (c) monitoring the response to treatment.

The clinical applications of tests of (a) subjective threshold of perception, for example, QST and (b) objective testing of regional sympathetic sudomotor abnormalities (STC) are presented within this chapter.

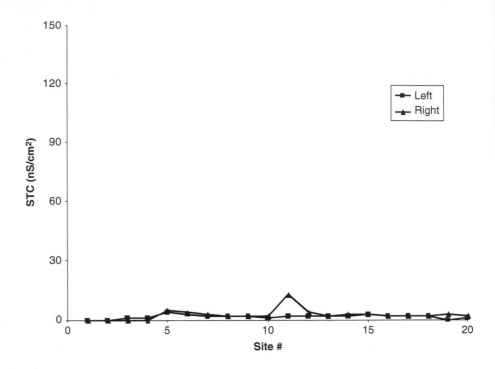

FIGURE 4

REFERENCES

1. Swanson AG, Buchan GC, Alvord EC Jr. Anatomic changes in congenital insensitivitiy to pain: absence of small primary sensory neurons in ganglia, roots and Lissauer's Tract. Arch Neurol 1965; 12:12.
2. Adams RA, Victor M. Diseases of the peripheral nerves. In: Adams RA, Victor M, eds. Principles of Neurology. 2nd ed. New York: McGraw-Hill Book Company, 1981:886–928.
3. Longmire DR. Classification of pain and pain syndromes. Pain Digest 1992; 2.
4. Merskey H, Bogduk N. Classification of Chronic Pain. Vol 2. Seattle, WA: IASP Press, 1994:211–212.
5. Kennedy LD. Laboratory investigations. In: Raj PP, ed. Pain Medicine: A Comprehensive Review. St. Louis, MO: Mosby, 1996:47–54.
6. Scadding JW. Neuropathic pain. In: Asbury AK, McKhann GM, McDonald WI, eds. Diseases of the Nervous System: Clinical Neurobiology. 2nd ed. Philadelphia, PA: WB Saunders Co, 1992:858–872.
7. Longmire DR, Jay GW, Boswell MV. Neuropathic pain. In: Cole BE, Boswell MV, eds. Weiner's Textbook of Pain Management: A Practical Guide for Clinicians. 7th ed. Boca Raton, FL: CRC Press, 2005:297–314.
8. Backonja M-M. Defining neuropathic pain. Anesth Analg 2003; 97:785–790.
9. Jay GW, Longmire DR. Neuropathic pain. In: Jay GW, ed. Chronic Pain. New York, NY: Informa HealthCare Publishers, 2007:145–192.
10. Longmire DR. Evaluation of the pain patient. In: Raj PP, ed. Pain Medicine: A Comprehensive Review. St. Louis, MO: Mosby, 1996:26–34.
11. Longmire DR. The medical pain history. Pain Digest 1991; 1:29–34.
12. Wiener S. Differential Diagnosis of Acute Pain by Body Region. New York: McGraw-Hill, 1993.

13. Melzack R. The McGill Pain Questionnaire. Major properties and scoring methods. Pain 1975; 1:275–299.
14. Haymaker W, Woodhall B. Peripheral Nerve Injuries. 2nd ed. Philadelphia, PA: Saunders, 1953.
15. Foerster O, Altenburger H, Kroll FW. Uber die Beziehungen des vegetativen Nervensystems zur Sensibilitat (1929) [On the relationships of the autonomic nervous system to sensibility (1929)]. In: Handwerker HO, Brune K, eds (translated by Dr. Biederman-Thorson). Deutschs-sprachige Klassiker der Schmerzforschung [Classical German Contributions to Pain Research], 1987:144–222.
16. Foerster O. The dermatomes in man. Brain 1983; 56:1–39.
17. Margolis RB, Tait RC, Krause SJ. A rating system for use with patient pain drawings. Pain 1986; 24:57–65.
18. Longmire DR. Bimodal dose–response to adjuvant use of tizanidine HCl in control of myofascial pain (Section 7.5). In: Staats PS, ed. Advancements in the Treatment of Neuromuscular Pain. CME Monograph. Baltimore, MD: Johns Hopkins University, Office of Continuing Medical Education, 2000:45–48.
19. Longmire DR, Krusz JC. Reduction of myofascial pain extent during adjunctive treatment with tizanidine hydrochloride: quantification using computer assisted drafting methods. In: Proceedings of the IX World Congress on Pain, International Association for the Study of Pain, Vienna, Austria, 1999:48–49. Abstract 154.
20. Valley MA. Pain measurement. In: Raj PP, ed. Pain Medicine: A Comprehensive Review. St. Louis, MO: Mosby, 1996:36–45.
21. Jensen MP, Karoly P. Self-report scales and procedures for assessing pain in adults. In: Turk DC, Melzack R, eds. Handbook of Pain Assessment. New York: Guilford Press, 1992:135–151.
22. Farrar JT, Young JP Jr, LaMoreaux L, et al. Clinical importance of changes in chronic pain intensity measured on an 11 point numerical pain rating scale. Pain 2001; 94:149–158.
23. Longmire NK, Longmire DR, Leak WD. Patient preferences for verbal numeric pain scales. Proc Am Pain Society 1991.
24. Longmire DR. The physical examination: methods and application in the clinical evaluation of pain. Pain Digest 1991; 2:136–143.
25. Dyck PJ, O'Brien PC. Approaches to quantitative cutaneous sensory assessment. Quantitative sensory testing: report of the Therapeutics and Technology Assessment Subcommittee of the American Academy of Neurology. Neurology 2003; 61:1628–1630.
26. Kelly KG, Cook T, Backonja M-M. Pain ratings at the thresholds are necessary for interpretation of quantitative sensory testing. Muscle Nerve 2005; 32:179–184.
27. Kennedy LD., Longmire DR,, Leak WD. The digital cold pressor test: method and potential application in clinical pain research. Proc Am Pain Society 1991.
28. Dyck PJ, Dyck PJ, Kennedy WR, et al. Limitations of quantitative sensory testing when patients are biased toward a bad outcome. Neurology 1998; 50:1213.
29. Fulton JF. Autonomic nervous system. In: Fulton JF, ed. Physiology of the Nervous System. 3rd ed. New York, NY: Oxford University Press, 1949:202–235.
30. Fulton JF. The hypothalamus and the autonomic nervous system. In: Fulton JF, ed. Physiology of the Nervous System. 3rd ed. New York, NY: Oxford University Press, 1949:236–265.
31. American Medical Association. CPT 2008: Current Procedural Terminology. Professional edition. Chicago, IL: American Medical Association, 2007:419.
32. Jay GW. The autonomic nervous system. In: Raj PP, ed. Pain Medicine: A Comprehensive Review. St. Louis, MO: Mosby, 1996:461–464.
33. Livingston KE. Personal communication, Neurosurgical Pain Service, Department of Neurosurgery, The Wellesley Hospital. Toronto, ON: University of Toronto, 1969–1971.
34. IASP Subcommittee on Taxonomy. Reflex sympathetic dystrophy (I-5). Pain 1986; (suppl 3):S29–S36.

35. Raj PP. Reflex sympathetic dystrophy. In: Raj PP, ed. Pain Medicine: A Comprehensive Review. St. Louis, MO: Mosby, 1996:466–464.
36. Livingston WK. Pain Mechanisms: A Physiologic Interpretation of Causalgia and Its Related States. New York: MacMillan, 1944.
37. Wilson P. Sympathetically maintained pain. In: Stanton-Hicks MD'A, ed. Sympathetic Pain. Boston, MA: Kluwer Academic Publishers, 1989.
38. Longmire DR, Stanton-Hicks M, Ranieri T, et al. Laboratory methods used in the diagnosis of sudomotor dysfunction and complex regional pain syndromes: a critical review. Pain Digest 1996; 6:21–29.
39. Low PA, Caskey PE, Tuck RR. Quantitative sudomotor axon reflex tests in normal and neuropathic subjects. Ann Neurol 1983; 14:573–580.
40. Kennedy WR, Navarro X. Evaluation of sudomotor function by sweat imprint methods. In: Low PA, ed. Clinical Autonomic Disorders: Evaluation and Management. Boston, MA: Little Brown & Company, 1993:253–261.
41. Shahani BT, Halperin JJ, Boulu P, et al. Sympathetic skin response: a method of assessing unmyelinated axon dysfunction in peripheral neuropathies. J Neurol Neurosurg Psychiatry 1984; 47:536–542.
42. Schondorf R. The role of the sympathetic skin response in the assessment of autonomic function. In: Low PA, ed. Clinical Autonomic Disorders: Evaluation and Management. Boston, MA: Little Brown & Company, 1993:231–242.
43. Fealey RD. The thermoregulatory sweat test. In: Low PA, ed. Clinical Autonomic Disorders: Evaluation and Management. Boston, MA: Little Brown & Company, 1993:217–229.
44. Brodal A. The autonomic nervous system. The hypothalamus. In: Brodal A, ed. Neurological Anatomy in Relation to Clinical Medicine. 3rd ed. New York, NY: Oxford University Press, 1981:698–787.
45. Longmire DR, Parris WCV. Selective tissue conductance in the assessment of sympathetically mediated pain. In: Parris WCV, ed. Contemporary Issues in Chronic Pain. Boston, MA: Kluwer Academic Publishers, 1991:147–160.
46. Longmire DR, Woodley WE. Clinical neurophysiology of pain-related sympathetic sudomotor dysfunction. Pain Digest 1993; 3:202–209.
47. Longmire DR. Sympathetic sudomotor testing in the clinical assessment of neuropathic pain. Pain Pract 2004:19–22.
48. Longmire DR, Woodley WE. Selective Tissue Conductance Meter, K874850A, Office of Device Evaluation, United States Department of Health and Human Services, Food and Drug Administration, 1988.
49. Longmire DR. An electrophysiological approach to the evaluation of regional sympathetic dysfunction: a proposed classification. Pain Physician 2007; 9:69–82.
50. Dyck PJ, Karnes J, O'Brien PC. Diagnosis, staging, and classification of diabetic neuropathy and association with other complications. In: Dyck PJ, Thomas PK, Asbury AK, eds. Diabetic Neuropathy. Philadelphia, PA: Saunders, 1987:36–44.
51. Thomas PK. Diabetic neuropathy: models, mechanisms and mayhem. Can J Neurol Sci 1992; 19:1–7.
52. Hilsted J, Low PA. Diabetic autonomic neuropathy. In: Low PA, ed. Clinical Autonomic Disorders: Evaluation and Management. Boston, MA: Little Brown & Company, 1993:423–443.
53. Lindblom U, Ochoa J. Somatosensory function and dysfunction. In: Asbury AK, McKhann GM, McDonald WI, eds. Diseases of the Nervous System: Clinical Neurobiology. 2nd ed. Philadelphia, PA: WB Saunders Co, 1992:213–228.

10

The Myofascial Pain Syndrome

Gary W. Jay

Clinical Disease Area Expert-Pain, Pfizer, Inc., New London, Connecticut, U.S.A.

The myofascial pain syndrome (MPS) has long been a clinical subject of interest as well as a diagnostic problem and dilemma. Historically, there have been many names for this clinical entity, which has led to a great deal of confusion. The older names included myofibrositis, myofascitis, fibromyositis, myogelosis, and fibrositis, to name a few. Fields (1) noted that many of the most common, persistent, and disabling pain problems are of musculoskeletal origin. He also noted that while the MPS was common, many therapists were unaware of its existence. Four years earlier, Travell and Simons (21) had published the criteria for diagnosing the MPS.

Unfortunately, the problem of the objectification and awareness of the MPS continues to the present day. The MPS is diagnostically challenging in that it has multiple guises, and many other clinical entities with supposedly specific diagnoses are actually secondary to the MPS.

THE DISORDER

The MPS has been defined by the International Association for the Study of Pain as a regional painful condition associated with the presence of trigger points (TRPs) (2). Myofascial trigger points (MTRPs) are loci of hyperirritability, which, when subjected to mechanical pressure, give rise to characteristic patterns of referred pain.

The MPS is a very common occurrence in pain clinic populations and may not be diagnostically straightforward. The diagnosis is basically a clinical one, as it is associated with normal radiological studies as well as having no diagnostic laboratory studies.

Yunus noted that one could not meaningfully study the etiology of a condition that is ill defined or nonspecific (3). Over the last decade, a great deal of clinical and scientific data have given greater definition to the MPS.

One study of 309 chronic pain patients revealed that the MPS with attendant TRPs was found in two-thirds of the patients and was found to be the most frequent clinical pain syndrome (4).

A more recent study found that there was general agreement across the specialties of pain management providers that the MPS was a legitimate diagnosis, with a high level of agreement regarding the signs and symptoms essential to or associated with the diagnosis of MPS (5).

Studies of the prevalence of the MPS have some difficulties when trying to compare them with each other. Specifically, differences in the criteria as well as the experience and skill of the examiners, along with different populations and variations of chronicity, can make diagnosis difficult.

The largest single tissue type in the body is skeletal muscle, which accounts for 50% of the body's weight (6). It should come as no surprise that substantial problems can be induced by difficulty in this system.

The term "myofascial pain syndrome" also appears to engender some confusion. Simons (7) notes that the term MPS has been used specifically with regard to a pain syndrome that is induced by TRPs found in the belly of a muscle, specifically, not scar, ligamentous or periosteal TRPs. The term has also been used generally to indicate many conditions that induce muscle pain without reference to and even in the absence of TRPs, making the MPS an ambiguous identifier. He suggests the use of the term "myofascial pain syndrome *due to trigger points*" to be more specific and the term "regional muscle pain syndrome" to be used as the more general term. It is thought that this is certainly correct—one of the major difficulties with the entire concept of MPS has been the lack of specifics relating to the diagnosis as well as the basic terminology of the disorder. In 1990, it was the Wolfe group (8) who developed specific criteria for the diagnosis of fibromyalgia. This has yet to be accomplished for the MPS with TRPs.

When reference is made to the MPS, in this chapter, it is specifically in reference to the myofascial pain syndrome with trigger points.

Clinically, the patient with an MPS may describe muscular pain, which is more frequently diffuse, but which can be localized. The attributes for this pain may be deep, dull, aching, and continuous. It is rare to have more neuropathic attributes such as burning, or vascular attributes such as throbbing.

The onset may be posttraumatic, following an acceleration/deceleration injury ("whiplash") or a slip and fall. It may begin insidiously, with the patient having worked at a desk on a computer for many hours or days. Many patients will report that they remember no inciting event. Indeed, as an MPS may be secondary to another medical problem, or even mimic another problem, its diagnosis may commonly be missed secondary to treatment of the purported primary problem (i.e., tooth pain which is secondary to referred pain from a MTRP).

Pain from MTRPs has been associated with tension-type headache and other forms of head and neck pain (9, 10). The ability to mimic other disorders has recently included a facial MPS, which presented as trigeminal neuralgia (11), as well as a subcutaneous TRP causing radiating postsurgical pain after dermatological surgery (referred pain extending down the arm ipsilateral to surgery secondary to a thoracic subcutaneous TRP) (12).

Aside from pain, other common complaints associated with an MPS may include muscle stiffness, fatigue, tenderness, weakness, sleep disorder, autonomic nervous system symptoms and even poor balance, dizziness, and ear pain (if more rostral musculature is affected).

When a patient is seen with a specific complaint, the differential diagnosis must include an MPS, if appropriate. More frequently, patients are referred to an ear, nose, and throat (ENT) specialist for complaints of ear pain or dizziness to which a full ENT workup can find no etiology. A great deal of time and money is spent before the TRPs in the sternocleidomastoid muscles, which can REFER these problems to the ear, are identified. Possibly, more common is the compliant of tooth pain (13), which leads to dental work, including tooth extraction, root canals, and more, with no effect. Referred pain from TRPs in the masseter and temporalis muscles are then identified.

DIAGNOSIS

A national survey of pain management providers found general agreement across specialists that MPS is a legitimate diagnosis that is distinct from the fibromyalgia syndrome (FMS). There was a high level of agreement regarding signs and symptoms essential to or associated with the diagnosis of MPS (14).

It has been noted that the MPS is seen more frequently in women than men, and it is most often seen in adults between the ages of 31 and 50, although TRPs have also been diagnosed in children and young adults (15, 16). Local and referred muscular pain from TRPs has been found to be a major factor in the majority of worker's compensation cases involving pain (17). Women, more frequently than men, appear to develop symptomatic myofascial pain (15).

To attain a correct diagnosis, a musculoskeletal examination should follow a general and neurological examination. This is what gives the most pertinent information regarding the presence or absence of an MPS. It is the author's preference to have a mirror in the examination room where the patient can use it to see what, if any, asymmetries are found.

The patient must be in a gown. You can then easily observe any physical asymmetries, such as finding one shoulder or one hip elevated. You can show this to the patients, who need to be educated from the start as to what is going on with them. Without such education, it is difficult for most patients to "just do what the doctor tells them." Patients read a lot and do a great deal of Internet surfing and read up on what they think or have been told their diagnosis is, and you must be prepared to show your patients exactly what findings cause you to make the diagnosis of an MPS.

Have the patient perform active cervical range of motion (ROM), or lumbosacral ROM in front of the mirror. Many of the patients have no prior idea how decreased their ROM may be.

As your patient, prior to the examination, should have drawn a pain picture which included the areas of pain, as well as numbness and tingling and/or weakness, you start with a good idea of where to look during the examination. However, the clinician must remember that when dealing with TRPs, the place you are initially looking at may be a zone of reference for the TRP(s) causing their chief complaint.

Pain is, after all, whatever the patient says it is. It is a symptom, not a diagnosis. It is up to the clinician, pain management specialist or not, to determine what the patient is talking about.

Therefore, the musculoskeletal examination must be as thorough as possible, with more care, if necessary, being given to the area of the origin of pain or etiology.

Recent research indicates that there is only modest genetic influence on the development of chronic musculoskeletal pain (18).

Pain related to chronic MPSs can induce disability from not only the attributes of the pain, but also from depression, sleep disturbances, other psychological and behavioral problems, and physical deconditioning secondary to lack of exercise (19).

Fricton et al. (20) studied 164 patients with the MPS and found that the mean duration of their pain was 5.8 years for men and 6.9 years for women, with an average of 4.5 clinicians having been seen in the past for their complaints of pain. This characterization of these patients has not changed in the years since Fricton's study was published.

TRP Examination

How does one go about finding a TRP, which is typically 2 to 5 mm in size? There are several techniques that can be utilized to go about this task.

Firstly, the patient must be warm and comfortable. If the patient is in a cold examination room, the general musculature will become tense, and a TRP examination may be futile. Secondly, the fingernails on the examiner's hands must be short, so as to avoid scrapping the patient's skin.

Flat palpation is the best way to begin, particularly, in large and smaller muscles that can be palpated from only one side. The fingers are slightly bent, with the fingertips perpendicular to the palm. The patient may be sitting or lying prone. The skin above the region of the suspected TRP is pushed to one side, and the fingertips slowly traverse the area. If the patient is warm and the muscle is relaxed, a taut band may be easily palpated, and the trigger point, likewise, is easily palpated. If the movement of the fingers is done too quickly (snapping palpation), it is likely to obtain a local twitch response (LTR), which is painful.

Pincer palpation can be used in muscles such as the sternocleidomastoid, which can be grasped between the thumb on one side of the muscle and the fingers on the other. A taut band can be palpated, as can the TRP, as the muscle is rolled between the fingers. This is helpful for obtaining a more discrete palpatory picture of the taut band and any TRPs. As the muscle is released from between the fingers, an LTR may be obtained.

Another important diagnostic exercise is to press directly over an active TRP, which may lead to the development/demonstration of referred pain. The pain should refer to the same place each time a specific TRP is compressed. It is helpful to know the typical TRP referral patterns found for different TRPs. This information is available in the superb "bible" of myofascial pain written by Travell and Simons (21, 22).

Pain related to MTRPs may be aggravated by pressure directly on the TRP; sustained and/or repeated contraction of the involved muscle; passively stretching the muscle; strenuous use of the muscle, particularly when it is in the shortened position; placing the involved muscle in a shortened position for prolonged period of time; and exposure to cold and drafts. MTRP pain may be decreased by short period of rest, moist heat applied directly to the TRP, slowly and passively stretching the involved muscles, short periods of light activity with movement, and by specific myofascial treatment (22).

Painful rolling of the skin is also frequently found.

Depending on the location of active TRPs, patients may develop a number of nonpainful symptoms of MTRPs. These may include pilomotor activity ("goose flesh"), changes in sudomotor activity (sweating), excessive lacrimation, and other autonomic signs and symptoms such as vasoconstriction causing one limb or region to appear "colder" to palpation, as well as dizziness. Dermatographia is the term for using the fingernail or a pencil to write or draw on the skin and, then, observe the areas become red and raised. This is seen most commonly on the skin over musculature affected by active TRPs, particularly over the muscles of the back, shoulders, neck, and torso. Depression and sleep disorders are also commonly seen.

Clinical accuracy in the determination of TRPs is not as easy as it sounds. Hsieh et al. (23) looked at the interrater reliability of the palpation of TRPs in the trunk, using as his examination group physiatrists and chiropractors. They were attempting to determine the interrater reliability of palpation of three characteristics of TRPs, the taut band, LTR, and referred pain. It was concluded that TRP palpation was not reliable for detecting taut bands and LTRs, but marginally reliable for referred pain, after training both physiatrists and chiropractors.

In another study, looking at the reliability of examination of patients with myofascial pain, chronic fibromyalgia and controls, both dolorimetry (algometry) and palpation were of sufficient reliability to discriminate control patients from patients with myofascial pain and fibromyalgia, but could not discriminate between patients with myofascial pain and fibromyalgia (24).

Gerwin et al. (25) reported two studies in which examiners looked at the distinctive features of the MPS, including a TRP in a taut band of muscle, the LTR, patterns of referred pain characteristic of specific TRPs, and the reproduction of the patient's pain during examination. In the first study, the attempt to establish interrater reliability failed. The second study by the same examiners included a training period, first, and was successful at establishing interrater reliability. Interestingly, while present, interrater reliability varied among the different features of the MPS.

More recently, Myburgh et al. (26) performed a review of the literature demonstrating reproducibility of manual palpation of TRPs and found the methodological quality of the majority of studies to be generally poor.

The importance of specific training as well as experience in the determination of the various aspects of the MPS, including taut bands and TRPs, is, therefore, not to be underestimated.

Differential Diagnosis of MTRPs and Other Disorders

Herniated disks in the cervical region may be assumed to cause arm pain that is secondary to TRPs in the supraspinatus and infraspinatus muscles. Cervical arthritis may also be a part of the differential diagnosis.

TRPs in the upper rectus abdominis musculature as well as the thoracic paravertebral muscles can cause mid back pain, frequently mimicking disk disease or herniation. Low back pain may be secondary to the lower aspects of the rectus abdominis muscles as well as the thoracolumbar paraspinal muscles. The piriformis muscle may also induce sciatic pain that may be assumed to be secondary to a herniated lumbar disk. Pain down the lateral aspect of the lower extremities may be diagnosed as a herniated disk; however, the presence of TRPs in the gluteus medius, tensor fascia, and even the gastrocnemius muscles must be evaluated.

The clinician should look for TRPs *after* performing an appropriate examination and performing spinal MRIs and/or electromyogram (EMG)/nerve conduction studies (NCVs). While TRPs are common, clinicians must first rule out other clinical causes of a problem. A caveat is that many times patients with a herniated disk(s) will also have a MPS with TRPs referring pain. Clinicians should first deal with the problem that may cause the most severe pathological difficulties. This does not mean that all patients with a herniated disk need to have surgery first. In fact, it may be clinically more appropriate to treat these patients conservatively with physical therapy (PT) and TRP injections. Clinically, it has been found that these patients may not need surgery over 80% of the time. The neurological indications that would mandate surgery include muscle weakness and atrophy, reflex changes and sensory changes including chronic, intractable pain. If clinicians can ameliorate the pain, and there are no other neurological abnormalities (even in the presence of a diminution of a reflex, not an absence), the need for surgery may be prevented for quite a while, if not be obviated.

Endocrine Disorders Associated with Myofascial Pain

It is not uncommon to find dozens of patients who present with muscle pain, spasm, and TRPs that are secondary to a primary endocrine disorder. The two most common are hypothyroidism and menopause. It is a good practice to perform a confirmatory laboratory test, and if clinical suspicions are correct, send the patient to an endocrinologist.

Some of the most common endocrine problems associated with myofascial pain include the following.

Hypothyroidism: secondary to a lack of thyroid hormone production [levothyroxine (T_4) and liothyronine (T_3)] secondary to a problem with the hypothalamic–pituitary–thyroid (HPT) axis. Clinically, patients are frequently overweight. Their eyelids may be puffy, their voice hoarse. The thyroid gland may be enlarged. Their muscles are stiff, tender, and, on occasion, weak. They may display muscle hypertrophy. TRPs are common. Their primary complaint may be diffuse muscle tenderness. The Achilles reflex may show delayed relaxation. Laboratory testing typically shows low serum thyroxine (T_4), free thyroxine index, and a high thyroid-stimulating hormone (TSH) level.

The most common complaints found in *hyperthyroidism* include muscle weakness and pain, TRPs, heat intolerance, increased sweating, thinning hair, increased appetite, emotional/mental difficulties, and sexual dysfunction. The physical findings may reveal a goiter, proptosis, loss of convergence, lid lag, increased deep tendon reflexes tachycardia, cardiac arrhythmias, and a fine, fast tremor of the hands/fingers. Laboratory findings include high levels of T_3, T_4, and free thyroxine index. The TSH is typically low.

Menopause, secondary to estrogenic insufficiency, may be difficult for the patient and associated with myofascial pain and TRPs, sweats, and "hot flashes." On occasion, muscle pain and/or joint pain may be the primary complaints. Associated symptoms may include anxiety, weakness, depression, emotional difficulties, and loss of libido. All of these symptoms typically improve with exogenous estrogen replacement.

"Male menopause," secondary to significant decreases in serum testosterone, may be associated with myofascial pain and TRPs, along with weakness and depression. Exogenous testosterone may relieve these symptoms.

Muscle weakness, wasting, spasm, and pain are frequently associated with *Cushing's disease* [secondary to an adrenocorticotropic hormone (ACTH) secreting tumor of the pituitary, with associated adrenal hyperplasia] as well as *Cushing's syndrome* (secondary to a primary adrenal tumor or ectopic production of ACTH). Other signs and symptoms include female facial hirsutism, round, red facies, purple abdominal striae, thin skin with easy bruising, thinning scalp hair, and osteoporosis. Hypertension and mild diabetes mellitus along with affective changes and spinal fractures (secondary to osteoporosis) may also be seen. Laboratory testing shows elevation of a 24-hour urinary free cortisol level, as well as a high morning plasma cortisol. Treatment includes surgical removal of the tumor and chemotherapy.

Primary adrenal insufficiency, or *Addison's disease,* may present with muscle pain, spasm or, on occasion, knee contractures. It can be associated with increased skin pigmentation on examination, low blood pressure, orthostatic hypotension, weakness, and cachexia. Laboratory testing can demonstrate abnormalities of the electrolytes, as well as an increased serum ACTH.

Pituitary–adrenal insufficiency typically is found to be caused by adrenal atrophy secondary to tumor, hemorrhage or even infarction of the pituitary. The presenting symptoms not infrequently include myofascial pain and TRPs. The examination should show poor muscle development, weakness, testicular atrophy, loss of libido, and an eunuchoid appearance.

Hypoparathyroidism, secondary to surgical damage or removal (or by spontaneous causation), may be associated with acute muscle spasms and even tetany secondary to decreased serum calcium. *Hyperparathyroidism* is associated with an increased level of serum calcium, secondary to increased serum parathyroid hormone. Muscle weakness, or myopathy, may be secondary to elevated calcium.

Perpetuating Factors

Once a myofascial pain syndrome with TRPs has manifested, there are a number of things that may perpetuate the syndrome. It is important to identify these mechanical and/or systemic problems and deal with them appropriately.

Mechanical factors may include tight collars, tight brassiere straps, carrying heavy purses or bags over the shoulders, compressing the hamstring muscle by the hard edges of chairs, and ergonomic problems associated with work, such as having a computer monitor that is too high, or a keyboard that is not properly placed or too difficult for a patient to utilize comfortably. These issues are relatively simple to correct. Ergonomic issues may be dealt with via an occupational therapist.

Postural abnormalities must be identified and corrected.

Other common problems include inherent structural inadequacies, such as the short leg syndrome (one leg shorter than another) and a small hemipelvis (secondary to an asymmetry in the height of the two halves of the pelvis).

Systemic perpetuating factors include endocrine or metabolic factors (discussed above), folic acid deficiency, and low iron levels. Muscle can also be stressed and show impaired healing secondary to toxic, inflammatory, and nutritional difficulties.

Chronic muscle pain associated with exercise intolerance may not be secondary to MPS (or even FMS). The differential diagnosis of the problem may include Lyme disease, deficiencies of vitamin D or even a mutation in the cytochrome b gene of mitochondrial DNA (mtDNA) (27, 28).

Psychological stressors are of equal importance in terms of perpetuating a myofascial problem. While the other perpetuating factors noted in this section may be found on examination or via laboratory testing, psychological problems may not "come out" easily, as a patient may have no understanding of the ability of such problems to be part of a *psychophysiological* muscle pain problem. This is one important reason for the utilization of an interdisciplinary treatment team that may be needed to deal with chronic myofascial, and other forms, of chronic pain.

The presence of unidentified psychological/psychophysiological factors will undermine appropriate treatment, and if unidentified, they will continue the patients' cycles of continued pain in spite of appropriate diagnosis and treatment of a physical problem such as an MPS. The "entire patient" must be treated, physically, mentally, and emotionally. Pain is, after all, a biopsychosocial problem.

PATHOPHYSIOLOGY

The *Neuromuscular Junction* is a synapse that depends on acetylcholine (ACh) as its main neurotransmitter. The nerve terminal receives energy via an action potential from the α-motoneuron, which opens the voltage gated calcium channels. Ionized calcium moves through these channels from the synaptic cleft into the nerve terminal. These channels are found on both sides of the nerve membrane, which releases packets of ACh in response to the ionized calcium. The production of packets of ACh is via a process which uses energy that is supplied by the mitochondria located in the nerve terminal.

When many packets of ACh are released essentially simultaneously, the amount of ACh overwhelms the cholinesterase (which metabolizes ACh) in the synaptic cleft and the ACh crosses the cleft and reaches the postjunctional membrane of the muscle fiber where the ACh receptors are found. The cholinesterase in the synaptic cleft will metabolize the ACh, which will end its action. This allows the synapse to again respond to another action potential.

When large numbers of vesicles of ACh are released simultaneously in response to an action potential that arrives at the nerve terminal, the postjunctional membrane is depolarized enough for it to reach its threshold for excitation. This will initiate an action potential that will be propagated by the surface membrane, the sarcolemma, throughout the specific muscle fiber.

The motor endplates link the terminal nerve fiber of a motoneuron to a muscle fiber. The endplate zone is the region where motor endplates innervate the fibers of the muscle, also called the motor points.

Myogelosis, an older term, describes small, typically circumscribed areas of firmness and tenderness to palpation found in a muscle or muscles associated with a patient's complaints of pain. This term is essentially synonymous with MTRPs. The focal tenderness, taut bands of muscle and nodules described in patients with myogelosis are also found to be associated with MTRPs.

A *taut band* is a grouping of tense muscle fibers that extend from a MTRP to the muscle's attachments. There are three associated features, including the absence of motor unit action potentials; severe, highly localized tenderness in the taut band at the MTRP; and the quick release of the taut band and MTRP associated tenderness by the inactivation of the TRP. Simons and Travell (21) felt that a local contracture, which was associated with nonelectrical, endogenous shortening of the sarcomere, was secondary to a local energy crisis in the muscle. They postulated that the energy crises would be secondary to the increased metabolic demand of the contractured sarcomeres in the presence of ischemia-induced hypoxia secondary to vigorous sustained contraction. This energy crisis would induce sensitization of contiguous nociceptors (29).

Gerwin reiterates that the entire muscle is not hard or in spasm; the tenderness is present over the hardened, taut band (27).

Simons noted shortened sarcomeres in the region of the MTRP with compensatory lengthening of sarcomeres (one of the repeating structural units of striated muscle fibrils) in the same fibers continuing to their attachments. This was associated with an expanded diameter of the shortened sarcomeres in the area of the MTRP with contiguous thinning of the fiber diameters beyond the MTRP, which was related to the increased firmness to palpation of the MTRP, itself (29, 30).

One of the clinical diagnostic criteria of an MTRP, the taut band, can also be found in patients without TRPs (31). This finding raises the question of whether a symptomatic MTRP represents an additional spread and "propagation" of TRP pathology from several contraction knots to more extensive involvement of more muscle fibers (22). The MPS in a single muscle with MTRPs may "metastasize" to involve other muscles which are both contiguous as well as in other regions of the body.

Active loci are multiple minute regions that exhibit spontaneous electrical activity (SEA), with endplate noise, in an MTRP that may be associated with spike activity characteristic of single fiber action potentials on electromyography. It was recognized that some of the endplates in MTRPs were abnormal, as the SEA was abnormal and resulted from an enormously increased release of ACh (29). It was noted by Simons that the active loci occurred predominantly in MTRPs and were the central dysfunction in the MTRP, and were also scattered among normal endplates throughout the MTRP (32). In humans, it was found that active loci are four times more common in TRPs than in the endplate zone outside of a TRP. Also, no active loci were found in the taut band outside of the endplate zone. The SEA type of auditory endplate electrical activity is related to MTRPs (22).

The electromyographic evidence has been variously interpreted, but it is thought by Simons that excessive ACh will induce increased and continuous electrical activity that produces a contraction knot (see below) (22). This will also create a higher voltage endplate potential which would be more readily detectable, and much more of the endplate region would be continuously active, electrically, not active intermittently at a few isolated miniscule locations. A contraction knot would increase the target size of the EMG needle. Normal miniature endplate potentials are more difficult to obtain (22).

An important feature of MTRPs, *Contraction Knots,* appeared on biopsy of dog muscle to be thick, enlarged, round muscle fibers with extremely contracted sarcomeres with corresponding swelling of the contiguous muscle fiber. Human biopsy showed on electronmicroscopy an excess of muscle A-band and lack of the I-band, on cross section. It was noted that the complete replacement of the I-band by the A-band only occurs in fully contracted sarcomeres (29).

The *LTR* is obtained by mechanical stimulation of an MTRP in a taut band of muscle. It is a transient, fast contraction of the palpable taut band of muscle fibers associated with an MTRP. The LTR may be provoked by mechanical/palpatory impact to the affected muscle, via needle penetration of the TRP and by snapping palpation of the TRP (see below) (33, 34). The LTR is a confirmatory clinical sign. Upon injection into an MTRP, the LTR is seen and this is indicative that the injection should be clinically effective. The LTR is typically and extremely painful when elicited, and it is a strong indication of the presence of an MTRP.

The relationship between the elicitation of a painful LTR from successful needling or injection of a TRP suggests that it may originate from stimulation of sensitized nociceptors in the region of the MTRP (35). The α-motoneurons associated with endplates with excessive ACh release appear to be responsive to the strong sensory spinal input from these sensitized nociceptors. Snapping palpation may induce an LTR in both the TRP palpated, as well as in the taut band of another muscle close by (22).

A patient who lost the LTR after a brachial plexus injury, which resulted in total loss of nerve conduction, was found to recover the LTR on EMG associated with the recovery of nerve conduction (36). This is consistent with rabbit literature that shows the LTR to be a direct spinal reflex (34).

Myofascial Trigger Points (MTRPs)

MTRPs are small, hyperirritable foci in muscles and fascia which are most typically found in a taut band of skeletal (striated) muscle. They can also be found in ligaments, tendons, skin, joint capsule, and periosteum. They may be localized to a single muscle or found in multiple muscle groups. When pressure is directed onto the active TRP, a local or referred pain pattern is obtained. The referred pain pattern will be consistent for a specific TRP. The "zone of reference" is the region of referred pain in an area distant from the TRP. Patients may also perceive paresthesias or numbness in the zone of reference. Compression of a latent TRP may also induce pain.

The areas of referred pain are not consistent with myotomal, dermatomal, or sclerotomal patterns. Kellgren's work (37) found this consistency after studying the specificity of muscular and ligamentous pain secondary to muscular injections of 0.1 to 0.3 mL of hypertonic saline.

Referred pain does tend to be segmental, in that the referred pain patterns are typically located in sites innervated by nearby or adjacent spinal cord segments (27).

A TRP may be formed, or activated, secondary to mechanical problems from muscle overload, which can be acute, sustained or repetitive. Nerve compression that can induce obvious neuropathic electromyographic changes is associated with an increased number of active MTRPs.

In summary, TRPs may be directly activated by work overload, muscle overwork fatigue, direct trauma, and radiculopathy (38). Indirect TRP activation can occur via other existing TRPs, visceral disease, joint dysfunctions, arthritic joints, and by stress/emotional distress (22).

There are six different classifications of TRPs (22):

Active MTRP is tender and, with direct compression, produces referred pain as well as referred motor phenomena and may induce autonomic phenomena; induces tenderness in the pain reference zone; it will mediate, after appropriate stimulation, an LTR; it is associated with a taut band of muscle; and other associated phenomena include muscle shortening, weakness, and decreased ROM (22).

Latent MTRP is painful only when directly palpated/compressed, but may have all the other clinical characteristics of an active TRP, including decreased ROM of the muscle, weakness, and muscle shortening. Referred pain is typically not seen (22). Of interest is the determination that nociceptive stimulation of latent TRPs can induce muscle cramping (39).

Primary MTRP is centrally located in the muscle; typically activated by an acute or chronic muscle work overload, or by repetitive overuse of the muscle in which it occurs; it is not secondary to TRP activity in another muscle (22).

Key MTRP is responsible for activating one or more satellite TRPs in its zone of reference; inactivation will also inactivate associated satellite TRPs (22).

Satellite MTRP is centrally located in the muscle; induced via mechanical or neurogenic stimulation by the activity of a key TRP; inactivated when the key TRP is inactivated; may be found in the key TRPs zone of reference, in an overloaded synergist that is substituting for the muscle in which the key TRP is found, in an antagonist muscle countering the increased tension of the key muscle, or in a muscle linked neurogenically to the key TRP (22).

Attachment TRP is found at the musculotendinous junction and/or where the muscle attaches to the bone; this induces an *enthesopathy* (see below) secondary to unrelieved tension/relative spasm of the taut band produced by a central TRP (22).

Enthesopathy is typically a well-circumscribed area of pain or tenderness found in the specific regions of muscle attachment: musculotendinous junctions or where tendons and ligaments attach to bone. This differs from the more diffuse TRP referred pain that may not be well localized. Enthesopathy may develop into *enthesitis*, which is typically posttraumatic in nature, found at muscle insertions, and can be associated, with continued muscle stress, with fibrosis and calcification (22).

The central MTRP is found at the center of muscle fibers and is associated with dysfunctional endplates in the motor endplate zone. Contraction knots cause the nodular findings on examination. Both local and referred pain are secondary to sensitized nociceptors via a local energy crisis. Finally, tension from contraction knots causes the taut band beyond the palpable nodule. These TRPs differ greatly in etiology from attachment TRPs, which are found in the attachment zone secondary to taut muscle band tension. An associated inflammatory reaction causes palpable induration, and local and referred pain are secondary to nociceptors sensitized by persistent taut band tension. The taut band at the attachment TRP is secondary to contraction knots in the central TRP.

Active TRPs may spontaneously convert to latent TRPs, and vice versa. Both active and latent TRPs can induce increased muscle tension, shortening of the muscle, and decreased ROM. These finding are most typically made on examination, as pain is the patients' primary complaint when active TRPs are palpated. Weakness is also seen, as the patient uses other, noninvolved muscles to perform routine tasks—while pain is a frequent complaint, latent TRPs which do not produce spontaneous pain may also cause weakness.

Shah and his group (39, 40) have found biochemical changes at the center of the TRP consisting of increased levels of calcitonin-gene–related peptide (CGRP), substance P, norepinephrine (NEP), interleukin 1 and 6, and tumor necrosis factor-α, all in association with a low pH of 3.0 to 4.0.

Trigger Point (TRP) Hypothesis

A TRP consists of many microscopic abnormal regions in extrafusal skeletal muscle fibers. The MPS with associated MTRPs is a *Neuromuscular Disease*.

As noted by Simon et al. (22), the integrated pathophysiology of an MTRP would include the following:

1. Excessive production and release of ACh at the myoneural junction (motor nerve terminal) during rest.
2. Association with sustained depolarization of the postjunctional membrane of the associated muscle fiber.
   a. Also associated with endplate noise (SEA).
3. Continued depolarization induces first a release of calcium ions that are not reabsorbed into the sarcoplasmic reticulum (SR), which then induces more and more extra SR calcium which is associated with continued sarcomere contracture, or shortening.
4. Continuous contractures inducing an increased need for energy at the site, which is further aggravated by the compression/constriction of small blood vessels by the continuous muscular contracture in the region, which will further increase an *energy crisis* by prohibiting appropriate oxygen and nutrients to flow from these vessels.
5. Increased demand for energy in the region (the MTRP) that has an impaired energy supply.
6. Release of algetic, sensitizing substances that would effect the autonomic, nociceptive, and nonnociceptive sensory nerves in the region, which, in turn, would increase production of ACh from the associated nerve endings.
7. Local sensitization from the algetic chemicals which would lead to sensitization of the associated spinal cord dorsal horn region, inducing continuous nociceptive impulses, which are sent rostrally.
   a. The spinal cord sensitization becomes self-sustaining, over time, secondary to continuous peripheral nociceptive information from the MTRP.
8. The continued release of algetic substances, which can contribute to the continued over-release of ACh from the nerve terminal, induces a vicious cycle of energy crisis, release of algetic substances, and release of more ACh.

In an extension of this hypothesis by Gerwin et al. (41), it is thought that muscle activity secondary to significant muscle stress which leads to muscle injury and capillary constriction is the initiating event. The muscle injury will induce a release of algetic substances, which stimulate muscle nociceptors. Sympathetic nervous system activation occurs in the evolving pathological state. Ischemia occurs from capillary contraction from the muscle contraction and causes hypoperfusion. The regional pH becomes acidic, which will inhibit acetylcholine-esterase (AChE). CGRP, which is released from nociceptors in the injured muscle, will also inhibit AChE, increases ACh release and up-regulates cholinergic receptors. This cascade leads to increased cholinergic activity with increased sarcomere hypercontraction, the formation of taut bands and increased frequency of miniature endplate potentials.

A Confluence of the Pathophysiological and the Clinical
It appears that tenderness and referred pain related to chronic musculoskeletal pain may well result from peripheral and central sensitization, which can then be instrumental in transitioning acute to chronic pain.

The fact that chronic musculoskeletal pain is associated with central sensitization has been noted in several recent studies including chronic whiplash-related pain (42, 43) and other forms of chronic myofascial pain (44–46).

It has also been noted that patients with referred hyperalgesia had experienced pain for at least six years, while patients in pain for six months had not developed hyperalgesia (47). Teleologically, it would take time for constant nociceptive input to induce central sensitization. Widespread musculoskeletal pain commonly begins with localized pain described as deep, also indicating that the development of central sensitization occurs over time (48).

Other studies appear to have found a relationship between the development of central sensitization and the number of clinically palpable TRPs in myofascial pain (49, 50). It is also noted that in the presence of central sensitization, low-intensity input could induce pain when a possible latent trigger point is activated; this may also indicate at least one causal relationship between a localized painful condition and its spread or development of generalized pain (48).

Sympathetic Aspects of Myofascial Pain

Referred pain from TRPs may be mediated by any of the four experimentally postulated mechanisms: (*i*) Convergence-projection, in which pain may be initiated by muscle nociceptors but then referred to another area served by other somatic receptors which converge on the same region of the spinothalamic tract. (*ii*) Convergence-facilitation in which impulses from one somatic zone are facilitated or amplified in the spinal cord by other activity originating in nociceptors from a TRP in another area of the body. (*iii*) Peripheral branching of primary afferent nociceptors in which the brain may misinterpret activity from nociceptors in one part of the body as originating from nerves coming from another part of the body. (*iv*) The last more relevant hypothesis is that of the sympathetic modulation of peripheral nociceptors including increased sympathetic modulation of peripheral nociceptors inducing increased sympathetic activity that causes an increase in substances which sensitize primary afferent nerve receptors in the area of referred pain as well as the site of initial peripheral sensitization. There are clinical correlations of this hypothesis, making it more clinically factual, which will be discussed below (63).

Sympathetically Maintained Pain

Sympathetically maintained pain, as described by Roberts (51), may begin after even minor soft-tissue or peripheral nerve trauma. The initial nociceptive impulses are transmitted via the unmyelinated C fibers to the Rexed layers in the dorsal horns, where they stimulate fibers of the wide-dynamic-range neurons and induce hypersensitivity in that region. The wide-dynamic-range neurons also become sensitized, or more responsive to all subsequent afferent stimuli.

Over time, the wide-dynamic-range neurons will continue to give a vigorous response to mechanical input from A-fiber mechanoreceptors. This may cause touch, or movement hypersensitivity or pain (allodynia). The wide-dynamic-range neurons are also directly connected to the lateral horn cells, which enervate sympathetic structures in the periphery. Studies documenting these concepts appear to explain the sometimes extreme sensitivity found in involved tissues, including nodularity (TRPs) found in painful myofascial areas, as well as vasomotor changes (14, 52–54).

The hypersensitivity reaction may also be induced in the area of trauma if nerves are injured. Compensatory pain and vasomotor symptoms of complex regional pain syndrome (CRPS, previously called reflex sympathetic dystrophy, or RSD) are dependent on local levels of NEP, which fluctuate, in part, by stress-induced increased sympathetic release of NEP (55). It has also been noted that the same increased response of the sympathetic nervous system occurs in the presence of uncontrolled stress, along with increased plasma ACTH (56).

A more recent study found that sympathetic vasoconstrictor activity is fully activated by painful stimulation of MTRPs (57).

Sympathetically Maintained Pain and the MPS

From the two entities, sympathetically maintained pain and the MPS, it is clinically possible, if not probable, that the multitudes of patients with soft-tissue injuries leading to MPSs who do not recover within a short period of time (1–3 months) of appropriate PT may have developed secondary sympathetically maintained pain.

Research data indicate that some receptors in skin and skeletal muscle can be influenced by sympathetic activity. It appears that the sympathetic influence on muscle receptors is functional in pathological states, but *not* under normal physiological conditions (58).

It has also been established that, with prolonged afferent input, central mechanisms may lead to skeletal muscle motor reactions, autonomic reactions, and distorted sensory phenomena including paresthesias and neurogenic pain (58).

Motoneurons, after changes in stimulation, may induce abnormal activity in thin myelinated and unmyelinated afferents from skeletal muscle and tendons, secondary to uncoordinated and tonic contraction (59).

Sympathetically maintained pain in many patients is not associated with tissue dysfunction (14, 60). It has been suggested that signs of sympathetic dystrophy seen in sympathetically maintained pain result from disuse atrophy and extreme muscular guarding behaviors, not sympathetic hyperfunction (61). Over time, the painful areas of sympathetically maintained pain do not expand (62).

Patients with the MPS also develop and maintain abnormal, guarded postures to prevent muscle stretch-induced pain. They also experience the expansion of the area of pain, secondary to this guarding, and the development of adjacent muscle spasm, pain and TRPs, which are associated with sympathetically maintained pain.

Other aspects of the MPS may be explained by sympathetically maintained pain, including painful skin rolling; hypersensitivity of the skin and muscles to touch and pressure; vasomotor changes including pallor, hyperemia, subjective coldness, and hyperhidrosis; and the marked central and neuropharmacological reactions to emotional stress.

Patients with the MPS also exhibit significant sleep abnormalities, typically an alpha intrusion into stage 4 sleep, also seen in asymptomatic patients with significant emotional stress, as well as depression. Serotonin and NEP are implicated in sleep pathophysiology and in depression.

The emotional or stress-related aspects noted above as possibly etiologic in the establishment of sympathetically maintained pain and/or CRPS are also frequently noted in patients with the MPS. As many of these patients experience trauma such as a motor vehicle accident, anxiety, fear, and stress, as well as the possible development of the posttraumatic stress disorder, emotional difficulties are prevalent. These admittedly situational stressors related to the trauma may be amplified by the loss of material goods, continued pain, loss of work, and, therefore, income as well as litigation, making them apparent "setups" for the development of sympathetically maintained pain.

Clinically speaking, how can the diagnoses of these two entities be differentiated? First, on examination the clinician will see painful skin rolling; dermatographia; hyperhidrosis, particularly on sudomotor, or sweat testing; and, on the face, scleral injection; lacrimation; ipsilateral rhinorrhea; even a partial Horner's syndrome, with ptosis and meiosis, but not anhidrosis. Further examination of the skin may reveal flushing over the painful areas, with associated warmth, and extreme sensitivity to palpation.

Also, treatment shows the various diagnoses. In cases of obvious myofascial pain with TRPs associated with CRPS, for example, a sympathetic block will decrease the pain, but not the elements of the MPS, which can then be treated appropriately with an excellent outcome.

TREATMENT

Conservative Care
Only after the clinical diagnosis of MPS has been made, and the physician has ruled out any endocrinopathies or other primary problems, can the patient begin therapy.

Patients who are injured (in a motor vehicle accident, slip and fall, or other injury) should be evaluated earlier rather than later. Initial examination must rule out spinal cord/nerve root problems, with an MRI performed if needed. In the presence of a nerve or nerve root injury, it will take at least three weeks before the EMG/NCV is positive from the acute injury. Examination should be neurologically and orthopedically within normal limits.

Palpable muscle spasm with associated tenderness is typically found. MPS with MTRPs does not immediately (most of the time) follow acute soft-tissue pain frequently given the acute diagnosis of cervical, thoracic, or lumbosacral strain/sprain.

However, not infrequently MTRPs and taut bands may be found in the patient with acute soft-tissue pain, but they may frequently have been preexisting (or of insidious onset) and may act as a physiological "setup" for the acute soft-tissue pain disorder, extending the injury and making it more severe.

The most conservative treatment approach is the initial use of medication. Acute muscle relaxants will not affect a preexisting MPS, nor will a nonsteroidal anti-inflammatory drug (NSAID). However, in the presence of an acute soft-tissue injury, these medications may be helpful. A simple muscle relaxant (see below) such as methocarbamol, metaxalone, or chlorzoxazone may be prescribed with the patients' understanding that they must be taken as directed to obtain a therapeutic plasma level.

NSAIDs such as ketoprofen or ibuprofen should be used to help a patient maintain their ability to function, as bed rest is not a beneficial treatment.

It may take at least 48 hours after a traumatic injury for the patients' resulting soft-tissue pain to maximize. This should be explained to them.

In cases of severe soft-tissue trauma, physical therapy (PT) may be necessary within a week of injury, when the initial tenderness has possibly remitted to some degree. The purpose of PT is to decrease edema, spasm and pain, and improve muscle pain/spasm and joint ROM.

Patients with MTRPs may need trigger point injections (TPIs). See *Chronic Pain* (63), chapter 7, in regards to the techniques of TPIs.

The majority of patients can be placed on appropriate medications, taught the appropriate muscle stretching exercises and, within several weeks, regain their preinjury status.

The most important reason to make the correct diagnosis and perform appropriate treatment as early as possible is to prevent the development of chronicity. Ten percent to fifteen percent of these patients may utilize/need 80% or more of the health care dollars needed to treat these then simple acute and subacute MPS conditions.

After the onset of MPS, pre- and/or postsoft-tissue injury, the development of chronicity may stem from (*i*) poor/inaccurate diagnosis; (*ii*) too much time passing prior to beginning care; (*iii*) poorly done PT; (*iv*) inappropriately recommended bed rest for days to weeks; (*v*) ignorance of the medical diagnosis of MPS; and (*vi*) iatrogenic overutilization of narcotic analgesics. After initial, acute trauma, narcotics may be used if needed to enable maintenance of function, for a 7- to 10-day period.

When patients with a chronic MPS are seen, prior to initiating treatment, they should be evaluated for depression, anxiety disorder, iatrogenic medication overutilization, and their psychosocial milieu must be detailed to enable the development of a full, appropriate individualized, interdisciplinary pain management program (63).

To hope to successfully provide therapy for the chronic MPS patient, all of the identified clinical-organic, psychological and psychosocial aspects of their pain problem must be treated simultaneously; most appropriately, in a full program provided under one roof.

The various aspects of treatment of MPS are as follows:

Medications

Simple analgesics are discussed in detail in chapter 2. They include aspirin and acetaminophen. These medications are frequently sold in combination with other drugs such as caffeine, which exerts no specific analgesic effects but may potentiate the analgesic effects of aspirin and acetaminophen. There are aspirin-caffeine combination drugs (Anacin) and aspirin, acetaminophen and caffeine combinations (Excedrin Extra-Strength, Excedrin Migraine and Vanquish). The recommended dosage is two tablets every six hours as needed.

The biggest problem is that taking aspirin, acetaminophen, or combination tablets daily or even every other day for a week or more (possibly less) can induce the problem of analgesic rebound headache (now called medication overuse headache, or MOH).

NSAIDs can be used, and include (see chap. 2)

- Ibuprofen
- Anaprox
- Ketoprofen

- Ketorolac
- Celecoxib

Muscle relaxants, also covered in detail in chapter 2, may be used, and include, for acute muscle spasm

- Carisoprodol
- Chlorzoxazone
- Metaxalone
- Methocarbamol
- Orphenadrine

For continued spasm (after 3 weeks), a trial of either of the following may be helpful. (See chap. 2 for details.)

- Clonazepam
- Tizanidine (64)

Antidepressant medications (ADMs) are also very useful, particularly the tricyclic antidepressants for pain, and if the patient feels denervated, selective serotonin reuptake inhibitors (SSRIs).

The TCA medication of choice is amitriptyline, a sedating tricyclic antidepressant. Like all of the tricyclics, it works in the synapse to decrease reuptake of serotonin and, (depending on the individual medication), NEP. Amitriptyline, unlike the other TCAs, also works to repair the damage in stage 4 sleep architecture. It is the most sedating tricyclic. The typical dosage is between 10 and 50 mg at night. The author has found it rare to need more than 20 or 30 mg at night.

Doxepin is also a very good tricyclic. Anticholinergic side effects such as sedation are reduced (but not by much) when compared to amitriptyline. It does *not* work on the sleep architecture. It is used at the same dosage levels of amitriptyline.

Notice that the tricyclics are not used in their antidepressant dosages, anywhere from 100 to 350 mg a day. Even though the doses are low, their effectiveness in the treatment of chronic posttraumatic tension-type headache is there.

The SSRIs include Prozac, Paxil, and Zoloft, among others. These medications are not typically sedating (although for some patients they may be) and with the exclusion of those patients, they are energizing. They should be given in the morning. Prozac and Paxil should start at 10 to 20 mg a day and can be increased to 60 to 80 mg. Zoloft should be given at 25 to 50 mg in the morning, up to 150 mg in divided doses. The doses should be divided, giving one when the patient gets up in the morning (around 7:00 am) and one at noon. Patients should understand that taking these medications later than noon can, in many cases, give them problems in sleeping.

The clinician can also safely combine 10 to 40 mg of Prozac or Paxil, or 50 mg of Zoloft given in the morning with a small dose of amitriptyline or doxepin (10–30 mg) at night. Inappropriate dosages of these two forms of medications can, rarely, induce the serotonin syndrome.

Norepinephrine/serotonin reuptake inhibitors (NSRIs) such as venlafaxine, and duloxetine may also be used. See chapter 26 for more information on ADMs.

A meta-analysis found that ADMs are more effective when compared to placebo in decreasing pain severity but not functional status in patients with chronic low back pain (65).

Tricyclic ADMs, such as amitriptyline, desipramine, and imipramine, for example, block the induction of long-term potentiation by inhibiting actions on NMDA receptors (66).

A randomized controlled trial (RCT) indicated that amitriptyline reduces the transmission of painful stimuli from myofascial tissue rather than by reducing overall pain sensitivity. It was felt that this effect was secondary to a segmental reduction of central sensitization in combination with peripheral antinociceptive actions (67). Topical (percutaneously applied) anesthetics may also be utilized (68).

Complimentary medical therapies have been used for the treatment of MPS. Studies supporting this are poor—they have only anecdotal effectiveness for the most part [acupuncture, biofeedback, ultrasound (US), lasers, massage]—but most are not rigorously investigated secondary to the poor research quality (lack of appropriate controls, sample sizes, and blending measures) (69).

TPI Therapy and Interventional Treatment (With Evidence-Based Medicine)

A systematic review, in the Cochrane database, indicates that there is little convincing clinical evidence regarding the effects of interventional therapy (facet joint and epidural, short- and long-term efficacy) for low back pain (70).

In a multicenter, randomized, controlled trial patients with MTRPs injected with sterile water reported a more painful treatment response than those injected with saline. Neither injectable showed a better clinical outcome in patients with chronic MPS (71).

Of interest is McNulty's study (72) showing increased needle EMG activity during stress, while two adjacent muscles remained electrically silent. These results suggest, at least, a mechanism by which emotional factors influence muscle pain, showing significant implications for the psychophysiology of pain with MTRPs.

A RCT indicated that needle EMG at TRPs on myofascial bands tended to improve symptoms. Needling these points elicits motor end plate activity and LTRs and induces far more relief than that seen when needling random points in the muscle (73).

A systematic review from the Cochrane database found that the efficacy of needling therapies (direct and indirect dry and wet needling) in the treatment of pain from MTRPs is neither supported nor refuted by research (23 trials, $N = 955$ patients) (74). In spite of objective clinical practice, this review showed no differences between TRP injections with various injectates or between wet or dry needling. In spite of this, the authors recommend that the method employed be the safest and most comfortable for a patient. Unfortunately, this form of equivocation appears to make so-called evidence-based medicine (EBM) systematic reviews less than, a "gold standard," clinically.

Botwin et al. (75) found benefit in performing TPIs into cervicothoracic musculature with the help of ultrasound (US) guidance, which was felt to reduce the potential for a pneumothorax by an inappropriately placed needle.

A systematic review (NIN Consensus Development Panel on Acupuncture) found acupuncture, or deep, dry needling, useful in the treatment of myofascial pain (and fibromyalgia) (76). A different randomized clinical trial found that Japanese acupuncture associated with heat will yield a modest pain reduction in patients with myofascial neck pain. Previous patient experience with acupuncture and their confidence in it helped to predict beneficial clinical outcomes (77).

Physical Therapy

Vapocoolants/Spray and Stretch

Ethyl chloride was the first vapocoolant thought to be a good conservative treatment for musculoskeletal pain with or without associated joint sprains (78). Travel and Rinzler (79) noted how best to utilize the vapocoolant to deactivate MTRPs. Problems existed with ethyl chloride: it could act as a general anesthetic; it was flammable; its vapor was toxic; and at 4% to 15% of vapor mixed with air, it was potentially explosive.

Travel (80) helped develop flouri-methane, a much safer alternative which, while possibly not as cold as ethyl chloride, was not flammable or explosive.

Spray and stretch, while a good adjunctive post-MTRP injection treatment, is also an alternative noninvasive approach to the treatment of MTRPs (78, 81, 82).

The purpose of the vapocoolant (or plain ice) is to provide an area of hypoesthesias around a TRP and associated shortened muscle, which would allow muscle stretching with less pain. Routinely, spray and stretch is performed until muscle length has been normalized.

Electrical Stimulation

Electrical stimulation (E-Stim) is frequently used to relieve muscle spasm and pain of MTRPs both pre- and post-TPI. Transcutaneous electrical nerve stimulation (TENS) is felt, at low frequencies (60–90 Hz), to work via the gate control theory, in the spinal cord. At the very low levels (1–4 Hz) galvanic or tetanizing current can work well to induce muscle relaxation. At both of these levels endogenous opiates are stimulated. High frequency TENS (up to 1000–2000 Hz) appears to have a more serotonergic system effect. Ultra-high frequency (15,000 Hz) TENS, which in the past was known as "cortical electrical stimulation" (CES), has been found to change the neurochemical milieu of the brain (82).

Phonophoresis and Iontophoresis

Electricity and US are used to move medication through the skin (83).

Stretching

Both active and passive stretching should begin early and proceed throughout treatment as a major part of all patients' home exercise program (84).

Soft-Tissue Treatment

There are varying forms of soft-tissue treatment (STT), including contraction and relaxation techniques (85, 86), muscle energy techniques, TRP pressure release, deep stroking massage, and myofascial release (86). Modalities, including therapeutic US, moist heat, high voltage galvanic stimulation and interferential current are also important, at least initially, in treatment (86).

Srbely et al. (87) reported that low-dose US evoked short-term segmental antinociceptive effects on TRPs.

One of the most frustrating problems seen is the administration of poor PT, which is one of the most common reasons for a patient referral to a tertiary care pain management center. Specifically, trying to strengthen a tight, contracted muscle in spasm will only potentiate the problem, and thus, guarantee the development of a chronic nonmalignant pain syndrome based on a chronic MPS.

Relaxation
There are various forms of relaxation training including muscular tense-relax (88, 89), autogenic training and biofeedback enhanced neuromuscular re-education and muscle relaxation (90, 91), and hypnosis and self-hypnosis.

Strengthening
As muscle relaxation occurs, strengthening is increased incrementally. Like stretching, strengthening should be part of every patient's home exercise program.

Psychological Treatment
There is absolutely no "one size fits all" psychological approach to the chronic pain patient. While many clinicians feel a behavioral management program is appropriate, utilizing the Fordyce (92) paradigm of behavior "modification" by not rewarding pain behaviors, most now favor cognitive behavioral therapy (CBT).

CBT involves restructuring of patients' maladaptive beliefs regarding their ability to cope with their pain or control it; the reduction of pain behaviors and building healthy behavioral patterns and relaxation training are also parts of this treatment strategy (93, 94).

These various aspects of the treatment of MPS should be applied to patients on an individualized, patient specific basis, whether the patient has acute soft-tissue pain/MPS or a chronic MPS.

EVIDENCE-BASED MEDICINE
One RCT (95) indicated that US gave no pain relief, but massage and exercise decreased the number and pain intensity of MTRPs.

A meta-analysis of the use of US therapy in musculoskeletal disorders (96) (from the Cochrane database) indicated that the results comparing US with sham-US were not significant, as the comparison of US with non-US treatment or no treatment was not undertaken. While finding an unimportant effect of US treatment, it was noted that there were "Problems in doing a meta-analysis of many different musculoskeletal diseases, where US may have a different impact. **However, although the pathogenesis varied, the cause of pain is to some extent always inflammation**" (96). (Bolded by author.) Finally, "no attempt was made to distinguish between acute and chronic disorders."

Several other systematic reviews from the Cochrane database were noted, both of which looked at transcutaneous electrical nerve stimulation (TENS).

One review tried to evaluate the effectiveness of TENS in chronic pain. Nineteen RCTs from 107 were evaluated. The "results of this review are inconclusive; the published trials do not provide information on the stimulation parameters, which are not likely to provide optimum pain relief, nor do they answer questions about long-term effectiveness" (97). Larger randomized studies were suggested.

Finally, another Cochrane Database systematic review looked at the efficacy of TENS in the treatment of chronic low back pain. Five trials were included ($N = 170$ patients receiving sham-TENS and $N = 251$ patients receiving active TENS). It was concluded that the results of the meta-analysis found no evidence to support the use of TENS in the treatment of chronic low back pain. It also notes that the meta-analysis "lacked data on how TENS effectiveness is affected by four important factors: type of application, site of application, treatment duration of TENS, optimal frequencies and intensities" (98).

The appropriateness of EBM guidelines based on poor experimental literature is questionable.

REFERENCES

1. Fields H. Pain. New York, NY: McGraw-Hill, 1987:209–229.
2. Mersky H, Bogduk N, eds. Classification of Chronic Pain: Descriptions of Chronic Pain Syndromes and Definition of Pain Terms, 2nd ed. Seattle, WA: IASP Press, 1994:47.
3. Yunus MB. Understanding myofascial pain syndromes: A reply. J Musculoske Pain 1994; 2(1):147–149.
4. Lidbeck J, Hautkamp GIM, Ceder RA, et al. Classification of chronic pain at a multidisciplinary pain rehabilitation clinic. Pain Res Manage 1998; 3(1):13–22.
5. Harden RN, Bruehl SP, Gass S, et al. Signs and symptoms of the myofascial pain syndrome: A national survey of pain management providers. Clin J Pain 2000; 16(1):64–72.
6. Clemente CD. Gray's Anatomy of the Human Body, 30th ed. Philadelphia, PA: Lea & Febiger, 1985:429.
7. Simons DG. Myofascial pain syndrome: One term but two concepts; A new understanding. J Musculoske Pain 1995; 3(1):7–13.
8. Wolfe F, Smythe HA, Yunus MB, et al. The American College of Rheumatology 1990 criteria for the classification of fibromyalgia. Arthritis Rheum 1990; 33:160–172.
9. Fernandez-de-las-Penas C, Simons D, Cuadrado ML, et al. The role of myofascial trigger points in musculoskeletal pain syndromes of the head and neck. Curr Pain Headache Rep 2007; 11(5):365–372.
10. Manolopoulos L, Vlastarakos PV, Georgiou L, et al. Myofascial pain syndromes in the maxillofacial area: A common but underdiagnosed cause of head and neck pain. Int J Oral Maxillofac Surg 2008; 37(11):975–984.
11. Yoon SZ, Lee SI, Choi SU, et al. A case of facial myofascial pain syndrome presenting as trigeminal neuralgia. Oral Surg Oral Med Oral Pathol Oral Radiol Endod 2009; 107(3):e29–e31.
12. Hendi A, Dorsher PT, Rizzo TD, et al. Subcutaneous trigger point causing radiating postsurgical pain. Arch Dermatol 2009; 145(1):52–54.
13. Kim ST. Myofascial pain and toothaches. Aust Endod J 2005; 31(3):106–110.
14. Tabmoush AL. Causalgia: Redefinition as a clinical pain syndrome. Pain 1981; 10:187–197.
15. Kraft GH, Johnson EW, LaBan MM. The fibrositis syndrome. Arch Phys Med Rehabil 1968; 49:155–162.

16. Sola AE, Rodenberger MS, Gettys BB. Incidence of hypersensitive areas in posterior shoulder muscles: A survey of two hundred young adults. Am J Phys Med 1955; 34:585–590.
17. Fricton JR, Awad EA, eds. Advances in Pain Research and Therapy, Vol 17. New York: Raven Press, 1990.
18. Kato K, Sullivan PF, Evengard B, et al. Importance of genetic influences on chronic widespread pain. Arthritis Rheum 2006; 54(5):1682–1686.
19. Moldofsky H, Scarisbrick P, England R, et al. Musculoskeletal symptoms and non-REM sleep disturbance in patients with "fibrositis syndrome" and healthy subjects. Psychosom Med 1975; 37:341–351.
20. Fricton JR, Kroening R, Haley D, et al. Myofascial pain syndrome of the head and neck: A review of clinical characteristics of 164 patients. Oral Surg 1985; 60:615–623.
21. Travell J, Simons D. Myofascial Pain and Dysfunction: The Trigger Point Manual. Baltimore, MD: Williams & Wilkins, 1983.
22. Simons DG, Travell JG, Simons LS. Travell & Simons' Myofascial Pain and Dysfunction: The Trigger Point Manual, Vol. 1, Upper Half of Body, 2nd ed. Baltimore, MD: Williams &Wilkins, 1999.
23. Hsieh CY, Hong CZ, Adams AH, et al. Interexaminer reliability of the palpation of trigger points in the trunk and lower limb muscles. Arch Phys Med Rehabil 2000; 81(3):258–264.
24. Tunks E, McCain GA, Hart LE, et al. The reliability of examination for tenderness in patients with myofascial pain, chronic fibromyalgia and controls. J Rheumatol 1995; 22(5):944–952.
25. Gerwin RD, Shannon S, Hong CZ, et al. Interrater reliability in myofascial trigger point examination. Pain 1997; 69(1–2):65–73.
26. Myburgh C, Larsen AH, Hartvigsen J. A systematic, critical review of manual palpation for identifying myofascial trigger points: Evidence and clinical significance. Arch Phys Med Rehabil 2008; 89(6):1169–1176.
27. Gerwin RD. A review of myofascial pain and fibromyalgia-factors that promote their persistence. Acupunct Med 2005; 23(3):121–134.
28. Andreu AL, Hanna MG, Reichmann H, et al. Exercise intolerance due to mutations in the cytochrome b gene of mitochondrial DNA. N Eng J Med 1999; 341(14):1037–1044.
29. Simons DG. Myofascial trigger points: The critical experiment. J Musculoske Pain 1997; 5(4):113–118.
30. Simons DG. Myofascial pain syndrome due to trigger points. In: Goodgold J, ed. Rehabilitation Medicine. St. Louis, MO: C.V. Mosby Co., 1988:686–723.
31. Wolfe F, Simons DG, Fricton J, et al. The fibromyalgia and myofascial pain syndromes: A preliminary study of tender points and trigger points in persons with fibromyalgia, myofascial pain syndrome and no disease. J Rheumatol 1992; 19:944–951.
32. Simons DG, Hong C-Z, Simons LS. Nature of myofascial trigger points, active loci. J Musculoske Pain 1995; 3(suppl. 1):62.
33. Simons DG, Dexter JR. Comparison of local twitch responses elicited by palpation and needling of myofascial trigger points. J Musculoske Pain 1995; 3(1):49–61.
34. Hong CZ, Torigoe Y. Electrophysiological characteristics of localized twitch responses in responsive taut bands of rabbit skeletal muscle. J Musculoske Pain 1994; 2(2):17–43.
35. Hong CZ. Lidocaine injection versus dry needling to myofascial trigger points: The importance of the local twitch response. Am J Phys Med Rehabil 1994; 73:256–263.
36. Hong CZ. Persistence of local twitch response with loss of conduction to and from the spinal cord. Arch Phys Med Rehabil 1994; 75:12–16.
37. Kellgren JH. A preliminary account of referred pains arising from muscle. Br Med J 1938; 2:325–327.
38. Travell JG. Myofascial trigger points: clinical view. In: Bonica JJ, Albe-Fessard D, eds. Advances in Pain Research and Therapy, Vol 1. New York: Raven Press, 1976:919–926.
39. Shah JP, Phillips TM, Danoff JV, et al. An in vivo microanalytical technique for measuring the local biochemical milieu of human skeletal muscle. J Appl Physiol 2005; 99(5):1977–1984.

40. Shah JP, Phillips TM, Danoff JV, et al. A novel microanalytical technique for assaying soft tissue demonstrates significant quantitative biochemical differences in 3 clinically distinct groups: normal, latent and active. Arch Phys Med Rehabil 2003; 84:A4.
41. Gerwin RD, Dommerhold J, Shah, JP. An expansion of Simons' integrated hypothesis of trigger point formation. Curr Pain Headache Rep 2004; 8(6):468–475.
42. Curatolo M, Petersen-Felix S, Arendt-Nielsen L, et al. Central hypersensitivity in chronic pain after whiplash injury. Clin J Pain 2001; 17:306–315.
43. Johansen MK, Graven-Nielsen T, Olesen AS, et al. Generalized muscular hyperalgesia in chronic whiplash syndrome. Pain 1999; 83:229–234.
44. Graven-Nielsen T, Arendt-Nielsen L, Svensson P, et al. Stimulus-response functions in areas with experimentally induced referred muscle pain: A psychophysical study. Brain Res 1997; 744:121–128.
45. Leffler AS, Kosek E, Lerndal T, et al. Somatosensory perception and function of diffuse noxious inhibitory controls (DNIC) in patients suffering from rheumatoid arthritis. Eur J Pain 2002; 6:161–176.
46. Svensson P, List T, Hector G. Analysis of stimulus-evoked pain in patients with myofascial temporomandibular pain disorders. Pain 2001; 92:399–409.
47. Leffler AS, Kosek E, Hansson P. The influence of pain intensity on somatosensory perception in patients suffering from subacute/chronic lateral epicondylalgia. Eur J Pain 2000; 4:57–71.
48. Arendt-Nielsen L, Graven-Nielsen T. Central sensitization in fibromyalgia and other musculoskeletal disorders. Curr Pain Headache Rep 2003; 7:355–361.
49. Carli G, SUman AL, Biasi G, et al. Reactivity to superficial and deep stimuli in patients with chronic musculoskeletal pain. Pain 2002; 100:259–269.
50. Bajaj P, Bajaj P, Graven-Nielsen T, et al. Trigger points in patients with lower limb osteoarthritis. J Musculoskel Pain 2001; 9:17–33.
51. Roberts WJ. A hypothesis on the physiological basis for causalgia and related pains. Pain 1986; 24:297–311.
52. Bonica JJ. Causalgia and other reflex sympathetic dystrophies. In: Bonica JJ, Liebeskind JC, Albe-Fessard DG, eds. Proceedings of the Second World Congress on Pain, Advances in Pain Research and Therapy, Vol 3. New York: Raven Press, 1970:141–166.
53. Van Houdenhove B, Basquez G, Onghena P, et al. Etiopathogenesis of reflex sympathetic dystrophy: A review and biopsychological hypothesis. Clin J Pain 1992; 8:300–306.
54. Bruel S, Carlson CR. Predisposing psychological factors in the development of reflex sympathetic dystrophy. Clin J Pain 1992; 8:287–299.
55. Ecker A. Norepinephrine in reflex sympathetic dystrophy: An hypothesis. Clin J Pain 1989; 5:313–315.
56. Breier A, Albus M, Pickar D, et al. Controllable and uncontrollable stress in humans. Alterations in mood and neuroendocrine and psychophysiological function. Am J Psychiatry 1987; 144:1419–1425.
57. Kimura Y, Ge HY, Zhang Y, et al. Evaluation of sympathetic vasoconstrictor response following nociceptive stimulation of latent myofascial trigger points in humans. Acta Physiol 2009. doi:10.1111/j.1748–1716.2009.01960.x.
58. Janig W. The sympathetic nervous system in pain: Physiology and pathophysiology. In: Stanton-Hicks M, ed. Pain and the Sympathetic Nervous System. Boston, MA: Kluwer Academic Publishers, 1990:17–90.
59. Mense S. Slowly conducting afferent fibers from deep tissues: Neurobiological properties and central nervous system actions. In: Progress in Sensory Physiology, Vol 6. New York, Springer Verlag, 1986:139–219.
60. Nathan PW. On the pathogenesis of causalgia in peripheral nerve injuries. Brain 1947; 70:145–170.
61. Ochoa JC, Torebjork E, Marchettini P, et al. Mechanisms of neuropathic pain. In: Fields HC, Dubner R, Cervero F, eds. Proceedings of the Fourth World Congress on Pain. Advances in Pain Research and Therapy, Vol 9. New York: Raven Press, 1985:431–450.

62. Loh L, Nathan PW. Painful peripheral states and sympathetic blocks. J Neurol Neurosurg Psychiat 1978; 41:664–671.
63. Jay GW. Chronic Pain. New York: Informa Healthcare, 2007:79–86.
64. Malanga G, Reiter RD, Garay E. Update on tizanidine for muscle spasticity and emerging indications. Expert Opin Pharacother 2008; 9(12):2209–2215.
65. Salerno SM, Browning R, Jackson JL. The effect of antidepressant treatment on chronic back pain: A meta-analysis. Arch Intern Med 2002; 162(1):19–24.
66. Watanable Y, Saito H, Abe K. Tricyclic antidepressants block NMDA receptor-mediated synaptic responses and induction of long-term potentiation in rat hippocampal slices. Neuropharmacology 1993; 32:479–486.
67. Bendtsen L, Jensen R. Amitriptyline reduces myofascial tenderness in patients with chronic tension-type headache. Cephalalgia 2000; 20(6):603–610.
68. Argoff CE. A review of the use of topical analgesics for myofascial pain. Curr Pain Headache Rep 2002; 6(5):375–378.
69. Harris RE, Clauw DJ. The use of complementary medical therapies in the management of myofascial pain disorders. Curr Pain Headache Rep 2002; 6(5):370–374.
70. Nelemans PJ, Bie RA de, Vet HCW de,et al. Injection therapy for subacute and chronic benign low back pain (Cochrane Review). In: The Cochrane Library, Issue 4, 2002. Oxford, Update Software.
71. Wreje U, Brorsson B. A multicenter controlled trial of injections of sterile water and saline for chronic myofascial pain syndromes. Pain 1995; 61(3):441–444.
72. NcNulty WH, Gevirtz RN, Hubbard DR, et al. Needle electromyographic evaluation of trigger point response to a psychological stressor. Psychophysiology 1944; 31(3):313–316.
73. Chu J. Does EMG (dry needling) reduce myofascial pain symptoms due to cervical nerve root irritation? Electromyogr Clin Neurophysiol 1997; 37(5):259–272.
74. Cummings TM, White AR. Needling therapies in the management of myofascial trigger point pain: A systematic review. Arch Phys Med Rehabil 2001; 82(7):986–992. (Cochrane Database Syst Rev 2002; 4:04414.)
75. Botwin KP, Sharma K, Saliba R, et al. Ultrasound guided trigger point injections in the cervicothoracic musculature: A new and unreported technique. Pain Physician 2008; 11(6):885–889.
76. NIN Consensus Development Panel on Acupuncture. JAMA 1998; 280:1518.
77. Birch S, Jamison RN. Controlled trial of Japanese acupuncture for chronic myofascial neck pain: Assessment of specific and nonspecific effects of treatment. Clin J Pain 1998; 14(3):248–255.
78. Kraus H. The use of surface anesthesia in the treatment of painful motion. JAMA 1941; 116:2582–2583.
79. Travel J, Rinzler SH. The myofascial genesis of pain. Postgrad Med 1952; 11:425–434.
80. Travel J. Office Hours: Day and Night. New York: World Publishing Company, 1968.
81. Tschopp KP, Gysin C. Local injection therapy in 107 patients with myofascial pain syndrome of the head and neck. Otorhinolaryngol Relat Spec 1996; 58(6):306–310.
82. Hong CZ. Considerations and recommendations regarding myofascial trigger point injection. J Musculoskeletal Pain 1994; 2(1):29–58.
83. Cassuto J, Liss S, Bennett A. The use of modulated energy carried on a high frequency wave for the relief of intractable pain. Int J Clin Pharmacol Res 1993; 13(4):239–241.
84. Kahn J. Principles and Practice of Electrotherapy, 2nd ed. New York: Churchill Livingstone, 1991.
85. Voss DE, Ionta MK, Myers BJ. Proprioceptive Neuromuscular Facilitation, 3rd ed. Philadelphia, PA: Harper & Row, 1985.
86. Simons DG, Travell JG, Simons LS. Myofascial pain and dysfunction: The Trigger Point Manual, Vol 1, Upper Half of Body, 2nd ed. Baltimore, MD: Williams & Wilkins, 1999:94–177.
87. Srbely JZ, Dickey JP, Lowerison M, et al. Stimulation of myofascial trigger points with ultrasound induces segmental antinociceptive effects: A randomized controlled study. Pain 2008; 139(2):260–266.

88. French AP, Tupin JP. Therapeutic application of a simple relaxation method. Am J Psychother 1974; 28:282–287.
89. Bernstein DA, Borkovee TD. Progressive Relaxation Training. Champaign, IL: Research Press, 1973.
90. Grzesiak RC. Biofeedback in the treatment of chronic pain. Curr Concepts Pain 1984; 2:3–8.
91. Nouwen A, Solinger JW. The effectiveness of EMG biofeedback training in low back pain. Biofeedback Self Regul 1979; 4:8–12.
92. Fordyce WE, Fowler RS, deLateur BJ. Application of behavior modification technique to problems of chronic pain. Behav Res Ther 1968; 6:105–107.
93. Turk DC, Meichenbaum D, Genest M. Pain and Behavioral Medicine: A Cognitive-Behavioral Perspective. New York: Guilford, 1983.
94. Ciccone DS, Grzesiak RC. Chronic musculoskeletal pain: A cognitive approach to psychophysiologic assessment and intervention. In: Eisenberg MG, Grzesiak RC, eds. Advances in Clinical Rehabilitation. Vol 3. New York: Springer, 1990:197–215.
95. Gam AN, Warming S, Larsen LH, et al. Treatment of myofascial trigger-points with ultrasound combined with massage and exercise—a randomized controlled trial. Pain 1998; 77(1):73–79.
96. Gam AN, Johannsen F. Ultrasound therapy in musculoskeletal disorders: A meta-analysis. Pain 1995; 63(1):85–91. (Cochrane Database Syst Rev 2002; 4:05520.)
97. Carroll D, Moore RA, McQuay HJ, et al. Transcutaneous electrical nerve stimulation (TENS) for chronic pain (Cochrane Review). In: The Cochrane Library, Issue 4, 2002. Oxford: Update Software.
98. Milne S, Welch V, Brosseau L, et al. Transcutaneous electrical nerve stimulation (TENS) for chronic low back pain (Cochrane Review). In: The Cochrane Library, Issue 4, 2002. Oxford: Update Software.

11

Piriformis Syndrome

Gary W. Jay

Clinical Disease Area Expert-Pain, Pfizer, Inc., New London, Connecticut, U.S.A.

THE DISORDER

Called in the past the "False L5-S1 pain syndrome," the piriformis syndrome is a controversial and underdiagnosed disorder. The author, who ran a tertiary care pain management center, found multiple cases of piriformis syndrome in patients with chronic low back pain, sometime lasting for years. Yet after diagnosis, appropriate treatment was very helpful and ofttimes mostly or totally ameliorated the patient's pain.

The diagnosis does remain one of exclusion, that is, one must rule out the more common causes of sciatic pain prior to determining this nondiscogenic sciatic pain pathoetiology. Even so, piriformis syndrome may encompass up to 5% of cases of low back, buttock, and leg pain (1).

Most commonly, these patients experience pain in the sciatic region. They also experience pain in the buttock, intolerance to sitting, tenderness to palpation of the greater sciatic notch, and pain with flexion, adduction, and internal rotation of the hip. They may limp and complain of ipsilateral lower extremity weakness.

DIAGNOSIS

The diagnosis was first named in 1947 (2). It is a relatively uncommon cause of buttock and leg pain, with or without electrodiagnostic or neurologic abnormalities.

Physical findings include tenderness in the sciatic notch and buttock pain on flexion, adduction, and internal rotation of the hip.

Imaging studies are rarely helpful, but one study shows MR neurography and interventional MRI in 239 consecutive patients with sciatica in whom standard diagnosis and treatment had failed. Final rediagnoses included piriformis syndrome (67.8%), distal foraminal nerve root entrapment (6%), ischial tunnel syndrome (4.7%), discogenic pain with referred leg pain (3.4%), pudendal nerve entrapment with referred pain (3%), distal sciatic entrapment (2.1%), sciatic tumor (1.7%), lumbosacral entrapment (1.3%), nerve root injury due to spinal surgery (1.3%), inadequate spinal nerve root decompression (0.8%), lumbosacral plexus tumor (0.4%), sacral fracture (0.4%), and no diagnosis (4.2%) (3).

Another study notes the finding of piriformis muscle hypertrophy on CAT scan (4).

The diagnosis is made following a complete history. One important question to ask during history is: "Do you feel like there is a tennis ball in the buttock that hurts when you sit on it?" This question is very sensitive for a positive response being associated with the piriformis syndrome.

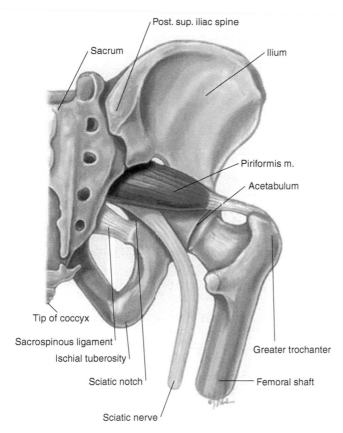

FIGURE 1 The piriformis muscle (Courtesy of Dr. Aaron Filler, Institute for Nerve Medicine. http://www.nervemed.com).

The physical examination shows local tenderness at the piriformis muscle. One way to find this muscle is to draw an imaginary line from the posterior superior iliac spine to the greater trochanter, and an intersecting line from the anterior superior iliac spine to the ischial tuberosity. The piriformis muscle would lie where the lines cross. (Fig. 1)

Some have recommended a pelvic or rectal examination and internal palpation of the piriformis muscle. Finally, range of motion tests, including passive internal rotation of the hip while in 0 degrees of flexion, may be painful. Passive external rotation and adduction while the hip is flexed to 90 degrees would also be expected to be both painful and limited.

Another manual test is a straight leg raising test, positive for buttock pain. Then the leg should be externally rotated; if symptoms diminish upon rotation, this is reported to be confirmation that the piriformis muscle is impinging on the sciatic nerve (5). Strength testing for the external rotators should be done while the patient is in a seated position. The manual muscle test for the piriformis with the hip flexed to 90 degrees would be resisted internal rotation. Also, remember to test the piriformis as an external rotator with the hip in 0 degrees flexion as the patient lies on his or her side or is prone. Finally, test hip rotation in both neutral and flexed positions (5).

Neurologic examination may be positive for both a diminished ipsilateral Achilles reflex as well as hypoesthesias in the lateral lower extremity in the region of the L5-S1, most commonly.

A limp may be seen ipsilaterally (secondary to weakness of the gluteus maximus muscle), along with weakness of the muscles enervated by the peroneal nerve, as well as the hamstrings (6).

PATHOPHYSIOLOGY

The piriformis muscle originates from the anterior surface of the second, third, and fourth sacral vertebrae and the capsule of the sacroiliac joint. The muscle goes lateral and exits the pelvis via the greater sciatic foramen, becomes tendinous, and inserts into the upper border of the greater trochanter (7).

The sciatic nerve travels behind the piriformis muscle about 85% of the time, anterior to the muscle about 10% of the time, and may go partially or totally through the piriformis muscle around 5% of the time.

The piriformis muscle is one of six external rotator muscles of the hip: piriformis, superior gemellus, obturator internus, inferior gemellus, obturator externus, and quadratus femoris. They all are anatomically close and work as a functional unit (8).

While the causes of sciatica are typically related to degenerative changes in the spin and disk lesions, secondary symptomatic sciatica may be induced by metastases to the vertebra, tuberculosis of the spine, tumors located inside the vertebral channel, as well as entrapment of the sciatic nerve by the piriformis muscle (9).

The piriformis syndrome can be secondary to trauma such as by injury post falls, as well as pyomyositis, dystonia musculorum deformans, and fibrosis after deep injections. It is also possible to develop the syndrome secondary to irritation of the sacroiliac joint or lump near the sciatic notch (9).

One study noted that posttraumatic piriformis syndrome was found in 14 patients who had a history of a blow to the buttock; all had pain in the buttock, intolerance to sitting, tenderness to palpation of the greater sciatic notch, and pain with flexion, adduction, and internal rotation of the hip (10).

TREATMENT

As always, start with conservative treatment. The use of anti-inflammatory medication may be useful. Some physicians combine this with a muscle relaxant. If needed, tizanidine, up to 12 mg at HS, may be used. If a patient is experiencing extreme pain that would prohibit physical therapy, the use of a mild analgesic taken an hour before the physical therapy treatment may be helpful. Some physicians also try anticonvulsant medications, which are not particularly helpful in this instance.

Physical therapy with associated home stretching exercise program is the treatment of choice. Goals include decreasing inflammation and associated pain and spasm. Cryotherapy may be helpful, along with gentle stretching exercises and electrical modalities.

Heat would be used later in treatment when more strenuous stretching exercises are needed.

Exercise is important, including passive stretching, soft tissue mobilization, and proprioceptive neuromuscular facilitation techniques are needed to restore the range of motion.

Functional activities are integral to any rehabilitation program and should start when appropriate. Typically, strength training would not begin too early in treatment.

Unfortunately, some patients fail conservative care or have such a long history of the disorder that they have no stomach for conservative care. In these cases, interventional treatment may be used initially.

The author would request the patient work in physical therapy TIW for three weeks. If no real progress ensued, an injection into the piriformis muscle would be made. This can be done with lidocaine 5% with or without steroid, or using botulinum toxin, 100 to 150 U if type A, or the equivalent units if using type B. This would be followed up with more physical therapy. In over a quarter century, no patient needed more than this; very few cases needed a follow-up injection.

Some physicians use either MRI or CAT scan–guided injections or fluoroscopy or ultrasound-guided interventional procedures (7).

For patients who desire, or who work with physicians who are more inclined, there are surgical options, including release of the piriformis tendon and sciatic neurolysis (10).

The piriformis muscle may be surgically released from the femur (11).

Surgery may also be performed to explore the sciatic nerve. A reported case indicates that such exploration found a fascial constricting band around the nerve as well as the piriformis muscle that lay anterior to the nerve (12).

REFERENCES

1. Papadopoulos EC, Khan SN. Piriformis syndrome and low back pain: a new classification and review of the literature. Orthop Clin North Am 2004; 35(1):65–71.
2. Robinson DR. Piriformis syndrome in relation to sciatic pain. Am J Surg 1947; 73:335–358.
3. Filler Ag, Haynes J, Jordan SE, et al. Sciatica of nondisc origin and piriformis syndrome: diagnosis by magnetic resonance neurography and interventional magnetic resonance imaging with outcome study of resulting treatment. J Neurosurg Spine 2005; 2(2):99–115.
4. Chen WS, Wan YL. Sciatica caused by piriformis muscle syndrome: report of two cases. J Formos Med Assoc 1992; 91(6):647–650.
5. Keskula DR, Tamburello M. Conservative management of piriformis syndrome. J Athl Train 1992; 27(2):102–110.
6. Synek VM. The piriformis syndrome: review and case presentation. Clin Exp Neurol 1987; 23:31–37.
7. Peng PWH, Tumber PS. Ultrasound-guided interventional procedures for patients with chronic pelvic pain—a description of techniques and a review of literature. Pain Physician 2008; 11:215–224.
8. Dalmau-Carola J. Myofascial pain syndrome affecting the piriformis and the obturator internus muscle. Pain Pract 2005; 5(4):361–363.
9. Kuncewicz E, Gajewska E, Sobieska M, et al. Piriformis muscle syndrome. Ann Acad Med Stetin 2006; 52(3):99–101.
10. Benson ER, Schutzer SF. Postraumatic piriformis syndrome: diagnosis and results of operative treatment. J Bone Joint Surg Am 1999; 81(7):941–949.
11. Foster MR. Piriformis syndrome. Orthopedics 2002; 25(8):821–825.
12. Sayson SC, Ducey JP, Maybrey JB, et al. Sciatic entrapment neuropathy associated with an anomalous piriformis muscle. Pain 1994; 59(1):149–152.

12 Fibromyalgia

Gary W. Jay

Clinical Disease Area Expert-Pain, Pfizer, Inc., New London, Connecticut, U.S.A.

THE DISORDER

Fibromyalgia syndrome (FMS) as a disorder has more than one sign or symptom and has the unfortunate problem of physicians and/or entire countries/cultures who either believe in the reality of the disorder or not.

Medicine has dealt with the problem of widespread musculoskeletal and soft tissue pain problems for centuries without having any definitive idea of specific diagnosis (1, 2). Gowers first used the term "fibrositis" in 1904 to describe what he felt was muscle pain secondary to inflammation (3). Traut (4) used the term fibrositis to describe generalized musculoskeletal aching, poor sleep, fatigue, and multiple tender points (TPs). The first controlled study of the clinical characteristics of the FMS was published by Yunus et al. (5). In this study, multiple symptoms including pain, poor sleep, fatigue, paresthesia, irritable bowel syndrome (IBS), and headaches, with multiple TPs, were found to be more common in fibromyalgic patients than in age-, sex-, and race-matched normal controls. This study brought the FMS to clinical consciousness. The multicenter criteria study performed by the American College of Rheumatology (ACR) helped establish the validity of FMS (6).

FMS, most simply, is characterized by chronic widespread musculoskeletal pain, stiffness, and tenderness to palpation at specific TPs (5–8). It has been classified as primary and concomitant (9).

Primary fibromyalgia indicates that there is no underlying or concomitant medical condition that might have contributed to a patient's pain. FMS is considered concomitant if another condition such as osteoarthritis, rheumatoid arthritis, systemic lupus erythematosus, or hypothyroidism is present and, in turn, contributes to a patient's pain or fatigue. There are no specific differences that exist between primary and concomitant FMS. When the concomitant condition is treated appropriately, there is no significant change in a patient's clinical picture of FMS. It is considered that the term secondary fibromyalgia should not be used instead of concomitant since there is no change in a patient's FMS after the successful treatment of the underlying condition (10). The concept of post-traumatic FMS has also been noted (38).

The diagnosis of FMS has been warily accepted, especially as there is no "gold standard" test that can confirm it. This, in association with the ever-growing numbers of patients given this diagnosis, who appear unable to work and frequently request disability, have made the diagnosis, to some, suspect (11). Others believe that FMS is a functional, or psychological problem, while still others do not believe FMS exists (12, 13).

Chronic widespread pain, a general diagnosis indicative of chronic generalized musculoskeletal pain (in the majority of cases) with no underlying diagnosis, with or without TPs, is an enormous problem. While between 14% and 26% of the American adult population suffers from chronic pain or arthritis, about 11% complain of chronic widespread pain (9, 14, 15). Generalized musculoskeletal pain, itself, encompasses between 10.6% and 17% of the adult population (16).

White et al. (17–20) felt that the patients classified as having FMS were clearly worse, in many ways, than patients who had chronic widespread pain but not FMS, and therefore, they considered FMS as a separate syndrome from chronic widespread pain.

While FMS patients seen at a tertiary care interdisciplinary pain center are mostly between 20 and 40 years of age, some studies have described FMS as occurring most commonly in women between 40 and 60 years of age (5, 6, 8). Roizenblatt et al. (21) and Yunus (22) have both described juvenile forms of FMS; FMS has also been noted to occur in the elderly (23).

Wolfe et al. (9) noted that the prevalence of FMS in Wichita, KS, was 2% in the community. Porter-Moffitt et al. found that the prevalence of FMS among women in the New York/New Jersey metropolitan area was 3.7%, with a higher rate among racial minorities (24). White et al. (25) found the prevalence of FMS in London, Ontario, Canada, to be 3.3%. In the Wichita study, the prevalence among women was 3.4% versus 0.5% in men. The London Ontario study also found a larger female prevalence: 4.9% in women compared to 1.6% in men.

A more recent Canadian study using the Canadian Community Health Survey, Cycle 1.1 (2000), found the Canadian prevalence rate to be 1.1%, with a 6:1 female-to-male ratio (26).

Weir et al. (27) found that patients with FMS (women more likely than men) were 2.14 to 7.05 times more likely to have at least one comorbid condition including depression, anxiety, headache, IBS, chronic fatigue syndrome, systemic lupus erythematosus and rheumatoid arthritis. In another study a high incidence of FMS was found in female, but not in male, migraine patients (28).

DIAGNOSIS

FMS is a common condition that has been associated with significant disability (29). Patients with FMS complain of widespread pain, frequently stating that they "hurt all over." Most of these patients also complain of stiffness (about 85%) (5), pain in the cervical region, the low back, and the major joints, as well as pain in their hands and feet and chest wall.

The patients should be evaluated to determine the presence or absence of widespread pain; pain on both sides of the body, pain above and below the waist, pain along the axial skeleton, and pain that has been constant and has lasted for at least three months, as well as (on examination) 11 of 18 TPs (Table 1). These pain criteria were developed by the ACR in their determination of the diagnostic classification of FMS (see later) (6).

The patients' pain and stiffness can be typically aggravated by overuse or under use/inactivity-induced deconditioning, weather (cold or humid), trauma, poor sleep, stress, and loud and/or continuous noise (5, 6). A subset of FMS patients complain of peripheral arthralgias, with some pain found on palpation, but no objective swelling, as one would expect with an inflammatory arthritis (30). Other common symptoms of FMS patients include severe fatigue, sleep difficulties, morning fatigue, or nonrestorative sleep, paresthesia, psychological

TABLE 1   Tender Point Regions Used in the Diagnosis of FMS[a]

1.   Suboccipital muscle
2.   Anterior cervical region at C6
3.   Upper Trapezius
4.   Supraspinatus muscle
5.   Parasternal at the second intercostals space
6.   Lateral epicondyle
7.   Upper outer quadrant of the gluteal muscles
8.   Greater trochanter
9.   Medial fat pad of the knee (or vastus medialis muscle)

[a]Each noted point is evaluated bilaterally.

distress, cognitive difficulties ("fibromyalgia fog"), and a swollen feeling in their distal extremities.

A recent paper notes that paresthesias of the upper limbs, hemorrhoids, and epistaxis should be considered common symptoms associated with FMS, secondary to "laxity of connective tissues" (31). About 50% of patients may also complain of neuritic type symptoms, including paresthesias (in 52%) and lancinating pain (about 50%). Restless legs syndrome is not uncommon (56%), nor are headaches (60%) (32). Fatigue is found to be moderate or severe in 75% to 90% of patients (5, 6). This may be secondary to poor sleep, excessive physical activity, deconditioning, or psychological factors (5, 33). Nonrestorative sleep is also common. Approximately 75% of FMS patients have sleep problems (7, 8). Morning fatigue is noted in 75% to 90% of patients (5, 6). Poor sleep is frequently a combination of initial insomnia, multiple nocturnal awakenings, light sleep, or restless legs syndrome and periodic limb movement abnormalities (10). Poor sleep correlated with fatigue and psychological distress as well as with increased pain (5, 6, 10, 33).

Moldofsky (34) noted diurnal variations in the pain of FMS patients. Their "worst" times were in the early morning, late afternoon, and evenings. They felt best between 10 AM and 2 PM. Seasonal effects were also noted, with FMS patients feeling better in spring and summer, but experiencing more pain and diminished energy and poor mood during November and March.

Psychological distress has also been correlated with increased severity of pain (19). Other associated features include headache, IBS, restless legs syndrome, "female urethral syndrome" or interstitial cystitis, thyroid disorder (typically hypothyroidism), and primary dysmenorrhea (6). FMS has also been reported to be associated with rheumatoid arthritis, osteoarthritis, systemic lupus erythematosus, and Sjögren's syndrome. It is important to note that these inflammatory conditions are not thought to cause FMS since appropriate treatment of these concomitant conditions does not decrease or ameliorate a patient's symptoms of FMS.

While there may be a higher occurrence of FMS with these disorders, the actual mechanistic relationship between them is unknown. It may be possible that in subgroups of FMS patients with these disorders, the concomitant problems, themselves, such as arthritis or other forms of peripheral inflammation, may be the initial source of continuous peripheral nociception to the central nervous system (CNS), which may lead to central sensitization with its associated neuroplastic changes yielding amplified pain and FMS.

The ACR's classification criteria for FMS was published in 1990 (6). It was not initially meant as diagnostic criteria, but has been used for this purpose. The FMS criteria included widespread pain for three months or more and the presence of 11 TPs among 18 specific TP sites (Table 1). Pain was to be found in all four body quadrants, including the limbs and the axial skeleton.

On clinical evaluation it appears that the number of TPs [which differ greatly from myofascial trigger points (MTRPs); TPs are discrete, palpable entities that do not refer pain] while clinically a reflection of the FMS criteria may not have a direct correspondence with a patient's level of disability. As a clinical measure, TPs appear to be a gross measure of a patient's discomfort and, possibly, a general or generic measure of the depths of a patient's FMS associated function in the same way a sedimentation rate is a general test that may indicate that there is something going on clinically but is not diagnostic. This is not meant to indicate that TPs are not extremely important in the diagnosis of FMS—they are. However, even during treatment that ameliorates a patient's symptoms, the clinical TP count may not change.

To to make the reliability of the TP count a more valid measure of a patient's overall pain and ability to function, more specific criteria have been found that attempt to more appropriately validate the severity of TP tenderness.

The tender point index (TPI) (35, 36) (also called the total myalgic score) is clinically simple to do. A possible problem is that it may incorporate some elements of a patient's subjective complaints. To obtain the TPI, the examiner sequentially presses the thumb or finger against the 18 TPs noted in the ACR criteria. The intensity should be equivalent to 4 kg/cm^2, or enough pressure be applied so as to cause the examiners thumbnail to blanch. With each site that is examined a tenderness severity scale is applied: non-tender = 0, tender without physical response = 1, tender plus wince or withdrawal = 2, exaggerated withdrawal = 3, and too painful to touch = 4. The myalgic score may also be done on a 0 to 3 basis. The sum of all the TP tenderness scores is the TPI. This measure may be repeated sequentially during treatment. The TPI has good interrater reliability with the average pain threshold, or APT.

Other typical clinical findings on examination include joint tenderness, but no swelling (unless there is coexistent osteoarthritis or rheumatoid arthritis), decreased range of motion of the neck and other joints secondary to pain, and even in the face of complaints of paresthesia, a normal neurological examination is found. Abnormal skin tenderness, possibly reflective of global hyperalgesia may be noted—another indication of a central pain disorder. The examiner may also find tenderness over the tibia (shin) and other bony regions.

Certain diseases can mimic FMS, but none have a sufficient number of TPs to satisfy the ACR criteria. These disorders may include arthritis, polymyalgia rheumatica, hypothyroidism, ankylosing spondylitis, disc herniation, and cardiothoracic pain (see later).

Yunus (37) notes a significant gender difference in patients with FMS, finding that only 10% of FMS patients are men. Women had more fatigue, nonrestorative sleep, a greater number of symptoms overall, and a greater number of TPs. Issues of anxiety and depression were not significantly different between men and women in several studies (38, 39). Yunus also notes that gender differences in FMS are due to a composite of biological, psychological, and sociocultural factors, with the relative contribution of each factor varying from patient to patient (37). Celentano et al. (40) note that women are more likely to consult a health care provider, therefore, utilize more medical resources and, finally, are more likely to report disability.

Finally, Yunus (37) describes hormonal differences that may affect gender differences in pain perception: estrogen modulates noradrenergic sensitivity to arterioles, cognitive function and mood, as well as serotonin tonus and vascular tone. Further, he notes that the rate of serotonin synthesis is 52% higher in men than women and that androgen seems to be protective in FMS.

PATHOPHYSIOLOGY
The pathophysiology of FMS is opined to be "central nervous system hypersensitivity." That being said, there are a number of abnormalities that have been found to be associated with the disorder. These issues are discussed in great depth in another book titled *Chronic Pain* (38). Because of the enormous amount of information, in this section we will just go into what is new since that book was published and summarize the rest.

While FMS is recognized as a biological–psychological–sociological problem associated with prolonged distress, myofascial pain, "pain behavior," anxiety, and depression, it is also associated with central sensitization, neuroendocrine, and autonomic nervous system dysfunction. It appears that the main problem is central in origin. It is the trigger or pathoetiology to the disorder that appears to be unknown.

Patients with FMS have psychophysiological evidence of hyperalgesia to mechanical, thermal, and electrical stimulation. This leads to the assumption of both peripheral and central nociceptive abnormalities. Peripheral nociceptive systems in the skin and musculature change significantly, with sensitization of vanilloid receptors, acid sensing ion channel receptors, and purino-receptors. Tissue modulators of inflammation and nerve growth factors can excite these receptors, leading to significant changes in pain sensitivity (39, 40). In FMS patients, however, there is no consistent evidence of inflammatory soft tissue abnormalities, leading the search for the pathoetiology to the CNS (40, 41).

Both abnormal temporal summation of second pain (wind-up) and central sensitization have been described in FMS. Both of these entities rely on CNS mechanisms. They occur after prolonged C-fiber nociceptive input and depend on the activation of specific nociceptive neurons and wide dynamic range neurons in the dorsal horn of the spinal cord. Other abnormal pain mechanisms associated include dysfunction of the diffuse noxious inhibitory controls. These pain inhibitory mechanisms rely on both spinal cord and supraspinal mechanisms, which both facilitate and inhibit pain (41).

Brain imaging techniques, which can detect neuronal activation after nociceptive stimulation, also give evidence for abnormal central pain mechanisms in FMS. Brain images have been shown to corroborate augmented pain experienced by FMS patients during experimental pain stimuli. Thalamic activity, for example, which contributes to pain processing, is found to be decreased in FMS patients (41). It has also been demonstrated that dysfunction of central pain mechanisms is not only secondary to neuronal activation but also, possibly, neuroglial cell activation, which appears to have an important role in the induction and maintenance of chronic pain (41).

The perceived pain in FMS patients appears to be related to biological–psychological–sociological factors, along with changes in the ANS and hypothalamic–pituitary–adrenal axis. FMS patients have demonstrated reduced

TABLE 2 Psychophysiological Abnormalities in Fibromyalgia (Summary)

1. Hyperalgesia to mechanical, thermal, and electrical stimulation
2. Central sensitization
3. Decreased (↓) sympathetic nervous system response to pain
4. Generalized diffuse pain to minimal mechanical pressure
5. Decreased perception (↓) of heat and cold pain but not perception thresholds

reactivity in the central sympathetic systems, which can be equated to changes or perturbations in the sympathetic–parasympathetic balance (42).

The evidence for central pain processing abnormalities in FMS patients is increasing, with research finding the following in these patients: hyperalgesia, allodynia, abnormal temporal summation of second pain, neuroendocrine abnormalities, ANS abnormalities, and activation of pain-related cerebral regions. Some studies have noted the characteristics of FMS, which are similar to a neuropathic pain syndrome, including characteristics such as hyperalgesia and the association of FMS with ineffective responses to many analgesics (43).

Clinical changes, possible evidence of the existence of FMS, can be divided into five different areas. Tables 2 to 6 summarize the findings in these areas:

1. Psychophysiological abnormalities (Table 2) (44–46)
2. Autonomic nervous system dysfunction (Table 3) (47–56)
3. Neurotransmitter dysfunction (Table 4) (57–105)
4. Neuroendocrine dysfunction (Table 5) (91, 106–126)
5. Cerebral abnormalities including functional cerebral abnormalities, CNS structural changes, and MR imaging of voxel-based morphometry (Table 6) (93, 127–144)

Muscle studies have not shown significant changes (145–152). Sleep disorders are also well known to have a part in the disorder in which nonrestorative sleep is one of the most common complaints, and an electroencephalographic abnormality (α–δ sleep abnormality) is seen in many, but not all, FMS patients (118, 153–158). Another study confirmed that women with FMS have significantly lower urinary cortisol compared to normal, healthy female controls (159).

Psychological abnormalities are also a known part of the disorder, including anxiety disorders, depression, and a more significantly poor quality of life than patients with other chronic pain disorders, including rheumatoid arthritis (24, 106, 160–195).

Other new information includes the hypothesis that FMS may be secondary to clinical endocannabinoid deficiency (196), which may explain why there is therapeutic benefit from exogenous and possibly endogenous (endo-) cannabinoids. CB1 (mostly central) cannabinoid receptors, along with opioid receptors,

TABLE 3 Autonomic Nervous System Abnormalities in Fibromyalgia (Summary)

1. Abnormal sympathetic function after stress in heart rate fluctuations
2. Decreased (↓) heart rate variability and loss of circadian variation of sympathetic/vagal balance
3. Increased (↑) noradrenergically evoked pain
4. Increased (↑) nocturnal sympathetic activity

TABLE 4   Neurochemical Abnormalities in Fibromyalgia (Summary)

1. Abnormal metabolism of serotonin
   a. Decreased (↓) serum levels
   b. Decreased (↓) cerebrospinal fluid (CSF) levels of 5-hydroxyindoleacetic acid (5-HIAA)
   c. Decreased (↓) platelet serotonin
2. Decreased (↓) serum β-endorphin concentration
3. Increased (↑) CSF Dynorphin
4. Increased (↑) CSF substance P (SP)
5. Increased (↑) CSF nerve growth factor in patients with primary fibromyalgia
6. Increased (↑) CSF calcitonin gene-related peptide (CGRP)
7. Decreased (↓) neuropeptide Y (NY)
8. Increased (↑) interleukin-6 and 8 (IL-6, IL-8)
9. Increased (↑) serum brain-derived neurotrophic factor (BDNF)
10. Gi protein hypofunction
11. Decreased (↓) dopamine and metabolites
12. Decreased (↓) endocannabinoid tonus

TABLE 5   Neuroendocrine Abnormalities in Fibromyalgia (Summary)

1. Hypothalamic–pituitary–adrenal axis changes
   a. Decreased (↓) 24-hour urinary free cortisol
   b. Decreased (↓) diurnal cortisol fluctuation and decreased (↓) evening cortisol levels
   c. Increased (↑) adrenocorticotrophic hormone (ACTH) response to corticotrophin releasing hormone (CRH)
   d. Decreased (↓) cortisol relative to increased (↑) ACTH
   e. Decreased (↓) release of ACTH after stimulation of interleukin-6
   f. Decreased (↓) growth hormone (GH)
   g. Decreased (↓) thyroid stimulating hormone to thyrotropin releasing hormone
   h. Decreased (↓) free triiodothyronine (T_3)

TABLE 6   Functional Cerebral Abnormalities, CNS Structural Changes, and MR Imaging of Voxel-Based Morphometry (MR-VBM) in Fibromyalgia (Summary)

1. Decreased (↓) levels of regional cerebral blood flow (rCBF) in thalamus and caudate nucleus via single photon-emission tomography
2. Bilateral cerebral activation to unilateral painful stimulation, with increased (↑) rCBF
3. Decreased (↓) Thalamic response to pain, via decreased (↓) rCBF
4. Decreased (↓) gray matter in the cingulate cortex, insular cortex, and medial frontal cortices
5. Decreased (↓) microstructural and volume changes in the central neuronal networks involved in both sensory discriminative and affective-motivational characteristics of pain, anxiety, memory, and stress response regulation

are found in many of the same areas of CNS pain perception, including the periaqueductal gray matter, the rostral ventromedial medulla, and the spinal cord (197, 198). A randomized controlled trial (RCT) demonstrated the effectiveness of nabilone—an orally administered cannabinoid currently approved for the management of nausea and vomiting during chemotherapy—in the treatment of FMS (65). Other cannabinoid studies have also shown some efficacy (199, 200).

Data appears to indicate that FMS is characterized by cortical or subcortical augmentation of pain processing (136) or centrally mediated, abnormal pain sensitivity (93, 137–139).

A voxel-based morphometric study was performed on patients who met the DSM-IV (*Diagnostic and Statistical Manual of Mental Disorders*, 4th edition) criteria—persistent and distressing chronic pain at one or more body sites which cannot be fully explained by a physiological process or somatic disorder. In the patient group, but not controls, the authors found significant gray matter decreases in the prefrontal, cingulate, and insular cortex—regions known to be involved in modulation of subjective pain experiences. Valet et al. noted that FMS patients met this criteria (140).

A similar study found that compared to normal healthy volunteers FMS patients had significantly less total gray matter volume and had a 3.3 times greater age-associated decrease in gray matter. FMS patients showed significantly less gray matter density compared to healthy controls in the cingulate cortex, insular cortex, and the medial frontal cortices as well as the parahippocampal gyri (141).

Another study showed changes in brain morphology in the right superior temporal gyrus and the left posterior thalamus (decreases in gray matter), and increased gray matter in the left orbitofronto cortex, the left cerebellum, and the bilateral striatum. All of these affected areas are known to be part of both the somatosensory system and the motor system (142). It has been hypothesized that prolonged nociceptive input to the CNS may induce functional and morphologic maladaptive processes, which could, then, further exacerbate the patients' experience of chronic pain (143).

By using both MR DTI (magnetic resonance diffusion–tensor imaging) and MR-VBM (MR imaging of voxel-based morphometry) in patients with FMS to determine microstructural and volume changes in the central neuronal networks involved in both sensory discriminative and affective-motivational characteristics of pain, anxiety, memory, and stress response regulation, it was found that FMS is associated with significant changes in cerebral microstructure of brain areas which are known to be functionally likened to the core symptoms of FMS. Lutz et al. also noted an association between the intensity of specific major FMS symptoms and the concurrent degree of structural tissue changes (144).

Central Sensitization
Central sensitization involves several neurophysiologic aspects, including enhanced spinal cord dorsal horn neuronal excitability associated with increased spontaneous neuronal activity, enlarged receptive fields, and an augmentation of stimuli transmitted by both large- and small-diameter primary afferent fibers. Activation of muscle nociceptors, more so than skin nociceptors, is much more likely to induce central sensitization (201).

The regions or laminae of the spinal cord dorsal horn (I and II) are involved in pain processing and the rostral transmission of nociceptive information. Excitatory neurons in the spinal cord are associated with various excitatory/algetic neurotransmitters including glutamate, substance P (SP), aspartate, vasoactive intestinal peptide, neurotensin, calcitonin gene–related peptide, and cholecystokinin, among others. This excitatory system is "down modulated" by inhibitory dorsal horn interneurons that produce γ-aminobutyric acid, which acts to inhibit nociceptive neurons.

Central sensitization may also be secondary to the activation of glial cells by neurotransmitters, cytokines or chemokines, and this may also contribute to the neurophysiological enhancement of CNS mechanisms that lead to central sensitization (201).

Another important process begins with peripheral nociceptive stimulation—the release of SP at the synapse in pre- and postsynaptic dorsal horn neurons, particularly in laminae II. The release of SP enables the removal of the magnesium block of the N-methyl-D-aspartate (NMDA) receptors, which allows excitatory amino acids such as glutamate and aspartate to activate the postsynaptic NMDA receptors. This process permits changes in cell membrane permeability, leading to the influx of calcium and further excitement of secondary neurons. An increased expression of NMDA receptors found in the skin of FMS patients was thought to be indicative of a possibly more generalized increase in other peripheral nerves (202). The activation of NMDA receptors currently appears to be very important for the induction and maintenance of central sensitization (203).

Opioid receptors are closely related to the NMDA receptors. Both have been detected on primary afferent neurons (204). Opioids can modulate NMDA receptor activity both directly and indirectly, the former aspect leading to the search for usable NMDA receptor antagonists, which can decrease opioid tolerance and, possibly, increase opioid potency.

The activation of NMDA receptors is linked to nitric oxide (NO) production (205). NO is a gaseous molecule that can diffuse into and activate adjacent neurons and glia (206). Its release in lamina I and II of the spinal cord dorsal horn, secondary to nociceptive activity, can, it has been postulated, induce the release of SP and calcitonin gene–related peptide from C-fibers—one mechanism of central sensitization, which would then be followed by further dorsal horn neuronal changes leading to hyperexcitability, hyperalgesia, and allodynia (207).

In another study, serum NO, catalase, and glutathione were measured. Serum glutathione and catalase levels were found to be significantly lower in FMS patients compared to healthy controls. No significant difference was found between the serum NO levels between the two groups. A correlation was noted between serum NO and pain, as well as a significant correlation between glutathione level and morning stiffness (208).

Repetitive stimulation of C-fibers will increase the discharges from second-order neurons in the spinal cord. This will induce pain amplification related to the temporal summation of second pain, or wind-up. Wind-up is a progressively increased response of the secondary dorsal horn neurons, which follows repeated and brief stimulation of the peripheral C-fibers: with each proceeding stimulus, the activated neuronal response increases and becomes stronger than after the prior stimulus. The NMDA receptors mediate wind-up, which is also inhibited by NMDA receptor antagonists. The concept of temporal summation in humans is similar to wind-up as demonstrated in animals (209). Wind-up has also been demonstrated in humans, with the further finding that wind-up results from a central, not a peripheral, pathophysiological mechanism, as input from C-fibers declines or stays the same with peripheral stimulus repetition (210, 211).

Clinically, first pain is typically described as sharp or lancinating, while second pain, most commonly seen in association with chronic pain, is described a dull, aching, or burning. Central sensitization may be relevant to FMS pain because it is frequently associated with extensive secondary hyperalgesia and allodynia. Psychophysiological studies, as noted above, show evidence that input to central nociceptive pathways are abnormally processed in FMS (44, 45). Ketamine, an NMDA receptor antagonist, has been shown in placebo-controlled studies to reduce both temporal summation and muscle pain, indicating the importance of NMDA receptors in the pathophysiology of FMS (72, 212).

Finally, Yunus questions the possibility of an "intrinsic" central sensitization in susceptible FMS patients, a *central sensitivity* rather than central sensitization, which would occur, possibly, without a peripheral nociceptive stimulus. He notes that this might occur secondary to defective inhibitory systems or a hyper-stimulated facilitatory pathway and/or generalized hyperexcitement of peripheral nociceptors (213).

FMS and MPS

Clinically, about 70% of FMS patients also have a local or regional myofascial pain syndrome (MPS) with associated MTRPs (214, 215). Initial trauma such as a slip and fall injury or a cervical strain/sprain from a motor vehicle injury ("whiplash") may induce a localized or regional MPS with associated MTRPs. The continuous barrage of nociceptive input from the peripherally located MTRPs centrally may induce central sensitization with the concurrent spread of pain to other areas. The central sensitization with abnormal sensory processing may, therefore, play an initiating role in the onset of FMS. There may be a subgroup of patients who have a genetic susceptibility to these phenomena. There may also be a subgroup of patients who are particularly sensitive to stressors, life events, and traumas (physical and emotional) as predisposing factors in the development of FMS.

Psychosocial factors may also play a role in a subgroup of patients with the FMS/MPS complex. The idea of major life events (death of a parent or spouse, divorce, etc.) and repeated life stressors being precipitating events leading to hypervigilance and chronic activation of the autonomic nervous system's "fight or flight" response may be reasonable (215). Looking at this group of factors, Bennett (216) felt that FMS could be a generalized form of complex regional pain syndrome/reflex sympathetic dystrophy. This might also lead to the possibility that in a subgroup of patients, sympathetically maintained pain may be an overlapping etiological factor in MPS and FMS. It appears possible that MPS and FMS may overlap. Patients with multiregional MPS may be mistakenly diagnosed with FMS. In at least one subgroup of patients, the development of MTRPs may be the first step in a final common pathway, leading to the onset or pathoetiology of more generalized muscle pain syndromes including FMS.

These mechanisms may help explain the frequently noted initial lack of significant physical peripheral damage being found that appears seemingly out of context in relation to the intensity of a patient's chronic pain. It may help to note Bennett's view that chronic pain is a continuous spectrum ranging from transient local pain to widespread allodynia (216).

Finally, continuous muscle pain in fibromyalgia and in myofascial pain, posttraumatic pain, pain from muscle overload, and inflammatory pain in rheumatic disorders may be a consequence of generalized pain hypersensitivity (217). Other predisposing factors may be functioning, particularly in fibromyalgia (218).

It appears that tenderness and referred pain related to chronic musculoskeletal pain may well result from peripheral and central sensitization, which can then be instrumental in transitioning acute to chronic pain. The fact that chronic musculoskeletal pain is associated with central sensitization has been demonstrated in several recent studies (219, 220).

While there are no gold standard tests that can be performed to confirm the diagnosis of FMS, there are enough known abnormalities in the neuroendocrine system, the autonomic nervous system, the neurotransmitter/neuropeptide systems, and the CNS, on a morphological basis, that this may not be so far in the future (Tables 3 to 6).

TREATMENT

General Comments

It is appropriate to evaluate the general treatment of FMS patients with an important caveat noted by Turk (221). He suggests that the myth of patient homogeneity—the thought that all patients with the same chronic pain syndrome are also similar in all associated variables—may be a reason for the lack of satisfactory treatment outcomes. He believes that patients should be split into subgroups that may have more meaningful outcomes and indicates that it may be appropriate to divide patients into subgroups on the basis of their psychosocial and behavioral characteristics.

Another important aspect of dealing with FMS is the problem of adherence to treatment. A recent study found that treatment adherence is influenced by patient–physician discordance as well as pain (clinical) and by distress (psychological factors) in women with FMS (222). If these issues could be improved, as a part of treatment or prior to treatment, there would be improvement in adherence to FMS treatment.

Pharmacological Treatment

Currently, three drugs pregabalin, duloxetine, and milnacipran have been approved by the FDA for the treatment of fibromyalgia (the last one was approved in January 2009). These will be discussed in detail later in the chapter. To date, no drugs have been approved in the European Union by the European Medicines Agency for the treatment of fibromyalgia.

The goal of pharmacological treatment is symptom amelioration, as it would rarely, if ever, totally obviate a symptom. Another key aspect is the importance of appropriate pharmacological treatment as a part of interdisciplinary treatment; the medications alone do not, clinically, provide the fullest form of relief (154, 155). Unfortunately, overmedication and indiscriminant polypharmacy frequently occurs. Physicians must be very familiar with all the pharmacological aspects of medications, particularly the side effects, as many FMS patients are very sensitive to medication effects and especially their side effects, particularly, those dealing with fatigue, sedation, and cognitive decrement.

In general, medications should be started "low and slow," with small doses increased gradually. It is not unusual to find effective medication dosages are lower than those noted in general medication textbooks. Some FMS patients are seemingly intolerant to almost all medications making them very resistant to pharmacological treatment. Nonpharmacological treatment should be encouraged for these patients. Another frequently seen problem is stopping a medication before it has had a pharmacological chance to help the patient.

Pharmacological treatment is utilized to help address the major FMS symptoms. For more detail on all forms of FMS treatment, see chap. 9 of *Chronic Pain* (38).

Analgesics

Pain is the most significant feature of FMS. While analgesic medications are not expected to totally eradicate FMS pain, they are palliative, that is, used to decrease pain enough to help patients improve with functional restoration.

In spite of the lack of peripheral or central inflammation, nonsteroidal anti-inflammatory drugs (NSAIDs) are the most common analgesics used (in about 90% of FMS patients) and corticosteroids are used in 24% of patients (223); this is in spite of the noted lack of efficacy of these medications (224–226). Acetaminophen and NSAIDs may be clinically effective when they are combined with centrally acting medications such as amitriptyline (AMI) (227). Some patients have found some relief with the use of these medications (228) while NSAIDs have not been found to be superior to placebo (224, 229). The efficacy of cyclooxygenase-2 inhibitors (Cox-2) has not been established in FMS (230). Only celecoxib remains on the market at this time, in this drug classification. The use of these medications does make surveillance for gastrointestinal symptoms imperative.

Tramadol appears to inhibit ascending pain pathways; it inhibits reuptake of norepinephrine and serotonin and it is also a μ-receptor agonist. In RCTs, tramadol has been shown to provide pain relief that is superior to placebo (227). It has been noted to be as effective as acetaminophen and codeine (231). Another RCT and other reports also indicate tramadol's efficacy (232, 233); at high dosages nausea, dizziness, as well as seizures have been noted (234).

The apparent pathophysiological aspects of peripheral and central sensitization and allodynia make the use of opioids appropriate in select patients with pain-limited functionality. There is no clinical evidence of the efficacy of opioids for the treatment of FMS (235). Short-acting opioids may be useful when taken 30 to 60 minutes prior to exercise or physical therapy for patients in whom pain prevents the treatment. Chronic, moderate- to high-dose opioid usage may induce problems with deep sleep as well as with the immune system (236). However, for select patients who need significant help to become functional and maintain their functionality, chronic opioid analgesic therapy may be indicated. Extended release opioids such as OxyContin, fentanyl percutaneous patches (Duragesic), or extended release morphine may be used. An opiate agreement must be used, and the patients told of the possibility of dependence. They should be monitored regularly to evaluate the patient's function as well as their appropriate use of the medication (237).

There are physician, patient, payer, and societal barriers to the appropriate utilization of opioids, including outmoded concerns about abuse, dependency, and tolerance, as well as underutilization, all secondary to poor education (238, 239) (see chapter 24).

Muscle relaxants may be useful, along with analgesics, to help deconditioned patients get through appropriate early and later exercise and rehabilitation. Tizanidine, a chronic muscle relaxant (at dosages of 0.5–3 mg/day), an α_2-adrenergic agonist, has been reported to help decrease pain in FMS patients (240).

Lidocaine injections to TPs have been noted in several studies to benefit the FMS patient (241, 242). Postinjection soreness is frequently great. Intravenous lidocaine appears to decrease pain and increase quality of life (243). A recent study indicates that injection therapy for FMS may be more effective if it focused less on TPs and more on trigger points found in association with MPS associated with FMS (244).

The use of NMDA receptor antagonists including ketamine (245) and dextromethorphan in the treatment of FMS needs more research (246). A recent study (247) found that patients with FMS showed abnormal wind-up during thermal and mechanical stimulation as compared to normal controls. Dextromethorphan reduced both thermal and mechanical wind-up and decreased stimulus intensity in both FMS patients and normal controls. Another study found that response to IV ketamine infusions was predictive of a response to oral dextromethorphan (248–250). Methadone, a narcotic with a long half-life, has a modest amount of NMDA receptor antagonism.

Antidepressants

New classes of antidepressants (ADM) and anticonvulsant medications (ACM) have created new opportunities for the treatment of chronic, nonmalignant pain. These drugs modulate pain by interacting with specific neurotransmitters and different ion channels. Newer antidepressants have been found to have varying degrees of effectiveness in the treatment of neuropathic pain (bupropion, venlafaxine, duloxetine). Older tricyclic antidepressants (TCAs) including amitriptyline (AMI), nortriptyline, and desipramine are also used for the treatment of neuropathic pain. The first-generation anticonvulsants (carbamazepine, valproic acid, and phenytoin) and newer anticonvulsants (gabapentin and pregabalin) are also effective in the treatment of neuropathic pain (251). TCAs have documented efficacy in the treatment of FMS. Duloxetine, an ADM, and pregabalin appear to have modest efficacy in patients with FMS (252).

Serotonin is involved in moderating pain, sleep, depression, and hypothalamic hormone release. The majority of the various types of antidepressant medications deal, at least partially, with serotonin reuptake.

Tricyclic Antidepressants

TCAs, particularly AMI, are known to be beneficial to the treatment of FMS as found in RCTs (226, 253–255). AMI is known to inhibit reuptake of both serotonin and norepinephrine. It is the most frequently prescribed medication for the treatment of FMS (256). One report indicates that only about a third of patients find significant clinical improvement with AMI (257). AMI is felt to have both central and peripheral analgesic effectiveness, as noted before. Common side effects include weight gain, constipation, dry mouth, sedation, and, in a small percentage of patients, agitation in, up to 20% of patients (258). Patients note decreased morning stiffness, better sleep, and increased energy with AMI (259). A more recent review of efficacy of AMI in the treatment of FMS shows it to be useful at doses of 25 mg/day for eight weeks or less. Higher dosages for longer times may not have been useful. However, more stringent RCTs with longer follow-up periods need to be done (260).

As noted above, treatment with a TCA should be started with a low dose (10 mg of AMI, for example) and be increased slowly. Antidepressant dosages (75–100 mg/day to 300 mg/day) are frequently too high for the FMS patient to tolerate. Nortriptyline (258), doxepin, as well as cyclobenzaprine may be used if patients do not respond to AMI (261). Imipramine has been noted to be ineffective (259).

Cyclobenzaprine, a tricyclic agent, while not decreasing pain in all studies, does help improve sleep and fatigue in other RCTs (262, 263). Another study, a double-blind, crossover study of CBP at two different strengths, finds improvements in the quality of sleep, anxiety, fatigue, stiffness, the number of TPs, and IBS (264).

Selective Serotonin Reuptake Inhibitors

Selective serotonin reuptake inhibitors (SSRIs), in general, have little analgesic effectiveness in FMS patients but do help with depression and sleep disorders (237, 265). RCTs have found a diminution of pain with fluoxetine (266) and citalopram (267). Sertraline has been found to both decrease pain and have no effect on pain (268). A recent study shows that FMS patients treated with sertraline had a better outcome in terms of pain, improved sleep, and decreased morning stiffness when compared to a group of FMS patients treated with physical therapy (269). Studies have found the combination of Fluoxetine and AMI to be more effective than either medication alone or placebo (270).

It must also be noted that the non-SSRIs (especially if there is a noradrenergic component) such as venlafaxine, nefazodone, and bupropion appear to be effective in FMS particularly in decreasing pain (271). Other, newer prominent noradrenergic or dopaminergic system effects may be more effective in reducing pain (272).

Selective Norepinephrine and Serotonin Reuptake Inhibitors

Duloxetine, a specific SNRI, was the second drug to be approved for the treatment of fibromyalgia by the FDA in June 2008. The drug was found to be efficacious in two pivotal 12-week studies including 874 patients (273–275). It has been found to show amelioration of pain, as opposed to being secondary to decreasing depression. The most common adverse events included nausea, dry mouth, constipation, decreased appetite, sleepiness, increased sweating, and agitation. It should be started at 20 mg daily and titrated to 60 mg twice daily over a two-week period. In some patients, 60 mg a day may be sufficient. It should not be used in patients with any type of hepatic insufficiency.

Venlafaxine appeared to be helpful in an open label trial, but not in an RCT (276).

Milnacipran, a norepinephrine serotonin reuptake inhibitor (NSRI), has been shown to have better analgesic properties, reportedly, than the SSRIs (277). This medication became the third to receive FDA approval for its use in the treatment of FMS. It was also found that milnacipran can relieve not only pain but other symptoms of FMS, including fatigue, sleep, and depression (48, 278). A recently published RCT shows the drug is efficacious at both 100 and 200 mg/day. The most commonly reported adverse events included nausea, headache, and constipation (279).

Mirtazapine (which selectively blocks 5-HT2 and 5-HT3 receptors) is a novel ADM. In an open-label study it was found to be effective in diminishing the pain of FMS (280).

Two evidence-based medicine (EBM) articles deal with the treatment of FMS with antidepressant medications (281, 282). The general consensus of both articles is that ADMs were efficacious in treating various symptoms of FMS, but one questioned if this action was independent of depression. More studies were felt to be needed.

Another study evaluated the RCT data for the use of ADMs and cognitive behavioral therapy for some of 11 somatic syndromes, including IBS, chronic back pain, headache, FMS, chronic fatigue syndrome, tinnitus, menopausal symptoms, chronic facial pain, noncardiac chest pain, interstitial cystitis, and chronic pelvic pain; this data was found to be either robust or too scanty to be useful (283).

Anticonvulsant Medications

It would make teleological sense that these medications may decrease pain from peripheral and/or central sensitization (284). Pregabalin, the first FDA approved drug for the treatment of fibromyalgia, was effective in FMS patients in the reduction of pain, sleep disturbance, and fatigue when compared to controls (285).

A 14-week study of 745 FMS patients, the most common adverse events were dizziness and somnolence, which resolved in the majority of patients who would continue on the drug. There were more after effects at the highest doses tested, 600 mg, but not a better efficacy than the 450 mg dose, so the 600 mg dose is not part of the approved fibromyalgia label. This data, which showed separation from placebo, was pooled with a second 14-week trial ($n = 1493$), which showed that pain and the patient global impression of change were improved on all doses of pregabalin utilized. The Fibromyalgia Impact Questionnaire (FIQ) showed improvement in the 450 and 600 mg dosages (286, 287).

Therapy should be initiated at 75 mg twice a day and increased to 150 mg twice daily over a seven-day period. Effects may be seen within a week. You may need to increase to 450 mg a day over another week. Adverse events typically include blurred vision, constipation, dizziness, drowsiness, edema, and weight gain. Out of 429 patients from another study, 249 entered an open-label trial for one year and showed sustained effects on pain measures, with just over 10% of patients reporting dizziness and approximately 10% reporting somnolence, peripheral edema, and weight gain (288).

The FREEDOM study, a 6-week open label trial followed by a 26-week placebo-controlled study, showed delay of loss of therapeutic response in the pain, function (via Fibromyalgia Impact Questionnaire (FIQ)), Patient Global Impression of Change (PGIC), sleep, and fatigue domains in the pregabalin treated patients (289).

Other Medications

Other types of medications have included 5-HT$_3$ receptor antagonists tropisetron and ondansetron (290–294); benzodiazepines including alprazolam, temazepam, and clonazepam (295, 296); atypical antipsychotics such as olanzapine (297); and sedative-hypnotics, including zolpidem and zopiclone, L-tryptophan, and even chlorpromazine, the latter of which is not recommended (118, 297–305).

Many other drugs have been used, including ribose (306), DHEA (dehydroepiandrosterone) (307), S-adenosylmethionine, a derivative of methionine (308, 309), L-tryptophan (305, 310), and calcitonin (311); none of these were found to be exceptionally helpful, with some noted as such in RCTs.

FMS patients with low levels of insulin-like growth factor-1 and who received daily injections of growth hormone (over nine months) had significant improvements in symptoms when compared to placebo (312). The injections are extremely, prohibitively expensive.

Dopaminergics

This drug group may become more important over time, as the rationale for its use is becoming more distinct.

Norepinephrine, the precursor of which is dopamine, evokes pain in FMS patients, supporting the hypothesis that FMS may be a form of sympathetically maintained pain syndrome (52).

It is considered that dopamine and dopamine subreceptors control a variety of important limbic system functions regarding the stress response (313). While there are no D$_3$ receptors in the brainstem, where autonomic arousal is generated, the limbic system is rich with dopamine receptors, including D$_3$.

Studies with another D$_3$ agonist, pramipexole, indicate that low doses of this drug would cause the limbic neurons to become less functional; as this is a gate for brainstem arousal, it would therefore be left "wide open," with arousal allowed to go unchecked (314). Excessive autonomic stimulation would induce sleep problems and other ANS problems. As doses of the drug increase, the neuronal concentration increases leading to postsynaptic neurotransmission becoming more significant than presynaptic transmission. A higher concentration of a D$_3$ agonist would increase limbic function to block the brainstem arousals. This central limbic control might help reverse other autonomic problems such as sleep problems. This may also help with induction of a decrement in pain perception secondary to a decrement in central hypersensitivity and decreased ANS arousal.

Both pramipexole and ropinirole have been found to be useful in the treatment of FMS (68, 315).

Blocks

Sphenopalatine blocks were ineffective in FMS and MPS patients (316). One study (317) reported beneficial effects of regional sympathetic blockade in FMS patients. Epidural opioid blockade at rest and after exercise was helpful (231).

Pharmacological Treatment of Associated Syndromes

Restless Legs Syndrome

Restless legs syndrome is typified by the perception of crawling sensations of the legs and strong urges to stretch noted early in the sleep cycle (318). This might also be associated with nocturnal myoclonus. Restless legs syndrome may respond to clonazepam (0.5–1.0 mg at bed time; L-dopa/carbidopa (10/100 mg at suppertime) or low-dose narcotics at bedtime (319, 320). Other dopamine agonists (pergolide, pramipexole) may also be effective (321, 322).

Fatigue

Fatigue, a very common problem with FMS, may be treated with antidepressant medications if it is secondary to depression. Tropisetron, a 5-HT3 receptor antagonist reportedly helps in FMS-related fatigue and chronic fatigue syndrome (291, 323, 324). Amphetamines, methylphenidate, as well as modafinil have been used to benefit some patients with severe fatigue. Dopaminergic agents amantadine and pemoline in addition to protriptyline and SSRIs may also prove beneficial.

Dysautonomia

The most common autonomic nervous system manifestation in FMS patients (about 33%) is neurally mediated hypotension (47, 51, 325–327). This is frequently associated with severe fatigue (326). Treatment includes increasing plasma volume (more fluids); increased salt intake; Florinef, a mineralocorticoid; avoidance of medications that increase hypotension (TCAs, antihypertensives); prevention of the ventricle–baroreceptor reflex (β-adrenergic antagonists or disopyramide); and minimize the efferent limb of the baroreceptor reflex (α-adrenergic agonists or anticholinergic agents (328).

Cold Intolerance

Many FMS patients have cold-induced vasospasm (329). Low-grade aerobic exercise helps as does treatment of dysautonomias and the use of vasodilators (calcium channel blockers), but these can potentially aggravate hypotension (330).

Cognitive Dysfunction

This is a common problem for FMS patients (331, 332). It may be associated with poor memory and concentration and lead to problems with employment. It appears to be related to the effects of chronic pain, depression, mental fatigue, and sleep disorders. Treatment of these various problems are needed: in some patients medication treatment of fatigue (see earlier in the chapter) may be helpful with this problem, which appears to be the result of 1 or more other FMS associated problem(s).

Complementary and Alternative Medical Therapies

A study from the Mayo clinic found, via a survey of 289 patients, that the 10 most common complementary and alternative medical therapies included exercise, spiritual healing (prayers), massage therapy, chiropractic therapy, vitamin C, vitamin E, magnesium, vitamin B complex, green tea, and weight loss programs (333).

Nonpharmacological Treatment

The nonpharmacological management of FMS patients is mostly based on empirical research, with only a few controlled studies (334). In a systematic review of mind–body therapies (MBT) for the treatment of FMS, MBT is more effective for some clinical outcomes as compared to being on a waiting, treatment as usual or placebo (335). However, when compared to active treatment, the results are largely inconclusive. Another study looked at complimentary medical treatment for FMS (336). This report indicated that the strongest data was found for mind–body therapies (biofeedback and cognitive behavioral therapy), especially when part of a multidisciplinary approach. The weakest data was for manipulative techniques (chiropractic and massage).

A meta-analysis of FMS treatment interventions found that the optimal intervention for FMS involved both medication management and nonpharmacological treatments (especially exercise and cognitive behavioral therapy) to help sleep and pain symptoms (337, 338).

Finally, a symptomatic review of RCTs of nonpharmacological FMS treatment interventions revealed the great difficulty noted and wide range of outcome measures, making conclusions across the studies very impractical, if possible (339). There was no strong evidence for any single intervention, although preliminary support of moderate evidence strength was noted for aerobic exercise.

Physical therapy

Physical therapy is a source of excellent adjunctive therapies for FMS patients. The most commonly used are the hands on treatments: massage, mobilization, stretching, and modalities (heat, ultrasound, electrical stimulation) (339). Most important are the various aspects of the home exercise program. However, no controlled studies with appropriate construction (number of patients, methodology) have confirmed efficacy of physical therapy in FMS patients.

One study documented the reduction of FMS-induced pain and SP along with improvements in sleep after massage therapy (340). In a double blind, placebo-controlled study, low-intensity infrared diode laser therapy was found to improve the number of TPs and global assessment scores (341). In an open study, TENS was found to provide transient benefit in 70% of 40 patients (342).

Exercise/fitness training

The majority of FMS patients show poor strength, flexibility, and aerobic fitness. Research has noted the benefits of exercise, including decreased perception of pain and lowered pain threshold (343, 344). The benefits of exercise for FMS patients, as well as in general, are based on reasonable scientific evidence (345, 346). The question is whether exercise may also have negative consequences. FMS introduces postexertional pain into the situation, secondary to central sensitization. Because of the elements of FMS pathophysiology, exercise may be both good and bad for FMS patients, as they would experience more postexertional pain compared to non-FMS patients (347–349). This is important to note, since it may be this problem and not a patient's lack of adherence to a rigorous exercise program that prevents patients from enduring long-term follow-up with exercise programs.

Deconditioning is very common in FMS patients and is associated with many FMS symptoms (237). Various types of exercise including stationary cycling, aerobic walking, and aerobic dance have been evaluated (350–354), and it has been determined that aerobic exercise three times a week can reduce TP tenderness (237, 355, 356). Strength training as well as aerobic exercise is associated with improvements in pain, TP counts, and disturbed sleep (354, 355, 357). As indicated, maintenance of exercise programs in FMS tends to be poor (358, 359).

Studies have shown exercise-related improvement of objective and subjective pain measurements in primary fibromyalgic patients (359–362). Systematic review (363) indicates that supervised aerobic exercise training will have beneficial effects on physical capacity and FMS symptoms. Strength training may also be beneficial. More research, per the authors, is needed. While positive RCTs have been reported (364) another study has shown that exercise is not helpful (365).

Chiropractics
Only limited evidence supports spinal manipulation in FMS patients (366).

Acupuncture
A published meta-analysis of acupuncture in the treatment of FMS found that this treatment modality is a useful adjunctive treatment for FMS on a short-term basis (367). Another study looked at FMS patients' treatment with acupuncture for six weeks and found decreased pain levels and number of TPs associated with increased serum serotonin and SP levels (368).

The National Institutes of Health consensus statement on acupuncture indicated that in some situations, including FMS, "acupuncture may be useful as an adjunct treatment or an acceptable alternative or may be included in a comprehensive management program" (369). It is worth remembering that if acupuncture works by stimulating the endogenous opiate system, it may not work as well in patients taking chronic daily narcotics.

Cognitive behavioral therapy
The primary goal of a cognitive behavioral therapy program is to help patients develop an active self-management approach to coping with their FMS. Typically, the program includes some or all of the following modalities: relaxation training, cognitive restructuring, meditation, aerobic exercise, stretching, pacing of activities, and patient and family education. The majority of published studies showed cognitive behavioral therapy to have some benefit (370–374). Some of the studies took place in interdisciplinary pain programs (375, 376). Finally, improvement was noted after periods of six months (375) to 30 months (373). Cognitive behavioral therapy appears to be a very useful adjunctive modality in the treatment, particularly the multidisciplinary treatment, of FMS.

Support groups and online chat rooms
Many patients learn more from speaking to other patients with similar problems than with physicians. This can be done via person-to-person interaction at local FMS support groups (to find one, look at http://www.arthritis.org) or online in less personable chat rooms. Unless "bad medicine" is being touted, these are typically helpful; "self-help" groups that have patients who only complain about everything tend to "turn off" many patients who need a more supportive environment.

Multidisciplinary treatment programs

One RCT shows the effectiveness of multidisciplinary rehabilitation in the treatment of FMS (377). Another study shows that while a relatively brief multidisciplinary pain program may be helpful for some FMS patients, a subgroup of patients need a more comprehensive program because of their very poor level of functioning (378).

Predictors of adherence to multimodal/multidisciplinary treatment program recommendations were found for both general and specific adherence: this was associated with lower pain posttreatment (379).

EVIDENCE-BASED MEDICINE

Please see above

REFERENCES

1. Reynolds MD. The development of the concept of fibrositis. J Hist Med Allied Sci 1983; 38:5–35.
2. Simons DG. Muscle pain syndrome-Part 1. Am J Phys Med 1975; 54:289–311.
3. Gowers WR. Lumbago: Its lessons and analogues. BMJ 1904; 1:117–121.
4. Traut EF. Fibrositis. J Am Geriatr Soc 1968; 16:531–538.
5. Yunus MB, Masi AT, Calabro JJ, et al. Primary fibromyalgia (fibrositis): Clinical study of 50 patients with matched normal controls. Semin Arthritis Rheum 1981; 11:151–171.
6. Wolfe F, Smythe HA, Yunus MB, et al. The American College of Rheumatology 1990 criteria for the classification of fibromyalgia. Report of the Multicenter Criteria Committee. Arthritis Rheum 1990; 33:160–172.
7. Goldenberg DL. Fibromyalgia syndrome: An emerging but controversial condition. JAMA 1987; 257:2782–2787.
8. Bengtsson A, Henriksson KG, Jorfeldt L, et al. Primary fibromyalgia. A clinical and laboratory study of 55 patients. Scand J Rheumatol 1986; 40:340–347.
9. Wolfe F, Ross K, Anderson J, et al. The prevalence and characteristics of fibromyalgia in the general population. Arthritis Rheum 1995; 38:19–28.
10. Yunus MB, Inanici F. Fibromyalgia syndrome: Clinical features, diagnosis and biopathophysiologic mechanisms. In: Rachlin ES, Rachlin IS, eds. Myofascial Pain and Fibromyalgia: Trigger Point Management, 2nd ed. St. Louis, MO: Mosby, 2002: 3–31.
11. Wolfe F. The fibromyalgia problem. J Rheumatol 1997; 24:1247–1249.
12. Barsky AJ, Borus JF. Functional somatic syndromes. Ann Intern Med 1999; 130:910–921.
13. Hadler NM. Fibromyalgia: La maladie est morte. Vive le malade! J Rheumatol 1997; 24:1250–1251.
14. Lawrence RC, Hochberg MC, Kelsey JL, et al. Estimates of prevalence of selected arthritic and musculoskeletal diseases in the United States. J Rheumatol 1989; 16:427–441.
15. Magni G, Marchetti M, Moreschi C, et al. Chronic musculoskeletal pain and depressive symptoms in the National Health and Nutrition Examination. I. Epidemiologic follow-up study. Pain 1993; 53:163–168.
16. White KP, Harth M. The occurrence and impact of generalized pain. Baillieres Clin Rheumatol 1999; 13:379–389.
17. White KP, Speechley M, Harth M, et al. Comparing self-reported function and work disability in 100 random community cases of fibromyalgia versus control in London, Ontario: The London Fibromyalgia Epidemiology Study. Arthritis Rheum 1999; 42:76–83.

18. White DP, Speechley M, Harth M, et al. The London Fibromyalgia Epidemiology Study: Comparing the demographic and clinical characteristics in 100 random community cases of fibromyalgia versus controls. J Rheumatol 1999; 26:1577–1585.

19. White KP, Harth M, Speechley M, et al. A general population study of fibromyalgia tender points in non-institutionalized adults with chronic widespread pain. J Rheumatol 2000; 27:2677–2682.

20. White DP, Harth M. Classification, epidemiology and natural history of fibromyalgia. Cur Pain Headache Reports 2001; 5:320–329.

21. Roizenblatt S, Tufik S, Goldenberg J, et al. Juvenile fibromyalgia: Clinical and polysomnographic aspects. J Rheumatol 1997; 24:579–585.

22. Yunus MB, Masi AT. Juvenile primary fibromyalgia syndrome. Arthritis Rheum 1985; 28:138–144.

23. Yunus MB, Holt GS, Masi AT, et al. Fibromyalgia syndrome among the elderly: comparison with younger patients. J Am Geriatr Soc 1988; 35:987–995.

24. Porter-Moffitt S, Gatchel RJ, Robinson RC, et al. Biopsychosocial profiles of different pain diagnostic groups. J Pain 2006; 7(5): 308–318.

25. White KP, Speechley M, Harth M, et al. The London Fibromyalgia Epidemiology Study: The prevalence of fibromyalgia syndrome in London, Ontario. J Rheumatol 1999; 26:1570–1576.

26. McNally JD, Matheson DA, Bakowsky VS. The epidemiology of self-reported fibromyalgia in Canada. Chronic Dis Can 2006; 27(1): 9–16.

27. Weir PT, Harlan GA, Nkoy FL, et al. The incidence of fibromyalgia and its associated comorbidities: A population-based retrospective cohort study based on International Classification of Diseases, 9th Revision codes. J Clin Rheumatol 2006; 12(3): 124–128.

28. Ifergane G, Buskila D, Simiseshvely N, et al. Prevalence of fibromyalgia syndrome in migraine patients. Cephalalgia 2006; 26(4): 451–456.

29. Bennett RM. Fibromyalgia and the disability dilemma. A new era in understanding a complex, multidimensional pain syndrome. Arthritis Rheum 1996; 39(10):1727–1634.

30. Reilly PA, Littlejohn GO. Peripheral arthralgic presentation of fibrositis/fibromyalgia syndrome. J Rheumatol 1992; 19:281–283.

31. Zoppi M, Maresca M. Symptoms accompanying fibromyalgia. Reumatismo 2008; 60(3):217–220.

32. McCain GA. Fibromyalgia and myofascial pain. In: Wall PD, Melzack R, eds. Textbook of Pain, 3rd ed. Edinburgh, UK: Churchill Livingstone, 1994:475–493.

33. Yunus MB, Inanici F, Aldag JC, et al. Fibromyalgia in men: Comparison of clinical features with women. J Rheumatol 2000; 27:485–490.

34. Moldofsky H. Chronobiological influences on fibromyalgia syndrome: Theoretical and therapeutic implications. Baillieres Clin Rheumatol 1994; 8:801–810.

35. Tunks E, McCain GA, Hart LE, et al. The reliability of examination for tenderness in patients with myofascial pain, chronic fibromyalgia and controls. J Rheumatol 1995; 22:944–952.

36. Russell IJ, Vipraio GA, Morgan WW, et al. Is there a metabolic basis for the fibrositis syndrome? Am J Med 1986; 81:50–56.

37. Yunus MB. Gender differences in fibromyalgia and other related syndromes. J Gend Specif Med 2002; 5(2):42–47.

38. Jay GW. Chronic Pain. New York: Informa Healthcare, 2007:91–106.

39. Wigers SH. Fibromyalgia—an update. Tidsskr Nor Laegeforen 2002; 122:1300–1304.

40. Smitherman SR. Peripheral and central sensitization in fibromyalgia: Pathogenetic role. Curr Pain Headache Rep 2002; 6(4):259–266.

41. Staud R. Evidence of involvement of central neural mechanisms in generating fibromyalgia pain. Curr Rheumatol Rep 2002; 4(4):299–305.

42. Malt EA, Olafsson S, Lund A, et al. Factors explaining variance in perceived pain in women with fibromyalgia. BMC Musculoskelet Disord 2002; 3:12–16.

43. Staud R, Domingo M. Evidence for abnormal pain processing in fibromyalgia syndrome. Pain Med 2001; 2(3):208–215.
44. Hurtig IM, Raak RI, Kendall SA, et al. Quantitative sensory testing in fibromyalgia patients and in healthy subjects: Identification of subgroups. Clin J Pain 2001; 17(4):316–322.
45. Granot M, Buskila D, Granovsky Y, et al. Simultaneous recording of late and ultralate pain evoked potentials in fibromyalgia. Clin Neurophys 2001; 112(10):1881–1887.
46. Montoya P, Sitges C, Garcia-Herrera M, et al. Reduced brain habituation to somatosensory stimulation in patients with fibromyalgia. Arthritis Rheum 2006; 54(6):1995–2003.
47. Martinez-Lavin M, Hermosillo AG, Mendoza C, et al. Orthostatic sympathetic derangement in subjects with fibromyalgia. J Rheumatol 1997; 24(4):714–718.
48. Martinez-Lavin M, Hermosillo AG, Rosas M, et al. Circadian studies of autonomic nervous balance in patients with fibromyalgia: A heart rate variability analysis. Arthritis Rheum 1998; 41:1966–1971.
49. Clauw DJ, Radulovic D, Heshmat Y, et al. Heart rate variability as a measure of autonomic function in patients with fibromyalgia (FM) and chronic fatigue syndrome (CSF) [abstract]. J Musculoske Pain 1995; 3(Suppl. 1):78.
50. Ozgocmen S, Yoldas T, Yigiter R, et al. R-R interval variation and sympathetic skin response in fibromyalgia. Arch Med Res 2006; 37(5): 630–634.
51. Bou-Holaigah I, Calkins H, Flynn JA, et al. Provocation of hypotension and pain during upright tilt table testing in adults with fibromyalgia. Clin Exp Rheumatol 1997; 15:239–246.
52. Martinez-Lavin M, Vidal M, Barbosa RE, et al. Norepinephrine-evoked pain in fibromyalgia. A randomized pilot study. BMC Musculoske Dis 2002; 3:2.
53. Marinus J, Van Hilten JJ. Clinical expression profiles of complex regional pain syndrome, fibromyalgia and a-specific repetitive strain injury: More common denominators than pain? Disabil Rehabil 2006; 28(6): 351–362.
54. Maekawa K, Clark GT, Kuboki T. Intramuscular hypoperfusion, adrenergic receptors, and chronic muscle pain. J Pain 2002; 3(4):251–260.
55. Bonnet MH, Arand DL. Heart rate variability: Sleep stage, time of night, and arousal influences. Electroencephalogr Clin Neurophysiol 1997; 102:390–396.
56. Naschitz JE, Mussafia-Priselac R, Kovalev Y, et al. Patterns of hypocapnia on tilt in patients with fibromyalgia, chronic fatigue syndrome, nonspecific dizziness, and neurally mediated syncope. Am J Med Sci 2006; 331(6):295–303.
57. Krieger DT, Rizzo F. Serotonin mediation of circadian periodicity of plasma 17-hydroxycorticosteroids. Am J Physiol 1969; 217:1703–1707.
58. Holms MC, Di Renzo G, Beckford U, et al. Role of serotonin in the control of secretion of corticotrophin releasing factor. J Endocrinol 1982; 93:151–160.
59. Wolfe F, Russell IJ, Vipraio G, et al. Serotonin levels, pain threshold and fibromyalgia symptoms in the general population. J Rheumatol 1997; 24:555–559.
60. Russell IJ, Michalek JE, Vipraio GA, et al. Serum amino acids in fibrositis/fibromyalgia syndrome. J Rheumatol 1989; 19(Suppl.):158–163.
61. Russell IJ, Michalek, Vipraio GA, et al. Platelet 3H-imipramine uptake receptor density and serum serotonin levels in patients with fibromyalgia/fibrositis syndrome. J Rheumatol 1992; 19:104–109.
62. Yunus MB, Dailey JW, Aldag JC, et al. Plasma tryptophan and other amino acids in primary fibromyalgia: A controlled study. J Rheumatol 1992; 19:90–94.
63. Yunus MB, Dailey JW, Aldag JC, et al. Plasma and urinary catecholamines in primary fibromyalgia: A controlled study. J Rheumatol 1992; 19:95–97.
64. Russell IJ, Vaeroy H, Javors M, et al. Cerebrospinal fluid biogenic amine metabolites in fibromyalgia/fibrositis syndrome and rheumatoid arthritis. Arthritis Rheum 1992; 35:550–556.
65. Russell IJ, Vipraio GA. Serotonin (5HT) in serum and platelets (PLT) from fibromyalgia patients (FS) and normal controls (NC) [Abstract]. Arthritis Rheum 1994; 37(Suppl.):S214.

66. Kang Y-K, Russell IJ, Vipraio GA, et al. Low urinary 5-hydroxyindole acetic acid in fibromyalgia syndrome: Evidence in support of a serotonin-deficiency pathogenesis. Myalgia 1998; 1:14–21.

67. Russell IJ, Vipraio GA, Acworth I. Abnormalities in the central nervous system (CNS) metabolism of tryptophan (TRY) to 3-hydroxy kynurenine (OHKY) in fibromyalgia syndrome (FS) [Abstract]. Arthritis Rheum 1993; 36:S222.

68. Holman AJ, Myers RR. A randomized, double-blind, placebo-controlled trial of pramipexole, a dopamine agonist, in patients with fibromyalgia receiving concomitant medication. Arthritis Rheum 2005; 52:2495–2505.

69. Yunus MB, Denko CW, Masi AT. Serum beta-endorphin in primary fibromyalgia syndrome: a controlled study. J Rheum 1986; 13(1):183–186.

70. Vaeroy H, Helle R, Forre O, et al. Cerebrospinal fluid levels of B-endorphin in patients with fibromyalgia (fibrositis syndrome). J Rheum 1988; 15:1804–1806.

71. Panerai AE, Vecchiet J, Panzeri P, et al. Peripheral blood mononuclear cell B-endorphin concentration is decreased in chronic fatigue syndrome and fibromyalgia but not in depression: Preliminary report. Clin J Pain 2002; 18(4):270–273.

72. Sorensen J, Bengtsson A, Backman E, et al. Pain analysis in patients with fibromyalgia. Effects of intravenous morphine, lidocaine and ketamine. Scan J Rheum 1995; 24(6):360–365.

73. Han JS, Xie CW. Dynorphin: Potent analgesic effect in spinal cord of the rat. Life Sci 1982; 31:1781–1784.

74. Vanderah T, Laughlin T, Lashbrook J, et al. Single intrathecal injections of dynorphin A or des-Tyr-dynorphins produce long lasting allodynia in rats: Blockade by MK-801 but not naloxone. Pain 1996; 68:275–281.

75. Laughlin TM, Vanderah T, Lashbrook JM, et al. Spinally administered dynorphin A produces long lasing allodynia: Involvement of NMDA but not opioid receptors. Pain 1997; 72:253–260.

76. Laughlin TM, Larson AA, Wilcox GL. Mechanisms of induction of persistent nociception by dynorphin. J Pharmacol Exp Ther 2001; 299(1):6–11.

77. Vaeroy H, Nyberg F, Terenius L. No evidence for endorphin deficiency in fibromyalgia following investigation of cerebrospinal fluid (CSF) dynorphin A and Met-enkephalin-Arg6-Phe7. Pain 1991; 46:139–143.

78. Coderre TJ, Katz J, Vaccarino AL, et al. Contribution of central neuroplasticity to pathological pain: Review of clinical and experimental evidence. Pain 1993; 52:259–285.

79. Tsigos C, Diemel LT, White A, et al. Cerebrospinal fluid levels of substance P and calcitonin-gene-related peptide: Correlation with sural nerve levels and neuropathic signs in sensory diabetic polyneuropathy. Clin Sci Colch 1993; 84:305–311.

80. Galeazza MT, Garry MG, Yost HJ, et al. Plasticity in the synthesis and storage of substance P and calcitonin gene-related peptide in primary afferent neurons during peripheral inflammation. Neuroscience 1995; 66:443–458.

81. Vaeroy H, Helle R, Forre O, et al. Elevated CSF levels of substance P and high incidence of Raynaud's phenomenon in patients with fibromyalgia: new features for diagnosis. Pain 1988; 32:21–26.

82. Russell IJ, Orr MD, Littman B, et al. Elevated cerebrospinal fluid levels of substance P in patients with the fibromyalgia syndrome. Arthritis Rheum 1994; 37:1593–1601.

83. Welin M, Bragee B, Nyberg F, et al. Elevated substance P levels are contrasted by a decrease in met-enkephalin-arg-phe levels in CSF from fibromyalgia patients. J Musculoskel Pain 1995; 3:4.

84. Bradley LA, Alberts KR, Alarcon GS, et al. Abnormal brain regional cerebral blood flow (rCBF) and cerebrospinal fluid (CSF) levels of substance P (SP) in patients and non-patients with fibromyalgia (FM). Arthritis Rheum1996; 39(suppl. 19):S212.

85. Russell IJ, Fletcher EM, Vipraio GA, et al. Cerebrospinal fluid (CSF) substance P (SP) in fibromyalgia: changes in CSF SP over time parallel changes in clinical activity [Abstract]. J Musculoske Pain 1998; 6(suppl. 2):77.

86. Schwarz MJ, Spath M, Muller-Bardorff H, et al. Relationship of substance P, 5-hydroxyindole acetic acid and tryptophan in serum of fibromyalgia patients. Neurosci Lett 1999; 259:196–198.

87. Lindsay RM, Harmar AJ. Nerve growth factor regulates expression of neuropeptides genes in adult sensory neurons. Nature 1989; 337:362–364.

88. Petty BG, Cornblath DR, Adornato BT, et al. The effect of systemically administered recombinant human nerve growth factor in healthy human subjects. Ann Neurol 1994; 36:244–246.

89. Giovengo SL, Russell IJ, Larson AA. Increased concentrations of nerve growth factor in cerebrospinal fluid of patient with fibromyalgia. J Rheumatol 1999; 26:1564–1596.

90. Vaeroy H, Sakurada T, Forre O, et al. Modulation of pain in fibromyalgia (fibrositis syndrome): Cerebrospinal fluid (CSF) investigation of pain related neuropeptides with special reference to calcitonin gene-related peptide (CGRP). J Rheumatol Suppl 1989; 19:94–97.

91. Crofford LJ, Pillemer SR, Kalogeras KT, et al. Hypothalamic-pituitary-adrenal axis perturbations in patients with fibromyalgia. Arthritis Rheum 1994; 37(11):1583–1592.

92. van Denderen JC, Boersma JW, Zeinstra P, et al. Physiological effects of exhaustive physical exercise in primary fibromyalgia syndrome (PFS): Is PFS a disorder of neuroendocrine reactivity? Scan J Rheumatol 1992; 21(1):35–37.

93. Pillemer SR, Bradley LA, Crofford LJ, et al. The neuroscience and endocrinology of fibromyalgia. Arthritis Rheum 1997; 40:1928–1939.

94. Yunus MB, Aldag JC, Dailey JW, et al. Interrelationships of biochemical parameters in classification of fibromyalgia syndrome and healthy normal controls. J Musculoske Pain 1995; 3(4):15–24.

95. Pall ML. Common etiology of posttraumatic stress disorder, fibromyalgia, chronic fatigue syndrome and multiple chemical sensitivity via elevated nitric oxide/peroxynitrite. Med Hypotheses 2001; 57(2):139–145.

96. Watkins LR, Milligan ED, Maier SF. Glial activation: a driving force for pathological pain. Trends Neurosci 2001; 24:450–455.

97. Kreutzberg GW. Microglia: A sensor for pathological events in the CNS. Trends Neurosci 1996; 19:312–318.

98. Raivich G, Bluethmann H, Kreutzberg GW. Signaling molecules and neuroglial activation in the injured central nervous system. Keio J Med 1996; 45:239–247.

99. Sarchielli P, ALberti A, Candeliere A, et al. Glial cell line-derived neurotrophic factor and somatostatin levels in cerebrospinal fluid of patients affected by chronic migraine and fibromyalgia. Cephalalgia 2006; 26(4):409–415.

100. Wallace DJ, Linker-Israeli M, Hallegua D, et al. Cytokines play an aetiopathogenetic role in fibromyalgia: A hypothesis and pilot study. Rheumatology 2001; 40:743–749.

101. Laske C, Stansky E, Eschweiler GW, et al. Increased BDNF serum concentration in fibromyalgia with or without depression or antidepressants. J Psychiatr Res 2007; 41(7):600–605.

102. Yaksh TL. Pharmacology and mechanisms of opioid analgesic activity. In: Yaksh TL, Lynch C III, Zapol WM, et al., eds. Anesthesia: Biologic Foundations. Philadelphia, PA: Lippincott-Raven, 1997:921–934.

103. Carter BD, Medzihradsky F. Go mediates the coupling of the mu opioid receptor to adenyl cyclase in cloned neural cells and brain. Proc Natl Acad Sci U S A 1993; 90:4062–4066.

104. Galeotti N, Ghelardini C, Zoppi M, et al. A reduced functionality of Gi proteins as a possible cause of fibromyalgia. J Rheumatol 2001; 28:2298–2304.

105. Galeotti N, Ghelardini C, Zoppi M, et al. Hypofunctionality of Gi proteins as aetiopathogenic mechanism for migraine and cluster headache. Cephalalgia 2001; 21:38–45.

106. Lentjes EG, Griep EN, Boersma JW, et al. Glucocorticoid receptors, fibromyalgia and low back pain. Psychoneuroendocrinology 1997; 22(8):603–614.

107. Crofford LJ, Demitrack MA. Evidence that abnormalities of central neurohormonal systems are key to understanding fibromyalgia and chronic fatigue syndrome. Rheum Dis Clin North Am 1996; 22:267–284.
108. Griep EN, Boersma JW, Lentjes EG, et al. Function of the hypothalamic-pituitary-adrenal axis in patients with fibromyalgia and low back pain. J Rheumatol 1998; 25:2125–1381.
109. McCain GA, Tilbe KS. Diurnal variation in fibromyalgia syndrome: A comparison with rheumatoid arthritis. J Rheumatol 1989; 19(suppl):154–157.
110. Riedel W, Kayka H, Neeck G. Secretory pattern of GH, TSH, thyroid hormones, ACTH, cortisol, FSH and LH in patients with fibromyalgia syndrome following systemic injection of the relevant hypothalamic-releasing hormones. Z Rheumatol 1998; 57(suppl 2):81–87.
111. Griep EN, Boersma JW, de Kloet ER. Altered reactivity of the hypothalamic-pituitary-adrenal axis in the primary fibromyalgia syndrome. J Rheumatol 1993; 20:469–474.
112. Torpy DJ, Papanicolaou DA, Lotsikas AJ, et al. Responses of the sympathetic nervous system and the hypothalamic-pituitary-adrenal axis to interleukin-6: A pilot study in fibromyalgia. Arthritis Rheum 2000; 43:872–880.
113. Leal-Cerro A, Povedano J, Astroga R, et al. The growth hormone (GH)-releasing hormone-GH-insulin-like growth factor-1 axis in patients with fibromyalgia syndrome. J Clin Endocrin Metabol 1999; 84:3378–3381.
114. Bagge E, Bengtsson BA, Carlsson L, et al. Low growth hormone secretion in patients with fibromyalgia—a preliminary report on 10 patients and 10 controls. J Rheumatol 1998; 25:145–148.
115. Adler GK, Manfredsdottir VF, Creskoff KW. Neuroendocrine abnormalities in fibromyalgia. Cur Pain Headache Reports 2002; 6:289–298.
116. Bennett RM, Clark SR, Burckhardt CS, et al. Hypothalamic-pituitary-insulin-like growth factor-1 axis dysfunction in patients with fibromyalgia. J Rheumatol 1997; 24(7):1384–1389.
117. Van Cauter E, Plat L, Copinschi G. Interrelations between sleep and the somatotopic axis. Sleep 1998; 21(6):553–566.
118. Moldofsky H, Scarisbrick P, England R, et al. Musculoskeletal symptoms and non-REM sleep disturbance in patients with "fibrositis" syndrome and healthy subjects. Psychosom Med 1975; 37:341–351.
119. Kato Y, Murakami Y, Sohmiya M, et al. Regulation of human growth hormone secretion and its disorders. Intern Med 2002; 41(1):7–13.
120. Anderson SM, Shah N, Evans WS, et al. Short-term estradiol supplementation augments growth hormone (GH) secretory responsiveness to dose-varying GH-releasing peptide infusions in healthy post-menopausal women. J Clin Endocrinol Metab 2001; 86(2):551–560.
121. Cordido F, Dieguez C, Casanueva FF. Effect of central cholinergic neurotransmission enhancement by pyridostigmine on the growth hormone secretion elicited by clonidine, arginine or hypoglycemia in normal and obese subjects. J Clin Endocrinol Metab 1990; 70(5):1361–1370.
122. Bennett RM, Cook DM, Clark SR, et al. Hypothalamic-pituitary-insulin-like growth factor-1 axis dysfunction in patients with fibromyalgia. J Rheumatol 1997; 24:1384–1389.
123. Neeck G, Riedel W. Thyroid function in patients with fibromyalgia syndrome. J Rheumatol 1992; 19:1120–1122.
124. Press J, Phillip M, Neumann L, et al. Normal melatonin levels in patients with fibromyalgia syndrome. J Rheumatol 1998; 25:551–555.
125. Korszun A, Sackett-Lundeen L, Papadopoulos E, et al. Melatonin levels in women with fibromyalgia and chronic fatigue syndrome. J Rheumatol 1999; 26:2675–2680.
126. Wikner J, Hirsch U, Wetterberg L, et al. Fibromyalgia: A syndrome associated with decreased nocturnal melatonin secretion. Clin Endocrinol 1998; 49(2):179–183.

127. Binder JR, Swanson SJ, Hammeke TE, et al. Determination of language dominance using functional MRI: A comparison with the Wada test. Neurology 1996; 46:978–984.
128. Mountz JM, Bradley LA, Modell JG, et al. Fibromyalgia in women. Abnormalities of regional cerebral blood flow in the thalamus and the caudate nucleus are associated with low pain threshold levels. Arthritis Rheum 1995; 38:926–938.
129. Lineberry CG, Vierck CJ. Attenuation of pain reactivity by caudate nucleus stimulation in monkeys. Brain Res 1975; 98:119–134.
130. Kwiatek R, Barnden L, Tedman R, et al. Regional cerebral blood flow in fibromyalgia: Single-photon-emission computed tomography evidence of reduction in the pontine tegmentum and thalami. Arthritis Rheum 2000; 43:2823–2833.
131. Bradley LA, Sotolongo A, Alberts KR, et al. Abnormal regional cerebral blood flow in the caudate nucleus among fibromyalgia patients and non-patients is associated with insidious symptom onset. J Musculoskeletal Pain 1999; 7:285–292.
132. Coghill RC, Talbot JD, Evans AC, et al. Distributed processing of pain and vibration by the human brain. J Neurosci 1994; 14:4095–4108.
133. Coghill RC, Sang CN, Maisog JM, et al. Pain intensity processing within the human brain: A bilateral, distributed mechanism. J Neurophysiol 1999; 82:1934–1943.
134. Cianfrini LR, McKendree-Smith NL, Bradley LA, et al. Pain sensitivity and bilateral activation of brain structures during pressure stimulation of patients with fibromyalgia (FM) is not mediated by major depression (DEP). Arthritis Rheum 2001; 44:S395.
135. Mountz JM, Bradley LA, Alarcon GS. Abnormal functional activity of the central nervous system in fibromyalgia syndrome. Am J Med Sci 1998; 315:385–396.
136. Gracely RH, Petzke F, Wolf JM, et al. Functional magnetic resonance imaging evidence of augmented pain processing in fibromyalgia. Arthritis Rheum 2002; 46(5):1333–1344.
137. Guedj E, Cammilleri S, Miboyet J, et al. Clinical correlate of Brain SPECT perfusion abnormalities in fibromyalgia. J Nucl Med 2008; 49(11):1798–1803.
138. Weigent DA, Bradley LA, Blalock JE, et al. Current concepts in the pathophysiology of abnormal pain perception in fibromyalgia. Am J Med Sci 1998; 315:405–412.
139. Pauli P, Wiedemann G, Nickola M. Pain sensitivity, cerebral laterality, and negative affect. Pain 1999; 80:359–364.
140. Valet M, Gundel H, Sprenger T, et al. Patients with pain disorder show gray-matter loss in pain-processing structures: A voxel-based morphometric study. Psychosom Med 2009; 71(1):49–56.
141. Kuchinad A, Schweinhardt P, Seminowicz DA, et al. Accelerated brain gray matter loss in fibromyalgia patients: Premature aging of the brain? J Neurosci 2007; 27(15):4004–4007.
142. Schmidt-Wilcke T, Luerding R, Weigand T, et al. Striatal grey matter increase in patients suffering from fibromyalgia—A voxel-based morphometry study. Pain 2007; 132:S109–S116.
143. Schmidt-Wilcke T. Variations in brain volume and regional morphology associated with chronic pain. Curr Rheumatol Rep 2008; 10(6):467–474.
144. Lutz J, Jager L, de Quervain D, et al. White and gray matter abnormalities in the brain of patients with fibromyalgia. Arthritis Rheum 2008; 58(12):3960–3969.
145. Elvin A, Siosteen AK, Nilsson A, et al. Decreased muscle blood flow in fibromyalgia patients during standardized muscle exercise: A contrast media enhanced colour Doppler study. Eur J Pain 2006; 10(2):137–144.
146. Kasikcioglu E, Dinler M, Berker E. Reduced tolerance of exercise in fibromyalgia may be a consequence of impaired microcirculation initiated by deficient action of nitric oxide. Med Hypotheses 2006; 66(5):950–952.
147. Yunus MB, Kalyan-Raman UP, Masi AT, et al. Electron microscopic studies of muscle biopsy in primary fibromyalgia syndrome: A controlled and blinded study. J Rheumatol 1989; 16:97–101.

148. Bengtsson A, Henriksson KG, Larsson J. Muscle biopsy in primary fibromyalgia: Light microscopical and histochemical findings. Scand J Rheumatol 1986; 15: 106.
149. Drewes AM, Andreasen A, Schroder HD, et al. Muscle biopsy in fibromyalgia. Scand J Rheumatol 1992; 94(suppl):20.
150. Bengtsson A, Henriksson KG, Larsson J. Reduced high-energy phosphate levels in the painful muscles of patients with primary fibromyalgia. Arthritis Rheum 1986; 29:817–821.
151. Simms RW. Fibromyalgia is not a muscle disorder. Am J Med Sci 1998; 315:346–350.
152. Simms RW. Is there muscle pathology in fibromyalgia syndrome. Rheum Dis Clin North Am 1996; 22:245–266.
153. Branco JC, Atalaia A, Paiva T. Sleep cycles and alpha-delta sleep in fibromyalgia syndrome. J Rheumatol 1994; 21:1113–1117.
154. Drewes AM, Gade J, Nielsen KD, et al. Clustering of sleep electroencephalopathic patterns in patients with the fibromyalgia syndrome. Br J Rheumatol 1995; 34:1151–1156.
155. Perlis ML, Giles DE, Bootzin RR, et al. Alpha sleep and information processing, perception of sleep, pain and arousability in fibromyalgia. Int J Neurosci 1997; 89:265–280.
156. Moldofsky H, Lue FA, Smythe HA. Alpha EEG sleep and morning symptoms in rheumatoid arthritis. J Rheumatol 1983; 10:373–379.
157. Moldofsky H, Saskin P, Lue FA. Sleep symptoms in fibrositis syndrome after a febrile illness. J Rheumatol 1988; 15:1701–1704.
158. Moldofsky H. Sleep and pain. Sleep Med Rev 2001; 5(5):385–396.
159. Izuierdo AS, Bocos Terraz P, Bancalero Flores JL, et al. Is there an association between fibromyalgia and below-normal levels of urinary cortisol? BMC Res Notes 2008; 1(1):134.
160. Ahles TA, Yunus MB, Masi AT. Is chronic pain a variant of depressive disease? The case of primary fibromyalgia syndrome. Pain 1987; 29:105–111.
161. Ahles TA, Khan SA, Yunus MB, et al. Psychiatric status of patients with primary fibromyalgia, patients with rheumatoid arthritis and subjects without pain: A blind comparison of DSM-III diagnoses. Am J Psychiatry 1991; 148:1721–1726.
162. Clark S, Campbell SM, Forehand ME, et al. Clinical characteristics of fibrositis. II. A "blinded", controlled study using standard psychological tests. Arthritis Rheum 1985; 28:132–137.
163. Kirmayer LJ, Robbins JM, Kapusta MA. Somatization and depression in fibromyalgia syndrome. Am J Psychiatry 1988; 145:950–954.
164. Hudson JI, Hudson MS, Pliner LF, et al. Fibromyalgia and major affective disorder: A controlled phenomenology and family history study. Am J Psychiatry 1985; 142:441–446.
165. Hudson JI, Goldenberg DL, Pope HG Jr, et al. Comorbidity of fibromyalgia with medical and psychiatric disorders. J Rheumatol Suppl 1992; 92:363–367.
166. Aaron LA, Bradley LA, Alarcon GS, et al. Psychiatric diagnoses in patients with fibromyalgia are related to health care-seeking behavior rather than to illness. Arthritis Rheum 1996; 39:436–445.
167. White KP, Nielson WR, Harth M, et al. Chronic widespread musculoskeletal pain with or without fibromyalgia: Psychological distress in a representative community adult sample. J Rheumatol 2002; 29:588–594.
168. Ahles TA, Yunus MB, Riley SD, et al. Psychological factors associated with primary fibromyalgia syndrome. Arthritis Rheum 1984; 27:1101–1106.
169. Dailey PA, Bishop GD, Russell IJ, et al. Psychological stress and the fibrositis/fibromyalgia syndrome. J Rheumatol 1990; 17:1380–1385.
170. Missole C, Toroni F, Sigala S, et al. Nerve growth factor in the anterior pituitary: Localization in mammotroph cells and cosecretion with prolactin by a dopamine-regulated mechanism. Proc Natl Acad Sci U S A 1996; 93:4240–4245.

171. Lindsay RM, Lockett C, Sternberg J, et al. Neuropeptide expression in cultures of adult sensory neurons: Modulation of substance P and calcitonin gene-related peptide levels by nerve growth factor. Neuroscience 1989; 33:53–65.

172. Goebel MU, Mills PJ, Irwin MR, et al. Interleukin-6 and tumor necrosis factor-alpha production after acute psychological stress, exercise and infused isoproterenol: Differential effects and pathways. Psychosom Med 2000; 62:591–598.

173. Davis MC, Zautra AJ, Reich JW. Vulnerability to stress among women in chronic pain from fibromyalgia and osteoarthritis. Ann Behav Med 2001; 23:215–226.

174. Adler GK, Kinsley BT, Hurwitz S, et al. Reduced hypothalamic-pituitary and sympathoadrenal responses to hypoglycemia in women with fibromyalgia syndrome. Am J Med 1999; 106:534–543.

175. Schatzberg AF, Rothschild AJ, Stahl JB, et al. The dexamethasone suppression test: Identification of subtypes of depression. Am J Psychiatry 1983; 140:88–91.

176. Banki CM, Bissette G, Arato M, et al. CSF corticotropin-releasing factor-like immunoreactivity in depression and schizophrenia. Am J Psychiatry 1987; 144:873–877.

177. Maes M, Lin A, Bonaccorso S, et al. Increased 24-hour urinary cortisol excretion in patients with post-traumatic stress disorder and patients with major depression, but not in patients with fibromyalgia. Acta Psychiat Scand 1998; 98:328–335.

178. Alexander RW, Bradley LA, Alarcon GS, et al. Sexual and physical abuse in women with fibromyalgia: Association with outpatients health care utilization and pain medication usage. Arthritis Care Res 1998; 11:102–115.

179. Goldberg RT, Pachas WN, Keith D. Relationship between traumatic events in childhood and chronic pain. Disabil Rehabil 1999; 21:23–30.

180. McBeth J, Macfarlane GJ, Benjamin S, et al. The association between tender points, psychological distress, and adverse childhood experiences: A community based study. Arthritis Rheum 1999; 42:1397–1404.

181. Boisset-Pioro MH, Esdaile JM, Fitzcharles MA. Sexual and physical abuse in women with fibromyalgia syndrome. Arthritis Rheum 1995; 38:235–241.

182. Fassbender K, Samborsky W, Kellner M, et al. Tender points, depressive and functional symptoms: Comparison between fibromyalgia and major depression. Clin Rheumatol 1997; 16:76–79.

183. Golding JM. Sexual-assault history and long-term physical health problems: Evidence from clinical and population epidemiology. Cur Dir Psychol Sci 1999; 8(6):191–194.

184. Leavitt F, Katz RS, Mills M, et al. Cognitive and dissociative manifestations in fibromyalgia. J Clin Rheumatol 2002; 8:77–84.

185. White KP, Nielson WR, Harth M, et al. Does the label "fibromyalgia" alter health status, function, and health service utilization? A prospective, within-group comparison in a community cohort of adults with chronic widespread pain. Arthritis Care Res 2002; 47(3):260–265.

186. Pelligrino MJ, Waylonis GW, Sommer A. Familial occurrence of primary fibromyalgia. Arch Phys Med Rehabil 1989; 70:61–63.

187. Buskila D, Neumann L. Fibromyalgia syndrome (FM) and nonarticular tenderness in relatives of patients with FM. J Rheumatol 1997; 24:941–944.

188. Offenbaecher M, Bondy B, de Jonge S, et al. Possible association of fibromyalgia with a polymorphism in the serotonin transporter gene regulatory region. Arthritis Rheum 1999; 42:2482–2488.

189. Martinez JE, Ferraz MB, Sato EI, et al. Fibromyalgia versus rheumatoid arthritis: A longitudinal comparison of the quality of life. J Rheumatol 1995; 22:270–274.

190. Henriksson CM. Longterm effects of fibromyalgia on everyday life. A study of 56 patients. Scand J Rheumatol 1994; 23:36–41.

191. Burckhardt CS, Clark SR, Bennett RM. Fibromyalgia and quality of life: A comparative analysis. J Rheumatol 1993; 20:475–479.

192. Wolfe F, Anderson J, Harkness D, et al. Work and disability status of persons with fibromyalgia. J Rheumatol 1997; 24:1171–1178.

193. Cathey MA, Wolfe F, Kleinheksel SM. Functional ability and work status in patients with fibromyalgia. Arthritis Care Res 1988; 1:25–33.
194. Lundberg G, Gerdle B. Tender point scores and their relations to signs of mobility, symptoms, and disability in female home care personnel and the prevalence of fibromyalgia syndrome. J Rheumatol 2002; 29:603–613.
195. Leidberg GM, Henriksson CM. Factors of importance for work disability in women with fibromyalgia: An interview study. Arthritis Care Res 2002; 47:266–274.
196. Russo EB. Clinical endocannabinoid deficiency (CECD): Can this concept explain therapeutic benefits of cannabis in migraine, fibromyalgia, irritable bowel syndrome and other treatment resistant conditions? Neuroendocrinol Lett 2004; 25:31–39.
197. Corchero J, Manzanares J, Fuentes JA. Cannabinoid/opioid crosstalk in the central nervous system. Crit Rev Neurobiol 2004; 16:159–172.
198. Salio C, Fischer J, Franzoni MF, et al. CB1-cannabinoid and mu-receptor co-localization on postsynaptic target in the rat dorsal horn. Neuroreport 2001; 12:3639–3692.
199. Skrabek RQ, Galimova L, Ethans K, et al. Nabilone for the treatment of pain in fibromyalgia. J Pain 2008; 9(2):164–173.
200. Ko G, Wine W. Chronic pain and cannabinoids: A survey study of current fibromyalgia treatment approaches together with an overview and case studies of a new "old" treatment approach. Pract Pain Manage 2005; 1:1–8.
201. Staud R, Smitherman ML. Peripheral and central sensitization in fibromyalgia: Pathogenetic role. Cur Pain Headache Reports 2002; 6:259–266.
202. Kim SH, Jang TJ, Moon IS. Increased expression of N-methyl-D-aspartate receptor subunit 2D in the skin of patients with fibromyalgia. J Rheumatol 2006; 33(4):785–788.
203. Woolf CJ, Thompson SW. The induction and maintenance of central sensitization is dependent on N-methyl-D-aspartic acid receptor activation; implications for the treatment of post-injury pain hypersensitivity states. Pain 1991; 44:293–299.
204. Stein C, Machelska H, Binder W, et al. Peripheral opioid analgesia. Curr Opin Pharmacol 2001; 1:62–65.
205. Brenman JE, Bredt DS. Synaptic signaling by nitric oxide. Curr Opin Neurobiol 1997; 7:374–378.
206. Schuman EM, Madison DV. Nitric oxide and synaptic function. Ann Rev Neurosci 1994; 17:153–183.
207. Aimar P, Pasti L, Carmignoto G, et al. Nitric oxide-producing islet cells modulate the release of sensory neuropeptides in the rat substantia gelatinosa. J Neurosci 1998; 18:10357–10388.
208. Sendur OF, Turan Y, Tasstaban E, et al. Serum antioxidants and nitric oxide levels in fibromyalgia: A controlled study. Rheumatol Int 2009; 29(6):629–633.
209. Price DD, Mao J, Frenk H, et al. The N-methyl-D-aspartate receptor antagonist dextromethorphan selectively reduces temporal summation of second pain in man. Pain 1994; 59:165–174.
210. Price DD, Hu JW, Dubner R, et al. Peripheral suppression of first pain and central summation of second pain evoked by noxious heat pulses. Pain 1977; 3:57–68.
211. Price DD. Characteristics of second pain and flexion reflexes indicative of prolonged central summation. Exp Neurol 1972; 37:371–387.
212. Graven-Nielsen T, Kendall SA, Henriksson KG, et al. Ketamine reduces muscle pain, temporal summation and referred pain in fibromyalgia patients. Pain 2000; 85:483–491.
213. Yunus MB, Inanici F. Clinical characteristics and biopathophyisological mechanisms of fibromyalgia syndrome. In: Baldry PE, ed. Myofascial Pain and Fibromyalgia Syndrome. London, UK: Churchill Livingstone, 2001:351–378.
214. Granges G, Littlejohn G. Prevalence of myofascial pain syndrome in fibromyalgia syndrome and regional pain syndrome: A comparative study. J Musculosk Pain 1993; 1(2):19–35.
215. Gerwin RD. A study of 96 subjects examined both for fibromyalgia and myofascial pain [Abstract]. J Musculoske Pain 1995; 3(suppl 1):21.

216. Bennett RM. Emerging concepts in the neurobiology of chronic pain: Evidence of abnormal sensory processing in fibromyalgia. Mayo Clin Proc 1999; 74:385–398.
217. Martinez-Lavin M. Is fibromyalgia a generalized reflex sympathetic dystrophy? Clin Exp Rheumatol 2001; 19:1–3.
218. Henriksson KG. Hypersensitivity in muscle pain syndromes. Curr Pain Headache Rep 2003; 7:426–432.
219. Sorensen J, Graven-Nielsen T, Hendriksson KG, et al. Hyperexcitability in fibromyalgia. J Rheumatol 1998; 25:152–155.
220. Wright A, Graven-Nielsen T, Davies, et al. Temporal summation of pain from skin, muscle and joint following nociceptive ultrasonic stimulation in humans. Exp Brain Res 2002; 144:475–482.
221. Turk DC. The potential of treatment matching for subgroups of patients with chronic pain: lumping versus splitting. Clin J Pain 2005; 21(1):44–55.
222. Dobkin PL, Sita A, Sewitch MJ. Predictors of adherence to treatment in women with fibromyalgia. Clin J Pain 2006; 22(3):286–294.
223. Melillo N, Corrado A, Quarta L, et al. Fibromyalgic syndrome: New perspectives in rehabilitation and management. A review. Minerva Med 2005; 96(6):417–423.
224. Arnold LM. Biology and therapy of fibromyalgia. New therapies in fibromyalgia. Arthritis Res Ther 2006; 8(4):212.
225. Wolfe F, Anderson J, Harkness D, et al. A prospective, longitudinal, multicenter study of service utilization and costs in fibromyalgia. Arthritis Rheum 1997; 40:1560–1570.
226. Goldenberg DL, Felson DT, Dinerman H. A randomized, controlled trial of amitriptyline and naproxen in the treatment of patients with fibromyalgia. Arthritis Rheum 1986; 29:1371–1377.
227. Yunus MB, Masi AT, Aldag JC. Short term effects of ibuprofen in primary fibromyalgia syndrome: A double blind, placebo controlled trial. J Rheumatol 1989; 16:527–532.
228. Clark S, Tindall E, Bennett RM. A double blind crossover trial of prednisone versus placebo in the treatment of fibrositis. J Rheumatol 1985; 12:980–983.
229. Ang D, Wilke WS. Diagnosis, etiology and therapy of fibromyalgia. Compr Ther 1999; 25:221–227.
230. Krsnich-Shriwise S. Fibromyalgia syndrome: an overview. Phys Ther 1997; 77:68–75.
231. Buskila D. Drug therapy. Baillieres Best Pract Res Clin Rheumatol 1999; 13:479–485.
232. Russell IJ, Kamin M, Sager D, et al. Efficacy of Ultram (Tramadol HCL) treatment of fibromyalgia syndrome: Preliminary analysis of a multi-center, randomized, placebo-controlled study. Arthritis Rheum 1997; 40(suppl 9):S117.
233. Rauck RL, Ruoff GE, McMillen JI. Comparison of tramadol and acetaminophen with codeine for long-term pain management in elderly patients. Curr Ther Res 1994; 55:1417–1431.
234. Biasi G, Manca S, Manganelli S, et al. Tramadol in the fibromyalgia syndrome: A controlled clinical trial versus placebo. Int J Clin Pharacol Res 1998; 18:13–19.
235. Russell IJ. Efficacy of ULTRAM (Tramadol Hcl) treatment of fibromyalgia syndrome (FMS): Secondary outcomes report. TPS-FM Study Group [Abstract]. J Musculoskeletal Pain 1998; 6(suppl 2):147.
236. Gasse C, Derby L, Vasilakis-Scaramozza C, et al. Incidence of first-time idiopathic seizures in users of tramadol. Pharacotherapy 2000; 20:629–634.
237. Leventhal LG. Management of fibromyalgia. Ann Intern Med 1999; 131:850–858.
238. Rospond RM, Spellman J. Fibromyalgia and the role of the pharmacist. U. S. Pharmacist. 1997; 22:41–52.
239. Brown RL, Fleming MF, Patterson JJ. Chronic opiod analgesic therapy for chronic low back pain. J Am Board Fam Pract 1996; 9:191–204.
240. The use of opiods for the treatment of chronic pain. A consensus statement from the American Academy of Pain Medicine and the American Pain Society. Clin J Pain 1997; 13:6–8.

241. Portenoy RK. Opioid therapy for chronic nonmalignant pain: A review of the critical issues. J Pain Symptom Manage 1996; 11:203–217.
242. McClain DA. The effects of Tizanidine HCL (Zanaflex®) in patients with Fibromyalgia. In: Jay GW, Drusz JC, Longmire DR, McLain DA, eds. Current Trends in the Diagnosis and Treatment of Chronic Neuromuscular Pain Syndromes. Am Academy of Pain Management. Precom International, August 2000.
243. Hong CZ, Hsueh TC. Difference in pain relief after trigger point injections in myofascial pain patients with and without fibromyalgia. Arch Phys Med Rehabil 1996; 77:1161–1166.
244. Yunus MB. Fibromyalgia syndrome: is there any effective therapy? Consultant 1996; 36:1279–1286.
245. Raphael JH, Southall JL, Treharne GJ, et al. Efficacy and adverse effects of intravenous lignocaine therapy in fibromyalgia syndrome. BMC Musculoskelet Disord 2002; 3(1):21.
246. Staud R. Are tender point injections beneficial: the role of tonic nociception in fibromyalgia. Curr Pharm Des 2006; 12(1):23–27.
247. Sorensen J, Bengtsson A, Ahlner J, et al. Fibromyalgia—are there different mechanisms in the processing of pain? A double blind crossover comparison of analgesic drugs. J Rheumatol 1996; 24:1615–1621.
248. Henriksson KG, Sorensen J. The promise of N-methyl-D-aspartate receptor antagonists in fibromyalgia. Rheum Dis Clinics North Am 2002; 28(2):1–7.
249. Stuad R, Vierck CJ, Robinson ME, et al. Effects of the N-methyl-D-aspartate receptor antagonist dextromethorphan on temporal summation of pain are similar in fibromyalgia patients and normal controls subjects. J Pain 2005; 6(5):323–332.
250. Cohen SP, Verdolin MH, Chang AS, et al. The intravenous ketamine test predicts subsequent response to an oral dextromethorphan treatment regimen in fibromyalgia patients. J Pain 2006; 7(6):391–399.
251. Maizels M, McCarberg B. Antidepressants and antiepileptic drugs for chronic noncancer pain. Am Fam Physician 2005; 71(3):483–490.
252. Scudds RA, McCain GA, Rollman GB, et al. Improvements in pain responsiveness in patients with fibrositis after successful treatment with amitriptyline. J Rheumatol 1989; 19(suppl):98–103.
253. Carette S, McCain GA, Bell DA, et al. Evaluation of amitriptyline in primary fibrositis. A double blind, placebo-controlled study. Arthritis Rheum 1986; 29(5):655–659.
254. Jaeschke R, Adachi J, Guyatt G, et al. Clinical usefulness of amitriptyline in fibromyalgia: The results of 23N-of-1 randomized controlled trials. J Rheumatol 1991; 18(3):447–451.
255. Maurizio SJ, Rogers JL. Recognizing and treating fibromyalgia. Nurse Pract 1997; 22:18–33.
256. Simms RW. Fibromyalgia syndrome: current concepts in pathophysiology, clinical features, and management. Arthritis Care Res 1996; 9:315–328.
257. Wallace DJ. The fibromyalgia syndrome. Ann Med 1997; 29:9–21.
258. Creamer P. Effective management of fibromyalgia. J Musculoskel Med 1999; 16:622.
259. Wysenbeek AJ, Mor F, Lurie Y, et al. Imipramine for the treatment of fibrositis: a therapeutic trial. Ann Rheum Dis 1985; 44:752–753.
260. Nishishinya B, Urrutia G, Walitt B, et al. Amitriptyline in the treatment of fibromyalgia: a systematic review of its efficacy. Rheumatology (Oxford) 2008; 47(12):1741–1746.
261. Reynolds WJ, Moldofsky H, Saskin P, et al. The effects of cyclobenzaprine on sleep physiology and symptoms in patients with fibromyalgia. J Rheumatol 1991; 18(3):452–454.
262. Bennett RM, Gatter RA, Campbell SM, et al. A comparison of cyclobenzaprine and placebo in the management of fibrositis. A double blind controlled study. Arthritis Rheum 1988; 31(12):1535–1542.
263. Carrette S, Bell MJ, Reynolds WJ, et al. Comparison of amitriptyline, cyclobenzaprine and placebo in the treatment of fibromyalgia. Arthritis Thrum 1994; 37(1):32–40.

264. Santandrea S, Montrone F, Sarzi-Puttini P, et al. A double-blind crossover study of two cyclobenzaprine regimens in primary fibromyalgia syndrome. J Int Med Res 1993; 21:74–80.
265. McCain GA. A cost-effective approach to the diagnosis and treatment of fibromyalgia. Rheum Dis Clin North Am 1996; 22:323–349.
266. Goldenberg D, Mayskiy M, Mossey C, et al. A randomized, double blind crossover trial of Fluoxetine and amitriptyline in the treatment of fibromyalgia. Arthritis Rheum 1996; 39(11):1852–1859.
267. Anderberg UM, Marteinsdottir I, von Knorring L. Citalopram in patients with fibromyalgia—a randomized, double-blind, placebo controlled study. Eur J Pain 2000; 4(1):27–35.
268. Alberts K, Bradley L, Alarcon G, et al. Sertraline hydrochloride alters pain threshold, sensory discrimination ability and functional brain activity in patients with fibromyalgia (FM): A randomized controlled trial. Arthritis Rheum 1998; 41(suppl):S259.
269. Gonzalez-Viejo MA, Avellanet M, Henrandez-Morcuende MI. A comparative study of fibromyalgia treatment: ultrasonography and physiotherapy versus sertraline treatment. Ann Readapt Med Phys 2005; 48(8):610–615.
270. Wolfe F, Cathey MA, Hawlet DJ. A double blind placebo controlled trial of Fluoxetine in fibromyalgia. Scand J Rheumatol 1994; 23:255–259.
271. Dwight MM, Arnold LM, O'Brien H, et al. An open clinical trial of venlafaxine treatment of fibromyalgia. Psychosomatics 1998; 39:14–17.
272. Clauw DJ. Treating fibromyalgia: Science vs. art. Am Fam Physician 2000; 62:1492–1494.
273. Arnold LM, Rosen A, Pritchett YL, et al. A randomized, double-blind, placebo-controlled trial of duloxetine in the treatment of women with fibromyalgia with or without major depressive disorder. Pain. 2005;119:5–15.
274. Russell IJ, Mease P, Smith T, et al. The safety and efficacy of duloxetine for the treatment of fibromyalgia syndrome in patients with or without major depressive disorder: results from a 6-month randomized, double-blind, placebo-controlled, fixed-dosed trial [Abstract #103]. J Musculoskel Pain 2007;15(suppl 13):58.
275. Chappell AS, Bradley LA, Wiltse C, et al. Duloxetine 6–120 mg versus placebo in the treatment of fibromyalgia syndrome. Program and abstracts of the American College of Rheumatology (ACR) 71 st Annual Meeting; November 6–11, 2007; Boston, Massachusetts. [Abstract #1543]
276. Zijlstra TR, Barendregt PT, van De Laar MA. Venlafaxine in fibromyaglia: Results of a randomized placebo-controlled double-blind trial. Arthritis Rheum 2002; 46: S105.
277. Rao SG, King T, Porreca F. Elucidation of the analgesic efficacy of Milnacipran n chronic pain. Presented at the International Association for the Study of Pain's Tenth World Congress on Pain, San Diego, CA, 2002.
278. Vitton O, Gendreau M, Gendreau J, et al. A double-blind placebo-controlled trial of milnacipran in the treatment of fibromyalgia. Hum Psychopharmacol. 2004; 19(suppl 1):S27–S35.
279. Clauw DJ, Mease P, Paolmer RH, et al. Milnacipran for the treatment of fibromyalgia in adults: A 15 week, multicenter, randomized, double-blind, placebo-controlled mutliple-dose clinical trial. Clin Ther 2008; 30(11):1988–2004.
280. Samborski W, Sezanska-Szpera M, Rybakowski JK. Open trial of Mirtazapine in patients with fibromyalgia. Pharacopsychiatry 2004; 37(4):168–170.
281. Arnold LM, Keck PE, Welge JA. Antidepressant treatment of fibromyalgia. A meta-analysis and review. Psychosomatics 2000; 41(2):104–113.
282. O'Malley PG, Balden E, Tomkins G, et al. Treatment of fibromyalgia with antidepressants: A meta-analysis. J Gen Int Med 2000; 15(9):659–666;Cochrane Database Syst Rev 2002; 4:05463.
283. Jackson JL, O'Malley PG, Kroenke K. Antidepressants and cognitive-behavioral therapy for symptom syndromes. CNS Spectr 2006; 11(3):121–122.

284. Wiffen P, Collins S, McQuay H, et al. Anticonvulsant drugs for acute and chronic pain (Cochrane Review). In: The Cochrane Library, Issue 4, 2002, Oxford: Update Software.

285. Duan R, Diri E, Young JP, et al. Efficacy of pregabalin monotherapy for relief of pain associated with fibromyalgia: time course and durability of pain results of a 14-week, double-blind, placebo controlled trial. Program and abstracts of the American College of Rheumatology (ACR) 71st Annual Meeting; November 6–11, 2007; Boston, Massachusetts. [Abstract #715]

286. Duan R, Florian H, Young JP, et al. Pregabalin monotherapy for management of fibromyalgia: analysis of two double-blind, randomized, placebo-controlled trials. Program and abstracts of the American College of Rheumatology (ACR) 71st Annual Meeting; November 6–11, 2007; Boston, Massachusetts. [Abstract #1524]

287. Crofford LJ, Rowbotham MC, Mease PJ, et al. Pregabalin for the treatment of fibromyalgia syndrome: Results of a randomized, double-blind, placebo-controlled trial. Arthritis Rheum 2005; 52(4):1264–1273.

288. Florian H, Young JP, Haig G, et al. Efficacy and safety of pregabalin as long-term treatment of pain associated with fibromyalgia: A 1-year, open-label study. Program and abstracts of the American College of Rheumatology (ACR) 71st Annual Meeting; November 6–11, 2007; Boston, Massachusetts. [Abstract #1523]

289. Simpson SL, Young JP, Haig G, et al. Pregabalin therapy for durability of meaningful relief of fibromyalgia. Program and abstracts of the American College of Rheumatology (ACR) 71st Annual Meeting; November 6–11, 2007; Boston, Massachusetts. [Abstract #1522]

290. Hrycaj P, Stratz T, Mennet P, et al. Pathogenic aspects of responsiveness to ondansetron (5-hydroxytryptamine type 3 receptor antagonist) in patients with primary fibromyalgia syndrome—a preliminary study. J Rheumatol 1996; 23:1418–1423.

291. Farber L, Stratz T, Bruckle W, et al. Efficacy and tolerability of tropisetron in primary fibromyalgia—a highly selective and competitive 5-HT3 receptor antagonist. German Fibromyalgia Study Group. Scand J Rheumatol 2000; 113(suppl):49–54.

292. Samborski W, Stratz T, Lacki JK, et al. The 5-HT3 blockers in the treatment of the primary fibromyalgia syndrome: A 10 day open study with Tropisetron at a low dose. Mater Med Pol 1996; 28:17–19.

293. Spath M, Stratz T, Neeck G, et al. Efficacy and tolerability of intravenous tropisetron in the treatment of fibromyalgia. Scand J Rheumatol 2004; 33(4):267–270.

294. Stratz T, Feibich B, Haus U, et al. Influence of tropisetron on th3e serum substance P levels in fibromyalgia patients. Scand J Rheumatol Suppl 2004; (119):41–43.

295. Russell IJ, Fletcher EM, Michalek JE, et al. Treatment of primary fibrositis/fibromyalgia syndrome with ibuprofen and alprazolam: A double blind, placebo-controlled study. Arthritis Rheum 1991; 34:552–560.

296. Hench PK, Cohen R, Mitler MM. Fibromyalgia: Effects of amitriptyline, temazepam and placebo on pain and sleep [Abstract]. Arthritis Rheum 1989; 32(suppl):S47.

297. Rico-Villademoros F, Hidalgo J, Dominguez I, et al. Atypical antipsychotics in the treatment of fibromyalgia: A case series with olanzapine. Prog Neuropsycholpharmacol Biol Psychiatry 2005; 29(1):161–164.

298. Moldofsky H, Scarisbrick P. Induction of neurasthenic musculoskeletal pain syndrome by selective sleep stage deprivation. Psychosom Med 1976; 38:35–44.

299. Moldofsky H. Sleep and musculoskeletal pain. Am J Med 1986; 81(suppl 3A):85–89.

300. Cote KA, Moldofsky H. Sleep Daytime symptoms, and cognitive performance in patients with fibromyalgia. J Rheumatol 1997; 24:2014–2023.

301. Drewes AM, Nielsen KD, Taagholt SJ, et al. Sleep intensity in fibromyalgia: Focus on the microstructure of the sleep process. Br J Rheum 1995; 34:629–635.

302. Moldofsky H, Lue FA, Mously C, et al. The effect of zolpidem in patients with fibromyalgia: A dose ranging, double blind placebo controlled, modified crossover study. J Rheumatol 1996; 23(3):529–533.

303. Drewes AM, Andreasen A, Jennum P, et al. Zopiclone the treatment of sleep abnormalities in fibromyalgia. Scan J Rheumatol 1991; 20(4):288–293.

304. Gronblad M, Nykanen J, Konttinen Y, et al: Effect of zopiclone on sleep quality, morning stiffness, widespread tenderness and pain and general discomfort in primary fibromyalgia patients. A double blind randomized trial. Clin Rheumatol 1993; 12(2):186–191.

305. Moldofsky H, Benz B, Luc F, et al. Comparison of chlorpromazine and L-tryptophan on sleep, musculoskeletal pain, and mood in fibrositis syndrome. Sleep Res 1976; 5:76.

306. Gebhart B, Jorgenson JA. Benefit of ribose in a patient with fibromyalgia. Pharmacotherapy 2004; 24(11):1646–1648.

307. Finckh A, Berner IC, Aubry-Rozier B, et al. A randomized controlled trial of dehydroepiandrosterone in postmenopausal women with fibromyalgia. J Rheumatol 2005; 32(7):1336–1340.

308. Tavoni A, Vitali C, Bombardieri S, et al. Evaluation of S-adenosylmethionine in primary fibromyalgia. A double blind crossover study. Am J Med 1987; 83(5A):107–110.

309. Tavoni A, Jeracitano G, Cirigloiano G. Evaluation of S-adenosylmethionine in secondary fibromyalgia: A double blind study [Letter]. Clin Exp Rheumatol 1998; 16(1):106–107.

310. Caruso I, Sarzi Puttinji P Cazzola M, et al. Double blind study of 5-hydroxytryptophan versus placebo in the treatment of primary fibromyalgia syndrome. J Int Med Res 1990; 18:201–209.

311. Bessette L, Carette S. Fossel AH,et al. A placebo controlled crossover trial of subcutaneous salmon calcitonin in the treatment of patients with fibromyalgia. Scand J Rheumatol 1998; 27:112–116.

312. Bennett RM, Clark SC, Walczyk J. A randomized, double blind, placebo controlled study of growth hormone in the treatment of fibromyalgia. Am J Med 1998; 104:227–231.

313. Wood PB. Fibromyalgia syndrome: A central role for the hippocampus: A theoretical construct. J Musculoskeletal Pain 2004; 12(1):19–26.

314. Dziedzicka-Wasylewska M, Ferrari F, Johnson RD, et al. Mechanisms of action of pramipexole: Effects on receptors. Rev Contemp Pharmacother 2001; 12(1–2):1–31.

315. Holman AJ. Treatment of fibromyalgia with the dopamine agonist ropinirole: A 14-week double-blind, pilot, randomized controlled trial with 14-week blinded extension. Arthritis Rheum 2004; 50(9)(suppl):A1870.

316. Janzen V, Scudds RA. Sphenopalatine blocks in the treatment of pain in fibromyalgia and myofascial pain. Laryngoscope 1997; 107:1420–1422.

317. Bengtsson A, Bengtsson M. Regional sympathetic blockade in primary fibromyalgia. Pain 1988; 33:161–167.

318. Yunus MB, Aldag JC. Restless legs syndrome and leg cramps in fibromyalgia syndrome: A controlled study. BMJ 1996; 312:1339.

319. Kaplan PW, Allen R, Bucholz DW, et al. A double blind, placebo-controlled study of the treatment of periodic limb movements in sleep using carbidopa/levodopa and propoxyphene. Sleep 1993; 16:713–716.

320. Becker PM, Jamieson AO, Brown WD. Dopaminergic agents in restless legs syndrome and periodic limb movements of sleep: Response and complications of extended treatment in 49 cases. Sleep 1993; 16:713–716.

321. Earley CJ, Yaffee JB, Allen RP. Randomized, double blind, placebo-controlled trial of pergolide in restless legs syndrome. Neurology 1998; 51:1599–1602.

322. Montplaisir J, Nicolas A, Denesle R, et al. Restless legs syndrome improved by pramipexole: a double blind randomized trial. Urology 1999; 52:938–943.

323. Spath M, Welzel D, Farber L. Treatment of chronic fatigue syndrome with 5-HT3 receptor antagonists-preliminary results. Scand J Rheumatol 2000; 113:72–77.

324. Guymer EK, Clauw DJ. Treatment of fatigue in fibromyalgia. Rheum Dis Clin North Am 2002; 28(2):367–378.

325. Martinez-Lavin M, Hermosillo AG. Autonomic nervous system dysfunction may explain the multisystem features of fibromyalgia. Semin Arthritis Rheum 2000; 29:197–199.

326. Karas B, Grubb BP, Boehm K, et al. The postural orthostatic tachycardia syndrome: A potentially treatable cause of chronic fatigue, exercise intolerance and cognitive impairment in adolescents. Pacing Clin Electrophysiol 2000; 23:344–351.

327. Raj SR, Brouillard D, Simpson CS, et al. Dysautonomia among patients with fibromyalgia: A non-invasive assessment. J Rheumatol 2000; 27:2660–2665.

328. Wilke WS, Fouad-Tarazi, Cash JM, et al. The connection between chronic fatigue syndrome and neurally mediated hypotension. Cleve Clin J Med 1998; 65:261–266.

329. Barkhuizen A. Rational and targeted pharmacologic treatment of fibromyalgia. Rheum Dis Clin North Am 28(2); 261–290.

330. Bennett RM, Clark SR, Campbell SM, et al. Symptoms of Raynaud's syndrome in patients with fibromyalgia. A study utilizing the Nielsen test, digital photo-plethysmography and measurement of platelet alpha 2-adrenergic receptors. Arthritis Rheum 1991; 34:264–269.

331. Sletvold H, Stiles TC, Landro NI. Information processing in primary fibromyalgia, major depression and healthy controls. J Rheumatol 1995; 22:137–142.

332. Landro NI, Stiles TC, Sletvold H. Memory functioning in patients with primary fibromyalgia an major depression and healthy controls. J Psychosom Res 1997; 42:297–306.

333. Wahner-Roedler DL, Elkin PL, Vincent A, et al. Use of complementary and alternative medical therapies by patients referred to a fibromyalgia treatment program at a tertiary care center. May Clin Proc 2005; 80(6):826.

334. Forseth K, Gran JT. Management of fibromyalgia: What are the best treatment choices? Drugs 2002; 6(4):577–592.

335. Hadhazy VA, Ezzo J, Creamer P, et al. Mind-body therapies for the treatment of fibromyalgia. A systematic review. J Rheumatol 2000; 27(12):2911–2918.

336. Berman BM, Swyers JP. Complementary medicine treatments for fibromyalgia syndrome. Baillieres Best Pract Res Clin Rheumatol 1999; 13(3):487–492.

337. White KP, Harth M. An analytical review of 24 controlled clinical trials for fibromyalgia syndrome (FMS). Pain 1996; 64(2):211–219.

338. Rossy LA, Buckelew SP, Dorr N, et al. A meta-analysis of fibromyalgia treatment interventions. Ann Behav Med 1999; 21:180–191.

339. Sim J, Adams N. Systematic review of randomized controlled trials of nonpharmacological interventions for fibromyalgia. Clin J Pain 2002; 18(5):324–336.

340. Rosen NB. Physical medicine and rehabilitation approaches to the management of myofascial pain and fibromyalgia syndromes. Baillieres Clin Rheumatol 1994; 8(4):881–916.

341. Field T, Diego M, Cullen C, et al. Fibromyalgia pain and Substance P decrease and sleep improves after massage therapy. J Clin Rheumatol 2002; 8(2):72–76.

342. Caballero-Uribe CV, Abuchaibe I, Abuchaibe S, et al. Treatment of tender points in patients with fibromyalgia syndrome (FMS) with therapeutic infrared laser ray. Arthritis Rheum 1997; 40(9)(suppl):S44.

343. Kaada B. Treatment of fibromyalgia by low-frequency transcutaneous nerve stimulation. Tidsskrift For Den Norske Laegeforening 1989; 109(29):2992–2995.

344. Guieu R, Blin O, Pouget J, et al. Nociceptive threshold and physical activity. Can J Neurol Sci 1992; 19:69–71.

345. Koltyn KF, Garvin AW, Gardiner RL, et al. Perception of pain following aerobic exercise. Med Sci Sports Exerc 1996; 28:1418–1421.

346. Schwarz L, Kindermann W. Changes in beta-endorphin levels in response to aerobic and anaerobic exercise. Sports Med 1992; 13:25–36.

347. Koltyn KF. Analgesia following exercise: A review. Sports Med 2000; 29:85–98.

348. Geel SE. The fibromyalgia syndrome: musculoskeletal pathophysiology. Semin Arthritis Rheum 1994; 23:347–353.

349. Watkins LR, Maier SF, Goehler LE. Immune activation: the role of proinflammatory cytokines in inflammation, illness responses and pathological pain states. Pain 1995; 63:289–302.

350. Bennett RM. The contribution of muscle to the generation of fibromyalgia symptomatology. J Musculoskeletal Pain 1996; 4:35–59.

351. McCain GA, Bell DA, Mai FM, et al. A controlled study of the effects of a supervised cardiovascular fitness training program on the manifestations of primary fibromyalgia. Arthritis Rheum 1988; 31:1135–1141.

352. Norregaard J, Lyddegaard JJ, Mehlsen J, et al. Exercise training in treatment of fibromyalgia. J Musculoskeletal Pain 1997; 5:71–79.

353. Nichols DS, Glenn TM. Effects of aerobic exercise on pain perception, affect and level of disability in individuals with fibromyalgia. Phys Ther 1994; 74:327–332.

354. Martin L, Nutting A, Macintosh BR, et al. An exercise program in the treatment of fibromyalgia. J Rheumatol 1996; 23:1050–1053.

355. Wigers SH, Stiles TC, Vogel PA. Effects of aerobic exercise versus stress management treatment in fibromyalgia. A 4.5 year prospective study. Scand J Rheumatol 1996; 25:77–86.

356. Jones KD, Burckhardt CS, Clark SR. A randomized controlled trial of muscle strengthening versus flexibility training in fibromyalgia. J Rheumatol 2002; 29:1041 1048.

357. Richards SC, Scott DL. Prescribed exercise in people with fibromyalgia: Parallel group randomized controlled trial. BMJ 2002; 325(7357):185.

358. Millea PJ, Holloway RL. Treating fibromyalgia. Am Fam Physician 2000; 62:1575–1582.

359. Gowans SE, Dehueck A, Voss S, et al. Six-month and one-year follow-up of 23 weeks of aerobic exercise for individuals with fibromyalgia. Arthritis Rheum 2004; 51(6):890–898.

360. Mannerkorpi K. Exercise in fibromyalgia. Curr Opin Rheumatol 2005; 17(2):190–194.

361. Da Costa D, Abrahamowicz M, Lowensteyn I, et al. A randomized clinical trial of an individualized home-based exercise programme for women with fibromyalgia. Rheumatology (Oxford) 2005; 44(11):1422–1427.

362. Maquet D, Croisier JL, Demoulin C, et al. Value of aerobic rehabilitation in the management of fibromyalgia. Rev Med Liege 2006; 61(2):109–116.

363. Busch A, Schachter CL, Peloso PM, et al. Exercise for treating fibromyalgia syndrome. Cochrane Database Syst Rev 2002; 3:CD003786.

364. Gowans SE, deHueck A, Voss S, et al. A randomized, controlled trial of exercise and education for individuals with fibromyalgia. Arthritis Care Res 1999; 12(2):120–128.

365. Ramsay C, Moreland J, Ho M, et al. An observer blinded comparison of supervised and unsupervised aerobic exercise regimen in fibromyalgia. Rheumatology 2000; 39(5):501–505.

366. Schneider M, Vernon H, Ko G, et al. Chiropractic management of fibromyalgia syndrome: A systematic review of the literature. J Manipulative Physiol Ther 2009; 32(1):25–40.

367. Berman BM, Ezzo J, Hadhazy V, et al. Is acupuncture effective in the treatment of fibromyalgia? J Fam Pract 1999; 48:213–218.

368. Sprott H, Franke S, Kluge H, et al. Pain treatment in fibromyalgia by acupuncture [letter]. Rheumatology Int 1998; 18(1):35–36.

369. NIH Consensus Conference. Acupuncture. JAMA 1998; 280:1518–1524.

370. Nielson WR, Walker C, McCain GA. Cognitive behavioral treatment of fibromyalgia syndrome: Preliminary findings. J Rheumatol 1992; 19:98–103.

371. Vlaeyen JW, Teeken-Gruben NJ, Goossens ME, et al. Cognitive educational treatment of fibromyalgia: a randomized trial. I. Clinical effects. J Rheumatol 1996; 23:1237–1245.

372. Goldenberg DL, Kaplan KH, Nadeau M. A controlled study of a stress-reduction, cognitive-behavioral treatment program in fibromyalgia. J Musculoskeletal Pain 1994; 2(2):53–66.

373. White KP, Nielson WR. Cognitive behavioral treatment of fibromyalgia syndrome: A followup assessment. J Rheumatol 1995; 22:717–721.

374. Singh BB, Berman BM, Hadhazy VA, et al. A pilot study of cognitive behavioral therapy in fibromyalgia. Altern Ther Health Med 1998; 4:67–70.
375. Turk DC, Okifuji A, Sinclair JD, et al. Interdisciplinary treatment for fibromyalgia syndrome: Clinical and statistical significance. Arthritis Care Res 1998; 11:186–195.
376. Mengshoel AM, Forseth KO, Haugen M. Multidisciplinary approach to fibromyalgia. A pilot study. Clin Rheumatol 1995; 14:165–170.
377. Lemstra M, Olszynski WP. The effectiveness of multidisciplinary rehabilitation in the treatment of fibromyalgia: a randomized controlled trial. Clin J Pain 2005; 21(2): 166–74.
378. Luedtke CA, Thompson JM, Postier JA, et al. A description of a brief multidisciplinary treatment program for fibromyalgia. Pain Manag Nurs 2005; 6(2):76–80.
379. Dobkin PL, Ionescu-Ittu R, Abrahamowicz M, et al. Predictors of adherence to an integrated multimodal program for fibromyalgia. J Rheumatol 2008; 35(11):2255–2264.

13 Low Back Pain and Sciatica: Pathogenesis, Diagnosis and Nonoperative Treatment

Anthony H. Wheeler

Pain and Orthopedic Neurology, Charlotte, North Carolina, U.S.A.

THE DISORDER

Like a modern skyscraper, the human spine defies gravity and defines us as vertical bipeds. It forms the infrastructure of a biological machine that anchors the kinetic chain and transfers biomechanical forces into coordinated functional activities. The spine acts as a conduit for precious neural structures and possesses the physiological capacity to act as a crane for lifting and a crankshaft for walking. Subjected to aging, it adjusts to the wear and tear of gravity and biomechanical loading through compensatory structural and neurochemical changes, some of which can be maladaptive and cause pain, functional disability, and altered neurophysiological circuitry. Some compensatory reactions are benign; however, some are destructive and interfere with the organism's capacity to function and cope. Spinal pain is multifaceted, involving structural, biomechanical, biochemical, medical, and psychosocial influences that result in dilemmas of such complexity that treatment application is often difficult or ineffective (1).

Low back pain (LBP) is the "most expensive, benign condition in industrialized countries" (2). Experts have estimated that approximately 80% of Americans will experience LBP during their lifetime (2–4). The annual prevalence of LBP ranges from 15% to 45% with a point prevalence that approximates 30% (5). Sixty percent of acute LBP sufferers recover in six weeks and up to 80% to 90% recover within 12 weeks; however, recovery of those remaining LBP patients is less certain (5). Of those individuals who remain disabled for more than six months, fewer than half return to work, and after two years of LBP disability, return to work is unlikely (5). Recent studies suggest that one-third to one-fourth of patients in a primary care setting may still have problems after one year (6, 7). Chronic LBP (cLBP) is the most common cause of disability in Americans under the age of 45 (8, 9). Each year 3% to 4% of the population is temporarily disabled, and 1% of the working-age population is totally and permanently disabled (2, 6, 10). LBP has been cited as the second most frequent reason to visit a physician for a chronic condition (6, 10–12), the fifth most common cause for hospitalization (6, 13–15), and the condition with the third highest frequency of surgical procedures performed (6, 13–15). The socioeconomic impact of cLBP is massive. Ironically, only a small minority of patients with cLBP and disability account for the majority of the economic burden (16–18).

Spinal Paradox: Definitions and Fundamental Dilemmas

Most commonly, diagnoses of acute painful spinal conditions are nonspecific, such as neck or back strain, although injuries may affect any of several pain-sensitive structures, which include the disk, facet joints, spinal musculature, and ligamentous support (19, 20). The origin of chronic back pain is often attributed to degenerative conditions of the spine; however, controlled studies have indicated that any correlation between clinical symptoms and radiological signs of degeneration is minimal or lacking (9, 19–23). Inflammatory arthropathy, metabolic bone conditions, and fibromyalgia are cited in some studies as the cause of chronic spine-related pain conditions (19, 20). Although disk herniation has been popularized as a cause of spinal and radicular pain, asymptomatic disk herniations on computed tomography (CT) and magnetic resonance imaging (MRI) are common (23–26). Furthermore, there is no clear relationship between the extent of disk protrusion and the degree of clinical symptoms (27). Degenerative change and injury to spinal structures produce lower back and leg pain that varies proportionally.

"Sciatica" describes leg pain that is localized in the distribution of one or more lumbosacral nerve roots, typically L4-S2, with or without neurological deficit (19, 20). However, physicians often refer to leg pain from any lumbosacral segment as sciatica. When a clear dermatomal distribution is unclear, the descriptive phrase "nonspecific radicular pattern" has been advocated. When initially evaluating a patient with lower back and leg pain, the physician must first determine that pain symptoms are consistent with common "activity-related" disorders of the spine resulting from the wear and tear of excessive biomechanical and gravitational loading that some traditionally describe as "mechanical" (20, 28, 29). Mechanical lumbar syndromes are typically aggravated by static loading of the spine (e.g., prolonged sitting or standing), by long lever activities (e.g., vacuuming or working with the arms elevated and away from the body), or by levered postures (e.g., bending forward) (20, 28, 29). Pain is reduced when the spine is balanced by multidirectional forces (e.g., walking or constantly changing positions) or when the spine is unloaded (e.g., reclining). Mechanical conditions of the spine, including disk disease, spondylosis, spinal stenosis, and fractures, account for up to 98% of LBP conditions, with the remaining cases due to systemic, visceral, or inflammatory disorders (1) (Table 1).

DIAGNOSIS

Overview

The natural history of spine-related pain is usually benign. However, prompt physician evaluation, including appropriate radiographic imaging, laboratory, and electrophysiological testing, is indicated in cases of persistent severe neurological deficit, intractable limb pain, suspicion of a systemic illness, or a change in bowel or bladder control (1).

In complex spinal disorders with chronic intractable pain and disability, provocative techniques (e.g., discography and facet injections) using needles or catheters that are fluoroscopically guided and directed at selective spinal structures or neural elements using irritant solutions (e.g., radio-opaque dyes) to provoke a characteristic pain pattern, followed by a local anesthetic to ablate it, can help identify spinal pain generators when performed properly by well-trained spinal interventionalists (1). When the cause of back pain is inconclusive, despite a thorough comprehensive diagnostic evaluation, including the cited interventional methods, a multidisciplinary evaluation combining surgical, medical, and

TABLE 1 Spinal Disorders: Mechanical Vs. Nonmechanical

Mechanical syndromes
Motion segment (discal and facet) degeneration
Myofascial and other muscular pain disorders
Discogenic pain with/without radicular symptoms
Radiculopathy due to structural impingement
Axial or radicular pain due to biochemical or inflammatory reaction to spinal injury
Motion segment/vertebral osseous fracture
Spondylosis with/without central or lateral canal stenosis
Macro- or microinstability of the spine with/without radiographic hypermobility or evidence of subluxation

Nonmechanical syndromes
Neurological syndromes
   Myelopathy or myelitis from intrinsic/extrinsic structural or vascular process
   Lumbosacral plexopathy (e.g., diabetes, vasculitis, malignancy)
   Polyneuropathy, acute, subacute, or chronic (e.g., chronic inflammatory demyelinating polyneuropathy, Guillain–Barré syndrome, diabetes)
   Mononeuropathy, including causalgia (e.g., trauma, diabetes)
   Myopathy, including myositis and various metabolic causes
   Dystonia: spinal segmental, lumbopelvic, or generalized
Systemic disorders
   Primary or metastatic neoplasms
   Osseous, discal, or epidural infection
   Inflammatory spondyloarthropathy
   Metabolic bone disease, including osteoporosis
   Vascular disorders such as atherosclerosis or vasculitis
Referred pain
   Gastrointestinal disorders (e.g., pancreatitis, pancreatic cancer, cholecystitis)
   Cardiorespiratory disorders (e.g., pericarditis, pleuritis, pneumonia)
   Disorders of the ribs or sternum
   Genitourinary disorders (e.g., nephrolithiasis, prostatitis, pyelonephritis)
   Thoracic or abdominal aortic aneurysm
   Hip disorders (e.g., injury, inflammation, or end-stage degeneration of joint and associated soft tissues—tendons, bursae, ligaments)

Source: Adapted from Ref. 28.

physical medicine and psychological subspecialists may help to better define peripheral and central pain generators and then to develop a new strategy or action plan (1).

The Spinal Lesion

The spinal lesion occurs when injury or disease adversely affects the capacity of the vertebral motion segment and its components, both contractile and noncontractile, to maintain normal function and manage normal biomechanical forces due to impending or actual tissue damage (1). The magnitude of actual or threatened tissue damage elicits an appropriate or parallel nociceptive stimulus that provokes the organism to behave or react protectively. Injuries are typically caused by singular or recurrent episodes of biomechanical overloading, particularly in cases of body movements performed when spinal and extremity muscles are fatigued; when muscle power is reduced; when truncal protective mechanisms are at fault; when errors occur due to poor neuromuscular coordination or cognitive dysfunction; when tasks have poor ergonomic design; or when movements are nonphysiological, such as simultaneous forward bending with twisting and lifting. Details of a specific event or trauma allow the practitioner to develop a thorough understanding of the biomechanics of the injury and, therefore, enable him to determine the likelihood of a mechanical pathogenesis. Identifying spinal pain and associated neurological symptoms as mechanical is the first most important diagnostic objective.

The Patient History

When interviewing a patient with spinal pain, it is important to establish the portion of the pain that is axial relative to its distribution in the ipsilateral (and contralateral) extremity. Cumulative microtrauma that occurs over time and injury-induced macrotrauma to spinal structures produce spinal and extremity pain in various combinations, but with similar characteristics. This process of aging and recurrent trauma is thought to cause progressive degeneration of spinal motion segments. Nevertheless, the presence of degenerative changes is typically seen in patients who complain of mechanical pain syndromes. Establishing that the patient's LBP is mechanical in character is the most important initial goal. Therefore, pain should be aggravated by static loading of the spine, long lever activities, and levered postures. Mechanical LBP is characteristically eased when the spine is balanced by multidirectional forces and when the spine is unloaded.

Neuropathic pain often occurs with limb involvement and is often characterized as thermal, jabbing, shooting, or like pins and needles, whereas nociceptive pain is usually described as dull and aching and is aggravated by biomechanical loading. Although, neuropathic pain may increase with exposure to increased biomechanical forces, it is usually worse at night or at rest and associated with other neurological symptoms such as reduced sensation or weakness. Determining the character of pain as neuropathic is helpful clinically but does not differentiate among the various neuropathic conditions that may be causative (30). The presence and location of neuropathic pain within the peripheral or central nervous system can be determined by neurological abnormalities found on physical examination. Neuropathic pain may also be seen in the thoracolumbar regions as a sign of cervical or thoracic myelopathy. Furthermore, the presence of allodynia and hyperalgesia are considered cardinal signs of neuropathic pain (30, 31). Allodynia is pain that results from a stimulus that does not normally evoke pain, whereas hyperalgesia is an exaggerated response to a stimulus that is normally not painful (1, 30, 31).

Following injury there is a critical period of time when historical recall is optimal and report of the details of an injury is most explicit. These details should be well documented to establish biomechanical influences, especially in cases of personal or work injury. It is important to request disclosure of any previous similar problems, compensation related or not. Physician evaluation of chronic or previously treated disorders requires examination of accumulated historical, diagnostic, and treatment data. After establishing the characteristics and behavior of the pain, any associated symptoms are determined through questioning by review of systems. Any systemic, neurological, or visceral dysfunction and any weight loss, fever, or other suspicious symptoms that would mitigate a mechanical cause should be scrutinized and investigated thoroughly (1).

Physical Examination

The purpose of the physical examination is to confirm or determine a working differential diagnosis of the anatomy and etiology of the patient's spinal pain and related symptoms. Observations of verbal and nonverbal pain behaviors suggesting "symptom magnification," and inconsistencies of requested tasks during the examination, nonphysiological findings, and other "red flags," which may suggest contributing psychological factors, should be documented. During the examination, it is essential to have the patient disrobed to view the spine. Open-back gowns leave the physician with only one view of the spine, and often, swimming attire is more appropriate for a complete 360-degree inspection of the trunk. Leg length discrepancy, pelvic obliquity, scoliosis, postural dysfunction with forward head and shoulders, or accentuated kyphosis should be noted. Physician preferences vary in regards to the importance that is attributed to testing range of motion; however, just asking the patient to move into forward bending is often the most worthwhile observation.

Observations with the patient standing should include body habitus, posture, stance, head–neck alignment, pelvic obliquity, spinal curvature, and a general overview of the contour, strength, and symmetry of truncal musculature. Next, the patient is asked to drop his or her head and shoulders forward, and then to move slowly into forward bending. Normal forward bending is revealed when the patient recruits from each cephalad segment to the level below, and so on, progressing from the cervical spine through the thoracic to the lumbar region where flexion of the hips completes the excursion into full flexion. Patients with significant mechanical back pain or lumbar segmental instability usually stop cephalad to caudal recruitment upon reaching the thoracolumbar junction or, in some cases, the injured lumbar segmental level. To continue forward bending, the patient braces the lumbar paraspinal muscles to protect the mechanically compromised segment en masse, and then completes forward bending through hip flexion. To rise back to an erect posture, recruitment occurs in the same manner but reversed, beginning with motion through the hips, followed by bracing the lumbar spine to stabilize the painful motion segment, then continuing from the cephalad segmental levels above the muscularly braced lumbar region. Movement may stop temporarily while surrounding muscles contract to brace the painful segment(s). When the area is sensed as secure by spinal neural mechanisms, cephalad segmental recruitment again commences completing the spine's excursion to the erect posture (1, 29). In cases of severe mechanical thoracolumbar pain and segmental instability with concomitant regional muscular spasm, the patient may be unable to demonstrate any flexion below the symptomatic spinal level. Any soft-tissue abnormalities and palpable tenderness should be recorded. Palpation of lumbar paraspinal, buttock, and other regional muscles should be performed early in the examination. The examiner should palpate pertinent truncal and limb-girdle muscles and make note of any areas that demonstrate superficial or deep muscle spasm, and trigger points, as well as any characteristic pattern(s) of referred pain.

Dissociation of physical findings from physiological or anatomical principles is key in patients when psychological factors are suspected to be influential. Examples of this phenomenon include nondermatomal patterns of sensory loss; nonphysiological demonstration of weakness (give-way weakness when not caused by pain or "ratchety weakness" related to simultaneous agonist and

TABLE 2   Low Back Pain: Diagnostic and Prognostic Red Flags

Pain unrelieved by rest or any postural modification
Pain unchanged despite treatment for 2 to 4 weeks
"Writhing" pain behavior
Colicky pain or pain associated with a visceral function
Known or previous cancer
Fever or immunosuppressed status
High risk for fracture (older age, osteoporosis)
Associated malaise, fatigue, or weight loss
Progressive neurological impairment
Bowel or bladder dysfunction
Severe morning stiffness as a primary complaint
Unable to ambulate or care for self
Nonorganic signs and symptoms
Dissociation between verbal and nonverbal pain behaviors
Compensable cause of injury
Out of work, disabled, or seeking disability
Psychological features, including depression and anxiety
Narcotic or psychoactive drug requests
Repeated failed surgical or medical treatment for LBP or other chronic illnesses

Abbreviation: LBP, low back pain.
Source: Adapted from Ref. 28.

antagonist muscular contraction); and dissociation between lumbar spine movements during the history or counseling sessions when compared to the patient's presentation during the examination (Table 2).

Waddell signs have been popularized as a physical examination approach to identify patients who have "nonorganic" or psychogenic embellishment of their LBP syndrome (32). Examination techniques proposed by Waddell consist of a series of maneuvers that would not normally cause pain, including simulated rotation of the hips en masse with the lumbar spine without allowing spinal rotation, light pressure upon the head, and gentle effleurage of superficial tissues. Additional signs are a dissociation between sitting and supine straight leg raising (SLR) and demonstration of nonphysiological weakness or sensory patterns by the patient (1, 32).

SLR is commonly used to determine the presence of sciatic nerve tension or irritability when patients experience lower extremity radicular symptoms. SLR is tested with the patient supine and should produce ipsilateral leg pain between 10 and 60 degrees to be declared positive. SLR that produces pain in the opposite leg signifies a high probability of disk herniation, and CT or MRI investigation should be considered, especially if neurological evidence for radiculopathy is present. Nonspecific complaints, overtly excessive pain behavior, patient contraction of antagonist muscles that limit the examiner's testing, or tightness of buttock and hamstring muscles are commonly mistaken examples of reported "positive" SLR. Reverse SLR, tested while the patient is prone, may elicit symptoms of pain by inducing neural tension upon irritated or compressed nerve roots in the mid to upper lumbar region. Additionally, this maneuver helps the clinician identify the presence of iliopsoas and/or quadriceps muscular tightness that contributes to chronic lumbar pain (1).

Neurological evaluation is performed to determine the presence/absence and level(s) of radiculopathy or myelopathy. Anatomical localization is derived through muscle and reflex testing combined with historical information obtained during the interview, and coupled with the absence of neurological symptoms or signs that would implicate cerebral or brainstem involvement. Consistent myotomal weakness and sensory findings that at least "seem to coincide" with segmental radiculopathy or polyradiculopathies should not be ignored (1).

Lower motor neuron versus upper motor neuron syndromes and the level of spinal dysfunction should be identified by the examining physician. Rectal examination is indicated in patients when myelopathy, especially cauda equina syndrome, is of diagnostic concern. Tone of the anal sphincter and the presence or absence of anal wink should be correlated with motor, sensory, and reflex findings in these cases. In all spinal examinations, a general overview of the patient's health must be confirmed by examination. Extremities affected by chronic pain may demonstrate abnormal skin with a rough, leathery texture or shiny skin with trophic changes including hair loss, edema, abnormal temperature, and discoloration (bluish, reddish, or brownish hues). These changes may infer the presence of chronic pain, sympathetic nervous system involvement, or vascular insufficiency. Knowledge of cardiovascular and peripheral vascular status obtained by examination is pivotal in cases of claudication or reduced exercise tolerance for determining a diagnostic and treatment plan (1) (Tables 2 and 3).

Diagnostic Strategies (Fig. 1)

When mechanical spine pain syndromes persist for 6 to 12 weeks despite adequate treatment, appropriate consultation and diagnostic imaging are indicated. Referral to a physician with expertise in spinal disorders should be considered before embarking on an expensive diagnostic workup. Appropriate consultation and diagnostic workup are urgently indicated at any point when an underlying serious etiology is suspected or with progressive neurological deficit. CT scanning is usually most effective when the spinal or neurological level is clear and when bony pathology is suspected (1, 38). MRI is more useful when the exact spinal or neurological level is unclear, when a pathological condition of the spinal cord or soft tissues is suspected, when an underlying infectious or neoplastic process is possible, or when an acute osseous process is suspected (1, 38). Contrast-enhanced MRI is more accurate for delineating recurrent postsurgical discal herniation (1, 38). Myelography is useful to clarify nerve root pathology, particularly in patients with previous spine surgery, degenerative scoliosis, dynamic neural compression, or with a metal fixation device in place (1, 38). CT myelography may be more informative for studying patients who have had multiple spinal operations or who have spinal stenosis (1, 38).

When limb pain predominates and imaging studies provide ambiguous information, clarification may be gained by electromyography, somatosensory evoked potentials, or selective nerve root blocks (1, 38). When axial and limb pain becomes chronic, a multidisciplinary evaluation may provide diagnostic and prognostic insight by uncovering unrecognized physical and psychosocial influences that may be contributing to prolonged pain and disability (1, 38). Refractory spinal pain may be further investigated using provocative interventional fluoroscopic techniques to identify which tissues are acting as pain generators.

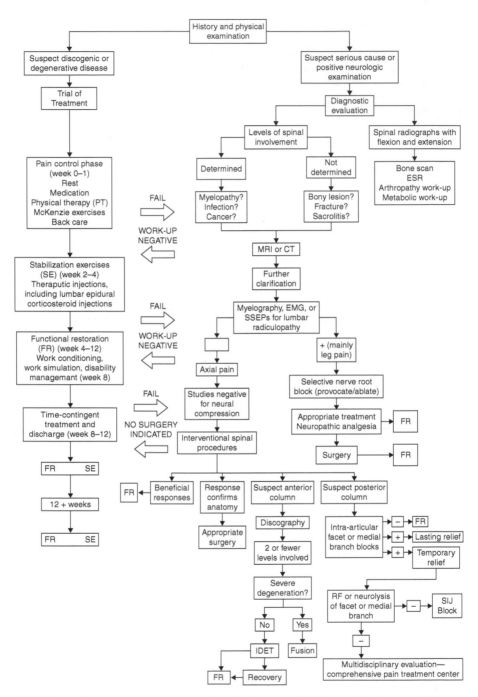

FIGURE 1 Algorithm for management of low back pain and sciatica. *Abbreviations*: ESR, erythrocyte sedimentation rate; MRI, magnetic resonance imaging; CT, computed tomography; SSEPs, somatosensory evoked potentials; RF, radiofrequency; IDET, intradiscal electrothermal therapy; SIJ, sacroiliac joint; FR, functional restoration (39).

Discography has remained controversial as a diagnostic procedure, but is still advocated by many to confirm a suspected discogenic source of pain (1, 38). Other commonly accepted indications for discography include assessment for surgical fusion, failed spine surgery, or percutaneous disk treatments (1, 38).

PATHOPHYSIOLOGY

A strictly pathoanatomic or mechanical explanation for spinal and radicular pain syndromes has proven inadequate (21, 27, 40, 41). In the setting of spinal injury, acute tissue damage to the spinal motion segment and associated soft tissues activates specific nociceptors that convey pertinent pain signals through peripheral neural pathways to the central nervous system (42, 43). These noxious afferent stimuli are converted from chemical to electrical neural messages within the spinal cord and then communicate cephalad to the brain stem, thalamus, and cerebral cortex (42, 43). Mechanical, thermal, and chemical stimuli activate peripheral nociceptors that transmit the pain messages through the lightly myelinated A-delta fibers and unmyelinated C fibers (42, 43). Nociceptors are present in the outer annulus fibrosis, facet capsule, posterior longitudinal ligament, associated muscles, and other structures of the spinal motion segment (42–45). Algogenic substances that are typically involved in tissue damage and are capable of inducing transduction peripherally include potassium, serotonin, bradykinin, histamine, prostaglandins, leukotrienes, and substance P (43). The afferent conduction of pain signals travels primarily through the dorsal root ganglion (DRG) to the dorsal horn of the spinal cord. The DRG contains cell bodies of primary afferent nociceptors and is a rich source of nociceptive chemical mediators including the neuropeptides substance P, calcitonin gene–related peptide, and vasoactive intestinal peptide (43). The DRG is mechanically sensitive and capable of independent pain transduction, transmission, and modulation. The dorsal horn is the initial major site for nociceptive modulation, which occurs in Rexed laminae I, II, and V of the substantia gelatinosa (42, 43). Pain reception at this level is subject to modification by other afferent stimuli arriving at the dorsal horn via A-beta fibers and/or by the descending endogenous opioid system. Subsequent to spinal cord influences, the resultant pain message travels cephalad by several routes to the brain where further modulation may occur. Pain perception is strongly influenced by psychological and environmental factors, as well as excitatory and inhibitory neurophysiological factors. These influences determine the final perception of pain, making each individual's pain experience unique and complex.

The pathophysiology of lumbosacral radicular pain is not fully understood. Unlike peripheral nerves, spinal nerve roots lack a well-developed intraneural blood–nerve barrier, which probably makes them more susceptible to becoming symptomatic from compression injury than peripheral nerves, and more vulnerable to neural compression as manifested by faulty bioelectric neural functioning, such as, conduction parameters; vascular compromise with ischemia, venous congestion, and endoneural edema formation; inflammatory and biochemical influences; and neural fibrosis with inadequate nutrition (1, 46, 47). Endoneural edema can be induced by increased vascular permeability caused by mechanical nerve root compression (47). Furthermore, elevated endoneural fluid pressure, caused by intraneural edema, can impede capillary blood flow and may cause intraneural fibrosis. Spinal nerve roots receive approximately

58% of their nutrition from surrounding cerebral spinal fluid; therefore, perineural fibrosis interferes with cerebral spinal fluid–mediated nutrition, which has been experimentally demonstrated to render nerve roots hyperesthetic and more sensitive to compressive forces (1, 47). Rapid onset of neural and vascular compromise is more likely to produce symptomatic radiculopathy than slow or gradual mechanical deformity (1, 47). Research has revealed that additional irritation appears to be caused by the nucleus pulposus cells in herniated discal tissue, which are capable of inducing local neural dysfunction and generating algogenic agents such as metalloproteases and cytokines, including tumor necrosis factor-α (1, 47). Therefore, the cause of symptomatic radiculopathy is more complex than just neural dysfunction from structural impingement and is often multifactorial (1, 47, 48).

In summary, an amalgam of pain messaging is integrated from nociceptive residua, algogenic factors, induced inflammatory pain and neuropathic stimuli; whereby involved spinal and neural tissues initiate nociception. Transduction occurs followed by transmission of the resultant noxious information through peripheral nerves to the spinal cord, where nociception is mediated and biased by numerous complex central mechanisms. This "spinal nociceptive model" is unique in proposing that various neurotransmitters and biochemical factors sensitize neural elements and spinal tissues within the motion segment, so that spinal pain is subsequently caused by normal biomechanical stresses that are harmless and were previously painless or asymptomatic gravitational loading movements or lifting tasks (1). It is unclear whether the biochemical changes that occur with spinal segmental degeneration are the consequence or cause of these painful conditions. However, chemical and inflammatory factors may create the environmental substrata through which biochemical stress and forces cause variable character and degrees of axial or limb pain, of pain intensity, of chronicity, and of disability (1). This spinal nociceptive model exists due to the failure of the "pathology model" to predict the cause of spinal pain that often leads to an ironic predicament. If diagnostic studies are unrevealing for a structural cause, physicians and patients alike often call into question whether the pain has a physical or psychological cause (1, 20).

The transition from acute tissue damage to a chronic pain state is influenced by both endogenous and exogenous factors, which alter function in the individual far beyond the initiating pathological process. Chronic spine-related pain may result from impaired tissue healing or persistent pathoanatomic instability (1, 21). When combined with nonphysical factors, a complex milieu of interwoven physiological, psychological, and social factors may result. Identification of contributing physical and nonphysical factors enables the treating physician to enact a comprehensive approach with the best chance for success; however, identifying these factors may also help physicians identify the prognosis as poor or identify cLBP that is not easily treatable by conventional medical resources or within reasonable cost-effective parameters. In some cases, cLBP disability may be driven by emotional, psychological, or psychosocial factors that cannot be influenced, and therefore, cannot be treated. These cases must be identified to reduce the burden of cost within the medical care system. cLBP differs from other disease categories due to its tendency to recur and its capacity to last for years or, in some cases, a lifetime (21). By definition, cLBP becomes refractory to treatment regardless of how efficiently or effectively the treatment is applied, and

TABLE 3   Factors That Influence Pain Perception and Chronicity

---

Psychological influences
Premorbid factors
  Depression
  Cognitive–affective dysfunction
  Anxiety or panic disorder
  Substance abuse
  At risk for personality disorders
  Predisposed to somatoform disorders
  Low intelligence
  Attribution and coping styles
Posttraumatic factors
  Persistent aberrant pain behaviors
  Exaggerated or prolonged psychophysiological reaction and symptoms
  Depression
  Panic or anxiety
  Posttraumatic stress disorder
  Somatoform pain disorder
  Symptom magnification
  Anger or hostility
  Loss of control or abnormal dependence on solicitous advisors
  Brain injury
Physical influences
  Medical illness that interferes with treatment, e.g., diabetes, heart disease, etc.
  Poor physical capacity for rehabilitation
  Failed surgery
  Comorbid neurological or musculoskeletal disorders
  Deconditioning syndrome
Psychosocial influences
  Compensated unemployment
  Out of work, disabled, or seeking disability
  Job dissatisfaction or conflicts
  Family or spousal dynamics
  Legal or adverse insurance influences
  Age-related factors
  Environmental stressors
  Limited education or vocational potential

Source: From Refs. 1, 33–37.

regardless of whether or not the applied treatments are cost-effective. Patients are not counseled regarding, any timeline or difficulty of treatment, or given any true perspective as to what criteria are used to judge an outcome as beneficial. Most clinical research studies use "return to work" as a measure of successful outcome. Patients are more likely to seek "pain relief" or "quality of life" as preferred outcomes. Ineffective, poorly applied treatment is not necessarily the primary cause of disappointing outcomes. The psychological, physical, and social environs that receive the condition may determine prognosis at onset, or these influences may combine with injury-related or posttraumatic variables that increase pain perception and lead to a chronic refractory condition. Table 3 summarizes some of these adverse influences. More comprehensive narratives and references that discuss the myriad of factors that act as barriers to LBP wellness can be found in the referenced materials (1, 33–37).

TREATMENT

Overview

Doubt remains regarding the relative efficacy and cost-effectiveness of surgical versus nonsurgical treatment approaches. An important longitudinal study was performed by the German neurologist Henrik Weber (49) who randomly divided patients with sciatica and confirmed disk herniations into operative and nonoperative treatment groups. The surgically treated group had significantly greater improvement at one-year follow-up; however, the groups showed no statistically significant difference in improvement at 4 to 10 years (49). Two more recent prospective cohort studies compared surgical and nonsurgical management of lumbar spinal stenosis and sciatica due to lumbar disk herniation (50, 51). For patients with severe symptoms, surgical treatment was associated with greater improvement and satisfaction, and although this distinction persisted, it narrowed between groups over time (50, 51). The rationale for nonoperative treatment of discal herniation has been supported by clinical and autopsy studies, which demonstrate that resorption of protruded and extruded disk material occurs over time (1, 50–54). Also, several studies that have correlated discal resorption on MR or CT imaging with successful nonoperative treatment in patients with symptomatic lumbar disk herniations and clinical radiculopathy (1, 52, 54). The greatest reduction in size typically occurred in patients who had the largest disk herniations.

In general, nonoperative treatment can be divided into three phases based on the duration of symptoms. Primary nonoperative care consists of passively applied physical therapy during the acute phase of soft-tissue healing (<6 weeks). Secondary treatment includes spine care education and active exercise programs during the subacute phase between 6 and 12 weeks with physical therapy–driven goals to achieve preinjury levels of physical function and return to work. After 12 weeks, if patients remain symptomatic, treatment focuses on interdisciplinary care using cognitive–behavioral methods to address physical and psychological deconditioning and resultant disability that typically develops as a result of chronic spinal pain and dysfunction (39).

When spinal pain persists into the chronic phase, therapeutic interventions shift from rest and applied therapies to active exercise and physical restoration. This shift is primarily a behavioral evolution with the responsibility of care passed from the doctor and therapist to the patient (1, 22). Bed rest should be used sparingly for chronic spinal pain to treat acute pain or a severe exacerbation of symptoms. In cases of cLBP, aggressive management of flare-ups may require therapeutic injections; manual therapy and other externally applied therapies should be used adjunctively to reduce pain, so that strength and flexibility training can continue. When spinal pain is chronic or recurrent, traction or other modalities, such as heat and ice, can be self-administered by patients for flare-ups to provide pain relief (1, 20, 22).

Rational physical, medical, and surgical therapies can be selected by determining the relevant pathoanatomy and causal pain generators. Acute spinal injuries are first managed by elimination of biomechanical stressors, including short-term rest, supplemented by physical and pharmacological therapies aimed directly at nociceptive or neuropathic lesion(s). The paradigm that best represents elimination of activity or causative biomechanical loading is bed rest. Bed rest is usually considered an appropriate treatment for acute back pain; however, two days of bed rest for acute LBP have been demonstrated to be as effective as seven days and resulted in less time lost from work (55). Prolonged bed rest can have deleterious physiological effects, and inactivity may reinforce abnormal illness behaviors; therefore, bed rest should be limited or avoided when treating chronic spinal conditions (1, 2).

Oral Pharmacology

Overview*
Rational pharmacology for the treatment of spinal pain is aimed at causative peripheral and central pain generators, determined by the types of pain under therapeutic scrutiny (e.g., neuropathic and/or nociceptive), and modified to deal with evolving neurochemical and psychological influences that occur with chronicity. In general, published research for evaluation of medication efficacy to treat back pain has demonstrated faulty methodology and inadequate patient/subject description (56). However, medications continue to be used adjunctive to other measures because of anecdotal reports, perceived standards of care, and by some supportive clinical research.

During the acute period of time following biomechanical injury to the spine, excluding fracture, subluxation, other serious osseous lesions, or significant neurological sequela, mild narcotic analgesics may assist patients in minimizing inactivity and safely maximizing gradual progression of activity, including prescribed therapeutic exercises. Nonsteroidal anti-inflammatory drugs (NSAIDs) and muscle spasmolytics used during the day or at bedtime may also provide benefit (1, 28, 29, 57).

Nonsteroidal Anti-inflammatory Drugs
NSAIDs contain both analgesic and anti-inflammatory properties, and therefore, may affect mediators of the pathophysiological process in addition to pain. Designed clinical trials have demonstrated NSAIDs to be useful as a treatment for pain; however, long-term use of NSAIDs should be avoided due to possible adverse renal and gastrointestinal side effects (1, 20, 56). A 2000 review and analysis of randomized and double-blind controlled trials of NSAIDs for LBP treatment revealed supportive evidence for short-term symptomatic relief in patients with acute LBP. Evidence for any benefit for cLBP or for any specific superiority of one NSAID was lacking (57). Therefore, the effects of these medications in the management of chronic musculoskeletal pain remain unclear, and no studies have demonstrated clear superiority over aspirin (1, 20). When using NSAIDs for treatment of cLBP, perceived ineffectiveness of the drug by the patient may sometimes require switching to different chemical families through sequential trials to identify a beneficial agent for that individual patient (1, 20).

Muscle Spasmolytics
Muscle spasmolytics or "relaxants" are traditionally used to treat painful musculoskeletal disorders, but share sedation and sometimes dizziness as common side effects; therefore, some clinicians prescribe them only at bedtime. Some muscle spasmolytics are also considered potentially addictive and have abuse potential, especially more traditional agents such as diazepam, butalbital, and

---

* *Note:* See selective chapters devoted to specific analgesic medications.

phenobarbital. Examples of commonly used muscle relaxants include cycloben-zaprine, carisoprodol, methocarbamol, chlorzoxazone, and metaxalone. Benzo-diazepines may be appropriate for concurrent anxiety states, and in these cases, clonazepam should be considered. Clonazepam operates via GABA-mediated mechanisms through internuncial neurons of the spinal cord to provide muscle relaxation (58). Another benzodiazepine, tetrazepam, showed strong evidence of efficacy, when compared to placebo, for improving short-term pain and mod-erate evidence for short-term improvement of muscle spasm, but any data for long-term use was lacking (59). A review and analysis of randomized or double-blinded controlled trials showed that muscle relaxants were effective for man-agement of LBP, but adverse side effects limited their utility (60). A similar com-prehensive meta-analysis of the effectiveness of cyclobenzaprine showed evi-dence to support short-term use (<4 days) citing modest benefit in early LBP, but with the same problematic side effects (61). Tizanidine is a central alpha-2-adrenoreceptor agonist that was developed for the management of spasticity due to cerebral or spinal cord injury, but also has demonstrated efficacy when com-pared to other muscle spasmolytics (62). Controlled clinical trials have demon-strated clinical efficacy of tizanidine, including reduced analgesic use and muscle spasm, in patients with acute neck and back pain (63, 64).

Neuropathic Analgesics

Conventional treatments for neuropathic pain usually consist of antiepilep-tic drugs (AEDs) or medications that share similar properties. Most AEDs act through one or more of four basic mechanisms, which probably accounts for their efficacy for treating neuropathic pain. These include inhibition of sodium channels, inhibition of calcium channels, regulation of levels or activity of the inhibitory transmitter GABA, or regulation of levels or activity of the excitatory amino acid glutamate (65, 66). These medications should be considered appro-priate for therapeutic trials in spinal conditions when nervous system structures are symptomatic, or for myofascial pain, which may also be a spinal-mediated disorder (65). Neuropathic pain often accompanies radiculopathy or myelopa-thy, and the neurologist may be asked for advice in the following cases: when a clear structural cause is absent; following complex or failed surgical treatment; or when surgical intervention is contraindicated (66). Carbamazepine is U.S. Food and Drug Administration (FDA) approved for trigeminal neuralgia and may have applications in neuropathic conditions characterized by brief, electri-cal, lancinating pains (66). Other available AEDs, lamotrigine, zonisamide, lev-etiracetam, tiagabine, and oxycabazepine, have shown promise in small studies for the treatment of headache and neuropathic pain (66).

Gabapentin and pregabalin have both received FDA approval for treat-ment of postherpetic neuralgia, a neuropathic condition characterized by burn-ing pain and allodynia (65, 66). Pregabalin has also achieved FDA approval for treatment of diabetic peripheral neuropathy and fibromyalgia (66). Anecdotally, these two medications are the most commonly used analgesic agents for spinal radicular pain in most clinical practices. Gabapentin has been demonstrated as effective in multiple double-blind, randomized, controlled studies for the treat-ment of multiple different types of neuropathic pain syndromes (65, 66). The most common reason for failure of these medications to alleviate or dampen spinal radicular pain is physician reluctance to increase either medication to a maximum tolerated safe dose per day that determines effectiveness. Evidence suggests that these anticonvulsants modulate voltage-gated calcium channels and decrease intracellular calcium influx (66). Topiramate has been used anecdotally in the treatment of complex regional pain syndrome type 1 (66) and can sometimes be substituted on a trial basis for spinal neuropathic pain when side effects of gabapentin or pregabalin, such as weight gain, fluid retention, ankle edema, sedation, or cognitive dysfunction, prohibit patient tolerance.

Antidepressants

Two systematic reviews found that antidepressants improved pain in cLBP sufferers, but did not improve functional outcome (59, 67). Tricyclic antidepressants (TCAs) are commonly used for chronic pain treatment to alleviate insomnia, enhance endogenous pain suppression, reduce painful dysesthesia, and to treat both headaches and neuropathic pain syndromes (1). TCAs possess the capacity to block serotonergic uptake, resulting in a potentiation of noradrenergic synaptic activity in the central nervous system brain stem–dorsal horn nociceptive-modulating system, and also act like local anesthetics as sodium channel blockers (1, 66, 68, 69). Selective serotonin reuptake inhibitors have not demonstrated similar efficacy to attenuate pain intensity (1, 66, 68–70). Venlafaxine and duloxetine are structurally novel antidepressants that have strong uptake inhibition of both serotonin and norepinephrine and anesthetic properties similar to the TCAs (1, 66, 68–70). See dedicated chapter(s) and text that describe these medications in detail.

Opioid Analgesics

Low-dose opioid medications may be useful for the treatment of spinal pain disorders, but long-term use may lead to aberrant behaviors such as drug abuse and addiction (1). Opioids may be helpful for activating an injured patient to participate in physical and psychological rehabilitation (1). Low-dose opioids are beneficial in patients with acute radiculopathy, particularly those cases that are pre- or postoperative. Occasionally, narcotic analgesics may be used to assist a person in acute exacerbation of chronic pain; however, continuous use of opioid analgesics for cLBP is usually reserved as a final treatment option.

Over the past decade, physicians have adopted a greater willingness to prescribe opioid analgesics for the treatment of refractory spinal pain and radiculopathy. The greater proportion of patients reclaim "what life they can." Inherent dangers include side effects such as respiratory depression or bowel obstruction, as well as addiction, naive withdrawal, and death from overdosage. Side effect profiles among long-acting opioids are similar, but cost is variable among current pharmaceutical offerings. Several principles apply to prescribing long-acting opioids for chronic pain. Medication should be taken in a time-contingent rather than pain-contingent manner and only provided by one prescribing physician and pharmacy. An agreement regarding the need and purpose of opioids, as well as medical necessity, should be signed by both patient and doctor and placed in the medical record. For chronic spinal pain, an independent program of spinal stabilization exercises should be considered mandatory as long as opioid prescriptions are requested. Achievement of physical, functional, vocational, recreational, and social goals is a better measure of medication efficacy than subjective estimates of pain relief (1).

Physical Therapy

Overview: Active Vs. Passive Therapy
Physical therapy for the spine may be divided into passive and active therapies. Passive therapies include modalities, such as ultrasound, electric stimulation, traction, heat and ice, and manual therapy. Passive modalities are most appropriate when used short-term with acute injury or an exacerbation of a chronic spinal problem. Traction has long been used to treat conditions of the spine. Acute pain or an exacerbation of chronic pain is the recommended indication. In the lumbar spine, at least 60% of the body weight must be applied to produce dimensional changes in the lumbar disk; however, no evidence exists that this reduces a disk herniation (19). A principle often advocated in chronic spine care is that such modalities be self-administered by the patient when possible (1).

Corsets and braces have been long used as adjuncts for treatment, though their efficacy has not been demonstrated by studies without methodological flaws. Brace users often report benefit from this prescription (1). Usually, rigid orthoses are more effective than a simple support aide (1). The primary mechanisms of action are unclear and probably differ based on variables including the type of brace, patient morphology, pathoanatomy, and spinal activities (1). Mechanisms of action are likely related to abdominal compression, but also to direct or indirect unloading of trunk muscles and to gross rather than intersegmental motion restriction. However, in a mixed population of back pain patients of variable duration, groups receiving lumbar supports showed no improvement when compared to control groups receiving other types of treatment (59).

Manual therapy includes passive stretching, soft-tissue mobilization, myofascial release, manual traction, muscle energy techniques, joint mobilization, and manipulation. Joint mobilization is a low-velocity passive stretch applied to a joint within or at the limit of its range. Manipulation uses a high-velocity thrust maneuver beyond a joint's restricted range of motion (71, 72). More controlled trials have been carried out to evaluate manipulation than any other nonoperative treatment measures (73). However, it is difficult to interpret these studies because of a variety of methodological issues. Manipulative therapy may vary due to the variable skill levels and techniques among different practitioners, that is, physiotherapists, osteopaths, physicians, and chiropractors. A recent systematic review showed evidence of a modest beneficial effect of spinal manipulation on cLBP when compared to sham interventions judged to have no efficacy; however, this effect was not greater than other usually applied therapies (74). Spinal manipulation is probably most beneficial for the treatment of acute axial spinal pain, without radiculopathy or neurological impairment (73).

Although back schools to educate and train patients have been popular internationally, they have been ineffective as a preventative measure (1, 75). With variation in class size and emphasis, these schools usually provide information to patients regarding anatomy, pathophysiology, ergonomics (i.e., correct postures and body mechanics), exercise programs, self-management techniques, psychology, and activities of daily living. Back schools have received high grades for patient satisfaction (1, 75) (94–96%); and in a prospective randomized controlled trial comparing back school education with exercise to exercise alone, the back school group showed significantly greater improvements in pain and disability

(76). Furthermore, at 16 weeks, the exercise-only group had reverted to their original level of disability, while the back-school group showed continued improvement (76). Other studies have also shown that LBP patients return to work sooner and seek less follow-up medical attention (1, 77). There is some evidence that supports improvement from back schools in short-term pain and functional outcomes, but any long-term benefits are unclear (59).

Therapeutic Exercise

Physicians commonly prescribe active therapeutic exercise for spinal pain; however, exercise interventions are often heterogeneous in their composition and application. Literature analysis reveals strong support for exercise therapy, but no evidence indicates superiority of any specific type of exercise compared to other approaches (78). Exercise therapy should be designed to improve posture, body core strength, and physical function. Because the spine functions as a crane, building posterior torso strength would seem to be a logical goal of any spinal exercise protocol. The intensity of exercise is typically increased gradually at fixed times over a targeted period of time (78). Patients vary in their inherent capacity to exercise; therefore, sometimes these "fixed" time periods must be renegotiated. Exercise protocols proceed independently, regardless of the presence of pain; however, in some cases, fear avoidance acts as an impediment, slows progression, and must be overcome. A pooled meta-analysis of a variety of exercises showed strong evidence for short-term improvement in pain and function when compared with no treatment (59). Improvement was also seen in the exercise group when compared to other conservative treatments (59).

Lumbar stabilization exercises were popularized by physicians and physiotherapists at the San Francisco Spine Institute in the 1980s and 1990s. Stabilization begins by teaching and then training the patient to obtain and sustain the spine in a posture with the least pain and potential risk for injury (79). In a neutral spine posture, the motion segment shares biomechanical forces across the three-joint complex, with the degree of lordosis determined by a combination of unloading pain generators, whether anterior or posterior column in location; load sharing between the anterior (intervertebral disks) and posterior column (facet joints); and establishing a safe "close-packed" or engaged status of the facets, which prevents nonphysiological movements that may cause further segmental injury (1). The patient is taught to maintain this position while surrounding muscles isometrically brace the spine. Extremity movements are performed while maintaining neutral spine postures in varied positions from supine to standing, and, eventually, using weight machines, free weights, or no resistance other than the weight of the arms and legs (79, 80). The goal of treatment is to maintain a neutral spine posture while performing general strengthening and flexibility exercise with the least amount of pain and injury potential while continuing to advance to increasingly complex daily or work-related activities (1, 79, 80).

Functional Restoration

To address deconditioning, Mayer and others have advocated functional restoration (FR), which uses a multidisciplinary and sports medicine approach to address industrial back injuries through a program of physical training to restore normal flexibility, strength, and endurance, and emphasizes the multifactorial nature of chronic back pain (2). FR programs, as advocated, are highly structured, interdisciplinary, and intensive (2). Programs consist of daily and intensive physical, psychological, and behavioral reconditioning with measured physical and functional progression (2). Patients participate in increasing levels of task-oriented rehabilitation and work simulation toward targeted goals. These programs characteristically run about four weeks, and patients are estimated as receiving over 100 hours of physical therapy (81). Physical training is usually coupled with cognitive–behavioral support, including didactic sessions and disability management, culminating in an exit evaluation that again measures physical and functional parameters correlated with consistency of effort in the form of a work–capacity assessment, which can be used to determine the patient's physical demand capacity for returning to work. There is moderate evidence that these programs improve pain and strong evidence that they improve function when compared with usual rehabilitation and other conservative care methods (59). A systematic review of long-term outcomes, for example, ≤5 years, showed strong evidence for long-term efficacy of intensive FR programs on quality of life and return to work. Programs with less intensive physical therapy demands, for example, <100 hours, did not demonstrate similar efficacy (81).

Therapeutic Spinal Interventional Techniques

Therapeutic Injections

Therapeutic injections of local anesthetics, corticosteroids, or other substances may be administered directly into painful soft tissues, facet joints, nerve roots, the epidural space, or intrathecally (1). Therapeutic injections have been advocated to alleviate acute pain or an exacerbation of chronic pain, help the patient maintain an ambulatory outpatient status, participate in a rehabilitation program, decrease the need for analgesics, or avoid surgery (1). Although injections into myofascial trigger points are widely advocated, a double-blind study evaluating local anesthetic versus saline (82) and a prospective randomized double-blind study evaluating dry needling versus groups in which lidocaine, corticosteroids, or vaporized coolants sprayed with acupressure were used showed no statistically significant differences in benefit between treatment groups (83). Two double-blind studies evaluating paravertebral injections of botulinum toxin A as a treatment for cLBP demonstrated statistically significant improvement in measures of pain and function in treatment groups when compared to controls who received saline injections. Improvements in both studies were statistically significant for up to eight weeks (84, 85).

Facet Joint Injections

Intra-articular Blocks

The superior and inferior articular processes of adjacent vertebral laminae join to form the facet joints, which are paired diarthrodial synovial articulations that share compressive loads and other biochemical forces with the intervertebral disk. Like other synovial joints, the facets react to trauma and inflammation by manifesting pain, stiffness, and dysfunction with secondary muscle spasm leading to joint stiffness, degeneration, and arthropathy (1). Boswell et al. systematically reviewed and analyzed published reports of clinical studies that included randomized and nonrandomized trials (both prospective and retrospective) that consisted of treatment with intra-articular injections of local anesthetic and corticosteroids (86, 87). On the basis of criteria that short-term relief is <6 weeks and long-term relief is 6 weeks, they found moderate evidence to support short-term and long-term relief (86, 87). Intra-articular injections of the facet joints are advocated by many experts as a method for diagnosis and treatment of spinal pain (1, 88). Although some physicians advocate facet injections as a treatment method, a large prospective study showed no long-term benefit (89). Therefore, despite the relative dearth of medical literature on the role of therapeutic intra-articular facet injections, which are costly and invasive, analysis of the best data currently available suggests that facet blocks have dubious therapeutic value when used in isolation; and there is no evidence that validates the procedure as a reliable method for inducing long-term pain relief. However, intra-articular facet injections are generally supported for their use as a diagnostic tool (1, 88).

Medial Branch Blocks
Medial branch blocks have traditionally been used for both diagnostic and prognostic purposes, but have limited value therapeutically. Using the same duration criteria as cited for intra-articular blocks, an evidence-based review of the available medical literature that evaluated the therapeutic effectiveness of median branch blocks showed moderate support for short-term and long-term relief of facet joint pain (88, 90).

Radiofrequency Medial Branch Neurotomy
Percutaneous radiofrequency (RF) neurotomy of the medial branches causes temporary denaturing of the nerves to the painful facet, but this effect may wear off when axons regenerate (1). In a 2002 review, Manchikanti et al. cite strong evidence that RF denervation provides short-term relief (<6 months) and moderate evidence for long-term relief (>6 months) of chronic thoracic and lumbar spine pain of facet origin (91). Improvement measures have not only included reduced pain, but also reduced functional disability and physical impairment. These systematic reviews of the evidence show strong support for both short-term and long-term benefit for RF medial branch neurotomy for the treatment of lumbar facet syndrome in chronic LBP patients (1, 88, 91). RF denervation showed improvement in patients who were treated following a diagnostic intra-articular facet block with local anesthetic (83). These improvements lasted up to two months; however, another study showed no long-term difference at 12 weeks when treatment was compared with controls (83). RF neurotomy, like all spinal interventions, is one treatment method in the toolbox. Most patients require spine care education and exercise in addition to the above-mentioned procedures.

Lumbar Epidural Injections
Lumbar epidural spinal injections (LESIs) are widely used with transforaminal, interlaminar, or caudal presentation combining corticosteroid and local anesthetic of varying volumes. An interlaminar entry is directed more closely to the site of assumed pathology and requires less volume of the injectate than a caudal route. However, the caudal entry is usually considered a safe approach with less risk for inadvertent dural puncture or neural trauma. Transforaminal injections

are more target specific and require the least volume of injectate to reach the presumed pathoanatomic site or primary pain generator by an approach through the ventral lateral epidural space (88).

When considering LESI, each approach has its advantages and disadvantages. The caudal approach requires a large fluid volume, thus greater dilution of the active ingredient within the injectate. Because the needle cannula is initially threaded at a relatively parallel plane to the spinal canal, there is greater risk of intravascular, subcutaneous, subperiosteal, or interosseous needle puncture. Disadvantages of the intralaminar approach can include dilution of the injectate; extraepidural or intravascular placement of the needle; preferential cranial and posterior flow of the solution; higher difficultly in postsurgical patients and below the L4-5 interspace; dural puncture; and spinal cord trauma. The transforaminal approach is difficult in the presence of postsurgical epidural adhesions, osseous fusion, or when hardware is present. Other risks include intraneural or intravascular injection and spinal cord trauma. The use of fluoroscopy to direct needle placement and observe contrast flow is now considered requisite to reduce potential adverse events (88).

An evidence synthesis by Datta et al. revealed limited evidence on the effectiveness of selective nerve root blocks as a diagnostic tool and cited moderate evidence for the diagnostic utility of transforaminal epidural injections in the preoperative evaluation of patients with negative or inconclusive imaging studies (92). Abdi et al. performed a systematic review looking at each epidural route as to its effectiveness. The evidence for lumbar transforaminal epidural steroid injections was strong for managing lumbosacral radicular pain on a short-term basis and moderate for long-term effectiveness; however, support was limited in managing lumbar radiculopathy pain that was present following surgery (93). Evidence was indeterminate in managing axial LBP (93). Evidence synthesis by Manchikanti demonstrated support for short-term and long-term pain relief when epidural injections were performed in a series, rather than a single injection. At present, there is strong literature support for the use of intralaminar corticosteroid epidural injections to provide short-term pain relief when treating cervical or lumbar radicular syndromes, even chronic cases, but this treatment is best reserved for use as an adjunctive therapy or during a flare-up of symptoms (88).

On the basis of the available evidence, the Therapeutics and Technology Assessment Subcommittee of the American Academy of Neurology found that epidural steroid injections may result in some improvement in radicular lumbosacral pain when assessed between two and six weeks following the injection, compared to control treatments. However, the magnitude of improvement was small, and no meaningful impact could be measured with regard to improved function, need for surgery, or pain relief beyond three months. The subcommittee concluded that the medical literature showed faulty methodology, in general, and there was insufficient evidence to support the use of LESIs in clinical practice (94).

Therefore, and in summary, the medical literature is flawed; and using this procedure depends on clinical judgment as to its rationale and safety, combining clinical experience with the chosen procedure. There is no clear evidence that these procedures will provide long-term pain relief or any benefit. Epidural injections may be useful as a method of pain control and may provide benefit that is adjunctive to other therapies. There is no evidence to support the use of

LESIs for axial LBP, but there is sketchy evidence to support the use of LESIs in patients with lumbosacral radiculopathy. Patients that benefit from short-term improvement would be appropriate in cases when a patient with refractory acute–subacute sciatica is awaiting a surgical procedure; or whereby exacerbation of chronic intermittent sciatica is pending further progress in physical therapy or the natural history of eventual improvement; or when a patient needs a temporary pain reduction to continue working with physiotherapy through stabilization exercises or an FR program; and lastly, for diagnostic purposes with the hope that short-term relief will make the patient more comfortable while determining further treatment. Other than exacerbation of a chronic condition that tends to relapse or fluctuate, the use of lumbar epidural corticosteroids seems to be at odds with the evidence presented. Furthermore, these injections provide even more limited benefit in patients who have failed surgery.

Intradiscal Therapies

Numerous procedures have been directed at the disk, which is presumed causative for many painful spinal and radicular syndromes. These have included chymopapain injections to achieve nucleolysis, percutaneous manual nucleotomy with nucleotome, thermal vaporization with laser, and percutaneous decompression with nucleotomy using coblation technology (nucleoplasty). Intradiscal electrothermal therapy (IDET) is a minimally invasive technique in which the annulus is subjected to thermomodulation (88). IDET is used with discography as a diagnostic procedure to demonstrate a concordant pain response. IDET is the most commonly used discal intervention, but remains a controversial treatment for cLBP (88). The largest randomized controlled trial was performed in a highly selected population and showed that IDET was effective in reducing pain and improving function when patients were carefully chosen (83, 88).

Spinal Cord Stimulation

The literature is inadequate to show support for spinal cord stimulation (SCS) in patients with failed back surgery or complex regional pain syndrome. There are no high-quality controlled studies to support the use of this intervention. Traditionally, radicular symptoms that respond, in part, to transcutaneous electrical nerve stimulation treatment would be candidates for a percutaneous trial of SCS. If successful, then a more permanently placed SCS can be pursued, which sometimes requires lumbar spine surgery (83).

Management Strategies

On the basis of the material presented, the author proposes the algorithm presented in Figure 1 as a framework for approaching the spinal pain patient. This algorithm may be useful as a guide.

REFERENCES

1. Wheeler AH, Murrey DB. Spinal pain: pathogenesis, evolutionary mechanisms, and management. In: Pappagallo M, ed. The Neurological Basis of Pain. New York: McGraw-Hill, 2005:421–452.
2. Mayer TG, Gatchel RJ. Functional Restoration for Spinal Disorders: The Sports Medicine Approach. Philadelphia, PA: Lea & Febiger, 1988.

3. Biering-Sorenson F. Low back trouble and a general population of 30-, 40-, 50-, and 60-year-old men and women. Dan Med Bull 1982; 29:289–299.
4. Damkot D, Pope M, Lord J, et al. The relationship between work history, work environment and low back pain in men. Spine 1984; 9:395–399.
5. Anderssen GBJ. Epidemiologic features of chronic low back pain. Lancet 1999; 354:581–585.
6. Anderssen GBJ. The epidemiology of spinal disorders. In: Frymoyer JW, ed. The Adult Spine: Principles and Practice. New York: Raven Press, 1997:93–141.
7. Nachemson Al, Waddell G, Norland AL. Epidemiology of neck and low back pain. In: Nachemson AL, Jonsson E, eds. Neck and Back Pain: The Scientific Evidence of Causes, Diagnoses, and Treatment. Philadelphia, PA: Lippincott Williams & Wilkins, 2000:165–187.
8. Kelsey JL, White AA. Epidemiology of low back pain. Spine 1980; 6:133–142.
9. Waddell G. A new clinical model for the treatment of low back pain. Spine 1987; 12:632–644.
10. Cunningham LS, Kelsey JL. Epidemiology of musculoskeletal impairments and associated disability. Am J Public Health 1984; 74:574–579.
11. National Center for Health Statistics. Limitations of Activity Due to Chronic Conditions, United States, 1974. 1977. Series 10, No. 111.
12. National Center for Health Statistics. Physician Visits, Volume and Interval Since Last Visit, United States, 1971. 1975. Series 10, No. 97.
13. National Center for Health Statistics. Surgical Operations in Short Stay Hospitals by Diagnosis, United States, 1978. 1982. Series 13, No. 61.
14. National Center for Health Statistics. Inpatient Utilization of Short Stay Hospitals by Diagnosis, United States, 1973. 1976. Series 13, No. 25.
15. National Center for Health Statistics. Surgical Operations in Short Stay Hospitals by Diagnosis, United States, 1973. 1976. Series 13, No. 24.
16. Spengler D, Bigos S, Martin N, et al. Back injuries in industry: a retrospective study. Overview and cost analysis. Spine 1986; 11;241–245.
17. Abenhaim L, Suissa S. Importance and economic burden of occupational back pain: a study of 2,500 cases representative of Quebeç. J Occup Med 1987; 29;670–674.
18. Engel C, Korff Mv, Katon W. Back pain in primary care: predictors of high health-care costs. Pain 1996; 65:197–204.
19. Frymoyer JW. Back pain and sciatica. N Engl J Med 1988; 318:291–300.
20. Argoff CE, Wheeler AH. Spinal and radicular pain syndromes. In: Backonja M-M, ed. Neurologic Clinics. Philadelphia, PA: WB Saunders, 1998:833–845.
21. Mooney V. Where is the pain coming from? Spine 1987; 12:754–759.
22. Wheeler AH, Hanley EN. Nonoperative treatment of low back pain: rest to restoration. Spine 1995; 20:375–378.
23. Modic MT, Brant-Zawadzki MN, Obuchowski N, et al. Magnetic resonance imaging of the lumbar spine in people without back pain. N Engl J Med 1994; 331:69–73.
24. Powell MC, Szypryt P, Wilson M, et al. Prevalence of lumbar disc degeneration observed by magnetic resonance in symptomless women. Lancet 1986; 2: 1366–1367.
25. Weinreb JC, Wolbrsht LB, Cohen JM, et al. Prevalence of lumbosacral intervertebral disc abnormalities on MR images in pregnant and asymptomatic nonpregnant women. Radiology 1989; 170:125–128.
26. Wiesel SW, Tsourmas N, Feffer HL, et al. A study of computer-assisted tomography. I. The incidence of positive CAT scans in an asymptomatic group of patients. Spine 1984; 9:549–551.
27. Haldeman S. Presidential Address, North American Spine Society: failure of the pathology model to model to predict back pain. Spine 1990; 15:718–724.
28. Wheeler AH. Diagnosis and management of low back pain and sciatica. Am Fam Physician 1995; 552(5):133–141.
29. Wheeler AH, Pathophysiology of Chronic Back Pain eMedicine from WebMD. Updateed April 27, 2009. Available at: http://emedicine.medscape.com/artoc;e/1144130-overview.

30. Galer B. Neuropathic pain of peripheral origin: advances in pharmacologic treatment. Neurology 1995; 45(suppl 9):S17–S25.
31. Backonja M-M, Galer BS. Pain assessment and evaluation of patients who have neuropathic pain. Neurol Clin 1998; 16:775–789.
32. Waddell G, McCulloch JA, Kummel E, et al. Nonorganic physical signs in low-back pain. Spine 1980; 5:117–124.
33. Wheeler AH. Evolutionary mechanisms in chronic low back pain and rationale for treatment. Am J Pain Manage 1995; 5:62–66.
34. Killian LE. Psychological barriers to recovery. In: Isernhagen SJ, ed. Work Injury Management and Prevention. Gaithersburg, MD: Aspen Inc., 1988:247–257.
35. Polatin PB, Kinny RK, Gatchel RJ, et al. Psychiatric illness in chronic low back pain. The mind and the spine which goes first? Spine 1993; 18:66–71.
36. Keefe FJ, Bedcham JC, Fillingim RB. The psychology of chronic back pain. In: Frymoyer JW, ed. The Adult Spine, Principles and Practice. New York: Raven Press, 1991:185–197.
37. Bigos S, Battie MC, Spengler DM, et al. A prospective study of work perceptions and psychosocial factors affecting the reports of back injuries. Spine 1991; 16:1–6.
38. The North American Spine Society's Ad Hoc Committee on Diagnostic and Therapeutic Procedures. Common diagnostic and therapeutic procedures of the lumbosacral spine. Spine 1991; 16:1161–1167.
39. Gatchel RJ, Mayer TG, Hazard RG, et al. Editorial: functional restoration. Pitfalls in evaluating efficacy. Spine 1992; 17:988–995.
40. Saal JA. The role of inflammation in lumbar pain. Physical medicine and rehabilitation. State Art Rev 1990; 4:191–199.
41. Weinstein J. The role of neurogenic and non-neurogenic mediators as they relate to pain and the development of osteoarthritis. The clinical review. Spine 1992; (suppl 10):356–361.
42. Fields HL. Pain. New York: McGraw-Hill, 1987.
43. Schofferman JA. Applied neurophysiology of pain. In: White AH, Schofferman JA, eds. Spine Care: Diagnosis and Conservative Treatment. St. Louis, MO: Mosby Press, 1995:23–26.
44. Cavanaugh JM, Weinstein JN. Low back pain: epidemiology, anatomy and neurophysiology. In: Wall PD, Melzack R, eds. Textbook of Pain. 3rd ed. London, UK: Churchill Livingstone, 1994:441–455.
45. Kuslich SD, Ulstrom CL, Michael CJ. The tissue origin of low back pain and sciatica: a report of pain response to tissue stimulation during operation on the lumbar spine using local anesthesia. Orthop Clin North Am 1991; 22:181–187.
46. Rydevik BL. The effects of compression on the physiology of nerve roots. J Manipulative Physiol Ther 1992; 1:62–66.
47. Olmarker K, Rydevik B. Pathophysiology of spinal nerve roots as related to sciatica and disc herniation. In: Herkowitz HN, Garfin SR, Balderston RA, et al., eds. Rothman-Simeone Studies: The Spine. Philadelphia, PA: WB Saunders, 1999:59–72.
48. Kang JD, Georgescu HI, MacIntyre-Larkin L, et al. Herniated lumbar intervertebral discs spontaneously produce matrix metalloproteinases, nitric oxide, interleukin-6 and prostaglandin E2. Spine 1996; 21(3):271–277.
49. Weber H. Lumbar disc herniation. A controlled, prospective study with ten years of observation. Spine 1983; 8:131–140.
50. Atlas SJ, Keller RB, Robson, et al. Surgical and nonsurgical management of lumbar spinal stenosis: four year outcomes from the maine lumbar spine study. Spine 2000; 25(5):556–562.
51. Atlas SJ, Keller RB, Chang Y, et al. Surgical and nonsurgical management of sciatica secondary to a lumbar disc herniation: five-year outcomes from the maine lumbar spine study. Spine 2001; 26(10):1179–1187.
52. Lindblom K, Hultqvist G. Absorption of protruded disc tissue. J Bone Joint Surg 1950; 32A:557–560.
53. Saal JA, Saal JS, Herzog RJ. The natural history of lumbar intervertebral disc extrusions treated non-operatively. Spine 1990; 15:683–686.

54. Komori H, Okawa A, Hirataka H, et al. Contrast-enhanced magnetic resonance imagining in conservative management of lumbar disc herniation. Spine 1998; 23:67–62.
55. Deyo RA, Diehl AK, Rosenthal M. How many days of bed rest for low back pain? A randomized clinical trial. N Engl J Med 1986; 315:1064–1070.
56. Deyo RA. Nonoperative treatment of low back disorders: differentiated useful from useless therapy. In: Frymoyer JW (ed-in-chief), Ducker TB, Hadler NM, et al., eds. The Adult Spine: Principles and Practice. Philadelphia, PA: Lippincott-Raven, 1997:1777–1793.
57. van Tulder MW, Scholten RJ, Koes BW, et al. Nonsteroidal anti-inflammatory drugs for low back pain: a systematic review within the framework of the Cochrane Collaboration Back Review Group. Spine 2000; 25(19):2501–2513.
58. Harkens S, Linford J, Cohen J, et al. Administration of clonazepam in the treatment of TMD and associated myofascial pain: a double-blind pilot study. J Craniomandib Disord 1991; 5:179–186.
59. van Tulder MW, Koes BW, Malmivaara A. Outcome of noninvasive treatment modalities on back pain: an evidence-based review. Eur Spine J 2006; 15:S64–S81.
60. van Tulder MW, Touray T, Furlan AD, et al. Muscle relaxants for nonspecific low back pain: a systematic review within the framework of the cochrane collaboration. Spine 2003; 28(17):1978–1992.
61. Browning R, Jackson JL, O'Malley PG. Cyclobenzaprine and back pain: a meta-analysis. Arch Intern Med 2001; 161(13):1613–1620.
62. Waldman SD. Recent advances in analgesic therapy—tizanidine. Pain Digest 1999; 9:40–43.
63. Berry H, Hutchinson DR. A multicenter placebo-controlled study in general practice to evaluate the safety and efficacy of tizanidine in acute low back pain. J Int Med Res 1988; 16:75–82.
64. Berry H, Hutchinson DR. Tizanidine and ibuprofen in acute low back pain: results of a multicenter double-blind study in general practice. J Int Med Res 1988; 16:83–91.
65. Rosenberg JM, Harrell C, Rishi H, et al. The effect of gabapentin on neuropathic pain. Clin J Pain 1997; 13:251–255.
66. Pappagallo M. Peripheral neuropathic pain. In: Pappagallo M, ed. The Neurological Basis of Pain. New York: McGraw-Hill, 2005:321–341.
67. van Tulder MW, Koes BW. Low back pain (chronic). Clin Evid 2006; 15:419–422.
68. Staiger T, Gastoer B, Sullivan M, et al. Systematic review of antidepressants in the treatment of chronic low back pain. Spine 2003; 28:2540–2545.
69. Watson CP. The treatment of neuropathic pain: antidepressants and opioids. Clin J Pain 2000; 16(suppl 2):S49–S55.
70. Pritchett YL, McCarberg BH, Watkin JG, et al. Duloxetine for the management of diabetic peripheral neuropathic pain: response profile. Pain Med 2007; 8:397–409.
71. Ottenbacher K, Difabio RP. Efficacy of spinal manipulation/mobilization therapy. A meta-analysis. Spine 1985; 10:833–837.
72. Triano J. Standards of care: manipulative procedures. In: White AH, Anderson R, eds. Conservative Care of Lower Back Pain. Baltimore, MD: Williams and Wilkins, 1991:159–168.
73. Shekelle PG. Spinal manipulation. Spine 1996; 19:858–861.
74. Assendelft W, Morton S, Yu E, et al. Spinal manipulation for low back pain: a meta-analysis of effectiveness related to other therapies. Ann Intern Med 2003; 138:871–881.
75. Moffett JA, Chase SM, Portek I, et al. A controlled, prospective study to evaluate the effectiveness of a back school in the relief of chronic low back pain. Spine 1986; 11:120–122.
76. Bergquist-Ullman M, Larsson U. Acute low back pain in industry. Acta Orthop Scand Suppl 1977; 17:1–150.
77. Hall H. Back School and Education. Non-operative Care of Lumbar Pain Syndromes. Boston, MA: North American Spine Society and Seton Medical Center, 1992:69–76.
78. van Tulder MW, Goossens M, Waddell G, et al. Conservative treatment of chronic low back pain. In: Nachemson AL, Jonsson E, eds. Neck and Back Pain: The Scientific

Evidence of Causes, Diagnoses, and Treatment. Philadelphia, PA: Lippincott Williams & Wilkins, 2000:271–304.

79. White AH. Stabilization of lumbar spine. In: White AH, Anderson R, eds. Conservative Care of Low Back Pain. Baltimore, MD: Williams & Wilkins, 1991:106–111.

80. Robison R. Low back school and stabilization: aggressive conservative care. In: White AG, Schofferman JA, eds. Spine Care: Diagnosis and Conservative Treatment. St. Louis, MO: Mosby Press, 1995:394–412.

81. Lurie JD. Evidence-based management of chronic low back pain. Adv Pain Manage 2000; 1(4):141–146.

82. Frost FA, Jessen B, Siggaard-Anderson J. A controlled, double blind comparison of mepivacaine injection versus saline injection for myofascial pain. Lancet 1980; 1:499–501.

83. Garvey TA, Marks MR, Wiesel SW. A prospective, randomized double-blind evaluation of trigger-point injection therapy for low back pain. Spine 1989; 14:962–964.

84. Foster L, Clapp L, Erickson M,et al. Botulinum toxin A and chronic low back pain: a randomized, double blind study. Neurology 2001; 56:1290–1293.

85. Knusel B, DeGryse R, Grant M, et al. Intramuscular injection of botulinum toxin type A (Botox) in chronic low back pain associated with muscle spasm [poster abstract]. American Pain Society Annual Meeting; November 5–8, 1998; San Diego, CA.

86. Boswell MV, Trescott AM, Datta S, et al. Interventional techniques: evidence-based practice guidelines in the management of chronic spinal pain. Pain Physician 2007; 10:7–111.

87. Boswell MV, Colson JD, Sehgal N, et al. A systematic review of therapeutic facet joint interventions in chronic spinal pain. Pain Physician 2007; 10:229–253.

88. Manchikanti L, Staats PS, Singh VJ, et al. Evidence-based guidelines for interventional techniques in the management of chronic spinal pain. Pain Physician 2003; 6:3–81.

89. Jackson RP, Jacobs RR, Montesano PX. Facet joint injection in low-back pain. Spine 1988; 13:966–971.

90. Manchikanti L, Pampati V, Bakhit CE, et al. Effectiveness of lumbar facet joint nerve blocks in chronic low back pain: a randomized clinical trial. Pain Physician 2001; 4:101–117.

91. Manchikanti K, Singh V, Vilims B, et al. Medial branch neurotomy in management of chronic spinal pain: systematic review of the evidence. Pain Physician 2002; 5:405–418.

92. Datta S, Everett CR, Trescott AM, et al. An updated systematic review of diagnostic utility of selective nerve root blocks. Pain Physician 2007; 10:113–120.

93. Abdi S, Datta S, Trescott AM, et al. Epidural steroids in the management of chronic spinal pain: a systematic review. Pain Physician 2007; 10:185–212.

94. Carmel A, Argoff CE, Samuels J, et al. Assessment: use of epidural steroid injections to treat particular lumbosacral pain. Neurology 2007; 68:723–729.

Neuropathic Low Back Pain

Joseph F. Audette, Joseph Walker III, and Alec L. Meleger

Department of Physical Medicine and Rehabilitation, Spaulding Rehabilitation Hospital, Harvard Medical School, Boston, Massachusetts, U.S.A.

Those who do not feel pain seldom feel that it is felt. ...
Dr. Samuel Johnson (1709–1784).

THE DISORDER

Low back pain (LBP) is the most common presenting complaint in pain and orthopedic specialty practices and is the second most common symptomatic complaint in a primary care setting with an annual prevalence of 15% to 20% in the United States (1). The most common cause of acute LBP is often described as nonspecific and is generally considered to have a mechanical etiology. Although disk herniation is often classified as a type of mechanical LBP (Table 1), it is, perhaps, the only commonly recognized cause of acute LBP that has neuropathic features. Chronic LBP is even less well understood, especially given the high prevalence of abnormal findings on imaging in populations of individuals without pain (2). In many ways, on a clinical level, the understanding of spine-related pain by most practicing physicians would not be alien to colleagues of Dr. Jason Mixter. In 1934, Mixter and Joseph S. Barr published an article on the intervertebral disk lesion as the source of sciatica in the *New England Journal of Medicine* (3). However, with the growth of knowledge over the last two decades about the neurophysiological mechanisms of persistent pain and the basic science of the neuropathic features associated with LBP, there is a need to translate this understanding into clinical practice, especially when the pain is chronic.

The current definition of neuropathic pain (NP) as proposed by the International Association for the Study of Pain (IASP) is "pain initiated or caused by a primary lesion or dysfunction of the nervous system" (4). Part of the problem with the proper classification of neuropathic LBP is that there is still debate about the IASP definition of NP, which has been criticized by many as vague, particularly with the use of the term "dysfunction" to describe nervous system pathology. The concern is that this opens the door to calling all chronic pain disorders neuropathic, even when there is no evidence of nerve damage or injury (5). To avoid such confusion, Woolf and Mannion have defined the following key features of NP: "The presence of a lesion, damage or disruption to some component of primary sensory neurons. The lesion may be in a peripheral nerve, the dorsal root ganglion or a dorsal root and may be the consequence of trauma, compression, tumor invasion, ischemia, inflammation, metabolic disturbances, nutritional deficits, cytotoxic agents and degenerative disorders" (6). However, there are a variety of clinical conditions that appear to have neuropathic features that do not, in any obvious way, involve injury or dysfunction of the peripheral

TABLE 1 Mechanical and Nonmechanical Causes of Low Back Pain

Mechanical	Nonmechanical
Lumbar strain or sprain	Neoplasia
Spondylolysis or degenerative arthritis	Metastatic carcinoma
Degenerative disk disease	Multiple myeloma
Facet arthopathy	Lymphoma
Diffuse idiopathic skeletal hyperostosis	Spinal cord tumors
Spondylolysis	Retroperitoneal tumors
Spondylolisthesis	Infection
Herniated disk	Osteomyelitis
Spinal stenosis	Septic discitis
Osteoporosis with compression fracture	Paraspinal or epidural abscess
Fractures	Endocarditis
Severe kyphosis	Inflammatory arthritis
Severe scoliosis	Ankylosing arthritis
Paget's disease	Reiter's syndrome
Sacroiliac joint dysfunction	Psoriatic spondylitis
Myofascial pain	Inflammatory bowel disease
	Polymyalgia rheumatica

Source: Modified from Ref. 1.

nervous system, making the definitive diagnosis of NP problematic. This is especially true in cases where the persistence of the pain, at least theoretically, suggests that there have been pathological neuroplastic changes in the central nervous system (CNS), despite the lack of visible signs of damage to the peripheral nervous system. Cases such as complex regional pain syndrome type I (reflex sympathetic dystrophy), fibromyalgia, irritable bowel syndrome, interstitial cystitis, and many cases of chronic LBP are often cited as being in this grey zone. However, as Bennett points out, prematurely excluding these types of cases for the reason that based on our current limited understanding of the etiology of these pain conditions we believe they do not meet criteria for NP may have adverse clinical implications. For example, such a strict interpretation of NP may lead one to not prescribe a helpful agent such as gabapentin for fibromyalgia or chronic LBP because there is no known nerve damage (7). Criteria that may be used to define NP and differentiate it from other types of pain without absolutely excluding clinical conditions in this grey zone could include the following:

1. Pain and abnormal sensory symptoms that persist beyond the normal healing period.
2. Presence, to a variable degree, of gross or subtle sensory neurological findings, potentially manifesting as either the absence of normal sensation or the presence of abnormally heightened sensation, or both.
3. Presence, to a variable degree, of other neurological signs, including motor or autonomic dysfunction.
4. The presence of NP would also not exclude the presence of other types of pain and pain mechanisms such as inflammatory pain or gross mechanical disruption of normal tissue often called nociceptive pain.

In this discussion, we hope to advance a clinical approach to LBP that is more in line with our modern understanding of NP. We will review the current understanding of both normal and pathological neuroanatomy of the lumbar spine. We will then outline how pathology in the different structures can lead to NP and cause common pain patterns seen in clinical practice. Finally, we will detail the available treatments for neuropathic LBP.

DIAGNOSIS

Evaluation of an individual with suspected neuropathic LBP must include a detailed medical history and review of systems in addition to a comprehensive physical and neurological examination to exclude primary peripheral neuropathies (8). The patient may report both positive sensory symptoms such as tingling or burning pain and negative sensory symptoms such as numbness. Psychological comorbidity and psychosocial stressors should be assessed to ensure the formulation of an optimal treatment plan. Finally, functional and quality-of-life assessment should be made to guide treatment goals.

Examination of Neuropathic LBP

Sensory, motor, and autonomic dysfunction should be thoroughly investigated during the physical examination. When performing the sensory component of the examination of neuropathic LBP, special attention should be given to the leg, inguinal region, gluteal region, and back. Often segmental facilitation is best assessed along the spine starting from the L1 dermatome just lateral to the spinous processes and working down the back to the sacral foramen. To properly assess the range of peripheral nerve dysfunction, light touch, pinprick, temperature, and vibration sensation should be assessed. Often there can be sensory deficits with one modality, such as loss of pinprick sensation, and exaggerated positive responses to another modality, such as pain with light touch. To help distinguish symptom amplification from reliable sensory dysfunction, there should be clear and repeatable findings in the affected area, while the subject is able to respond normally in an unaffected area. In addition to findings of allodynia and hyperalgesia, one can look for signs of cutaneous C-fiber dropout by applying hot water in a plastic bag over the skin and comparing the time it takes to withdraw to an unaffected area. With the loss of C fibers, the withdrawal latency will be prolonged. Summation can also be assessed by repeatedly applying the same pinprick stimulus with the same force and having the patient report the changing pain intensity. The normal nervous system tends to accommodate to repeated painful stimuli, whereas an individual with a facilitated nervous system will report increasing pain intensity. Other findings of autonomic dysfunction such as abnormal skin temperature, local areas of cutaneous trophedema, and hair loss should be looked for. In addition to weakness, muscle irritability in a specific myotome, including trigger points, spontaneous muscle fasciculations, and cramps, should also suggest more subtle segmental nerve dysfunction. If abnormal sensory or motor findings are found along a certain dermatome or myotome, then the corresponding dermatome along the related spine segments should be checked for hyperalgesia and allodynia. Strong correlation between the distal and proximal abnormal sensory and motor findings is more supportive of specific segmental nerve root dysfunction and facilitation.

PATHOPHYSIOLOGY

Normal Anatomy of the Lumbar Spine

Musculoskeletal Anatomy

The lumbar spine consists of five separate lumbar vertebrae and links the thoracic vertebral column to the sacrum. Each vertebra consists of a vertebral body, paired sets of transverse processes, laminas, pedicles, superior and inferior articular processes, and a single spinous process. An intervertebral foramen is formed anteriorly by the posterior aspect of the vertebral body and intervertebral disk, superiorly and inferiorly by the adjacent pedicles, and posteriorly by the superior and inferior articular processes of the respective facet joints. Each intervertebral disk consists of a centrally placed, semifluid nucleus pulposus and a peripheral, collagen-rich annulus fibrosus. The annulus is made up of strong collagen fibers that form highly ordered concentric rings and surround the disk nucleus. Each lumbar facet joint is formed by a superior articular process of the caudally positioned vertebra and an inferior articular process of the overlying adjacent vertebra. This joint is a typical synovial joint consisting of an articular cartilage, synovium, and an encapsulating fibrous capsule.

An extensive ligamentous network is present and adds extra stability to the lumbar spine. The vertebral bodies are held together by anterior and posterior longitudinal ligaments, which run vertically along the anterior and posterior aspects of the vertebral column, respectively. The lamina and the spinous processes are interconnected with the help of ligamentum flavum, interspinous, and supraspinous ligaments. A thick iliolumbar ligament connects the vertebral bodies and the transverse processes of the L5 vertebra to the respective ilia bilaterally.

Another set of ligaments play less of a structurally functional role and are called transforaminal, intertransverse, and mamillo-accessory ligaments (Fig. 1). Transforaminal ligaments are present almost uniformly at all levels of the lumbar spine and are classified as intra- or extraforaminal. They can compartmentalize the respective neuroforamina by crossing superiorly or inferiorly in a horizontal or oblique fashion, thus placing them in close proximity to the exiting neurovascular elements (9). The intertransverse ligaments connect the ipsilateral transverse processes and consist of dorsal and ventral leafs where the latter is pierced by the nerve branches en route to the psoas muscle and the exiting ventral ramus (10). The mamillo-accessory ligament forms a bridge between the mamillary and accessory vertebral processes under which medial branch of the dorsal ramus passes on its way to innervating the respective lumbar facet joint. This ligament has been shown to have tendencies toward partial or complete ossification in older populations (11).

There is an impressive array of muscles surrounding the lumbar spine. Posteriorly, the erector spinae, multifidi, interspinales, and intertransversarii mediales muscles aid in lumbar rotation and extension. The quadratus lumborum, located laterally, plays a major role in lateral flexion with the anterolaterally positioned large psoas muscle providing only minimal biomechanical effect.

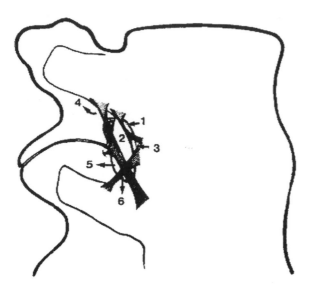

FIGURE 1 Schematic diagram showing attachments of the ligaments and the effect on partitioning the neural foramen: 1, compartment for the spinal artery; 2, compartment for the vertebral ramus of the spinal nerve; 3, compartment for the recurrent meningeal nerve, which also transmits a small branch of the segmental artery; 4, tunnels transmitting the medial division of the dorsal primary ramus with accompanying vessels; 5, tunnels transmitting the lateral division of the dorsal primary ramus with accompanying vessels; 6, compartment for the veins.

Neural Anatomy

The spinal cord, which typically terminates at the L2 vertebral level, sends out dorsal and ventral roots, which combine at the level of the respective neuroforamina and form exiting lumbar spinal nerves. The ventral root carries mainly motor fibers, and the sensory root transmits sensory fibers from the spinal nerve to the spinal cord. Immediately prior to the junction with the ventral root, the dorsal root forms the dorsal root ganglion, which contains cell bodies of the root's ascending sensory fibers.

Upon exiting the intervertebral foramen, the spinal nerve splits into a ventral and a dorsal ramus. The ventral ramus eventually becomes part of the lumbosacral plexus, which provides motor and sensory innervation to the iliopsoas, gluteals, and muscles and skin of the lower extremity. The ventral ramus also sends off two other important branches, a grey rami communicantes, which connects the ventral ramus to the sympathetic trunk, and the sinuvertebral nerve, which reenters via an intervertebral foramen and innervates the anterior dura mater, posterior longitudinal ligament, as well as posterior aspects of the intervertebral disk and the vertebral body. A dorsal ramus typically subdivides into three branches: medial, intermediate, and lateral. The lateral branch of the lumbar dorsal ramus innervates the skin and the underlying iliocostalis muscle (12, 13). The intermediate branch innervates the lumbar portion of the longissimus muscle (14, 15). The medial branch nerve innervates the multifidi, facet joints, and supra-/interspinous ligaments (16). (Fig. 2)

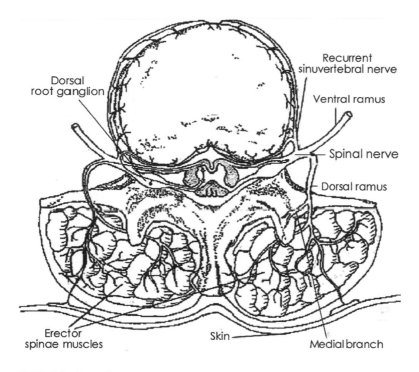

Dorsal
root ganglion

Recurrent
sinuvertebral nerve

Ventral ramus

Spinal nerve

Dorsal ramus

Erector
spinae muscles

Skin

Medial branch

FIGURE 2 Normal neuroanatomy of the lumbar spine.

The innervation of the intervertebral disk and the vertebral body periosteum is anatomically more complex. In a nonpathological state, only the outer third of the annulus fibrosus carries sensory nerve endings (17). The posterior aspect of the annulus and the adjacent periosteum are innervated by the posterior nerve plexus derived from the sinuvertebral nerves. The anterior nerve plexus formed by the two sympathetic trunks innervates the anterior annulus/periosteal complex (18). Both of these plexi are also connected by a lateral nerve plexus, formed by the branches of grey rami communicantes, and innervate the lateral portion of the intervertebral disk and the vertebral body (19). Recent research has also suggested that at least some of the sensory innervation of the lower lumbar disks is controlled in a multisegmental fashion by the more proximal dorsal root ganglions, which receive their afferent input via the ascending sympathetic trunks (20). This can explain why an L5/S1 disk protrusion can symptomatically present with an ipsilateral groin pain referral pattern.

Pathological Anatomy of the Lumbar Spine

Entrapment Neuropathy

Entrapment of nerve tissue at the spinal level can be subdivided into paraspinal, extraforaminal, intraforaminal, subarticular, or lateral recess and central types. The putative pathophysiologic mechanisms of mechanical entrapment include microvascular ischemia, venous congestion, and possible demyelinating or axonal injury of the nerves involved. The subsequent inflammatory cascade with the additional secretion of inflammatory neuropeptides from degenerated disks and facet joints can lead to sensitization and lowering of the pain threshold of the nerves and dorsal root ganglia involved. In addition, the nervi nervorum constitute the intrinsic innervation of nerve sheaths. There is evidence in animal models that even when the mechanical or chemical irritation is insufficient to sensitize the large nerve trunk, it can be sufficient to cause alteration in the sensitivities of the nervi nervorum and result in an entrapment neuropathy and the development of NP along that segment (21, 22).

Paraspinal entrapment, a less-recognized clinical entity, has been suggested and reported in several studies and case reports. One large cadaveric study found a relatively frequent, age-related occurrence of an ossified mamillo-accessory ligament leading study authors to consider the possibility of entrapment neuropathy involving the medial branch of the dorsal ramus, which passes underneath this ligament (11). Lumbar nerve root compression by a combination of an intertransverse ligament and a vertebral osteophyte has been reported in one case as well.

As a result, extraforaminal entrapment neuropathy of the exiting spinal nerve may be caused not only by major mechanical derangement of the lumbar spinal anatomy, including far lateral intervertebral disk protrusions (herniations), facet joint cysts, and hypertrophic facet joints, but also by more subtle degenerative changes that may affect the nervi nervorum (Fig. 3). Likewise, various branches of the spinal nerve such as the ventral and dorsal rami, the grey ramus communicans, and the sinuvertebral nerve can be potentially entrapped by the outer intraforaminal ligaments (23).

An intraforaminal entrapment neuropathy can affect both the exiting spinal nerve and the dorsal root ganglion and is caused by the pathological narrowing of the involved neuroforamen. Common causes of this type of entrapment include facet joint pathology, intraforaminal disk protrusion, vertebral osteophytes, intraforaminal ligaments, severe degenerative disk disease, and a high-level spondylolisthesis leading to clinically significant loss in vertical and anteroposterior neuroforaminal dimensions, respectively.

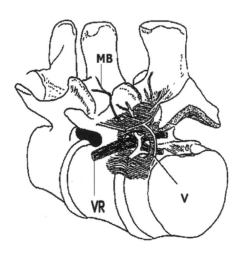

FIGURE 3 Illustration of the fascial planes through which the VR and MB of the dorsal ramus must pass in the extraforaminal space of the lumbar spine. *Abbreviations*: V, vein; VR, ventral ramus; MB, medial branch.

Structural narrowing of the subarticular or lateral recesses (lateral recess entrapment neuropathy) can involve the exiting spinal nerve, a descending spinal nerve that exits at the level below, a combination of both, or a sinuvertebral nerve. This can be caused by a far lateral disk protrusion, a large diffuse disk bulge, facet joint or ligamentum flavum hypertrophy, facet joint cyst, spondylolisthesis, Tarlov cyst, or a combination of these.

Depending on the level of a central entrapment neuropathy, the nerve tissue of the conus medullaris, which is the distal part of the spinal cord terminating at the L2 vertebral level, or the nerve roots of the cauda equina can be affected. The most common central entrapment neuropathy is of the degenerative type, which clinically presents as neurogenic claudication or spinal stenosis. A combination of hypertrophic facet joints, thickening of the ligamentum flavum, and degenerative protrusion of the intervertebral disk most commonly causes this structural entrapment. Other possible etiologies are higher grades of spondylolisthesis, congenital narrowing of the central canal, epidural lipomatosis as well as the more ominous causes including neoplasm, spinal abscess, or hematoma.

Another possible and controversial cause of entrapment neuropathy is iatrogenic in nature and could be due to postlaminectomy or postdiscectomy epidural scar formation leading to potential entrapment of sensory nerve tissues that occupy the central spinal canal. One study showed direct association of radicular pain incidence and the amount of such postoperative fibrosis (24).

Neuropathic Discogenic Pain

In a normal intervertebral disk, only the outer portion of the annulus fibrosis receives sensory innervation. Histochemical studies of the degenerated disks have shown extensive nerve fiber ingrowth into the middle third and even the inner third of the diseased annulus (25). The nociceptive properties of at least some of these nerves have been suggested by the presence of substance P, vasoactive intestinal peptide, calcitonin gene–related protein immunoreactivity (26, 27). A combination of the inflammatory neuropeptides present within the degenerated disk together with abnormal mechanical pressure loads experienced by an incompetent annulus can lead to both chemical and mechanical sensitization and stimulation of these thin unmyelinated nerve fibers.

Neuropathic ischemic pain microvascular insufficiency has been implicated as one of the putative mechanisms in the development of peripheral neuropathic states such as diabetic neuropathy. Cadaveric evidence also suggests strong association between aorto-spinal arterial atherosclerosis and history of chronic LBP with degenerative disk disease (28). It is plausible that local tissue ischemia can lead to pathological changes of the spinal neural elements leading to aberrant sensory transmission of nociceptive and nonnociceptive stimuli.

The Facilitated Segment

Peripheral Nervous System

The neuroanatomy of nociception can be organized into three distinct but connected domains: the peripheral sensory apparatus, the spinal cord, and the brain. Starting in the periphery, small fiber sensory axons that respond to various types of noxious input are referred to as nociceptors. There are two main nerve types that carry pain and temperature information from cutaneous structures, the small, high-threshold unmyelinated C fibers, and the larger, thinly myelinated, A-delta fibers. Similar sensory afferents are found in muscle; however, in muscle, both thinly myelinated and unmyelinated fiber types (groups III and IV) convey a dull aching sensation when activated in contrast to skin nociceptors. In addition to nociceptors responding to mechanical pain and temperature input, the release of chemical substances in damaged tissue such as protons, histamine, bradykinin, serotonin, vasoactive polypeptide, and a whole array of others can also lead to nociceptor sensitization (6).

Spinal Cord

The sensory nerves from the periphery enter via the dorsal root ganglion and synapse primarily in laminas I–IV of the dorsal horn gray matter, with laminas I and II receiving the bulk of the nociceptive input from the skin, and laminas IV and V from muscle. It is in laminas IV and V that wide dynamic range (WDR) second-order neurons reside. Unlike second-order neurons in laminas I and II that have an on-off response to sensory input, the WDR neurons have a graded response to sensory input. Under pathological conditions, windup can occur in the second-order WDR neurons found in laminas IV and V, and low-frequency input can lead to high-frequency output. This heightened firing pattern of WDR neurons in the CNS is believed to be one of the factors involved with chronic pain (29). Another unique feature of WDR second-order neurons is that there is convergence of sensory information from the afferents of skin, muscle, viscera, tendons, and joints (30). This opens the door to understanding how persistent afferent drive from one damaged structure or sensitized nerve in the segment, for example, a facet joint or an entrapped medial branch nerve as it passes through scarred or shortened fascia and ligaments, can cause neuroplastic changes in a WDR neuron that also receives input from the skin and muscle in that segment. The presence of a facilitated WDR neuron, fueled by the afferent drive of an underlying joint injury or subtle nerve entrapment, can then help to explain the common clinical finding in such cases where minimal sensory stimulation of skin (allodynia or hyperalgesia) or muscle (myofascial irritability) in the region of the facet can produce an exaggerated pain response, even when there has been no direct injury to that tissue.

Chronic Pain

Current research suggests that chronic pain may be the result of pathological neuroplastic changes of the peripheral and CNS. Changes in intracellular signal transduction, gene expression, receptor and ion channel density, and depolarization thresholds contribute to a peripheral sensitization and central windup phenomenon in the pain pathway. In addition, chronic damage, irritation, or facilitation of a sensory neuron at any point, even at the level of the dorsal horn, can lead to the retrograde release of neurotransmitters such as substance P and calcitonin gene–related peptide into peripheral tissue such as skin and muscle. In theory, this "neurogenic inflammation" can cause a cascade of chemical releases by mast cells, endothelium, and so on that inappropriately signal tissue "damage" or "inflammation," which, in turn, can act in a feed forward manner to increase the peripheral and central facilitation of the sensory terminal (6). Positive symptoms can then result not only from changes in the injured primary sensory neurons but also in segmentally related, noninjured tissues affecting multiple structures in that segmental level. Eventually, this facilitation can spread the longer such abnormalities persist, leading to transynaptic changes in neurons at multiple segments and levels of the CNS, causing more widespread pain (31).

Clinical Causes of Neuropathic LBP

NP of Muscle Origin

Myofascial pain syndrome (MPS) is a common, yet often underrecognized, presenting cause of chronic LBP. The pain associated with MPS is thought to be due to the firing of both low-threshold group III and high-threshold group IV muscle nociceptive afferents (30). These nociceptors are believed to be activated by pH changes in the muscle due to transient ischemia (32). This theory, however, does not explain why many individuals without pain also have taut muscle bands, called latent trigger points, which would fit criteria for MPS except that they lack pain at rest. One explanation is that the pain associated with an active trigger point depends on segmental central sensitization at the level of the spinal cord, which can lead to both pain at rest and abnormal muscle irritability (33). Recent work at NIH using an in vivo microdialysis technique suggests that the discomfort felt with active myofascial trigger points is due to release of neuropeptides into the muscle by the muscle nociceptors, so called neurogenic inflammation (34). In the absence of direct trauma to the muscle, the best explanation for the presence of neurogenic inflammation in the muscle would be the presence of a facilitated segment, where the primary lesion is in a segmentally related structure such as a facet, disk, or related nerve entrapment.

Annular Tears

Annular tears are the most common cause of axial discogenic pain, and in cases of extensive fissuring involving the outer disk perimeter, a frequent cause of radicular symptoms. These tears are either traumatic or degenerative in nature and, in a significant number of patients, can undergo spontaneous resolution after about 24 to 30 weeks. In the minority of patients, however, these tears do not resolve and progress to a state of chronic degenerative disk disease. Pathological evidence shows abnormal presence of granulation tissue, thickly innervated with nociceptive nerve fibers, which can extend from the nucleus to the outer periphery of the degenerated disk potentially leading to the development of chronic axial LBP (27). Annular tears may also lead to the leakage of a multitude of inflammatory mediators (e.g., phospholipase A2 and interleukins) from the center of the involved disks into the epidural space with the subsequent induction of an inflammatory response around the exiting adjacent spinal nerve roots causing NP (35). Signs of nerve dysfunction include positive sciatic dural tension signs (slump test or straight leg raising test), reflex changes along with minor numbness, and weakness along the dermatomal territory of the affected nerve. Given that there is no mechanical spinal irritation of the nerve, profound weakness or bladder and bowel dysfunction are extremely rare.

Disk Prolapse

Disk prolapse results from central nuclear material herniation through a disrupted posterior annulus into the epidural space. Depending on the size, position, and the number of levels involved, there may be single or multiple compressed spinal roots producing symptoms of LBP and lumbar radiculopathy, the latter typically carrying a higher level of discomfort. Significant central disk herniations can produce myelopathy by direct compression of the spinal cord if above L2, or bladder, bowel, and sexual dysfunction (and a saddle anesthesia) by compression of the cauda equina and should be emergently evaluated. A less common foraminal disk extrusion involves the extrusion of disk material laterally, into the neural foramen, causing compression of the residing dorsal root ganglion. Clinically, this presents with mostly leg pain that is exacerbated with standing and lumbar extension.

Spinal Stenosis

The normal lumbar canal diameter is >12 mm in the AP plane and >77 mm^2 in cross-sectional area. When there is a 50% reduction in cross-sectional area in animal models, motor and sensory deficits are produced. A diameter of <10 mm represents absolute stenosis (36). Spinal canal stenosis may be congenital but is most commonly of the acquired variety that is secondary to a variety of age-related factors, including progressive degenerative changes. Congenitally short pedicles are associated with the development of the acquired form of spinal stenosis earlier in life. Spondylolisthesis, postsurgical scarring, and Tarlov's cysts are less common causes of acquired spinal stenosis (37). The mechanism of pain is thought to be due to neurogenic claudication by mechanical irritation, followed by vascular ischemia and venous congestion of the nerves as they traverse the narrowed canal. Patients suffering from spinal stenosis classically can present with normal neurological examination and with bilateral or unilateral leg pain occurring upon ambulation or with prolonged standing.

Foraminal Stenosis

Foraminal stenosis is the narrowing of one or more neural foramina in the spine. Symptoms may be associated with axial or sciatic type back pain, particularly with prolonged standing or walking due to relative decrease in the foraminal diameter upon assumption of an upright posture as explained by intrinsic neuroforaminal biomechanics. NP arises from nerve root irritation with referral to the buttocks or leg. Facet joint arthritis, osteophytosis, degenerative disk disease with loss of disk height, and spondylolisthesis are all associated features of this not uncommon source of back and leg pain. The patient can present with either radicular or neurogenic claudication on clinical examination.

Spondylolisthesis

This is found most commonly in the lumbar spine and occurs when one vertebra slips anteriorly (more common) or posteriorly relative to the other vertebrae. By convention, the behavior of the more cephalad one relative to its subjacent neighbor guides the description of this malalignment and is usually due to a defect in the pars interarticularis. Other causes include degenerative, congenital (dysplastic), pathological, or posttraumatic types. There are five grades described on the basis of percent of vertebral slippage: grade I: <25% displacement of vertebral body; grade II: 25% to 50% displacement of vertebral body; grade III: 50% to 75% displacement of vertebral body; grade IV: 75% to 100% displacement of vertebral body; grade V: spondyloptosis or a complete vertebral anterior dislocation (38). Such vertebral slippage can lead to a combination of either central, lateral recess or foraminal stenosis with subsequent clinical presentation of neurogenic claudi-cation or a radicular pattern of pain. Presence of spondylolisthesis, especially if the involved segment exhibits abnormal mobility on flexion–extension imaging, can lead to early onset of degenerative disk disease as well.

Spondylolysis

Spondylolysis, or a defect in the pars interarticularis, is thought to result from a combination of "weak" or poorly mineralized bone and repetitive normal trauma of bipedal ambulation or participation in various athletic activities during child-hood and the adolescent growth spurt. Predisposing familial conditions for spondylolysis include Marfan syndrome, osteogenesis imperfecta, osteopenia, spina bifida occulta, scoliosis, Scheuermann disease, and other inherited condi-tions. Often participation in sports such as gymnastics, weight lifting, wrestling, and/or football at an early age with repetitive exposure to rotation, flexion–extension, and hyperextension can cause fracture of the pars interarticularis. Free nerve endings believed to play a role in nociception have been isolated from the pars interarticularis defects of symptomatic adults (39). Presence of spondyloly-sis can lead, in a significant number of cases, to the development of spondylolis-thesis. Patients with spondylolysis without spondylolisthesis typically present with axial LBP exaggerated with extension maneuvers.

Lumbar Facet Arthropathy

Lumbar facet arthropathy describes osteoarthritis of the lumbar apophyseal syn-ovial joints and is virtually universal after age 60 years. Pain can be related to potential osteophytic irritation of the nervi nervorum of the medial branch nerves, capsular distension, inflammatory synovitis, entrapment of synovial villi between two articular processes, or actual nerve root impingement by osteo-phytes. Pain is centered in the hips, buttocks, or thighs, but at times can extend below the knees and is typically aggravated by hyperextension (40, 41). Facet arthropathy may be associated and contribute to synovial cysts, degenerative disk disease, central canal stenosis, and foraminal stenosis.

Epidural Adhesions

Epidural adhesions and arachnoiditis can develop following spinal surgery and infections of the meninges, leading to adhesions that form around the lumbar spinal nerve roots, causing chronic irritation and sciatica. There is no correlation between the extent of surgery and the amount or density of adhesions formed. Ionic, water-based contrast agents used for antecedent myelography are asso-ciated with adhesions. The most common presentation is that of chronic LBP and radicular or nonradicular leg pain, which may simulate spinal stenosis and polyneuropathy.

Piriformis Syndrome

Piriformis syndrome is a commonly underdiagnosed cause of buttock pain and scixatica caused by the compression and irritation of the sciatic nerve by the pir-iformis muscle.

The piriformis muscle originates at the sides of the sacral bone and inserts onto the posterior part of the greater trochanter of the femur. It externally rotates the leg with the leg straight, and abducts the hip with the hip bent at 90 degrees.

The sciatic nerve was traditionally felt to pass through the piriformis muscle in 10% of the population with possible compression and irritation of the sciatic nerve due to contraction and shortening of the muscle. With recent advances in MRI neurography, our understanding the piriformis muscle leading to nondiscogenic causes of sciatica may have to be amplified. In a recent study of 239 consecutive patients who presented with sciatica but had normal or nondiagnostic lumbar MRIs, MR neurography and interventional MR imaging led to a final rediagnosis of piriformis syndrome in 67.8% of the patients. The diagnostic efficacy of MR neurography revealed that piriformis muscle asymmetry and sciatic nerve hyperintensity at the sciatic notch exhibited a 93% specificity and 64% sensitivity in distinguishing patients with piriformis syndrome from those without who had similar symptoms ($p < 0.01$) (42).

Referred Pain

Referred pain can come from pathology in structures other than disks and nerves such as the zygapophysial joints, sacroiliac joints, hip joint and muscles, spinal paravertebral muscles, and spinal ligaments. Referred pain often presents as deep buttock or leg ache, sometimes with mild tingling, but rarely with any of the other sensory or motor signs of nerve dysfunction such as numbness, allodynia (pain due to a stimulus that does not normally provoke pain, such as light touch), hyperalgesia (an increased response to a stimulus that is normally painful such as pinprick or hot sensation), or weakness. It occurs because the nerve supply to the area of reference and that of the culprit pain generator share embryological origins.

TREATMENT

Treatment should focus on treating the whole person and not just the pain problem. The goal should be to optimize the patient's chances of making a functional recovery in rehabilitation by improving exercise tolerance, mood, and sleep, with the use of invasive and other nonpharmacological therapies as appropriate (43) (Table 2). In general, when the pain is chronic, a biobehavioral approach is essential; and cognitive–behavioral treatments should be viewed as important complements to the various treatments listed (44). Medications play an essential role in the treatment of neuropathic LBP, and the following principles should be applied:

1. Minimize side effects
2. Minimize medications that could cause dependency issues
3. Avoid cognitive impairment
4. Avoid organ toxicity
5. Use of rational polypharmacy, when appropriate, directed at different components of the pain presentation

While a number of drugs and complementary treatments may decrease NP symptoms in some patients, the FDA has only formally approved five medications for the treatment of NP (Table 3).

Given the similarities in the pathophysiology of the above diagnoses, the indications have been extrapolated, and as a result, neuropathic back pain is often treated using the above medications or a combination thereof. It is

TABLE 2 Common Nonpharmacological Treatment Options

Condition	Treatment options	Comments
Annular tears, disk prolapse, spondylolisthesis, and epidural adhesions		Treatment would vary depending on presence or absence of radicular symptoms
	Spine exercises	Directional preference
	Thermal modalities	
	Epidural steroid injection	Transforaminal and interlaminar
	Chemonucleolysis	Used in Europe
	Intradiscal electrothermy	Poor evidence
	Percutaneous nucleoplasty	Poor evidence
	Spinal cord stimulation	
	Acupuncture/TENS therapy	For associated muscle spasm
	Spine surgery	
Spinal stenosis and foraminal stenosis		
	Spine exercises	Flexion preference
	Thermal modalities	
	Epidural steroid injections	Transforaminal and interlaminar
	Acupuncture/TENS therapy	For associated muscle spasm
	Spine surgery	
Facet arthropathy, segmental rigidity		
	Spine exercises	Directional preference
	Thermal modalities	
	Facet joint injections	If synovial cyst present, percutaneous aspiration and steroid injection is indicated
	Radiofrequency ablation	If medial branch blocks successful
	Transforaminal epidural	If suspect nerve root impingement or irritation
	Joint manipulation	
	Acupuncture/TENS therapy	For associated muscle spasm
	Spine surgery	
Epidural adhesions, failed back syndrome		
	Transforaminal epidural	
	Lysis of adhesions	Transforaminal and caudal approach
	Spinal cord stimulation	
Vertebral compression fractures		
	Vertebroplasty	
	Thermal modalities	
Piriformis syndrome and myofascial pain		
	Stretching and strengthening program	
	Thermal modalities	

TABLE 2   (Continued)

Condition	Treatment options	Comments
	Trigger point injections	
	Botulinum injections	
	Transforaminal epidural	If segmental facilitation is suspected
	Facet or sacroiliac joint manipulation or injection	If underlying joint dysfunction is suspected
	Acupuncture/TENS therapy	
Sacroiliac joint dysfunction	Stabilization exercises	
	Joint manipulation	
	Joint injection	

Abbreviation: TENS, transcutaneous electrical nerve stimulation.
Source: From Ref. 43.

important to note, however, that there is little comparative literature, which makes broad statements about one drug being superior to another difficult.

In 2007, Dworkin et al. (45) explored the evidence base of analgesics in the management of NP. Their first-line recommendations included the five medications mentioned in Table 3, but also included serotonin–norepinephrine reuptake inhibitor antidepressant venlafaxine, tramadol, and opioids (Table 4). Other medications that are frequently used but have minimal supportive evidence include non-steroidal antiinflammatory medications and selective serotonin reuptake inhibitors (46, 47). In general, the numbers needed to treat for both tricyclic antidepressants and anticonvulsants are between 2.5 and 5 (47, 48).

When choosing medications, familiarity with both the type of NP and the basic mechanisms of action of the various drug choices can provide some structure to treatment (49). For example, better medication selection can be made if one can, within reason, use clinical findings and history to distinguish whether an individual has one or a combination of the following:

1. Sensitized peripheral nociceptor (the presence of hyperalgesia)
2. Altered central processing of pain or the windup phenomenon (summation of sensory input)
3. Loss of descending pain modulation and loss of inhibitory neurons in the dorsal horn with C-fiber dropout and phenotypic switching of A-beta fibers (allodynia, segmental widening of pain, and/or bilateral findings)
4. Altered sympathetic activation (trophedema, temperature changes)

TABLE 3   Food and Drug Agency Approved Neuropathic Medications

Generic name	Trade name	Original indication	Date of approval
Carbamazepine	Tegretol	Trigeminal neuralgia	
Gabapentin	Neurontin	Postherpetic neuralgia	2002
Transdermal lidocaine	Lidoderm	Postherpetic neuralgia	
Duloxetine	Cymbalta	Diabetic neuropathy	2004
Pregabalin	Lyrica	Diabetic neuropathy and postherpetic neuralgia	2004

TABLE 4   Dworkin et al. Recommendations for Treatment of Neuropathic Pain

First line	Second line	Others
Nortriptyline, desipramine	Opioids and tramadol	Other anticonvulsants
Gabapentin, pregabalin		Other antidepressants
Opioids + tramadol		Capsaicin
Topical lidocaine patch		α_2-agonists
Duloxetine, venlafaxine		

Source: From Ref. 45.

    With this approach, a patient with signs and symptoms suggestive of NP that fit into category 1 above may respond better to a topical lidocaine patch, mexiletine, or an anticonvulsant with known sodium channel blocking properties, such as topiramate or lamotrigine, rather than gabapentin. Individuals with NP that fits into category 3 may respond better to antidepressants and may have little or no response to a topical patch. In general, most patients will manifest with some combination of the four classes, and so rational polypharmacy often makes sense. Table 5 lists the medications available for the treatment of neuropathic LBP in light of Dworkin's recommendations. As mentioned above, of those listed, only the tricyclic antidepressants, selective serotonin and norepinephrine reuptake inhibitors, gabapentin, pregabalin, tramadol, topical lidocaine 5%, and opioids have strong support in the literature for effectiveness (45). The others listed have the promise of potential benefit with either case reports or a single, randomized control trial to support their use (8,48).

Opioid Medications in the Treatment of Neuropathic LBP

As recently as 1995, opioid analgesics were not recommended in the treatment of NP for three reasons: (*i*) a common belief that NP did not respond well to opioids, (*ii*) that opioids had a high potential for abuse, and (*iii*) a general lack of consensus data on their efficacy (50–52). In more recent years, there has been an emergence of studies that dispel our previously held beliefs (53). In addition to the growing body of medical literature on opioid use for chronic pain, the addictions literature is also studying this phenomenon. We argue that physicians must be fluent in both bodies of literature in order to treat the "whole" patient, rather than simply the patient's physical pain. The physician is responsible for treating the pain while taking every precaution to prevent opioid addiction.

    To date, the most commonly used opioid with the most research backing its usage is methadone (54–57). However, given the unique properties of methadone including its variably long half-life (6–150 hours), the risk for cardiac toxicity, especially when combined with other agents that can influence NP such as TCAs, physicians must proceed very carefully when prescribing this medication (54,58). Gilron (2005) showed that morphine and gabapentin work better in combination than individually in treating NP (59). In a study comparing opioids and tricyclic antidepressants in postherpetic neuralgia, Raja et al. found that both medications were more effective than placebo and that different patients responded differently to the medications (60). Unfortunately, we have no data to help us understand the long-term effects of opioids on chronic pain. Most studies reported opioid results for patients receiving them for a short duration of time, ranging from four to eight weeks (53). This lack of long-term data is especially concerning in the case of opioid pain management as there is some concern that

TABLE 5 Drug Treatment of Neuropathic Low Back Pain

Drug	Starting dose	Dose range	Usual dose schedule	Major drug classifications and drug specific characteristics and issues
First line				
Antidepressants				
TCAs				Prolonged QT interval, urinary retention, sedation
Nortriptyline	10 mg	10–150 mg	Once in the evening	Moderate adverse effects
Desipramine	10 mg	10–150 mg	Once in the evening	Fewer adverse effects
Selective serotonin norepinephrine reuptake inhibitors				
Venlafaxine	37.5 mg	150–375 mg	Once or twice daily	
Duloxetine	20 mg	40–60 mg	Once or twice daily	
Anticonvulsants				
Carbamazepine	200 mg	1000–1600 mg	Twice daily	Highly protein bound, liver metabolism (adverse effects: aplastic anemia, hepatic)
Gabapentin	100 mg	1800–3600 mg	Three or four times	<3% protein bound, not metabolized (adverse effects: cognitive)
Pregabalin	150 mg	150–600 mg	Two or three times	Dizziness, somnolence, dry mouth
Topical medication				
Lidocaine 5% patch		Up to 3 patches	12 hr	Potentiates cardiac toxicity from mexiletine
Opioids				
Opioids	5–10 mg	30–188 mg	Varies	Somnolence, constipation, mood alterations, risk of tolerance, and dose escalation
Tramadol	50 mg	50–100 mg	Every 4–6 hr	Not to exceed 400 mg/day
Second line				
Opioids	5–10 mg	30–188 mg	Varies	Somnolence, constipation, mood alterations, risk of tolerance, and dose escalation
Tramadol	50 mg	50–100 mg	Every 4–6 hr	Not to exceed 400 mg/day
Third line (others)				
Antidepressants				
Amitriptyline	10 mg	10–150 mg	Once in the evening	More adverse effects
Anticonvulsants				

Medication	Starting dose	Dose range	Frequency	Comments / adverse effects
Oxcarbazepine	300 mg	1200–2400 mg	Twice daily	Moderately protein bound, liver metabolism (adverse effects: leukopenia, thrombocytopenia)
Valproic Acid	250 mg	500–1000 mg	Twice daily	Adverse effects: hepatic failure, thrombocytopenia, pancreatitis
Phenytoin	100 mg	300–500 mg	Once daily	Adverse effects: gum hypertrophy, osteomalacia, lymphadenopathy, hepatotoxicity, blood dyscrasias
Lamotrigine	25 mg	200–600 mg	Once or twice daily	Moderate protein bound, liver metabolism (adverse effects: Stevens–Johnson syndrome, paresthesias)
Topiramate	25 mg	100–800 mg	Once or twice daily	17% protein bound minimal liver metabolism (adverse effects: cognitive, renal stones, glaucoma)
Levetiracetam	250 mg	1000–3000 mg	Once or twice daily	<10% protein bound, minimal liver metabolism (adverse effects: cognitive)
Tiagabine	2 mg	4–56 mg	Two to four times daily	
Clonazepam	0.5 mg	1.5–20 mg	One to three times daily	Adverse effects: cognitive, blood dyscrasias
Antiarrhythmic				
Mexiletine	150 mg	300–1200 mg	Twice daily	Adverse effects: gastrointestinal, hepatic, arrhythmia
α_2-agonist				
Clonidine	0.1 mg	0.3–2.4 mg	One to three times daily	Hepatic
Tizanidine	2 mg	8–36 mg	One to three times daily	Hepatic
Topical medication				
Capsaicin 0.075%		Up to three patches	Three times daily	Rash
Doxepin 5%		Up to three patches	Three times daily	Potential systemic side effects similar to TCAs

Abbreviation: TCAs, tricyclic antidepressants.

prolonged use can, in some cases, lead to a worsening of pain due to tolerance and opioid-induced hyperalgesia (61, 62).

When prescribing opioids for pain, physicians must take extra steps to ensure patient compliance and minimize patient misuse and/or abuse of the substance. This has been detailed at length elsewhere and the reader is encouraged to read the listed references (63–66).

Nonpharmacological Approaches

We have discussed the various pharmacological treatments available to patients suffering from chronic neuropathic back pain. To date, there are no conclusive studies that strongly support a particular nonpharmacological treatment definitively for NP. Yet, there is a growing body of research on two types of treatment: extension-based exercise and acupuncture. As with most treatments of chronic pain conditions, these modalities are likely most effective when combined with appropriate medications and, when appropriate, cognitive and behavioral strategies.

Extension-based exercise, also known as the McKenzie approach, emphasizes patient education regarding posture and self-treatment. The treatment is based upon pain-relieving movements. The goal of the McKenzie approach is to cause centralization of the NP (67). In terms of neuropathic LBP, the goal of McKenzie approach is to have progressive regression of radiating leg pain to the point that the source is solely in the low back. Petersen (2002) studied subacute LBP using the McKenzie approach and found that there is a strong tendency for reduction in low back and leg pain at two months (68). Physicians should note that the McKenzie approach may also be applicable to discogenic pain.

Acupuncture is another complementary treatment that physicians may prescribe to patients. The literature on acupuncture is scarce when it comes to NP. However, as mentioned in the *Clinical Guidelines* published by the American Pain Society and the American College of Physicians, there was a moderate net benefit to this modality for the treatment of chronic LBP, which, as we have discussed above, may have neuropathic features (69).

CONCLUSIONS

The treatment of LBP can be challenging in part because of the lack of a clear theory about the causes, especially when the pain has become chronic. Although biobehavioral and rehabilitation-based therapies are important, in many cases, patients fail to make progress because of unremitting, functionally limiting pain. Based on the discussion above, we hope that clinicians will become more aware that NP is often present in LBP; and early assessment and institution of appropriate treatment could prevent the devastation of severe, persistent NP.

REFERENCES

1. Atlas SJ, Deyo RA. Evaluating and managing acute low back pain in the primary care setting. J Gen Intern Med 2001; 16(2):120–131.
2. Jensen MC, Brantzawadzki MN, Obuchowski N, et al. Magnetic resonance imaging of the lumbar spine in people without back pain. N Engl J Med 1994; 331(2):69–73.
3. Parisien RC, Ball PA. William Jason Mixter (1880–1958). Ushering in the "dynasty of the disc." Spine 1998; 23(21):2363–2366.
4. Merskey H, Bogduk N. Classification of Chronic Pain. Seattle, WA: IASP Press, 1994.

5. Backonja M-M. Defining neuropathic pain. Anesth Analg 2003; 97(3):785–790.
6. Woolf CJ, Costigan M. Transcriptional and posttranslational plasticity and the generation of inflammatory pain. Proc Natl Acad Sci U S A 1999; 96(14):7723–7730.
7. Bennett GJ. Neuropathic pain: a crisis of definition? Anesth Analg 2003; 97(3):619–620.
8. Mendell JR, Sahenk Z. Painful sensory neuropathy. N Engl J Med 2003; 348(13):1243–1255.
9. Park HK, Rudrappa S, Dujovny M, et al. Intervertebral foraminal ligaments of the lumbar spine: anatomy and biomechanics. Childs Nerv Syst 2001; 17(4–5):275–282.
10. Hirsch C, Lewin T. Lumbosacral synovial joints in flexion–extension. Acta Orthop Scand 1968; 39(3):303–311.
11. Maigne JY, Maigne R, Guerinsurville H. The lumbar mamillo-accessory foramen—a study of 203 lumbosacral spines. Surg Radiol Anat 1991; 13(1):29–32.
12. Johnston HM. The cutaneous branches of the posterior primary divisions of the spinal nerves, and their distribution in the skin. J Anat Physiol 1908; 43:80–91.
13. Maigne JY, Lazareth JP, Guerin Surville H, et al. The lateral cutaneous branches of the dorsal rami of the thoraco-lumbar junction. An anatomical study on 37 dissections. Surg Radiol Anat 1989; 11(4):289–293.
14. Bogduk N, Wilson AS, Tynan W. The human lumbar dorsal rami. J Anat 1982; 134(Mar):383–397.
15. Bradley KC. Anatomy of backache. Aus N Z J Surg 1974; 44(3):227–232.
16. Bogduk N. The nerve supply to the human lumbar vertebral column. 2. The dorsal rami. J Anat 1981; 132(Mar):316.
17. Malinsky J. The ontogenetic development of nerve terminations in the intervertebral discs of man. (Histology of intervertebral discs, 11th communication). Acta Anat (Basel) 1959; 38:96–113.
18. Groen GJ, Baljet B, Drukker J. Nerves and nerve plexuses of the human vertebral column. Am J Anat 1990; 188(3):282–296.
19. Bogduk N. Clinical Anatomy of the Lumbar Spine and Sacrum, 3rd ed. New York: Churchill Livingstone, 1997.
20. Ohtori S, Takahashi Y, Takahashi K, et al. Sensory innervation of the dorsal portion of the lumbar intervertebral disc in rats. Spine 1999; 24(22):2295–2299.
21. Bove GM, Light AR. The nervi nervorum—missing link for neuropathic pain? Pain Forum 1997; 6(3):181–190.
22. Sauer SK, Bove GM, Averbeck B, et al. Rat peripheral nerve components release calcitonin gene-related peptide and prostaglandin E-2 in response to noxious stimuli: evidence that nervi nervorum are nociceptors. Neuroscience 1999; 92(1):319–325.
23. Amonookuofi HS, Elbadawi MG, Fatani JA. Ligaments associated with lumbar intervertebral foramina.1. L1 to L4. J Anat 1988; 156:177–183.
24. Ross JS, Robertson JT, Frederickson RCA,et al. Association between peridural scar and recurrent radicular pain after lumbar discectomy: magnetic resonance evaluation. Neurosurgery 1996; 38(4):855–861.
25. Freemont AJ, Peacock TE, Goupille P, et al. Nerve ingrowth into diseased intervertebral disc in chronic back pain. Lancet 1997; 350(9072):178–181.
26. Coppes MH, Marani E, Thomeer R, et al. Innervation of "painful" lumbar discs. Spine 1997; 22(20):2342–2349.
27. Peng B,, Wu W,, Hou S,,et al. The pathogenesis of discogenic low back pain. J Bone Joint Surg Br 2005; 87B(1):62–67.
28. Kauppila LI. Prevalence of stenotic changes in arteries supplying the lumbar spine. A postmortem angiographic study on 140 subjects. Ann Rheum Dis 1997; 56(10):591–595.
29. Woolf CJ, Salter MW. Neuroscience—neuronal plasticity: increasing the gain in pain. Science 2000; 288(5472):1765–1768.
30. Graven-Nielsen T, Mense S. The peripheral apparatus of muscle pain: evidence from animal and human studies. Clin J Pain 2001; 17(1):2–10.
31. Woolf CJ. Dissecting out mechanisms responsible for peripheral neuropathic pain: implications for diagnosis and therapy. Life Sci 2004; 74(21):2605–2610.

32. Hong CZ, Simons DG. Pathophysiologic and electrophysiologic mechanisms of myofascial trigger points. Arch Phy Med Rehabil 1998; 79(7):863–872.
33. Audette JF, Wang F, Smith H. Bilateral activation of motor unit potentials with unilateral needle stimulation of active myofascial trigger points. Am J Phy Med Rehabil 2004; 83(5):368–374.
34. Shah JP, Phillips T, Danoff JV, et al. An in vivo microanalytical technique for measuring the local biochemical milieu of human skeletal muscle. J Appl Physiol 2005; 99(5):1977–1984.
35. Omarker K, Myers RR. Pathogenesis of sciatic pain: role of herniated nucleus pulposus and deformation of spinal nerve root and dorsal root ganglion. Pain 1998; 78(2):99–105.
36. Arnoldi CC, Brodsky AE, Cauchoix J, et al. Lumbar spinal stenosis and nerve root entrapment syndromes—definition and classification. Clin Orthop Relat Res 1976; (115):4–5.
37. Kirkaldy-Willis WH, Paine KWE, Cauchoix J, et al. Lumbar spinal stenosis. Clin Orthop Relat Res 1974; (99):30–50.
38. Wiltse LL, Newman PH, Macnab I. Classification of spondylolysis and spondylolisthesis. Clin Orthop Relat Res 1976; (117):23–29.
39. Schneiderman GA, McLain RF, Hambley MF, et al. The pars defect as a pain source—a histologic-study. Spine 1995; 20(16):1761–1764.
40. Dreyer SJ, Dreyfuss PH. Low back pain and the zygapophysial (facet) joints. Arch Phys Med Rehabil 1996; 77(3):290–300.
41. Fukui S, Ohseto K, Shiotani M, et al. Distribution of referred pain from the lumbar zygapophyseal joints and dorsal rami. Clin J Pain 1997; 13(4):303–307.
42. Beatty RA. Piriformis syndrome. J Neurosurg Spine 2006; 5(1):101–101.
43. Nachemson AL, Jonsson E. Neck and Back Pain: The Scientific Evidence of Causes, Diagnosis, and Treatment. Philadelphia, PA: Lippincott Williams & Wilkins, 2000:1–495.
44. Turk DC. Cognitive–behavioral approach to the treatment of chronic pain patients. Reg Anesth Pain Med 2003; 28(6):573–579.
45. Dworkin RH, O'Connor AB, Backonja M, et al. Pharmacologic management of neuropathic pain: evidence-based recommendations. Pain 2007; 132(3):237–251.
46. Staiger TO, Gaster B, Sullivan MD, et al. Systematic review of antidepressants in the treatment of chronic low back pain. Spine 2003; 28(22):2540–2545.
47. Collins SL, Moore RA, McQuay HJ, et al. Antidepressants and anticonvulsants for diabetic neuropathy and postherpetic neuralgia: a quantitative systematic review. J Pain Symptom Manage 2000; 20(6):449–458.
48. McQuay HJ, Tramer M, Nye BA, et al. Systematic review of antidepressants in neuropathic pain. Pain 1996; 68(2–3):217–227.
49. Dworkin RH, Backonja M, Rowbotham MC, et al. Advances in neuropathic pain—diagnosis, mechanisms, and treatment recommendations. Arch Neurol 2003; 60(11):1524–1534.
50. Arner S, Meyerson BA. Lack of analgesic effect of opioids on neuropathic and idiopathic forms of pain. Pain 1988; 33(1):11–23.
51. Davies HTO, Crombie IK, Lonsdale M, et al. Consensus and contention in the treatment of chronic nerve-damage pain. Pain 1991; 47(2):191–196.
52. Clark CM, Lee DA. Prevention and treatment of the complications of diabetes-mellitus. N Engl J Med 1995; 332(18):1210–1217.
53. Eisenberg E, McNicol ED, Carr DB. Efficacy and safety of opioid agonists in the treatment of neuropathic pain of nonmalignant origin—systematic review and meta-analysis of randomized controlled trials. JAMA 2005; 293(24):3043–3052.
54. Fishman SM, Wilsey B, Mahajan G, et al. Methadone reincarnated: novel clinical applications with related concerns. Pain Med 2002; 3(4):339–348.
55. Gagnon B, Almahrezi A, Schreier G. Methadone in the treatment of neuropathic pain. Pain Res Manag 2003; 8(3):149–154.
56. Altier N, Dion D, Boulanger A, et al. Management of chronic neuropathic pain with methadone: a review of 13 cases. Clin J Pain 2005; 21(4):364–369.

57. Morley JS, Bridson J, Nash TP, et al. Low-dose methadone has an analgesic effect in neuropathic pain: a double-blind randomized controlled crossover trial. Palliat Med 2003; 17(7):576–587.
58. Pearson EC, Woosley RL. QT prolongation and torsades de pointes among methadone users: reports to the FDA spontaneous reporting system. Pharmacoepidemiol Drug Saf 2005; 14(11):747–753.
59. Gilron I, Weaver DF. Morphine, gabapentin, or their combination for neuropathic pain—the authors reply. N Engl J Med 2005; 352(25):2651–2651.
60. Raja SN, Haythornthwaite JA, Pappagallo M, et al. Opioids versus antidepressants in postherpetic neuralgia—a randomized, placebo-controlled trial. Neurology 2002; 59(7):1015–1021.
61. Chang G, Chen L, Mao JR. Opioid tolerance and hyperalgesia. Med Clin North Am 2007; 91(2):199–211.
62. Cohen SP, Christo PJ, Wang S, et al. The effect of opioid dose and treatment duration on the perception of a painful standardized clinical stimulus. Reg Anesth Pain Med 2008; 33(3):199–206.
63. Katz NP, Adams EH, Benneyan JC, et al. Foundations of opioid risk management. Clin J Pain 2007; 23(2):103–118.
64. Katz NP, Sherburne S, Beach M, et al. Behavioral monitoring and urine toxicology testing in patients receiving long-term opioid therapy. Anesth Analg 2003; 97(4):1097–1102.
65. Passik SD, Kirsh KL, Whitcomb L, et al. A new tool to assess and document pain outcomes in chronic pain patients receiving opioid therapy. Clin Ther 2004; 26(4):552–561.
66. Fishman SM, Kreis PG. The opioid contract. Clin J Pain 2002; 18(4):S70–S75.
67. Donelson R, Aprill C, Medcalf R, et al. A prospective study of centralization of lumbar and referred pain—a predictor of symptomatic discs and anular competence. Spine 1997; 22(10):1115–1122.
68. Petersen T, Kryger P, Ekdahl C, et al. The effect of McKenzie therapy as compared with that of intensive strengthening training for the treatment of patients with subacute or chronic low back pain—a randomized controlled trial. Spine 2002; 27(16):1702–1708.
69. Chou R, Huffman LH. Nonpharmacologic therapies for acute and chronic low back pain: a review of the evidence for an American pain Society/American college of physicians clinical practice guideline. Ann Intern Med 2007; 147(7):492–504.

15 Interstitial Cystitis

Neel Shah
UMDNJ New Jersey Medical School, Newark, New Jersey, U.S.A.

Hossein Sadeghi-Nejad
UMDNJ New Jersey Medical School, Newark; Hackensack University Medical Center, Hackensack; and VA NJ Health Care System, East Orange, New Jersey, U.S.A.

Robert Moldwin
Pelvic Pain Center, The Arthur Smith Institute for Urology; Long Island Jewish Medical Center, New Hyde Park, New York, U.S.A.

THE DISORDER

Interstitial cystitis (IC) is a chronic bladder disorder typified by irritative voiding symptoms, bladder-based pelvic pain/discomfort, and no readily identifiable cause such as urinary tract infection or bladder cancer. Symptoms are chronic and often debilitating. IC is a condition that can be seen in all age groups, although it usually strikes patients in their 20s to 40s, their most otherwise productive years. From its first description in 1808 by Philip Syng Physick, to Hunner's description of the "elusive ulcer" in 1914, to today's current research, the cause of IC remains unknown. Once thought to be a rare condition largely restricted to females, recent studies suggest over 1 million afflicted individuals in the United States with a female-to-male ratio of 5:1 (1). The larger number of male IC patients being diagnosed may relate to its overlap with prostatitis syndromes (2).

Classification

IC may be divided into ulcerative (or "classical") and nonulcerative (or "nonclassical") forms. The ulcerative form of IC accounts for less than 10% of patients (3). Erythematous regions, or what have been termed "Hunner's ulcers or patches," can be seen upon routine cystoscopic examination. Histopathology of these regions usually demonstrates a panmural infiltrate of chronic and acute inflammatory cells. The vast majority of IC patients have nonulcerative disease, essentially presenting with bladder-based symptoms, negative urine studies, and a negative cystoscopic examination.

The term "interstitial cystitis" implies an interstitial inflammatory infiltrate, a finding that is not identified in most patients. As such, calls for a change in IC nomenclature have arisen over the past several years. The International Continence Society suggested using the term "painful bladder syndrome" to denote a syndrome where pain is perceived to be derived from the bladder irrespective of inflammatory events (4). The European Society for the Study of Interstitial Cystitis recently recommended that the term IC be replaced by "bladder pain syndrome" (5). According to the European Society for the Study of Interstitial

Cystitis, the name of IC/bladder pain syndrome should be reserved only for patients with typical cystoscopic findings (see "Other Diagnostic Tests" section). Regardless of the evolving nomenclature, as mentioned above, IC is often divided into Hunner's ulcer (classic) and nonulcer disease. This subdivision may be clinically significant, as differences have been noted in the age distribution, clinical presentation, histopathology, and response to treatment modalities (6, 7).

DIAGNOSIS

The National Institute of Diabetes and Digestive and Kidney Diseases developed criteria for the diagnosis of IC in 1987 and 1988 (8). These criteria were established for research purposes and typically identified patients with moderate to severe symptoms. Unfortunately, many clinicians used these criteria in their clinical practices and likely missed the diagnosis of IC in an estimated 60% of cases (9).

In clinical practice today, the diagnosis of IC is largely made on the basis of the correct clinical presentation and the lack of any other definable pathology that might cause those symptoms. Patients may present with symptoms that have been present for years, having seen multiple clinicians without receiving any diagnosis to account for their condition. Many have been treated with various medications including anticholinergic agents, antibiotics, or analgesics with little success. Patients usually present with the symptom cluster of urinary frequency, urgency, and pelvic pain/discomfort. Patient descriptions or voiding diaries usually demonstrate low-volume, frequent voids with accompanying nocturia. Patients usually describe that their frequency is very much dependent upon the mounting pelvic discomfort or frank pain that occurs with bladder filling. Urgency, a term that is frequently linked to the overactive bladder patient, is usually described by the IC patient as the mounting need to use bathroom facilities, not for fear of urine loss, but to relieve the pelvic pain.

Dyspareunia in the female IC patient is common either as a consequence of impact against the anterior vaginal wall (in the region of the bladder) or on the basis of comorbid conditions such as vulvodynia or pelvic floor muscle spasm. Most IC patients will report a premenstrual flare in symptoms, but many experience a decline in urinary symptoms during their menstrual flow (10).

In addition, a sexual, gynecological, psychological, and gastrointestinal history should be elicited. Other disorders such as endometriosis, irritable bowel syndrome, overactive bladder, recurrent urinary tract infections, prostatitis, or malignancy may have overlapping symptoms with IC (11). In conjunction with the history, symptom surveys such as the Pelvic Pain and Urgency/Frequency Symptom Scale and the O'Leary–Sant Symptom and Problem Index may help monitor symptoms during therapy. The physical exam should include a thorough pelvic examination in women and a digital rectal examination in men. Physical examination is usually unrevealing, but bladder tenderness as assessed through the anterior vaginal wall is often identified. Careful attention on physical examination should be structured to exclude other disease states, that is, vaginitis, urethral diverticulum, pelvic floor muscle spasm, and urinary retention. A urinalysis and urine culture is mandatory to exclude other urological disease. Although hematuria is often identified in the classical form of IC, this finding mandates a more aggressive urological evaluation for other diseases, that is, renal stones, urological tumors. A urine specimen may be sent for cytological analysis when deemed clinically appropriate, such as in smokers or patients over 40 years of age. Urine may be assessed for acid-fast bacilli if sterile pyuria is documented. Radiographic imaging is performed based upon the clinician's discretion.

Other Diagnostic Tests

Once the clinical features have been identified and no other pathology has been found, a diagnosis of IC can be made. Other diagnostic tests, none of which can "make" the diagnosis alone, can be employed particularly in cases where the diagnosis is still questioned. Office cystoscopy may be useful to exclude other diseases of the bladder, such as cancer, bladder stones, or the presence of Hunner's ulcer disease (12).

Cystoscopy with bladder hydrodistention has been the "gold standard" in the diagnosis of IC. This procedure is typically performed under anesthesia. Cystoscopic examination is then performed with the irrigant entering the bladder at a final high pressure of 80 cm H_2O. The irrigant is subsequently released and the volume is measured to determine the "anesthetic bladder capacity." This typically varies between 800 and 1200 cc in non-IC patients, but most IC patients will have a lower capacity. Additionally, the release of the irrigant is usually followed by the production of glomerulations, small submucosal hemorrhages that are typically seen through the bladder wall. While cystoscopy with hydrodistention is identified as part of the National Institute of Diabetes and Digestive and Kidney Diseases diagnostic criteria, it is not considered mandatory to diagnose IC. Bladder hydrodistention has certain limitations as a diagnostic test. Glomerulations have been noted in asymptomatic women undergoing tubal ligation (13). Conversely, patients with symptoms of IC may have initial negative findings at the time of bladder hydrodistention (14). In younger women with a clinical diagnosis of IC, three of the four women who had normal findings at the time of the initial hydrodistention were noted on subsequent procedures to have findings consistent with IC.

A provocative, office-based maneuver that may aid in the diagnosis of IC is the potassium sensitivity test (15). As noted in "Pathophysiology" section, IC patients are believed to have an alteration of their bladder surface mucin, leading to increased mucosal permeability. The basis of this test is that in the IC patient, potassium ions introduced into the bladder will be absorbed into the underlying bladder wall and stimulate nerves (C-fibers and A-delta fibers), thereby increasing symptoms. Some speculate that this response is simply due to potassium's contact with the urothelial nerve–like surface. Nevertheless, the sensitivity and specificity of the procedure approach 70% and 60%, respectively (16). False-positive results may occur with cystitis, while false-negative responses may occur if the patient has had prior therapy (11). The relatively low sensitivity and specificity, as well as the often significant discomfort to the patient, may limit the value of this test.

Another approach to evaluation of the bladder as a "pain generator" is to apply an anesthetic directly into the bladder, in much the same fashion as the clinician might perform a diagnostic nerve block. Identification of a decline in symptoms with this "intravesical anesthetic challenge" suggests the bladder as a source of pain. Additionally, a reduction in symptoms implies that various intravesical anesthetic solutions may be used therapeutically. Solutions employed have usually consisted of either alkalinized lidocaine or lidocaine–bupivacaine combinations (17, 18).

Urinary Markers

Of the potential urinary markers, antiproliferative factor (APF) holds the most promise. APF is a sialoglycopeptide found in the bladder urine, not renal pelvic urine, of patients with IC and has been shown to inhibit bladder epithelial cell proliferation (19). APF induces normal, cultured bladder epithelial cells to have increased permeability and changes in cell adhesion (20). In comparing multiple urine markers for IC, Erickson et al. reported that APF was significantly elevated in the IC group and, most consistently, separated the IC patients from the control group (21). When compared to a control group, APF activity was significantly more in IC patients, with both a sensitivity and a specificity greater than 90% (22). In one study of 100 males, men with IC had significantly more APF activity compared to asymptomatic men or those with chronic prostatitis (23).

PATHOPHYSIOLOGY

Theories of pathogenesis abound for this enigmatic condition. As IC symptoms often overlap with bacterial cystitis, investigators have explored the role of chronic infection as a causative factor. Studies have attempted to isolate bacteria, fungi, or viruses without consistent results (24). A recent study found an incidence of 46% of positive PCR for bacterial ribosomal RNA gene, yet no difference was found between IC patients and controls (25). More recently, Al-Hadithi et al. examined bladder biopsies from both IC patients and controls, looking for the presence of bacterial or viral DNA sequences using PCR (26). In 92 patients with IC, there was no evidence of the persistence of bacterial or viral DNA in the bladder.

Traditionally, the bladder urothelium has been viewed as a static and passive barrier whose role was to limit entry of toxins into the suburothelial space. However, recent data suggest that the urothelial surface may have neurosecretory properties with the presence of receptors attributed to neurons, such as purinoreceptors (P2X), and ability to release neurotransmitters such as adenosine triphosphate (ATP) and nitric oxide (NO) (27, 28). ATP, acting at the P2X receptors, is implicated in bladder sensation and pain in both normal and abnormal bladder function (29, 30). Given that IC is a hypersensory condition, it would be expected that there is an upregulation of this pathway. Studies have demonstrated higher ATP levels in urine samples of patients with IC compared to controls and an increased expression of P2X receptors (27,31).

Another factor that may play a role in IC pathogenesis includes neural inflammation/upregulation. This theory was based on observations that patients with IC were found to have an increase in nerves in bladder submucosal tissue with accompanying perineuritis (32). In the normal response to bacteria or toxins, there is a local recruitment of defenses allowing the bladder to clear the insult. However, in IC, this can become maladaptive. In patients with IC, certain gene products, such as nerve growth factor (NGF), are upregulated and elevated (33). Elevated NGF may be responsible for the continued hyperalgesia, even after the original inciting agent is removed (33). With continued organ insult, bladder afferent nerve fibers can become sensitized, that is, hyper-excitable. Urothelial mechanosensitive A-gamma and C-fibers respond to distension and code for urgency and bladder contraction (29). As the bladder begins to distend in IC, these sensitized nerve fibers discharge at lower bladder volumes, leading to lower cystometric bladder values and increased urgency (29). In chronic visceral disorders, sensitization may not only be limited to afferent neurons. Second-order neurons in the spinal cord and supraspinal neurons can have altered excitability that can also contribute to the continued pain (29,34). Moreover, rat and mice studies suggest that there may be a neural convergence between afferent inputs of the colon and bladder, possibly explaining why patients with IC may complain of irritable bowel syndrome, and vice versa (35).

One of the most popularized theories of IC pathogenesis is a defect of the bladder's mucosal lining (36). Normally, the bladder is highly impermeable to urine and its constituents based upon its complex histology and the bladder mucin that lines its surface. The bladder surface mucin is composed of proteoglycans and glycoproteins and is often referred to as the glycosaminoglycan or "GAG" layer. Compared to controls, patients with IC had absorbed significantly more urea after bladder instillation of concentrated urea (15). Studies have also shown that patients with IC have decreased urinary GAG excretion and bladder biopsies revealing disrupted GAG arrangement (37). Absorption of various urinary constituents such as potassium and urea in the face of bladder surface mucin abnormalities has been speculated to cause nerve stimulation and other downstream inflammatory events. Further support for this theory is that administration of pentosan polysulfate sodium (PPS), a synthetic compound similar to GAG, often alleviates patients' symptoms (38).

TREATMENT

General Management Strategies
Although symptom remission is possible, IC is a chronic and often debilitating condition that is not truly "curable." Prior to initiation of therapy, the physician should set realistic goals of symptom improvement for the patient and align them with the patient's expectations. Management should begin with conservative measures and proceed to more aggressive therapies as clinically indicated. There is no "set" protocol for the treatment of IC and patients may benefit from a single agent or multimodal therapy. The benefit, limitations, and side effects of the treatment regimen should be explained, fostering a more productive therapeutic relationship between the physician and the patient.

Conservative Therapy
Prior to initiating medical therapy, patients with IC may benefit first from modification of risk factors. One modifiable risk factor is diet. In a survey of 104 IC patients, 90% of patients responded that certain foods exacerbated their bladder symptoms (39). Caffeine, alcohol, citrus fruits, artificial sweeteners, and hot peppers were the most commonly reported items. Data from the Boston Area Community Health Survey demonstrate the relationship of medications, as well as both medical and psychosocial problems, with symptoms of IC (40, 41). In men, only depression was associated with painful bladder symptoms. In women, depression, history of urinary tract infections, chronic yeast infections, hysterectomy, and certain medications such as calcium channel blockers and cardiac

glycosides were associated with painful bladder symptoms (41). In addition, patients with a history of abuse and stress were more likely to experience painful bladder symptoms (40). These results suggest that a multidisciplinary approach combining medical and psychological treatment may be necessary.

Medical Therapies

Pentosan Polysulfate Sodium

PPS is the only oral agent approved in the United States for the treatment of IC. PPS is a heparin sulfate analog, one of the GAGs normally found on the bladder surface. PPS presumably improves IC symptoms by enhancement of an abnormal and permeable bladder surface; however, the amount of drug that reaches the urine appears to be quite low (42). Another theory of PPS clinical activity is its potential role in inhibiting mast cell function (43). The usual dosage of PPS is 100 mg three times daily. In a meta-analysis, PPS was more efficacious than placebo in terms of pain, urgency, and frequency (44). In a double-blind, randomized study, Nickel et al. compared 300 mg of PPS to higher dosages of 600 and 900 mg (45). Although symptom scores improved at all dose ranges, this effect related to duration of treatment as opposed to the dose. Fifty percent of patients responded at 32 weeks. Despite favorable studies, Sant et al. conducted a prospective, randomized study comparing PPS and hydroxyzine to placebo (46). In this study, neither agent compared to placebo achieved a statistically significant outcome. However, this study was felt to be "underpowered" due to poor patient accrual. Adverse effects are typically mild and include reversible alopecia, diarrhea, nausea, headache, and rash.

Amitriptyline

Amitriptyline is a tricyclic antidepressant that has been reported to ameliorate IC symptoms. Its mechanism of action includes blockade of acetylcholine receptors and H_1-histaminergic receptors, inhibition of reuptake of released serotonin and norepinephrine, and mast cell stabilization. The usual starting dose is 10 to 25 mg and can be titrated to 75 to 100 mg. In a double-blind, prospective, placebo-controlled study, 48 patients with IC were treated with amitriptyline (47). After four months of treatment and with initial dosage of 25 mg with escalation to a maximum of 100 mg, there was a significant improvement in mean symptom score, urgency, and pain. In a subsequent long-term study, 94 patients were treated with a mean dose of 55 mg of amitriptyline for a 20-month period (48). The response rate was 64%, with an overall 46% good/excellent patient satisfaction. However, there was a 31% dropout rate attributed to side effects. These are usually anticholinergic in nature and may include weight gain, fatigue, palpitations, constipation, urinary retention, dry mouth, and decrease in libido. The dose should be titrated slowly to balance symptom reduction with adverse effects. If a patient is on amitriptyline for psychiatric purposes, it is important to titrate the medication in conjunction with the psychiatrist.

Hydroxyzine

Hydroxyzine is a histamine H_1 receptor antagonist. It can inhibit neuronal activation of mast cells and suppress mast cell degranulation. Typically, dosing starts at 25 mg at bedtime and can be increased to 75 mg as tolerated. In an initial series, a 40% reduction in symptoms scores was noted (49). In addition, patients with concurrent migraines, irritable bowel syndrome, or allergies, noted a decrease in these symptoms. A prospective study, comparing PPS or hydroxyzine versus placebo, did not show a significant effect of this agent (46). However, this was an underpowered study with poor patient accrual.

Cimetidine
Cimetidine, an H2 antagonist, has been shown to have a therapeutic effect in IC patients (50). In a 36-patient placebo-controlled study, those receiving cimetidine had a significantly improved suprapubic pain and decreased nocturia compared to placebo (51). The dose for cimetidine is typically 600 mg daily in divided doses.

Gabapentin
Initially used as an anticonvulsant, gabapentin also has been efficacious in treating neuropathic pain conditions such as diabetic neuropathy and postherpetic neuralgia. Although its mechanism is unclear, gabapentin may have an antinociceptive effect by modulating calcium channels, enhancing endogenous opioid release, and having activity at the N-methyl-D-aspartate (NMDA) receptor (52). Initially, gabapentin is started at 100 mg daily and can be titrated to 3600 mg divided three times daily. Serum levels do not need to be monitored and a common side effect is drowsiness. Its efficacy in IC treatment is limited to small trials (53, 54).

Intravesical Agents/Options
Intravesical therapy has an expanding role in the management of IC. It can be used as primary therapy in IC for patients who would prefer treatment that targets the "source" directly. Intravesical treatment can act as bridging therapy during the interval before oral agents take effect. In combination with conservative therapies and types of intravesical agents, an enhanced therapeutic effect can be achieved. For patients who fail conservative therapy including oral medication, this represents another nonsurgical option.

Dimethylsulfoxide
Dimethylsulfoxide (DMSO) is an FDA-approved intravesical therapy for the treatment of IC. Its therapeutic benefit may be due to anti-inflammatory, analgesic, bacteriostatic, or muscle relaxant properties (55). The typical regimen is an initial dose of 50 mL weekly for six to eight weeks followed by maintenance doses of 50 mL every two weeks for up to 12 months. Upon the first few instillations, patients may experience a flare-up of pain and irritative voiding symptoms. This is expected and typically resolves after the third or fourth instillation. A 50% to 70% response rate has been reported in the literature (56). In clinical practice, a DMSO "cocktail" is usually used and is composed of agents that may each have a theoretical benefit to the patient. Other agents typically added to the DMSO include sodium bicarbonate, heparin sodium, a steroid (often hydrocortisone or triamcinolone), and an antibiotic. Anecdotal reports suggest better patient tolerance and clinical improvements with the "cocktail" (57).

Other Intravesical Therapies

Two neurotoxins, resiniferatoxin and capsaicin, have been employed as potential treatments for IC. Currently, there is no data supporting the use of capsaicin. In a meta-analysis, Mourtzoukou et al. concluded that, although well tolerated, the efficacy of resiniferatoxin still remains questionable (58). Clorpactin and silver nitrate are two other agents that have been used, but both are caustic. Caution is advised when administering these agents, as they can result in ureteral and bladder scarring. Intravesical bacillus Calmette-Guerin (BCG) has also been investigated as a potential treatment. After 34 weeks in a randomized, controlled trial, overall response rates to both BCG and placebo were low; and there was no statistically significant difference in response rate between the BCG and placebo groups (59).

Anesthetic Agents

As discussed earlier, intravesical anesthetic agents may have a role in diagnosis as well as a therapeutic benefit. In 2001, Henry et al. demonstrated that alkalized intravesical lidocaine is safely absorbed into the bladder at sufficient levels with accompanying decrease in acute pain scores in patients with IC (17). In 2005, Parsons et al. reported that an intravesical solution 40,000 U heparin, 1% lidocaine, and 8.4% sodium bicarbonate resulted in an immediate and durable decrease in pain and urgency of IC patients. The 1% lidocaine can be titrated to 2% in patients who did not respond initially (18). Nickel et al. performed a randomized, double-blind study in 2008 comparing effects of instilled lidocaine solution buffered with 8.4% sodium bicarbonate solution to placebo (60). After three days of instillation, there was a significant improvement in bladder symptoms in patients completing instillation of the lidocaine solution. These effects lasted beyond the treatment period without any evidence of lidocaine toxicity.

Botulinum Toxin

BoNT/A (botulinum toxin A) has been used for the treatment of a number of pain syndromes, bladder overactivity, and lower urinary tract dysfunction. It may have an antinociceptive effect on afferent neurotransmission and has been shown to reduce bladder levels of NGF (61). In 2008, Giannantoni et al. evaluated the one-year efficacy of a total of 200 U BoNT/A (10 U BoNT/A per site) injected at the trigone and lateral walls in patients with painful bladder symptoms and urinary frequency unresponsive to conventional treatments (62). A total of 15 patients were prospectively studied, with 13 reporting a subjective improvement of pain at one and three months follow-up and significantly decreased urinary frequency. At five months of follow-up, bladder pain returned in 11 patients, and at 1 year, bladder pain recurred in all patients. In addition, BoNT/A did result in impaired detrusor contractility in 9 of the 15 patients. Therefore, prior to this procedure, patients should be counseled on the possible need to perform clean intermittent catheterization postoperatively and demonstrate ability to perform this task. IC patients with urethral pain may not be candidates for this procedure. BoNT/A is not FDA approved for treatment of IC.

Surgical Options

For many patients who have failed conservative, oral, and intravesical treatment, surgical management may offer relief of IC symptoms. However, it must always be borne in mind that IC is a nonmalignant condition and temporary remission is possible. With this under consideration, a decision to proceed with surgical management must be made with great care and in tandem with the patient.

Hydrodistention

In addition to its diagnostic value, cystoscopy with hydrodistention has a therapeutic benefit. Following bladder distension, Ottem et al. reported 56% of patients experiencing symptom reduction for a mean duration of two months (63). Erickson et al. reported only a 30% reduction in symptom score in a minority of patients (64). Although the exact mechanism by which symptom improvement occurs is unknown, bladder distension may influence bladder sensory nerves and also have an anti-inflammatory effect. Hydrodistention is relatively safe. However, complications such as hematuria and bladder perforation can occur. If bladder perforation is noticed intraoperatively, it is usually managed conservatively with catheter drainage. Although very rare, a more serious complication is bladder necrosis (65, 66). Patients will present with severe, intractable abdominal pain and require surgical intervention. Since most patients derive no therapeutic benefit from the procedure and, when benefit occurs, it is usually short lived, hydrodistention is often reserved for patients who have failed other more conservative forms of care.

Sacral Neuromodulation

Sacral neuromodulation has been used successfully in the treatment of severe urge urinary incontinence, neurogenic detrusor hyperreflexia, and pelvic pain. Although the mechanism is not clearly defined, it is believed that both the afferent and efferent pathways are affected leading to improved bladder function. Twenty-five patients with refractory IC were prospectively evaluated with sacral nerve stimulation (67). Of these, 17 patients qualified for permanent sacral nerve stimulator implantation after these patients showed greater than 50% improvement in frequency, nocturia, voided volume, and average pain. At a mean follow-up of 14 months, these patients showed a significant improvement in mean voided volume, pain, nocturia, and frequency. Of note, there was a higher success rate for test stimulation using the quadripolar lead versus the unipolar lead. This may be due to decreased dislodgement and better stimulation of the S3 nerve root of the quadripolar lead. No infectious or mechanical complications were reported. At this time, IC is not an approved indication for sacral neuromodulation.

Transurethral Resection and Coagulation

Patients with focal inflammatory lesions of the bladder wall (Hunner's ulcers) may be amenable to endoscopic resection or fulguration of these lesions. These procedures are usually employed only when more conservative forms of care have failed. In a series of 103 patients with classic IC, 259 transurethral resections (TURs) of visible lesions were performed with 92 patients reporting improved symptoms (68). Of these patients, 40% had continued relief after three years and after three or more TUR procedures.

Laser ablation is a reasonable endourologic alternative to TUR. In 2001, Rofeim prospectively studied 24 patients with classic IC undergoing ablative Nd:YAG laser ablation of Hunner's lesions (69). After a period of 23 months, patients reported significant improvement in pain, nocturia, urgency scores, and mean voiding interval. However, 11 patients experienced relapse, requiring additional treatment. In addition, forward scatter of the laser can cause unrecognized thermal injury to bowel.

Role of Urinary Diversion

After failed conservative measures and continued disabling symptoms, reconstructive surgery should be contemplated. One technique employed is supratrigonal cystectomy with substitution enterocystoplasty. In this procedure the trigone, ureteral orifices, and bladder neck are retained, while the remaining diseased bladder is excised. This allows for preservation of the ureteral antireflux mechanism. The bladder is then enlarged, preferably with an ileocecal segment (70). Using criteria including relief of symptoms, stable renal function, and successful reconstruction, long-term success rates of substitution cystoplasty have ranged from 25% to 96% (71). Patient selection is vital for success. Poor results may occur in those with an increased preoperative bladder capacity under anesthesia (72). On the other hand, improved outcomes are seen in patients with classic IC compared to nonulcer disease (7,73). In addition, patients with a history of urethral pain may not be suitable candidates due to the possibility of postoperative urethral catheterization (70). A second option is subtrigonal cystectomy with substitution enteroplasty. In contrast to the supratrigonal approach, only a small remnant of bladder neck is retained and bilateral ureteral reimplantation is necessary. In a comparison between the two techniques, Linn et al. reported similar relief of symptoms in the two groups (74). However, there was an increased need for clean intermittent catheterization in patients who underwent subtrigonal cystectomy. A third technique is supravesical diversion. The urinary diversion can be noncontinent, that is, ileal conduit, or continent, that is, Kock pouch. The question to perform a cystectomy or leave the bladder in situ is debatable. Despite the removal of the bladder, patients still may experience pelvic pain (75). On the other hand, the defunctionalized, retained bladder can lead to chronic infections (76). A fourth technique is augmentation enterocystoplasty (AC). In 2005, Blaivas et al. reported failed AC in a subset of seven IC patients (77). Given this experience, the authors conclude that AC has no role in the surgical management of IC.

CONCLUSION

Although there are many viable theories, the pathogenesis of IC remains largely unknown. The diagnosis of IC remains challenging as many other disease processes have common presentations. While there are no effective curative agents, a number of well-tolerated therapies are available, which can contain and improve patient symptoms. With increasing awareness and prevalence of IC, continued basic and clinical research is needed to further our knowledge of IC.

REFERENCES

1. Clemens JQ, Link CL, Eggers PW, et al. Prevalence of painful bladder symptoms and effect on quality of life in black, Hispanic and white men and women. J Urol 2007; 177:1390–1394.

2. Forrest JB, Nickel JC, Moldwin RM. Chronic prostatitis/chronic pelvic pain syndrome and male interstitial cystitis: enigmas and opportunities. Urology 2007; 69: 60–63.

3. Simon LJ, Landis JR, Erickson DR, et al. The interstitial cystitis data base study: concepts and preliminary baseline descriptive statistics. Urology 1997; 49:64–75.

4. Abrams P, Cardozo L, Fall M, et al. The standardisation of terminology of lower urinary tract function: report from the Standardisation Sub-committee of the International Continence Society. Am J Obstet Gynecol 2002; 187:116–126.

5. van de Merwe JP, Nordling J, Bouchelouche P, et al. Diagnostic criteria, classification, and nomenclature for painful bladder syndrome/interstitial cystitis: an ESSIC proposal. Eur Urol 2008; 53:60–67.

6. Koziol JA, Adams HP, Frutos A. Discrimination between the ulcerous and the nonulcerous forms of interstitial cystitis by noninvasive findings. J Urol 1996; 155:87–90.

7. Peeker R, Fall M. Toward a precise definition of interstitial cystitis: further evidence of differences in classic and nonulcer disease. J Urol 2002; 167:2470–2472.

8. Gillenwater JY, Wein AJ. Summary of the National Institute of Arthritis, Diabetes, Digestive and Kidney Diseases Workshop on Interstitial Cystitis, National Institutes of Health, Bethesda, Maryland, August 28–29, 1987. J Urol 1988; 140:203–206.

9. Hanno PM, Landis JR, Matthews-Cook Y, et al. The diagnosis of interstitial cystitis revisited: lessons learned from the National Institutes of Health Interstitial Cystitis Database study. J Urol 1999; 161:553–557.

10. Powell-Boone T, Ness TJ, Cannon R, et al. Menstrual cycle affects bladder pain sensation in subjects with interstitial cystitis. J Urol 2005; 174:1832–1836.

11. Forrest JB, Moldwin R. Diagnostic options for early identification and management of interstitial cystitis/painful bladder syndrome. Int J Clin Pract 2008; 62:1926–1934.

12. Braunstein R, Shapiro E, Kaye J, et al. The role of cystoscopy in the diagnosis of Hunner's ulcer disease. J Urol 2008; 180:1383–1386.

13. Waxman JA, Sulak PJ, Kuehl TJ. Cystoscopic findings consistent with interstitial cystitis in normal women undergoing tubal ligation. J Urol 1998; 160:1663–1667.

14. Shear S, Mayer R. Development of glomerulations in younger women with interstitial cystitis. Urology 2006; 68:253–256.

15. Parsons CL, Zupkas P, Parsons JK. Intravesical potassium sensitivity in patients with interstitial cystitis and urethral syndrome. Urology 2001; 57:428–432; discussion 32–33.

16. Chambers GK, Fenster HN, Cripps S, et al. An assessment of the use of intravesical potassium in the diagnosis of interstitial cystitis. J Urol 1999; 162:699–701.

17. Henry R, Patterson L, Avery N, et al. Absorption of alkalized intravesical lidocaine in normal and inflamed bladders: a simple method for improving bladder anesthesia. J Urol 2001; 165:1900–1903.

18. Parsons CL. Successful downregulation of bladder sensory nerves with combination of heparin and alkalinized lidocaine in patients with interstitial cystitis. Urology 2005; 65:45–48.

19. Keay SK, Szekely Z, Conrads TP, et al. An antiproliferative factor from interstitial cystitis patients is a frizzled 8 protein-related sialoglycopeptide. Proc Natl Acad Sci U S A 2004; 101:11803–11808.

20. Zhang CO, Wang JY, Koch KR, et al. Regulation of tight junction proteins and bladder epithelial paracellular permeability by an antiproliferative factor from patients with interstitial cystitis. J Urol 2005; 174:2382–2387.

21. Erickson DR. Urine markers of interstitial cystitis. Urology 2001; 57:15–21.

22. Keay S, Zhang CO, Marvel R, et al. Antiproliferative factor, heparin-binding epidermal growth factor-like growth factor, and epidermal growth factor: sensitive and specific urine markers for interstitial cystitis. Urology 2001; 57:104.

23. Keay S, Zhang CO, Chai T, et al. Antiproliferative factor, heparin-binding epidermal growth factor-like growth factor, and epidermal growth factor in men with interstitial cystitis versus chronic pelvic pain syndrome. Urology 2004; 63:22–26.

24. Keay S, Schwalbe RS, Trifillis AL, et al. A prospective study of microorganisms in urine and bladder biopsies from interstitial cystitis patients and controls. Urology 1995; 45:223–229.
25. Heritz DM, Lacroix JM, Batra SD, et al. Detection of eubacteria in interstitial cystitis by 16S rDNA amplification. J Urol 1997; 158:2291–2295.
26. Al-Hadithi HN, Williams H, Hart CA, et al. Absence of bacterial and viral DNA in bladder biopsies from patients with interstitial cystitis/chronic pelvic pain syndrome. J Urol 2005; 174:151–154.
27. Tempest HV, Dixon AK, Turner WH, et al. P2X and P2X receptor expression in human bladder urothelium and changes in interstitial cystitis. BJU Int 2004; 93:1344–1348.
28. Sun Y, Chai TC. Up-regulation of P2×3 receptor during stretch of bladder urothelial cells from patients with interstitial cystitis. J Urol 2004; 171:448–452.
29. Nazif O, Teichman JM, Gebhart GF. Neural upregulation in interstitial cystitis. Urology 2007; 69:24–33.
30. Kumar V, Chapple CR, Surprenant AM, et al. Enhanced adenosine triphosphate release from the urothelium of patients with painful bladder syndrome: a possible pathophysiological explanation. J Urol 2007; 178:1533–1536.
31. Sun Y, Keay S, De Deyne PG, et al. Augmented stretch activated adenosine triphosphate release from bladder uroepithelial cells in patients with interstitial cystitis. J Urol 2001; 166:1951–1956.
32. Christmas TJ, Rode J, Chapple CR, et al. Nerve fibre proliferation in interstitial cystitis. Virchows Arch A Pathol Anat Histopathol 1990; 416:447–451.
33. Lowe EM, Anand P, Terenghi G, et al. Increased nerve growth factor levels in the urinary bladder of women with idiopathic sensory urgency and interstitial cystitis. Br J Urol 1997; 79:572–577.
34. Urban MO, Gebhart GF. Supraspinal contributions to hyperalgesia. Proc Natl Acad Sci U S A 1999; 96:7687–7692.
35. Malykhina AP, Qin C, Greenwood-van Meerveld B, et al. Hyperexcitability of convergent colon and bladder dorsal root ganglion neurons after colonic inflammation: mechanism for pelvic organ cross-talk. Neurogastroenterol Motil 2006; 18: 936–948.
36. Teichman JM, Moldwin R. The role of the bladder surface in interstitial cystitis/painful bladder syndrome. Can J Urol 2007; 14:3599–3607.
37. Hurst RE, Moldwin RM, Mulholland SG. Bladder defense molecules, urothelial differentiation, urinary biomarkers, and interstitial cystitis. Urology 2007; 69:17–23.
38. Parsons CL. Prostatitis, interstitial cystitis, chronic pelvic pain, and urethral syndrome share a common pathophysiology: lower urinary dysfunctional epithelium and potassium recycling. Urology 2003; 62:976–982.
39. Shorter B, Lesser M, Moldwin RM, et al. Effect of comestibles on symptoms of interstitial cystitis. J Urol 2007; 178:145–152.
40. Link CL, Pulliam SJ, Hanno PM, et al. Prevalence and psychosocial correlates of symptoms suggestive of painful bladder syndrome: results from the Boston area community health survey. J Urol 2008; 180:599–606.
41. Hall SA, Link CL, Pulliam SJ, et al. The relationship of common medical conditions and medication use with symptoms of painful bladder syndrome: results from the Boston area community health survey. J Urol 2008; 180:593–598.
42. Erickson DR, Sheykhnazari M, Bhavanandan VP. Molecular size affects urine excretion of pentosan polysulfate. J Urol 2006; 175:1143–1147.
43. Chiang G, Patra P, Letourneau R, et al. Pentosanpolysulfate (Elmiron) is a potent inhibitor of mast cell histamine secretion. Adv Exp Med Biol 2003; 539:713–729.
44. Hwang P, Auclair B, Beechinor D, et al. Efficacy of pentosan polysulfate in the treatment of interstitial cystitis: a meta-analysis. Urology 1997; 50:39–43.
45. Nickel JC, Barkin J, Forrest J, et al. Randomized, double-blind, dose-ranging study of pentosan polysulfate sodium for interstitial cystitis. Urology 2005; 65:654–658.
46. Sant GR, Propert KJ, Hanno PM, et al. A pilot clinical trial of oral pentosan polysulfate and oral hydroxyzine in patients with interstitial cystitis. J Urol 2003; 170: 810–815.

47. van Ophoven A, Pokupic S, Heinecke A, et al. A prospective, randomized, placebo controlled, double-blind study of amitriptyline for the treatment of interstitial cystitis. J Urol 2004; 172:533–536.
48. van Ophoven A, Hertle L. Long-term results of amitriptyline treatment for interstitial cystitis. J Urol 2005; 174:1837–1840.
49. Theoharides TC. Hydroxyzine in the treatment of interstitial cystitis. Urol Clin North Am 1994; 21:113–119.
50. Seshadri P, Emerson L, Morales A. Cimetidine in the treatment of interstitial cystitis. Urology 1994; 44:614–616.
51. Thilagarajah R, Witherow RO, Walker MM. Oral cimetidine gives effective symptom relief in painful bladder disease: a prospective, randomized, double-blind placebo-controlled trial. BJU Int 2001; 87:207–212.
52. Phatak S, Foster HE Jr. The management of interstitial cystitis: an update. Nat Clin Pract Urol 2006; 3:45–53.
53. Hansen HC. Interstitial cystitis and the potential role of gabapentin. South Med J 2000; 93:238–242.
54. Sasaki K, Smith CP, Chuang YC, et al. Oral gabapentin (neurontin) treatment of refractory genitourinary tract pain. Tech Urol 2001; 7:47–49.
55. Hohlbrugger G, Lentsch P, Pfaller K, et al. Permeability characteristics of the rat urinary bladder in experimental cystitis and after overdistension. Urol Int 1985; 40:211–216.
56. Sant GR, LaRock DR. Standard intravesical therapies for interstitial cystitis. Urol Clin North Am 1994; 21:73–83.
57. Ghoniem GM, McBride D, Sood OP, et al. Clinical experience with multiagent intravesical therapy in interstitial cystitis patients unresponsive to single-agent therapy. World J Urol 1993; 11:178–182.
58. Mourtzoukou EG, Iavazzo C, Falagas ME. Resiniferatoxin in the treatment of interstitial cystitis: a systematic review. Int Urogynecol J Pelvic Floor Dysfunct 2008; 19:1571–1576.
59. Mayer R, Propert KJ, Peters KM, et al. A randomized controlled trial of intravesical bacillus calmette-guerin for treatment refractory interstitial cystitis. J Urol 2005; 173:1186–1191.
60. Nickel JC, Moldwin R, Lee S, et al. Intravesical alkalinized lidocaine (PSD597) offers sustained relief from symptoms of interstitial cystitis and painful bladder syndrome. BJU Int 2009; 103:910–918.
61. Smith CP, Radziszewski P, Borkowski A, et al. Botulinum toxin a has antinociceptive effects in treating interstitial cystitis. Urology 2004; 64:871–875; discussion 5.
62. Giannantoni A, Porena M, Costantini E, et al. Botulinum A toxin intravesical injection in patients with painful bladder syndrome: 1-year followup. J Urol 2008; 179:1031–1034.
63. Ottem DP, Teichman JM. What is the value of cystoscopy with hydrodistension for interstitial cystitis? Urology 2005; 66:494–499.
64. Erickson DR, Kunselman AR, Bentley CM, et al. Changes in urine markers and symptoms after bladder distention for interstitial cystitis. J Urol 2007; 177:556–560.
65. Grossklaus DJ, Franke JJ. Vesical necrosis after hydrodistension of the urinary bladder in a patient with interstitial cystitis. BJU Int 2000; 86:140–141.
66. Zabihi N, Allee T, Maher MG, et al. Bladder necrosis following hydrodistention in patients with interstitial cystitis. J Urol 2007; 177:149–152; discussion 52.
67. Comiter CV. Sacral neuromodulation for the symptomatic treatment of refractory interstitial cystitis: a prospective study. J Urol 2003; 169:1369–1373.
68. Peeker R, Aldenborg F, Fall M. Complete transurethral resection of ulcers in classic interstitial cystitis. Int Urogynecol J Pelvic Floor Dysfunct 2000; 11:290–295.
69. Rofeim O, Hom D, Freid RM, et al. Use of the neodymium: YAG laser for interstitial cystitis: a prospective study. J Urol 2001; 166:134–136.
70. van Ophoven A, Oberpenning F, Hertle L. Long-term results of trigone-preserving orthotopic substitution enterocystoplasty for interstitial cystitis. J Urol 2002; 167:603–607.

71. Nielsen KK, Kromann-Andersen B, Steven K, et al. Failure of combined supratrigonal cystectomy and Mainz ileocecocystoplasty in intractable interstitial cystitis: is histology and mast cell count a reliable predictor for the outcome of surgery? J Urol 1990; 144:255–258; discussion 8–9.
72. Webster GD, Maggio MI. The management of chronic interstitial cystitis by substitution cystoplasty. J Urol 1989; 141:287–291.
73. Rossberger J, Fall M, Jonsson O, et al. Long-term results of reconstructive surgery in patients with bladder pain syndrome/interstitial cystitis: subtyping is imperative. Urology 2007; 70:638–642.
74. Linn JF, Hohenfellner M, Roth S, et al. Treatment of interstitial cystitis: comparison of subtrigonal and supratrigonal cystectomy combined with orthotopic bladder substitution. J Urol 1998; 159:774–778.
75. Baskin LS, Tanagho EA. Pelvic pain without pelvic organs. J Urol 1992; 147:683–686.
76. Adeyoju AB, Thornhill J, Lynch T, et al. The fate of the defunctioned bladder following supravesical urinary diversion. Br J Urol 1996; 78:80–83.
77. Blaivas JG, Weiss JP, Desai P, et al. Long-term followup of augmentation enterocystoplasty and continent diversion in patients with benign disease. J Urol 2005; 173:1631–1634.

Chronic Prostatitis/Chronic Pelvic Pain Syndrome—A Urologist's Perspective

Richard A. Watson

Touro University College of Medicine & Hackensack University Medical Center, Hackensack, New Jersey; and UMDNJ New Jersey Medical School, Newark, New Jersey, U.S.A.

Hossein Sadeghi-Nejad

UMDNJ New Jersey Medical School, Newark; Hackensack University Medical Center, Hackensack; and VA NJ Health Care System, East Orange, New Jersey, U.S.A.

THE DISORDER

Chronic prostatitis (CP) or chronic pelvic pain syndrome (CPPS), formerly known as prostatodynia, refers to any unexplained pelvic pain experienced in men. Often this pain is associated with irritative voiding symptoms and/or pain located in the groin, genitalia, or perineum in the absence of pyuria and bacteriuria.

The NIH describes four categories of prostatitis, as follows:

Type I—Acute bacterial prostatitis
Type II—Chronic bacterial prostatitis
Type III—Chronic abacterial prostatitis, that is, CPPS categorized as either type IIIa (inflammatory CPPS) or type IIIb (noninflammatory CPPS)
Type IV—Asymptomatic inflammatory prostatitis

Of these, CPPS comprises the category: "NIH prostatitis type III." No pus cells (WBC) or bacteria are seen on microscopic analysis of a clean-catch urine specimen. However, excess WBCs or bacteria may be seen on Gram stain and culture of expressed prostatic secretions (EPS).

A distinction is currently made between patients with excess WBCs in their prostatic secretions (chronic abacterial prostatitis, type IIIa) and those with normal prostatic secretions (chronic abacterial type IIIb). However, the clinical value of this distinction has been challenged, since the discriminating factor is merely the number of WBCs seen on a single smear of prostatic secretions. This number may vary widely within the same specimen and even more so from one sample to the next, even though the samples are taken from the same patient, without remedial intervention. Furthermore, asymptomatic controls, who are devoid of any evidence of pelvic pathology, have also been found to have a significant number of WBCs in their prostatic secretions. The subcategorization into types IIIa and IIIb does not have a major clinical impact as diagnosis and treatment options are not significantly altered (1).

DIAGNOSIS

The typical patient is a young- to middle-aged man who presents with a variable array of chronic, irritative, and/or obstructive voiding symptoms, accompanied by moderate to severe pain in the pelvis, lower back, perineum, and/or genitalia. Symptoms parallel those experienced by persons with chronic bacterial and nonbacterial prostatitis. (Refer to the sections in this text dealing specifically with those diagnoses for complete details.)

Sexual and/or ejaculatory dysfunction—most especially, pain upon or immediately following ejaculation, as well as premature ejaculation—is the symptom that initially brings many men to seek medical attention. The subject is difficult to discuss for many patients and may not be brought up in the interview at all unless directly addressed by the physician (1).

Chronic Prostatitis Symptom Index (NIH-CPSI): To facilitate history taking and to establish a more uniform standard, a U.S. National Institutes of Health (NIH) collaborative panel has proposed the NIH-CPSI. This index employs a series of nine questions that contain 21 items to assess pertinent history in a standardized and quantifiable format.

Pain symptoms (four questions): In the past week:

- Have you experienced any pain between your rectum and testicles, and/or in your testicles, and/or in the tip of your penis, and/or below your waist?
- Have you experienced pain or burning upon urination or pain or discomfort during or after sexual intercourse?
- How often have you had pain in any of the above areas over the last week?
- Which number (2–12) best describes your average pain or discomfort on the days that you had it?

Urinary symptoms (two questions): Over the past week, how often:

- Have you had the sensation of not emptying your bladder completely after you finished urinating?
- Have you had to urinate again less than two hours after you finished urinating?

Impact of symptoms (two questions): Over the past week, how much:

- Have your symptoms kept you from doing the kinds of things you would usually do?
- How much did you think about your symptoms?

Quality of life: If you were to spend the rest of your life with your symptoms just the way they have been during the last week, how would you feel about that?

Physical Findings

No physical finding is pathognomonic. Examination of the genitalia is usually normal, despite the fact that patients often complain of associated discomfort in the scrotal and perineal area. On occasion, palpable induration of the epididymis may be present.

Digital rectal examination may reveal a tight anal sphincter. When the anal sphincter tone is hyperactive, an underlying spastic neuropathy must be excluded. The hyperactivity may otherwise indicate an intrinsic hyperirritability of the pelvic floor musculature, which may be amenable to medical and biofeedback therapies.

The prostate and adjacent tissues may be moderately or severely tender, and the gland, itself, may be slightly congested or boggy. However, the presence of a small, relatively firm gland does not exclude the possibility of CP/CPPS. Extreme tenderness upon gentle palpation of the prostate should raise suspicion for acute bacterial prostatitis or even a prostatic abscess.

Further Diagnostic Testing

The foremost objective of the complete physical examination and further diagnostic testing is to exclude other diagnoses. The differential is formidable—prostate cancer, chronic urethritis/meatitis, granulomatous prostatitis, acute bacterial prostatitis and prostatic abscess or cyst, anal fissure, anorectal tumors, bladder cancer, carcinoma in situ of the urinary bladder, coccydynia, colovesical fistula, cystitis—bacterial, nonbacterial, and interstitial, fistula-in-ano, gonococcal infections and other sexually transmitted infections, hemorrhoids, inflammatory bowel disease, distal ureteral calculi, myofascial pain syndrome, seminal vesiculitis, Reiter's syndrome, tuberculosis of the genitourinary system, urethral cancer, urethral diverticulum, syringocoele (cystic dilatation of bulbourethral gland ducts), pelvic neuropathy—either primary or secondary, and urethral strictures. These many differential diagnoses—and this list is, by no means, complete—reveal the conundrum of diagnosing CPPS/CP. Because the diagnosis is one of exclusion, in theory, this diagnosis cannot be made until all of these alternatives have been definitively excluded. Demonstration of these specific clinical findings is often hampered by practical factors such as time, patience, and medical resources (1).

One example would be differentiating between CP/CPPS and interstitial cystitis in the male. A detailed review of the diagnosis of interstitial cystitis is presented thoroughly in the chapter on interstitial cystitis. The distinction between CP/CPPS and interstitial cystitis is particularly challenging in that both conditions are diagnoses of exclusion, that is, two separate "wastebasket" diagnoses. No diagnostic test can be used to definitively establish or to exclude the diagnosis of CP/CPPS or interstitial cystitis. In fact, there is at least the theoretical possibility that a given patient could actually have both conditions concurrently. Cystoscopy under anesthesia may include a bladder biopsy and possible bladder hydrodistension when there is a high index of suspicion to confirm the diagnosis (1,2).

The symptoms of interstitial cystitis closely parallel those of CP/CPPS (3). Most of the patients with interstitial cystitis, in one large series, were initially referred for urological evaluation with an initial diagnosis of CCPS/CP (54%) or of benign prostatic hyperplasia (23%). Their presenting symptom was most often only mild discomfort in the suprapubic area. However, their symptoms rapidly worsened; within less than three years, they had marked suprapubic pain, severe dysuria, and debilitating urinary frequency, during both daytime and nighttime. Sexual dysfunction was an issue for 60% of these men, with painful ejaculation being the most frequently expressed symptom. Low-back pain, perineal pain, and testicular pain were reported by 50% of these patients. Symptoms were so severe that total cystectomy was performed as a last resort in two of these patients (3).

The point at which the physician empirically recommends for a given patient with CP/CPPS, an empirical trial therapy specific for interstitial cystitis is based on the physician's judgment. For example, therapies such as pentosan sulfate (Elmiron) and intravesical instillations of dimethyl sulfoxide have yielded success in selected patients with CP/CPPS. (Details regarding the various interstitial cystitis therapies are beyond the scope of this article. For further information, turn to the chapter on interstitial cystitis.) The diagnostician should keep this diagnosis in mind when evaluating a patient with refractory CPPS/CP.

Similarly, other diagnoses also must be excluded. For another example, the distinction between chronic urethritis and CP/CPPS can prove problematic (4). Of the seven symptoms evaluated in the NIH-CPSI, three symptoms are common to both populations: penile pain, urinary frequency, and dysuria. The remaining four symptoms are typical of CP/CPPS alone: perineal pain, pain in the testicles, pain in the suprapubic area, and pain upon ejaculation. Conversely, urethral discharge was characteristic of nongonococcal urethritis (NGU) but was not specifically reported in cases of CP/CPPS. Urethral WBCs were identified in all patients with NGU and in 50% of those with CP/CPPS (4).

Most importantly, any risk of underlying cancer must be addressed thoroughly and up front. Transitional cell cancer and carcinoma in situ of the bladder are deadly masqueraders. Prostate cancer can also manifest as symptoms that suggest CP/CPPS. Neoplasms of the rectum and GI tract and rare tumors of other pelvic organs have first manifested as irritative prostatic symptoms. Benign prostatic hyperplasia and obstructive uropathy also manifest in this manner. All of these life-threatening diagnoses must be carefully considered when diagnosing CP/CPPS.

Older men who experience the symptoms of CP/CPPS for the first time may understandably be concerned that these symptoms represent underlying cancer of the bladder or prostate, but they may be reluctant to openly voice this anxiety. Ignoring these possibilities in patients with CP/CPPS may eventually prove to be a fatal mistake. However, to subject every patient to a physically and financially exhaustive gauntlet of tests and procedures is also clearly inappropriate. Tailoring the diagnostic workup to meet the needs of a specific patient is a skill that defies textbook codification. The art of medicine comes into play in deciding, together with the patient, which possibilities to pursue and how vigorously to pursue each of them.

Reassuring the patient about the nonmalignant nature of the pathology is critical when the work-up is complete and cancer has been excluded as a possible diagnosis (1).

Standard teaching has been that men with CP/CPPS have no increased risk of prostate cancer. However, a study from Case Western Reserve reveals that patients who underwent an initial prostate biopsy that was negative for cancer but positive for CP were at higher risk of subsequently developing cancer than were men who underwent prostate biopsy that was negative both for cancer and for prostatic inflammation (5). The researchers do not recommend any change in current recommendations, pending confirmatory studies. The recommendations for prostate cancer screening are currently undergoing close scrutiny; the CP/CPPS patients should nonetheless follow the standard recommendations as they apply to general population (1,6).

Laboratory Evaluation

Urinalysis and Urine Culture

No test unequivocally proves or disproves the diagnosis of CP/CPPS. Many laboratory tests are aimed at identifying an alternate diagnosis. The presence of pyuria and/or bacteriuria supports a diagnosis of bacterial prostatitis. The presence either of an inordinate number of WBCs and/or bacteria on Gram stain or of a heavy, nearly pure growth of bacterial pathogens on culture indicates a diagnosis of bacterial prostatitis. However, contamination from the urethra, from an external site, or from a source of infection in the upper urinary tract can lead to a false-positive result, while errors in collection or processing can lead to a false-negative result.

Prostate-Specific Antigen

The prostate-specific antigen (PSA) level is often elevated in men with acute bacterial prostatitis and may also be modestly elevated in those with CP/CPPS. PSA testing in men with CP/CPPS symptoms may be helpful in distinguishing between chronic bacterial prostatitis (PSA value is often elevated) and CP/CPPS (PSA value usually within reference range); however, this conjecture has yet to be tested in a well-controlled clinical trial (7).

Urinary Cytology

Voided urine cytologies, while not routine, should be readily considered whenever the index of suspicion is at all elevated—for instance, patients who either have had a long history of smoking, or have had occupational exposure to known toxins, or exhibit persistent microhematuria. When such a patient is undergoing cystoscopy, bladder-wash cytology may be obtained. Carcinoma in situ of the bladder (CIS) may resemble normal epithelium or appear as an erythematous, velvety patch of mucosa (1).

Radiographic Studies

Because no diagnostic radiological finding has proven definitive, all imaging studies (intravenous pyelography, videocystourethrography, CT scan, magnetic resonance imaging, ultrasonography of the scrotum, transrectal ultrasonography of the prostate, etc.) are aimed at excluding the presence of other, more definable and treatable causes of the patient's symptoms.

None of these studies warrants automatic application to every case of CP/CPPS. A cost-effective diagnostic algorithm should be individualized for each patient suspected of having CP/CPPS, incorporating only laboratory tests and radiographic procedures which are appropriate to that specific patient's problem.

Diagnostic Office Procedures

Prostatic Massage (Diagnostic) and the Third Voided Midstream Urine Specimen

In the absence of a positive urinalysis and/or culture, prostatic massage may produce secretions *per urethram*—EPS. Gram stain and culture of the EPS have been used to distinguish between bacterial and abacterial prostatitis and to guide selection of appropriate antibiotics. In many cases, however, no prostatic secretion flows from the meatus after massage. In these cases, Stamey recommends obtaining the first 10 mL of voided urine, immediately following massage—a "VB_3" (third voided midstream urine specimen) urine specimen—and submitting it for Gram stain and culture, as a substitute for the EPS. If there is a significant increase in WBCs or bacteria in the VB_3 specimen, compared to the initial urinalysis, this differential further implicates the prostate as the source of the pyuria and related symptoms. While the Stamey approach is still taught widely in medical school and residencies, this maneuver is much less widely practiced by clinical urologists today. Nickel suggests that a simplified premassage and postmassage urine smear and culture may prove more efficacious (8).

The NIH Chronic Prostatitis Cohort Study, in reviewing the screening results from 488 men with CP/CPPS, found, discouragingly, that there was no reliable correlation between the leukocyte counts or the bacterial counts and the degree of symptomatology, whether the analysis was performed on the EPS, the VB_3, or the ejaculate. The authors concluded that factors other than leukocytes and bacteria must contribute to symptom development in men with CPPS (9). (Refer to the section on chronic bacterial prostatitis for further details.)

Most urologists have abandoned the practice of personally evaluating a "wet prep" slide under a microscopic in their own office. However, relying on a distant laboratory for the report of a Gram stain performed on a dried specimen precludes making the diagnosis of Trichomonas urethritis/prostatitis, since the organism is detectable neither on air-dried slide nor by routine culture techniques.

Videourodynamics

Videourodynamic evaluation may uncover evidence of a spastic dysfunction of the bladder neck and prostatic urethra. Nickel contends that dysfunctional voiding and intraprostatic reflux of urine may be initiating factors in the onset of CP/CPPS (8).

Findings of spastic hyperactivity of the pelvic musculature in the absence of a definable underlying neuropathy suggest the presence of either an idiopathic neural etiology or an acquired functional voiding disorder.

Clinical researchers at Columbia University have discovered that an important subset of patients, who had been treated unsuccessfully for symptoms of chronic abacterial prostatitis for more than 10 years yet remained unresponsive to long-term antibiotic and α-blocker therapies, were actually experiencing pseudodyssynergia (a contraction of the external sphincter during voiding). This condition was documented on the basis of electromyography and fluoroscopy findings. Patients thus identified responded to treatment with biofeedback and behavior modification in 83% of cases (10).

Myofascial pain syndrome has been postulated as a cause for CPPS/CP. Even in the face of clinical apparent inflammation of the prostate gland, itself, a reflex triggering of spasm in the musculature of the pelvic floor can be a secondary, but clinically significant, source of the compounded symptomatology (11).

Beyond helping to detect occult neuropathies, urodynamic evaluation of patients with CP/CPPS may lead to a better understanding of the underlying voiding dysfunctions that are peculiar to certain select subsets of patients with this condition. Additionally, by subcategorizing patients with CP/CPPS based on the presence and the nature of abnormal urodynamic findings, an improved rationale for case-specific therapies may be forthcoming (12).

Flow Rate
Formal flow rate studies often show intermittency of flow and weakening of the urinary stream with a diminished peak urinary flow rate. The urethral pressure profile typically shows a high maximum urethral closing pressure.

Cystoscopy
Findings are often entirely normal, or, at most, reveal only nonspecific findings of minimal-to-mild inflammation and congestion in the area of the trigone and prostatic urethra. The main purpose of this intervention is, as with other procedures discussed above, to help rule out the presence of other causes of the patient's symptoms.

Cystoscopy may be performed in an outpatient setting after urethral injection of lidocaine (Xylocaine) jelly. However, cystoscopy under general or regional anesthesia or under conscious sedation offers several advantages:

1. As a rule, patients with CP/CPPS tend to be hypersensitive with a low pain tolerance. When the patient is unable to cooperate fully, endoscopic inspection is compromised.
2. General or regional anesthesia allows for more comfortable performance both of cold-mucosal cup biopsies to rule out carcinoma in situ and of hydrodistension of the bladder to rule out interstitial cystitis. (If hydrodistension is planned, it is important to complete hydrodistension before performing cold-cup biopsies, in order to minimize the risk of extravasation and bladder rupture during the hydrodistension.
3. Minor pathology, such as an annular stricture of the urethra or a prostatic polyp, can be treated at the same time. A sharp eye is needed to detect the opening in the proximal bulbar urethra of a symptomatic syringocoele (13).

Anal Sphincter Electromyography and/or Sphincter Function Profiles
These studies during cystometrography detect reflex reactivity and may uncover the presence of hypertonicity of the pelvic floor musculature. Such tension may be a sign of underlying myofascial pain syndrome. Pelvic floor activity during cystometrography can also be monitored via perianal surface electrodes. While such experimental evaluations are not yet part of the standard urological armamentarium, they are available at select centers (7).

PATHOPHYSIOLOGY
A comprehensive update, surveying relevant articles on this topic (2), categorizes the numerous pathophysiologic mechanisms implicated as the potential etiology of CPPS.

Special signaling molecules called *cytokines*, which are produced by WBCs (and by other cells), may play a role. While certain cytokines stimulate an inflammatory reaction, others inhibit inflammation. Moreover, the same cytokine may act as either an inciting influence or an inhibiting influence at different sites under varying conditions. Tissue necrosis factors, interleukins, interferons, and epithelial neutrophil-activating factors are but a few of these cytokines. To complicate matters, each of these terms indicates a whole, separate family of closely related molecules, not a single agent. Pelvic pain and inflammation in CP/CPPS patients may be linked to an imbalance in the complex network of proinflammatory cytokines and endogenous cytokine inhibitors (1). *Genetic predisposition* to CP/CPPS may be the result of differences in DNA sequences at chromosomal sites that regulate the production and action of these various cytokines. *Autoimmunity* has long been suspected of playing a role in the development of CP/CPPS. *Testosterone* levels have been shown to protect against inflammation within the prostate. Perhaps a low testosterone level (or, more likely, a breakdown in the mechanism whereby testosterone inhibits prostatic inflammation) may be at work in some men with CP/CPPS. *Abnormal functioning of the nervous system*, at the local level and/or within the CNS, may also play a role in the development of CP/CPPS. Nerve growth factor affects the number and sensitivity of pain transmitting pelvic nerves and may have an effect on CP/CPPS symptom development (1). *Psychological stress and depression* have long been associated with CP/CPPS flare-ups. This observation has led some researchers to mistakenly conclude that CP/CPPS is "all in your head" or that such mental stress results in a lower psychological threshold for the same objective degree of pain. Local production of cytokines such as interleukin-10 and interleukin-6 in the pelvis may be influenced by psychological stress and depression, factors that can lead to worsening of CP/CPPS symptoms which, in turn, can adversely affect a patient's mental health and thus result in a vicious cycle (1).

Occult Bacteria
Some cases of "abacterial" prostatitis may not actually be abacterial. Recent data suggest that gram-positive bacteria, which have traditionally been dismissed as normal florae in prostatic fluid cultures, may not be so normal in men with CP/CPPS. Normal defense mechanisms allow healthy men to render these bacteria harmless—mere microbial "hitchhikers." However, these defense mechanisms may be defective in men with CP/CPPS. Based on this theory, despite the absence of pathogenic bacteria, patients with CP/CPPS may at times find relief following antibiotic therapy (1).

Bacteria
A role for fastidious bacteria (i.e., bacteria that cannot be isolated on standard culture media) in the development of CP/CPPS has recently been suggested (3). Among the fastidious organisms that have been implicated are *Chlamydia trachomatis*, the genital mycoplasmas (i.e., *Ureaplasma urealyticum, Mycoplasma hominis, Mycoplasma genitalium*), a protozoan (i.e., *Trichomonas vaginalis*), *Neisseria gonorrhoeae*, genital tract viruses (e.g., herpes simplex virus types 1 and 2, and cytomegalovirus), fungi, anaerobic bacteria, and gram-positive bacteria.

Propionibacterium acnes
Intriguing findings suggest that persistent microbial infection with an indolent, but persistent, organism that is difficult to detect and difficult for the host to eradicate may act as an etiologic agent for CP/CPPS and also for the subsequent

development of prostate cancer (14). The presence of *P. acnes* could be detected only via sophisticated gene-sequencing and polymerase chain reaction technology. *P. acnes* cannot be identified using routine histology, Gram stain, or culture techniques. Preliminary findings suggest that chronic abacterial prostatitis may, in certain cases, actually be due to an occult, chronic, bacterial infection. Further, persistence of this smoldering infection may lead to the development of some prostate cancers.

Identification of effective methods to eradiacate these bacteria may lead to both care and possible prevention in at least some cases of CP and prostate cancer (1).

Escherichia coli

E. coli infection is a common cause of acute bacterial prostatitis. However, select strains of these bacteria may have developed a cloaking defense that allows them to conceal their activity and to resist antibiotic therapy. Biofilms develop when large numbers of bacteria embed in a microscopic slime layer called the exopolysaccharide matrix. Entrenched within this biofilm layer, the bacteria may resist antibacterial treatment, counter the human body's natural defenses, and defy detection by routine culture techniques. By forming these biofilms within the prostate, *E. coli* and related bacterial pathogens may cause chronic, treatment-resistant prostatitis. In some cases, they may also be the cause of chronic abacterial prostatitis. Future development of CP/CPPS following and episode of acute prostatitis may be prevented with a prolonged (4–6 week) course of an appropriate antibiotic with good prostate tissue penentrability preventing the bacteria from forming a biofilm (1,15).

TREATMENT

Prostatic massage (therapeutic): The physician places a finger rectally over the back of the prostate gland (just the same as is when performing a routine prostate examination) and presses firmly and methodically down upon the entire surface gland, working from the lateral edge centrally. The goal is to break up congestion within the prostatic ducts that have become plugged with inspissated material and to express the released secretions into the urethra.

The success of prostate massage in providing symptomatic relief is controversial (16). Despite little evidence-based medicine to recommend it, regularly repeated prostatic massages have been employed in the past, particularly for patients with large, congested glands. Nevertheless, some patients find that massage provides temporary relief worth the awkwardness and discomfort of the maneuver itself (17).

Symptomatic relief for some patients may still be achieved with prostate massage, but the practice has been largely abandoned by most contemporary urologists (1).

Therapeutic ejaculation: The role of frequent ejaculation in either producing or reducing CP/CPPS symptoms remains controversial. Patients with enlarged, symptomatically congested glands are often advised that regular sexual intercourse may alleviate their symptoms. There is not much scientific evidence for the claim, but most patients find this recommendation more tolerable than serial prostate massages (1).

Sitz baths: Sitz baths may provide partial relief from acute exacerbations. A hot water bath in a deep tub seems to provide better overall temporary relief than a shallow perineal dip (1).

Medication

Antibiotics

CP/CPPS should, by definition, exclude men with a proven bacteriologic etiology. Therefore, antibiotics are theoretically inappropriate for the treatment of this condition. Nevertheless, most practitioners are inclined to initiate at least one trial of long-term antibiosis. Evidence-based research finds limited validation for the use of antibacterials, even in the face of chronic bacterial prostatitis, let alone for abacterial CP/CPPS. Cure rates, based on sterilization of the prostatitic secretions, even for this more specific indication, ranged from 0% to 90% and correlated poorly with symptomatic responses. Limited evidence from retrospective studies suggests that quinolones [e.g., ciprofloxacin (Cipro), levofloxacin (Levaquin)] may be more effective than trimethoprim–sulfamethoxazole (Bactrim, Septra). Absent a well-documented bacterial culture, this recommendation must be weighed against the significant cost differential between these two options (1).

While antibiotics should have a very limited role in therapy for this condition, in desperation to do something for the distraught patient, multiple courses of antibiotics are frequently prescribed, often for extraordinarily protracted periods. Some patients are maintained on long-term, low-dose regimens, such as one capsule of trimethoprim–sulfamethoxazole (Septra DS) daily; and occasionally, patients experience symptomatic relief on these regimens. Recent studies suggest that, beyond the placebo effect, certain antibiotics may actually be providing an objective anti-inflammatory and/or analgesic benefit to these patients.

In screening for a bacterial etiology, the finding of gram-positive organisms has often been dismissed as a contaminant. However, small studies have found evidence to suggest that anaerobes and gram-positive aerobes, even coagulase-negative staphylococci, may, in fact, be pathogens, and appropriate antibiotic therapy has proven effective in select cases (18).

The goals of pharmacotherapy are to reduce morbidity and to prevent complications.

Keep in mind that no antibiotic regimen has been proven categorically efficacious in the treatment of CP/CPPS. According to E. M. Meares, "Antibacterial agents are neither effective nor indicated in the treatment of nonbacterial prostatitis" (19–21). A trial of antibiotics may be considered if *U. urealyticum* or *C. trachomatis* infection is suspected (1).

In a vigorous attempt to clarify the presence of bacteria in the uncontaminated prostate tissue of men with CP/CPPS, researchers in Seattle performed digitally guided, transperineal prostate biopsies in 118 subjects with CP/CPPS and in 59 control subjects. They found no difference in the rates of positive cultures (38% vs. 36%) and concluded that, while the prostatic colonization of bacteria within the prostate is not uncommon, particularly in older men, prostatic bacteria are probably not etiologically involved in the symptoms in most men with CP/CPPS (22).

In approaching the antibiotic option, remember that no antibiotic is free of complications. In justifying an empirical trial of antibiotics for CP/CPPS, many practitioners comment that at least antibiotics cannot hurt. As a grim reminder of the rare but devastating consequences attendant to the casual use of such antibiotics, this author has consulted for subsequent treatment for a CP/CPPS patient who suffered life-threatening complications from a failed liver/kidney transplantation that was necessitated by his extremely adverse reaction to a course of trimethoprim–sulfamethoxazole. When multiple prescriptions are provided for the latest recommended antibiotics, cost considerations can become a major factor (1).

Muscle Relaxants

Tension myalgia of the pelvic floor muscles, combined with overall stress-related psychological tension, can be partially relieved with muscle relaxants (19–21).

α-Adrenergic blockers: These agents have become a mainstay in the symptomatic treatment of this condition (23–25). By relieving the secondary smooth muscle spasm within the bladder neck and prostatic urethra, they afford greater comfort in voiding. The dosage should be titrated progressively and administered at night to minimize the main adverse effect of orthostatic hypotension. The final dose must be individualized to meet the patient's needs. While the antihypertensive agent has been administered to patients already taking other blood pressure medications, it is wise to coordinate the addition of this medication with the primary care physician or cardiologist who is prescribing the patient's other antihypertensive medications. Special caution is appropriate when prescribing this medication for frail, elderly men at high risk of injurious falling.

One study has suggested an advantage for α-blockers in combination with antibiotics over antibiotic therapy alone in the treatment of chronic bacterial prostatitis (25). Again, as with other medications, remember that the use of α-adrenergic blockade is not approved by the U.S. Food and Drug Administration for the treatment of CP/CPPS.

Surgery

Transurethral Resection of the Prostate

A widely held opinion among urologists is that transurethral resection of the prostate (TURP) should be restricted to patients who have experienced extreme, persistent symptoms over a protracted period, with no relief from nonoperative interventions. TURP, even when contemplated as an approach of last resort, should be offered only by experienced resectionists and then only with the clear understanding that symptomatic relief is not guaranteed. Indeed, symptoms might even worsen and might be compounded by the added burdens of erectile dysfunction and urinary incontinence.

When TURP is undertaken, completing a thorough resection of all tissues, down to the capsule, is essential. The concern is that residual tissue, partially coagulated, will lead to obstruction of the ductal drainage from prostatic acini, further exacerbating the patient's already intolerable symptoms (26).

Radical Prostatectomy

This extreme measure should be reserved for the most desperate of cases, if at all (27).

Consultation

Pain Management

Experts in the field of pain management may be able to assist with providing significant symptomatic relief. No analgesics are specifically appropriate in the treatment of CP/CPPS. Standard, mild analgesics such as acetaminophen (Tylenol), aspirin, and ibuprofen are well within the purview of the urologist's (and indeed the primary care physician's) domain of management. Keep in mind that the patient's analgesic needs are likely to fluctuate. Often, encouraging the patient to maintain a long-term, low-level intake of a minor analgesic (such as acetylsalicylic acid or acetaminophen three times a day) diminishes his need for more potent analgesics. Both patient's and physician's fear of analgesic abuse or addiction often lead to *under* medication, causing unnecessary pain and suffering. Be quick to invite consultation from specialists at an established pain management center.

Clinicians at Washington University have documented the beneficial impact that a coordinated, multidisciplinary approach between the urologist and the pain management team can have on improving the quality of life for many of these patients. These patients are often dismissed too easily, and their complaints are trivialized. Symptomatic patients can be encumbered by pain as devastating as that caused by cancer, neurologic diseases, and other conditions that merit a vigorous approach to effective pain management.

Psychiatry/Psychology

Frequently, patients with CP/CPPS are stereotyped as being high-strung, hypochondriacal, and even neurotic. Experiencing the daily torment of uncontrolled pelvic pain, urinary dysfunction, erectile dysfunction, and social embarrassment can understandably lead to profound psychological sequelae. Many patients encounter frustrated, dismissive, and unhelpful physicians in their quest for care, compounding their frustration, depression, and despair. A sympathetic, constructive attitude by the physician can do much to alleviate this strain.

Moreover, a mild relaxant such as diazepam (Valium), prescribed judiciously, may help your patient adjust to his condition and, at the same time, relax the spasm of the pelvic floor muscles, providing objective relief. The prescription of psychotropic medications should be undertaken with caution, however, and rarely without consultation from a psychiatrist. Reassure your patient that his condition is real and that his suffering is not imaginary. A psychiatrist and/or psychologist who is particularly interested in helping these patients can be a valuable member of the treatment team that includes the primary care physician, the urologist, and the pain management experts.

Andrology

A specialist in Andrology should be consulted for management of any attendant symptoms of erectile dysfunction. Specialists at Stanford University found that 92% of men with refractory CP/CPPS reported related erectile dysfunction, including problems with decreased libido (66%), pain upon ejaculation (56%), and ejaculatory dysfunction (31%) (28). Often, men are reluctant to volunteer problems they are facing in this regard. It is important to encourage open discussion of these issues from the outset. Questionnaires, such as the CPSI and International Index of Erectile Function, provide an apercu for patients to raise issues in this sensitive area. Active participation on the part of patient's partner should be strongly encouraged early in counseling and treatment process (29).

Many remedies and treatments are available, including sildenafil, vacuum devices, injection and intraurethral therapies, and penile implants; a physician would be profoundly remiss to not broach the topic and its treatment possibilities. A review of this topic by Sadeghi-Nejad and Seftel brings attention to the linkage of CP/CPPS to sexual dysfunction (30).

Physical Medicine

Lately, authorities have appreciated that in many cases, the symptoms formerly attributed to CP/CPPS may actually reflect pelvic floor spasm and chronic pelvic pain that is not prostatic in origin. In light of this, physiotherapists may provide an important role in helping to distinguish diagnostically and to ameliorate therapeutically neuromuscular-based symptoms. For example, patients with palpable myofascial tenderness in the rectal area are often unable to relax their pelvic floor musculature. This dysfunction of the pelvic floor muscles (i.e., Levator syndrome) is objectively documentable. Moreover, modulation based therapies such as biofeedback, alpha blockers, and sacral nerve stimulation have been used successfully to achieve symptom relief (1).

More recently, men with refractory CP/CPPS were treated at Stanford University with one month or more of trigger point release/paradoxical relaxation training, in order to release trigger points in their pelvic floor musculature. Clinical success—markedly or moderately improved symptoms—was achieved in 70% of the patients (28).

The presence of documented inflammation of the prostate and urethra does not exclude the presence of neuromuscular spasm of the pelvic floor. It is unclear whether the spasm (secondary to dysfunctional voiding and urinary tract infections) or the infection are the initial triggers for the chronic cycle of pain and pelvic spasms (1). In either case, both the infection and the spasm must be treated concurrently to achieve long-term relief in these difficult cases. While the urologist is best suited to address the prostatic inflammation, coordination with an interested physiotherapist for the management of biofeedback and nerve-root stimulation may often prove worthwhile.

Diet

The influence of diet on this condition varies. Traditionally, CP/CPPS patients have been warned to avoid excessive intake of prostate irritants, such as tobacco (smoking), coffee, tea, soda (cola drinks and diet drinks may be especially irritating), caffeine, spicy foods, and alcohol. Reassure your patient that none of these items is known to cause actual physical damage or to worsen the long-term prognosis. Nevertheless, responsible limitation of these items may help to control the day-to-day symptoms. Conversely, a glass or two of wine or sherry may actually lessen nocturia symptoms. Alkalinization of the urine seems to help some patients. A teaspoonful of baking soda (sodium bicarbonate) in a tall glass of warm water taken at bedtime may help reduce nighttime symptoms. However, caution patients regarding the risk of an excessive sodium load with higher intakes, especially in those receiving treatment for hypertension, fluid retention, or congestive heart failure. A potassium-based alkalinizer, such as potassium citrate (Urocit K), may prove more efficacious under these circumstances. Conversely, Stephen W. Leslie, MD, has found that some of his patients have very alkaline urine, which can also be irritating and result in discomfort and dysuria.

Further Outpatient Care

Voiding and Environmental Impact Diaries
A voiding diary is recommended for CP/CPPS patients (1).

In the *voiding diary*, record (*i*) the time and approximate amount of each void and (*ii*) the time and amount of each fluid intake. This record helps distinguish between urinary frequency (voiding normal amounts of urine over a 24-hour period, but in small, frequent voids) versus polyuria (voiding excessive amounts of urine each day overall).

In this light, objectively monitoring the patient's response to your advice to drink large quantities of water each day is often valuable. The general agreement is that dehydration should be avoided, because good hydration contributes to overall well-being and may dilute the concentration of the urinary irritants that exacerbate symptoms. On the other hand, advising a patient who is already seriously impaired by excessive daytime and nocturnal frequency and urgency to maximally increase his intake of fluid seems counterintuitive.

While the same advice might be interpreted by one patient as meaning 1 to 2 qt of fluid each day, another might take it to mean 1 to 2 gal! Information from a voiding diary can help guide your patient safely between the dangers of too much and too little daily fluid intake.

In the *environmental impact record*, every incident of living is detailed, both on "Bad Days"—those on which symptoms flare up markedly, and on "Good Days"—when symptoms are unusually quiescent. All incidents of daily living are recorded, including but not limited to the type, time, and amount of food and beverage intake. Patients should also chart exercise performed or lack of activity, including bike-riding, long car rides, and prolonged sitting or standing. They should include incidents of sexual stimulation and whether or not they resulted in ejaculation. They should also note a lack of sexual stimulation. Patients should record any unusual physical or emotional stress. Exposure to allergens such as animals, dust, or pollen can also be charted. After a series of "good days" and "bad days" have been recorded, patients can review these recordings with their treating physician to search out patterns in diet, exposures, or activity that seem to lead to either amelioration or exacerbation of symptoms. The patient should have a clear understanding that this exercise is not undertaken as a curative maneuver, but rather as a means for the patient to have better control over the condition and gain insight into some of the factors that may affect the symptoms (1).

EVIDENCE-BASED MEDICINE

The "British Medical Journal Clinical Evidence Handbook," an international resource of the best available evidence for effective health care, categorizes the treatment of CPPS/CP (31):

- "Likely to be beneficial"
  ○ α-Blockers
- "Unknown effectiveness"
  ○ 5α-Reductase inhibitors
  ○ Allopurinol
  ○ Biofeedback
  ○ Mepartricin
  ○ Nonsteroidal anti-inflammatory drugs
  ○ Pentosan polysulfate
  ○ Quercetin
  ○ Sitz baths
  ○ Transurethral microwave thermotherapy
- "Unlikely to be beneficial"
  ○ Oral antibiotic drugs
  ○ Prostatic massage

Resources for Patients

The following Web sites are helpful for both patients and physicians:

- Prostatitis Foundation

  provides extensive, patient-oriented information, newsletter, and reference data.
  Prostatitis Foundation
  1063 30th Street Box 8
  Smithshire, Illinois 61478
  fax 1-309-325-7184
  voice mail 1-888-891-4200
     http://www.prostatitis.org/
- Chronic Prostatitis/Chronic Pelvic Pain Syndrome Network
     http://www.chronicprostatitis.com/
- British Prostatitis Support Association offers information and encouragement from abroad.
     http://www.bps-assoc.org.uk/info.cfm

Resources for Physicians

"Chronic Pelvic Pain Syndrome and Prostatodynia" e-Medicine http://www.emedicine.com/MED/topic1922.htm provides online information (1).

CP/CPPS presents an excellent up-to-date overview of this topic (32).

"Campbell's Urology" is the mainstay of urological information regarding this topic (33).

Future Directions

Ultimately, a cure for CP/CPPS will be found by those who make clinical distinctions among cases rather than those who bundle all cases into one category.

Clinical investigators who are able to recognize within this hapless conglomeration discrete subsets of patients whose symptoms and findings can be proven to relate to a single, common etiologic factor will achieve meaningful success in treatment. Identification of a given causal factor and development of an effective remedy against it will provide a cure for that particular subset of patients with CP/CPPS. Hopefully, over time, individualized cures (as opposed to one single panacea for all CP/CPPS) will be achieved progressively for one subset of patients after another.

The key to success lies in the wider encouragement and the more effective funding of well-designed clinical, bench-top, and translational research projects. Public awareness of the prevalence of this condition, its devastating effects in terms of personal suffering, and its remarkable financial impact needs far greater promotion.

Funding for research from both private and public sectors needs to be increased. The patients who experience this condition and the physicians who care for them must be more effective in demanding improvement in both immediate care and long-term research (34).

What to Tell Your Patients

The most important aspect of treatment is that monotherapy is usually not successful; multimodal therapy is required. This includes addressing pain, voiding symptoms, and quality-of-life issues. What is needed is a combined biopsychosocial approach, which goes beyond just prescribing medications (32).

Treating a patient with CP/CPPS challenges even the most compassionate physician. The patient is often understandably tense, wary, and defensive. Most patients have already encountered frustration and rejection under the prior care of several unsympathetic physicians. These patients often approach new physicians with an off-putting combination of unrealistic hopes for a cure and suspicion related to past treatment failures. The physician and the patient should approach treatment as a "team" with well defined goals and objectives to minimize disappointments along the way (1).

CP/CPPS is a well-established condition notorious for the pain and disability it causes. It is a condition, not a disease or syndrome. As is true for other chronic conditions, such as arthritis, CP/CPPS, while treatable, is not curable. While no known cure exists for CP/CPPS, a variety of treatments, individualized for each patient, can often make this condition more bearable. Over time, this condition may improve or stabilize on its own.

Because CP/CPPS is a diagnosis of exclusion, it is essential to review the patient's records and perform a thorough physical examination to eliminate the possibility that another, more treatable disease is causing these symptoms. Assure your patient that only those diagnostic tests that hold a reasonable chance of producing a significant result will be recommended, while avoiding excessive testing.

Many medications and other forms of treatment can help alleviate the symptoms of CP/CPPS. However, it is important to be patient, trying only one or two new treatments at a time, and giving each enough time to take effect. Do not overwhelm the patient with an unreasonable number of simultaneous treatments, which only cause excessive inconvenience and expense. Simultaneous treatments might actually work against one another, and the adverse effects of these treatments might cause more, rather than fewer, problems for the patient.

Reassure your patient that CP/CPPS is a real physical condition; his problem is not merely an imagined one. However, this devastating condition inevitably leads to severe psychological stress. Therefore, it makes sense to suggest medications to help calm the patient and to offer consultation with a psychiatrist or psychologist. A mental health-care professional who has a special interest in this area can prove very beneficial. Again, it is important for the patient to understand that a referral for psychiatric consultation does not imply that he is insane or that his symptoms are imaginary or psychosomatic. Rather, psychiatric counseling and medication may help him to deal more effectively with the emotional and interpersonal consequences of this devastating illness.

Also, reassure the patient that his CP/CPPS symptoms are not a sign of cancer. CP/CPPS is not a life-threatening condition, it is not a venereal disease, and it is not contagious. Explain that the patient did not acquire this condition from someone else nor will he pass it on to anyone.

Remind the patient that he is not alone. Many men experience this problem. Local and national support groups can provide additional information and encouragement. Caution him that, while there are numerous very worthwhile sources of information on the Internet, there is also a thicket of scam artists and quackery. Suggest that he check with his treating physician before mailing away for a "secret formula" or embarking on a cruise to a clinic in the Philippines.

Agree on a schedule of planned follow-up visits performed regularly, as frequently as appropriate management of symptoms dictates. These scheduled appointments minimize the need for emergency visits and telephone calls, while providing comfort and creating trust between doctor and patient.

The urologist should always institute treatment in close communication with the patient's primary care physician, who remains the mainstay of care.

Remind the patient that he is free to seek the advice of other physicians and health-care providers, while he is under your urological care. However, the patient must keep his treating physician informed of all other treatments and medications tried, including alternative medicines and home remedies.

Assure the patient that you take his problem very seriously and that every effort will be made, with his cooperation, to minimize the problems that this condition causes. The patient–physician relationship should be a partnership formed to gain control of this condition and allow the patient to enjoy life more fully.

ACKNOWLEDGMENT

"Chronic Pelvic Pain Syndrome and Prostatodynia" (e-Medicine) has served as the base reference for much of the material presented in this review. It continues to provide updated information on this and related topics (1).

REFERENCES

1. Watson R, Irwin R. Chronic Pelvic Pain Syndrome and Prostatodynia. e-Medicine 2007. Available at: http://emedicine-medscape.com/article/437745-overview. Accessed October 2009.
2. Miller JL, Rothman I, Bavendam TG, et al. Prostatodynia and interstitial cystitis: one and the same? Urology 1995; 45(4):587–590.

3. Forrest JB, Schmidt S. Interstitial cystitis, chronic nonbacterial prostatitis and chronic pelvic pain syndrome in men: a common and frequently identical clinical entity. J Urol 2004; 172(6 pt 2):2561–2562.
4. Krieger JN, Riley DE. Chronic prostatitis: Charlottesville to Seattle. J Urol 2004; 172(6 pt 2):2557–2560.
5. MacLennan GT, Eisenberg R, Fleshman RL, et al. The influence of chronic inflammation in prostatic carcinogenesis: a 5-year followup study. J Urol 2006; 176(3):1012–1016.
6. Caire AA, Sun L, Robertson CN, et al. Public Survey and Survival Data Do Not Support Recommendations to Discontinue Prostate-specific Antigen Screening in Men at Age 75. [Epub ahead of print]. Urology Oct 6, 2009.
7. Pansadoro V, Emiliozzi P, Defidio L, et al. Prostate-specific antigen and prostatitis in men under fifty. Eur Urol 1996; 30(1):24–27.
8. Nickel JC. Practical approach to the management of prostatitis. Tech Urol 1995; 1(3):162–167.
9. Schaeffer A, Stern J. Chronic prostatitis. Clin Evid 2002; (8):864–871.
10. Kaplan SA, Santarosa RP, D'Alisera PM, et al. Pseudodyssynergia (contraction of the external sphincter during voiding) misdiagnosed as chronic nonbacterial prostatitis and the role of biofeedback as a therapeutic option. J Urol 1997; 157(6):2234–2237.
11. Zermann D, Ishigooka M, Doggweiler R. Chronic Prostatitis: a myofascial syndrome? Infect Urol 1999; 12:82–92.
12. Theodorou C, Konidaris D, Moutzouris G, et al. The urodynamic profile of prostatodynia. BJU Int 1999; 84(4):461–463.
13. Watson RA, Lassoff MA, Sawczuk IS, et al. Syringocele of Cowper's gland duct: an increasingly common rarity. J Urol 2007; 178(1):285.
14. Cohen RJ, Shannon BA, McNeal JE, et al. *Propionibacterium acnes* associated with inflammation in radical prostatectomy specimens: a possible link to cancer evolution? J Urol 2005; 173(6):1969–1974.
15. Soto SM, Smithson A, Martinez JA, et al. Biofilm formation in uropathogenic *Escherichia coli* strains: relationship with prostatitis, urovirulence factors and antimicrobial resistance. J Urol 2007; 177(1):365–368.
16. Ateya A, Fayez A, Hani R, et al. Evaluation of prostatic massage in treatment of chronic prostatitis. Urology 2006; 67(4):674–678.
17. Nickel JC, Alexander R, Anderson R, et al. Prostatitis unplugged? Prostatic massage revisited. Tech Urol 1999; 5(1):1–7.
18. Lowentritt JE, Kawahara K, Human LG, et al. Bacterial infection in prostatodynia. J Urol 1995; 154(4):1378–1381.
19. Meares EM Jr. Prostatitis. Med Clin North Am. 1991; 75(2):405–424.
20. Meares E. Non-specific infections of the genitourinary tract. In: Tanagho E, McAninch J, eds. Smith's General Urology. 14th ed. Norwalk, CT: Appleton & Lange, 1995:231–234.
21. Meares E. Prostatitis and related disorders. In: Walsh PC, Retik AB, Vaughn ED, et al., eds. Campbell's Urology. 7th ed. Philadelphia, PA: WB Saunders, 1998:285–286.
22. Lee JC, Muller CH, Rothman I, et al. Prostate biopsy culture findings of men with chronic pelvic pain syndrome do not differ from those of healthy controls. J Urol 2003; 169(2):584–587; discussion 587–588.
23. Nickel JC. Role of alpha1-blockers in chronic prostatitis syndromes. BJU Int 2008; 101(suppl 3):11–16.
24. Mishra VC, Browne J, Emberton M. Role of alpha-blockers in type III prostatitis: a systematic review of the literature. J Urol 2007; 177(1):25–30.
25. Barbalias GA, Nikiforidis G, Liatsikos EN. Alpha-blockers for the treatment of chronic prostatitis in combination with antibiotics. J Urol 1998; 159(3):883–887.
26. Smart CJ, Jenkins JD, Lloyd RS. The painful prostate. Br J Urol 1975; 47(7):861–869.
27. Davis BE, Weigel JW. Adenocarcinoma of the prostate discovered in 2 young patients following total prostatovesiculectomy for refractory prostatitis. J Urol 1990; 144(3):744–745.

28. Anderson RU, Wise D, Sawyer T, et al. Sexual dysfunction in men with chronic prostatitis/chronic pelvic pain syndrome: improvement after trigger point release and paradoxical relaxation training. J Urol 2006; 176(4 pt 1):1534–1538; discussion 1538–1539.
29. Rosen RC, Cappelleri JC, Gendrano N III. The International Index of Erectile Function (IIEF): a state-of-the-science review. Int J Impot Res 2002; 14(4):226–244.
30. Sadeghi-Nejad H, Seftel A. Sexual dysfunction and prostatitis. Curr Urol Rep 2006; 7(6):479–484.
31. Erickson B, Jang T, Schaeffer A. Chronic Prostatitis. London, UK: BMJ Publishing Group, 2007:281–282.
32. Pontari MA. Chronic prostatitis/chronic pelvic pain syndrome. Urol Clin North Am 2008; 35(1):81–89; vi.
33. Nickel JC. Inflammatory conditions of the male genitourinary tract: prostatitis and related conditions, orchitis and epididymitis. In: Wein A, Kavoussi L, Novick A, et al., eds. Campbell–Walsh Urology. 9th ed. Philadelphia, PA: WB Saunders, 2007.
34. Bartoletti R, Cai T, Dinelli N, et al. Prevalence, incidence estimation, risk factors and characterization of chronic prostatitis/chronic pelvic pain syndrome in urological hospital outpatients in Italy: results of a multicenter case-control observational study. J Urol. 2007; 178:2415.

17 Female Chronic Pelvic Pain

Frank F. Tu and Sangeeta Senapati

NorthShore University HealthSystem, Evanston, and Pritzker School of Medicine, Chicago, Illinois, U.S.A.

Gregory Goldstein and Alexandra Roybal

Northwestern University, Evanston, Illinois, U.S.A.

THE DISORDER

Chronic pelvic pain (CPP) is a frustrating clinical condition affecting roughly 9 million women each year. The American College of Obstetricians and Gynecologists defines the disorder as noncyclic lower abdominal pain persisting for at least six months with enough severity to cause functional incapacity or require medical or surgical care. Pain is localized in the anatomic pelvis, which includes the anterior abdominal wall below the umbilicus, the lumbosacral back, and the buttocks (1).

Although it affects both women and men, CPP is widely considered a gynecologic disorder. Approximately 15% to 20% of women aged 18 to 50 years have CPP lasting for at least one year. As many as 25% to 50% of these women will have multiple diagnoses (2). Demographic differences do not appear to predict higher risk of developing this disorder. While CPP is more common among reproductive-age women, it can present at any age.

Causes of pain may be difficult to attribute to a single origin. For example, sources of pain can be visceral or somatic. Visceral origins of CPP arise in reproductive, genitourinary, vascular, and gastrointestinal regions of the body. Somatic sources include the pelvic bones, ligaments, muscles, skin of the abdomen and perineum, and fascia. Women suffering from CPP often experience multiple pelvic symptoms, such as dysmenorrhea (81% vs. 58% in controls) and dyspareunia (41% vs. 14% in controls) (3). This is likely due to organ cross-sensitization, where pain in one pelvic structure impacts the afferent output from another structure. Further complicating the evaluation are central influences on pain expression: nearly half of women seen in tertiary CPP clinics have experienced serious trauma such as sexual or physical abuse, although the cause and effect relationship is unclear (4). Not surprisingly, many women with CPP suffer from coexisting depression, anxiety, sleep disorders, sexual dysfunction, and trouble with relationships.

CPP is a costly disorder physically, financially, and emotionally. The psychosocial ramifications of CPP manifest as physical pain, change in mood, and disturbances in social activities, reducing a woman's overall quality of life. CPP in the United States has been estimated to cost over $2 billion annually in direct and indirect costs (5). In that study, 15% of women reported lost time for paid work, and 45% could not work as efficiently.

DIAGNOSIS

Approximately two-thirds of women suffering from CPP do not undergo diagnostic testing and are never referred to a specialist for diagnosis or treatment (3). A thorough history and physical examination are central to the efficient management of a woman with CPP. The clinician begins the evaluation by characterizing the location, quality, severity, inciting and palliating factors, and timing of pain symptoms. Certain features, such as cramping, pain with intercourse, bladder symptoms, diarrhea, or constipation, suggest visceral dysfunction—the duration and onset of painful menses, if present, may point to endometriosis. If none of these features is present, focal somatic pain may be more likely. Review of previous surgical, medical, and social history can identify potential triggers for pain. Previous accidents or surgeries should be considered as potential initiators of the current pain problem; one notable example is urological procedures in younger children, which have been associated with subsequent development of voiding dysfunction and pain in adulthood. Childhood involvement in high-intensity activities such as gymnastics or ballet may predispose women to pelvic girdle issues. Current and past sexual habits and satisfaction should be gently queried. Previous pregnancies and contraceptive histories must be detailed as well as a history of vaginal and pelvic infections. Operative reports and pathology reports from any gynecologic surgical procedure should potentially be obtained, particularly if a questionable history of endometriosis is made.

A patient's general history should note any health problems throughout her life, particularly with regard to concomitant mood issues or pain disorders. Use of illicit drugs and alcohol abuse must be evaluated in women considering chronic opioid use. Evaluation of the social and occupational history can identify work-related stress and whether adequate support from family exists.

Physical examination should focus on the back, abdomen, and pelvis, but assessment for systemic disease is, of course, prudent. This evaluation is useful in ruling out other acute, emergent causes of pelvic pain, such as appendicitis or inflammatory bowel disease. We prefer to evaluate the musculoskeletal and lumbosacral peripheral nerve function prior to the gynecologic examination, as these are often ignored by general women's health practitioners. The examination should be concerned with both the somatic and the visceral tissues of the abdomen, back, hips, and pelvis. The single-digit examination consists of superficial and deep palpation and can differentiate between superficial allodynia and myofascial pain of the abdominal wall, versus deeper visceral pain. If focal areas of muscle spasm are present, trigger point injections may help determine if the pain is predominantly of somatic origin.

In addition to the physical examination, selected laboratory studies should be obtained in order to exclude other disease processes. Beyond a routine pregnancy test in reproductive-age women, a complete blood count and pelvic cultures should be taken to rule out pelvic inflammatory disease. Imaging studies should be conducted on all patients with a pelvic examination suggestive of infection or a pelvic mass. Ultrasonography can assist in identifying the origin of the mass as uterine, adnexal, gastrointestinal, or from the bladder. While magnetic resonance imaging and ultrasound are good tests for characterizing suspected uterine disorders and pelvic masses such as endometriomas, they are not particularly good as a nonspecific screening tool in CPP. Pelvic CT is most advantageous in identifying intra-abdominal infection or bowel issues and, therefore, is best used to confirm diagnoses suggested by the examination. In certain patients, transfundal retrograde venography or MR venograms can image the pelvic venous system to determine if pelvic varicosities or pelvic congestion syndrome is present.

In the presence of symptoms suggestive of bowel or bladder pathology, selective cystoscopy or colonoscopy may be needed, particularly when occult bleeding is noted. Endometriosis can rarely infiltrate into both organs, in which case magnetic resonance imaging may be helpful. Diagnostic pelvic laparoscopic evaluation ideally should focus on those patients with prominent visceral pain, such as painful periods, or pain readily reproducible on internal examination of the pelvic organs. When pathology is found, some 90% of diagnoses will be either endometriosis or adhesions (6). A major advantage of this approach is the ability to treat identified problems at the time of diagnosis. The surgeon must be careful not to overlook atypical or subtle areas of disease, ideally performing a biopsy on all suspicious lesions to rule out endometriosis. Conscious laparoscopic pain mapping, performed under local anesthesia, has been suggested as a way to allow patients to identify focal intra-abdominal pain generators, but remains unproven in its generalizability or efficacy.

PATHOPHYSIOLOGY
The cerebral representation of the abdominal and pelvic structures is heavily overlapping with some 70% of central neurons having responsiveness to multiple different loci (7). Unfortunately, gynecologic surgeons are trained to focus on individual internal organ pathology without an appreciation of associated somatic tissue dysfunction (8). The consequence of such a narrow focus is often elusive diagnoses and imprecise treatment regimens.

Neuropathic Origin
Pelvic pain generators are characterized as being either somatic or visceral (9). Pelvic somatic structures such as bones, joints, muscles, and skin pass afferents to the central nervous system via first-order neurons synapsing in the dorsal horn of the lower thoracic, lumbar, and sacral spinal cord (10). The dull, achy quality of deep muscle pain often overlaps with the presentation of visceral pain. Conversely, visceral pain is conveyed to the central nervous system through afferents embedded in or lining internal structures of the pelvis (i.e., bladder, ureter, ovaries, etc.) This cramping type of pain is transmitted through sensory and motor fibers of the autonomic nervous system (10). Pelvic pain frequently presents without evidence of physical tissue injury, suggesting the possibility of nonnociceptive pain. Experimentally induced injury to the dorsal horn of animals, for example, results in alterations in pain processing in response to noxious stimulation of the abdominal and pelvic organs (11). Spinal cord processing of painful stimuli from abdominal and visceral organs also is modulated by descending inhibitory neurons (12). Contributions from cingulate cortex and other limbic centers may explain the observed emotional component seen in CPP and related visceral disorders, and may be one pathway by which abuse and trauma influence expression of pelvic pain (4,13).

TABLE 1   Contributors to CPP

Gynecologic	Adenomyosis, adhesions, dysmenorrhea, endometriosis, leiomyoma, ovarian cysts, pelvic inflammatory disease, pudendal neuralgia, vulvodynia
Gastrointestinal	Chronic appendicitis, diverticulitis, inflammatory bowel disease, irritable bowel syndrome
Urological	Painful bladder syndrome/interstitial cystitis, urethral syndrome
Musculoskeletal/other	Fibromyalgia, pelvic floor myalgia, pelvic varicosities, trigger points

Abbreviation: CPP, chronic pelvic pain.

Variety of Causes

In a 1999 study, Zondervan et al. found that in over 5000 women diagnosed with CPP, 37.7% of the cases were related to the gastrointestinal tract, 30.8% were urinary, and 20.2% gynecologic (14). Table 1 summarizes some of the more common causes.

Gynecologic

Gynecologists tend to see the most women with pelvic pain. Endometriosis, where endometrial tissue invades into the pelvic peritoneum, ovaries, or adjacent tissues, may affect up to 10% of women of reproductive age (15). While most menstruating women will spill endometrial cells into the peritoneal cavity, development of this disease is complex, encompassing defects in immune surveillance, enhanced angiogenesis, and aberrant expression of cellular adhesion molecules (16). Pain, including dysmenorrhea and dyspareunia, likely relates to direct tissue inflammation and scarring, activating peritoneal and visceral afferents. A closely related condition, adenomyosis, involves uterine endometrium invading into the adjacent uterine musculature, or myometrium. Both conditions can be asymptomatic in many women, however.

Ovarian cysts, whether functional or persistent, can also cause pain. When they grow above 5 cm and remain persistent, they are generally removed to prevent ovarian torsion and to rule out occult malignancy. Examples of benign ovarian cysts include endometriomas; teratomas; fibromas; and serous and mucinous cystadenomas, which must be distinguished from the malignant subtypes: borderline, adenocarcinomas, and sex-cord stromal tumors.

Uterine leiomyoma can also be associated with pelvic pain, and occur in 70% to 80% of premenopausal women (17). These benign tumor growths from the myometrium likely cause pain from ischemia or local inflammation, although many smaller tumors will never be symptomatic.

Pelvic inflammatory disease affects up to a million women annually in the U.S. and is generally a polymicrobial infection, often following initial infection with gonorrhea or chlamydia. Notably, the latter two can readily be treated with antibiotics, but chronic pelvic inflammatory disease can lead to chronic pain from severe tubal damage and adhesions, affecting up to one-third of women initially diagnosed (18).

Perineal pain syndromes including vulvodynia and pudendal neuralgia may be present in 20% of pelvic pain patients (19). These cutaneous pain syndromes are poorly understood but may arise following initial nociceptive pain (yeast infection), trauma, peripheral nerve fiber proliferation, and failure of normal homeostatic mechanisms to restore baseline pain sensitivity, resulting in neuroinflammation and central sensitization (20). They frequently present with concomitant pelvic floor muscle spasm.

Musculoskeletal
Studies suggest that between 20% and 90% of women with CPP display myofascial dysfunction. Pelvic floor pain dysfunction is associated both with dyspareunia and with visceral pain dysfunction of the bladder. Pelvic pain patients display enhanced pressure–pain threshold sensitivity in the pelvic floor (21). Postulated causes of such dysfunction may include mechanical strain, injury following childbirth, or tonic activation in relation to postural issues or centrally mediated autonomic changes from trauma.

Gastrointestinal/Genitourinary
Irritable bowel syndrome and painful bladder/interstitial cystitis frequently overlap with other causes of pelvic pain (endometriosis, vulvodynia, musculoskeletal pain) and are discussed in chapter 15. Of note, enhanced bladder urothelial sensitivity has been seen in 80% of endometriosis patients, suggesting overlapping aberrations in pain processing (22).

Vascular
The role of pelvic varicosities in pelvic pain etiology remains highly controversial. Some clinicians believe that sluggish blood flow in the iliac, ovarian, and uterine veins may be a source of nociception; indeed, in one Turkish study, venous distention was the only identifiable pathology in 30% of CPP patients (23). This is countered by evidence that many asymptomatic women also have the same radiographic appearance on magnetic resonance venography. More studies are clearly needed.

Adhesions and Postoperative Neuropathic Pain
Following selected abdominal procedures such as cesarean section or hysterectomy, 30% to 40% of women may report persistent pain, which is often attributed to scar formation (24, 25). Conscious pain mapping demonstrates that many, but not all, intra-abdominal adhesions can be pain sensitive. Thus, the exact role of adhesions in CPP remains unclear, as in many cases the presentation resembles neuropathic pain. Nerve impingement or transection from abdominal or pelvic incisions also can occur following such procedures.

TREATMENT
A comprehensive approach to treating CPP considers the psychosocial, sexual, and somatic aspects of a patient (26, 27). The previously mentioned Dutch randomized, controlled trial comparing somatic, psychological, dietary, environmental, and physiotherapeutic treatment versus only laparoscopy found the multimodal arm to be more effective in reducing pelvic pain symptoms (28). This comprehensive approach also may provide a cure in selected cases of CPP, particularly musculoskeletal. For long-standing pain of years' duration, patients' expectations of cure may need to be modified to accept pain management and optimal quality of life (1). Figure 1 displays a proposed systematic treatment

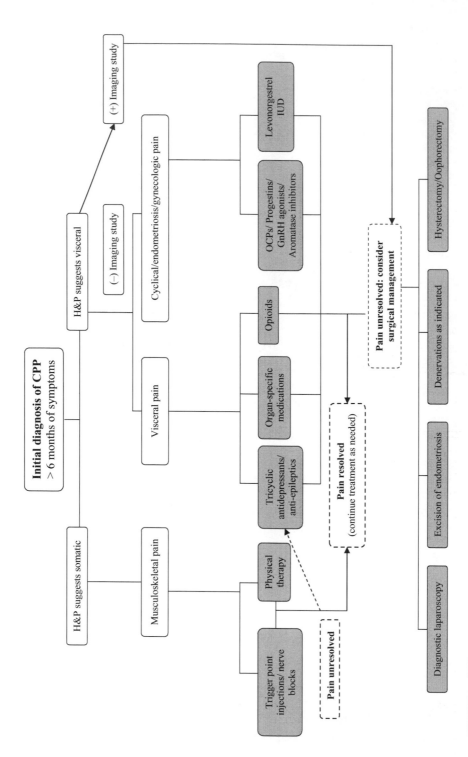

FIGURE 1 CPP treatment algorithm. *Abbreviation:* CPP, chronic pelvic pain.

guideline. We break down treatments into medical, procedural, and integrative approaches, roughly.

Medical Management

Cyclic pelvic pain often responds well to sex hormone modulation. Hormonal therapy impacts on nociception likely include alterations in pain sensitivity as well as direct inhibition of ovarian or uterine inflammation related to ovulation or menses. Oral contraceptives are the best-tolerated initial approach for hormonal suppression. In one small, Italian, randomized, controlled trial, oral contraceptives were found to show effectiveness for endometriosis-associated pain (29). Notably, they do slightly increase the risk of venous thromboembolism, particularly in women with undetected thrombophilias. Similarly, randomized, controlled trials have demonstrated moderate improvement in pelvic pain symptoms following both gonadotropin-releasing hormone agonist treatment and oral progestins (30, 31). Prolonged gonadotropin-releasing hormone agonist therapy can cause bone loss, mood changes, and menopausal symptoms, so women may require hormone replacement therapy with estrogen or progesterone, and bone density monitoring. In some women, progestins are associated with irregular bleeding, fluid retention, and modest weight gain. Insertion of a progestin-contained intrauterine device may be an alternative with fewer side effects, as the systemic absorption is largely limited to the pelvis (32, 33). Danocrine, a once-popular androgenic treatment, is less commonly used today because of virilizing side effects.

Neuromodulating agents are also used increasingly for CPP, particularly when associated with painful bladder syndrome/interstitial cystitis or irritable bowel syndrome where hyperalgesia or allodynia is present. Randomized, controlled trials show that tricyclic antidepressants (TCAs) and antiseizure drugs provide significant pain relief (average changes in visual analog pain intensity > 4/10) for women with CPP up to two years after initiating therapy (34, 35). We find that amitriptyline or nortriptyline dosed between 10 and 100 mg nightly, or gabapentin dosed 300 to 900 mg three times daily are often crucial adjuncts for treatment of visceral pain, chronic musculoskeletal pain, as well as vulvar pain. Related agents such as topiramate, lamotrigine, duloxetine, and pregabalin likely may be effective for some women, but published studies are limited. The gynecologic community only recently has begun to embrace use of such neurological agents. Side effects for these agents include dizziness and sedation. The anticholinergic properties of TCAs also can cause constipation, dry eyes, and dry mouth, usually in a dose-dependent fashion. Individuals with a cardiac history or who are over age 50 should consider obtaining a pretreatment electrocardiogram because of the effects of TCAs on the cardiac conducting system.

By the time CPP has been diagnosed, nonsteroidal anti-inflammatory medications have usually failed as monotherapy but may still be useful as adjuncts. Opioids are widely accepted for treatment of chronic pain because of their fast-acting, potent capacity to relieve pain (36). Sadly, no long-term data exists to support use of opioids for CPP. In addition to risks of tolerance and addiction, chronic opioid use may affect pituitary function, impairing fertility and inducing a relative menopausal state (37). For each patient, the relative benefit–risk balance must be assessed, and ideally, opioids are limited for short-term usage to bridge patients into other therapies.

Procedural Treatments: Surgery, Nerve Excision, and Nerve Blocks

One-third of laparoscopies in the United States are performed for an indication of pelvic pain. Surgical removal of endometriosis reduces pain with stable results in over 60% of women at up to five-year follow-up (38, 39). For severe intractable pain, hysterectomy appears effective in 75% of women one year after surgery; success rates drop to 60% when no identifiable pathology is noted (suggesting more central neurological pain) (40). This does eliminate future childbearing and should be used sparingly, only after multimodal therapy has been attempted. Little evidence exists for repeated removal of functional ovarian cysts or leiomyoma as an effective treatment for CPP; and randomized, controlled trials indicate that surgical adhesiolysis is no better than diagnostic laparoscopy in reducing abdominal/pelvic pain in women with adhesions (41).

Nerve-directed therapy can be helpful with focal pain syndromes. Localized nerve blocks and trigger point injections, including pudendal nerve blocks, have limited evidence to support their use. However, they may prove helpful for diagnosis, facilitating physical therapy by relieving pain and, occasionally, resolving focal pain. In a related fashion, bladder cocktails combining local anesthetics, anti-inflammatory drugs, and steroids are frequently used for chronic management of painful bladder syndrome. For vulvodynia, chronic application of topical anesthetic agents often proves effective (42).

Neuroablative procedures are often a treatment of last resort. Clinical trials involving severe dysmenorrhea and endometriosis-associated CPP suggest that presacral neurectomy improves central midline CPP, but it runs a small risk of inducing chronic constipation or irritative urinary voiding (43). Laparoscopic uterine nerve ablation, while less effective for dysmenorrhea, is generally easier to perform by less-skilled surgeons (44).

Behavioral Modification

For both chronic somatic and visceral pain syndromes, a combination of musculoskeletal treatment, dietary manipulation, and psychotherapy can afford meaningful improvements in symptoms. This chapter can only highlight some of these promising strategies, which, undeniably, need much more systematic study. Physical therapy seeks to improve pelvic stability, core strength, and muscle spasm and can alleviate problems of the female pelvic floor, bony pelvic girdle, abdominal core deconditioning, and ligamentous pelvic instability. Evidence that probiotics for irritable bowel syndrome and dietary restrictions in painful bladder syndrome can influence symptom flares suggests that dietary approaches can be relevant for pelvic pain syndromes (45, 46). Finally, for patients with concomitant depression, anxiety, insomnia, or poor coping, cognitive–behavioral strategies are a crucial component of a successful management program (see the associated chaps. 19 and 23).

REFERENCES

1. Howard FM. Chronic pelvic pain. Obstet Gynecol 2003; 101(3):594–611.
2. Zondervan K, Barlow DH. Epidemiology of chronic pelvic pain. Baillieres Best Pract Res Clin Obstet Gynaecol 2000; 14(3):403–414.
3. Zondervan KT, Yudkin PL, Vessey MP, et al. The community prevalence of chronic pelvic pain in women and associated illness behaviour. Br J Gen Pract 2001; 51(468):541–547.

4. Meltzer-Brody S, Leserman J, Zolnoun D, et al. Trauma and posttraumatic stress disorder in women with chronic pelvic pain. Obstet Gynecol 2007; 109(4):902–908.

5. Mathias SD, Kuppermann M, Liberman RF, et al. Chronic pelvic pain: prevalence, health-related quality of life, and economic correlates. Obstet Gynecol 1996; 87(3):321–327.

6. Howard FM. The role of laparoscopy in chronic pelvic pain: promise and pitfalls. Obstet Gynecol Surv 1993; 48(6):357–387.

7. Berkley KJ. A life of pelvic pain. Physiol Behav 2005; 86(3):272–280.

8. Selfe SA, Van Vugt M, Stones RW. Chronic gynaecological pain: an exploration of medical attitudes. Pain 1998; 77(2):215–225.

9. Lamvu G, Steege JF. The anatomy and neurophysiology of pelvic pain. J Minim Invasive Gynecol 2006; 13(6):516–522.

10. Gunter J. Chronic pelvic pain: an integrated approach to diagnosis and treatment. Obstet Gynecol Surv 2003; 58(9):615–623.

11. Wang J, Kawamata M, Namiki A. Changes in properties of spinal dorsal horn neurons and their sensitivity to morphine after spinal cord injury in the rat. Anesthesiology 2005; 102(1):152–164.

12. Wilder-Smith CH, Schindler D, Lovblad K, et al. Brain functional magnetic resonance imaging of rectal pain and activation of endogenous inhibitory mechanisms in irritable bowel syndrome patient subgroups and healthy controls. Gut 2004; 53(11):1595–1601.

13. Levy BS. Nonsurgical management of chronic pelvic pain. J Am Assoc Gynecol Laparosc 1997; 4(5):551–556.

14. Zondervan KT, Yudkin PL, Vessey MP, et al. Patterns of diagnosis and referral in women consulting for chronic pelvic pain in UK primary care. Br J Obstet Gynaecol 1999; 106(11):1156–1161.

15. Cramer DW, Missmer SA. The epidemiology of endometriosis. Ann N Y Acad Sci 2002; 955:11–22; discussion 34–36, 396–406.

16. Giudice LC, Kao LC. Endometriosis. Lancet 2004; 364(9447):1789–1799.

17. Day Baird D, Dunson DB, Hill MC, et al. High cumulative incidence of uterine leiomyoma in black and white women: ultrasound evidence. Am J Obstet Gynecol 2003; 188(1):100–107.

18. Ness RB, Soper DE, Holley RL, et al. Effectiveness of inpatient and outpatient treatment strategies for women with pelvic inflammatory disease: results from the Pelvic Inflammatory Disease Evaluation and Clinical Health (PEACH) Randomized Trial. Am J Obstet Gynecol 2002; 186(5):929–937.

19. Stanford EJ, Koziol J, Feng A. The prevalence of interstitial cystitis, endometriosis, adhesions, and vulvar pain in women with chronic pelvic pain. J Minim Invasive Gynecol 2005; 12(1):43–49.

20. Haefner HK, Collins ME, Davis GD, et al. The vulvodynia guideline. J Low Genit Tract Dis 2005; 9(1):40–51.

21. Tu FF, Fitzgerald CM, Kuiken T, et al. Comparative measurement of pelvic floor pain sensitivity in chronic pelvic pain. Obstet Gynecol 2007; 110(6):1244–1248.

22. Chung MK, Chung RP, Gordon D. Interstitial cystitis and endometriosis in patients with chronic pelvic pain: the "evil twins" syndrome. JSLS 2005; 9(1):25–29.

23. Soysal ME, Soysal S, Vicdan K, et al. A randomized controlled trial of goserelin and medroxyprogesterone acetate in the treatment of pelvic congestion. Hum Reprod 2001; 16(5):931–939.

24. Brandsborg B, Nikolajsen L, Hansen CT, et al. Risk factors for chronic pain after hysterectomy: a nationwide questionnaire and database study. Anesthesiology 2007; 106(5):1003–1012.

25. Loos MJ, Scheltinga MR, Mulders LG, et al. The Pfannenstiel incision as a source of chronic pain. Obstet Gynecol 2008; 111(4):839–846.

26. Peters AA, Van Den Tillaart SA. The difficult patient in gastroenterology: chronic pelvic pain, adhesions, and sub occlusive episodes. Best Pract Res Clin Gastroenterol 2007; 21(3):445–463.

27. Steege JF, Stout AL, Somkuti SG. Chronic pelvic pain in women: toward an integrative model. Obstet Gynecol Surv 1993; 48(2):95–110.
28. Peters AA, van Dorst E, Jellis B, et al. A randomized clinical trial to compare two different approaches in women with chronic pelvic pain. Obstet Gynecol 1991; 77(5):740–744.
29. ACOG Practice Bulletin No. 51. Chronic pelvic pain. Obstet Gynecol 2004; 103(3):589–605.
30. Ling FW. Randomized controlled trial of depot leuprolide in patients with chronic pelvic pain and clinically suspected endometriosis. Pelvic Pain Study Group. Obstet Gynecol 1999; 93(1):51–58.
31. Farquhar CM, Rogers V, Franks S, et al. A randomized controlled trial of medroxyprogesterone acetate and psychotherapy for the treatment of pelvic congestion. Br J Obstet Gynaecol 1989; 96(10):1153–1162.
32. Fortney JA, Feldblum PJ, Raymond EG. Intrauterine devices. The optimal long-term contraceptive method? J Reprod Med 1999; 44(3):269–274.
33. Chi IC. The progestin-only pills and the levonorgestrel-releasing IUD: two progestin-only contraceptives. Clin Obstet Gynecol 1995; 38(4):872–889.
34. Sator-Katzenschlager SM, Scharbert G, Kress HG, et al. Chronic pelvic pain treated with gabapentin and amitriptyline: a randomized controlled pilot study. Wien Klin Wochenschr 2005; 117(21/22):761–768.
35. Walker EA, Sullivan MD, Stenchever MA. Use of antidepressants in the management of women with chronic pelvic pain. Obstet Gynecol Clin North Am 1993; 20(4):743–751.
36. Portenoy RK. Current pharmacotherapy of chronic pain. J Pain Symptom Manage 2000; 19(suppl 1):S16–S20.
37. Bondanelli M, Ambrosio MR, Franceschetti P, et al. Effect of delta-opioid receptor agonist deltorphin on circulating concentrations of luteinizing hormone and follicle stimulating hormone in healthy fertile women. Hum Reprod 1998; 13(5):1159–1162.
38. Tu FF, Beaumont JL. Outpatient laparoscopy for abdominal and pelvic pain in the United States 1994 through 1996. Am J Obstet Gynecol 2006; 194(3):699–703.
39. Abbott JA, Hawe J, Clayton RD, et al. The effects and effectiveness of laparoscopic excision of endometriosis: a prospective study with 2–5 year follow-up. Hum Reprod 2003; 18(9):1922–1927.
40. Hillis SD, Marchbanks PA, Peterson HB. The effectiveness of hysterectomy for chronic pelvic pain. Obstet Gynecol 1995; 86(6):941–945.
41. Swank DJ, Swank-Bordewijk SC, Hop WC, et al. Laparoscopic adhesiolysis in patients with chronic abdominal pain: a blinded randomised controlled multi-centre trial. Lancet 2003; 361(9365):1247–1251.
42. Zolnoun DA, Hartmann KE, Steege JF. Overnight 5% lidocaine ointment for treatment of vulvar vestibulitis. Obstet Gynecol 2003; 102(1):84–87.
43. Zullo F, Palomba S, Zupi E, et al. Effectiveness of presacral neurectomy in women with severe dysmenorrhea caused by endometriosis who were treated with laparoscopic conservative surgery: a 1-year prospective randomized double-blind controlled trial. Am J Obstet Gynecol 2003; 189(1):5–10.
44. Chen FP, Chang SD, Chu KK, et al. Comparison of laparoscopic presacral neurectomy and laparoscopic uterine nerve ablation for primary dysmenorrhea. J Reprod Med 1996; 41(7):463–466.
45. Whorwell PJ, Altringer L, Morel J, et al. Efficacy of an encapsulated probiotic Bifidobacterium infantis 35624 in women with irritable bowel syndrome. Am J Gastroenterol 2006; 101(7):1581–1590.
46. Shorter B, Lesser M, Moldwin RM, et al. Effect of comestibles on symptoms of interstitial cystitis. J Urol 2007; 178(1):145–152.

18 Cancer Pain

Judith A. Paice

Cancer Pain Program, Division of Hematology–Oncology, Feinberg School of Medicine, Northwestern University, Chicago, Illinois, U.S.A.

THE DISORDER

Cancer remains one of the most common life-threatening illnesses seen today, with approximately 1.5 million new cases diagnosed in the United States each year. Cancer is the cause of death for over one-half million people. Furthermore, this is a global problem as 6.6 million people die from cancer around the world annually. Cancer pain is relatively common and is greatly feared. The prevalence of cancer pain ranges from 14% to 100%, with approximately 20% to 75% reporting pain at the time of diagnosis and 23% to 100% of those with advanced disease experiencing pain (1). As people are diagnosed with cancer earlier and have greater access to more effective, life-prolonging and, in some cases, curative treatments, the prevalence of pain will likely increase. Another factor leading to increased rates of pain is the use of more neurotoxic anticancer therapies.

Despite its prevalence, cancer pain remains underrecognized, often with disastrous results. The consequences of inadequate cancer pain relief include increased physiological stress, diminished immunocompetence, decreased functional status, and potential enhanced risk for the complications of immobility, such as pneumonia and thromboembolism, as well as diminished survival (2). Neuronal plasticity along with hyperalgesia and allodynia can occur. Additionally, pain most certainly leads to social isolation, despair, and ultimately impaired quality of life. Finally, caregivers and loved ones suffer distress long after observing their family member in pain. Those at particular risk for undertreatment of pain include children, older adults, minorities, those individuals from lower socioeconomic groups and the uninsured, women, non–English-speaking patients, and those with a history of substance abuse (3, 4).

DIAGNOSIS

Universal screening of all patients with cancer should be conducted during any encounter with the health-care system, including presentation at clinic or when hospitalized (5). Any indication of the presence of pain warrants a comprehensive assessment, since this is an essential first step to determining the etiology of the pain and developing a treatment plan. Assessment includes a detailed pain history, with attention to the past and current medication history, along with careful physical assessment. Awareness of the presence of other symptoms is critical, as fatigue, dyspnea, constipation, and mood disturbances are common and should be addressed when developing a plan of care. Assessment of functional impairment also contributes to the treatment plan, leading to consults for physical and occupational therapy, along with teaching regarding safety measures (e.g., assistive devices, need for caregivers in the home).

Diagnostic evaluation (e.g., MRI, CT, laboratory testing) may be ordered if it will contribute to the treatment plan and is consistent with the goals of care. For example, in patients with more advanced disease at the end of life, testing may yield little data that will inform the analgesic regimen and may instead lead to greater discomfort.

Assessment Tools

Several assessment tools have been validated for use in cancer populations, most notably the Brief Pain Inventory, which is available in numerous languages. The Brief Pain Inventory, a clinically useful pain assessment tool that has been used extensively in people with cancer, includes a diagram to note the location of pain, questions regarding pain intensity (current, average, worst using a 0–10 rating scale), as well as items that gauge impairment due to pain. Other tools incorporate assessment of multiple symptoms common in cancer including the Edmonton Symptom Assessment Scale, the M.D. Anderson Symptom Inventory, and the Memorial Symptom Assessment Scale (6–8).

PATHOPHYSIOLOGY

Because of the heterogeneous nature of cancer pain, there is no one pathophysiological mechanism. Broadly, most cancer pain syndromes related to the tumor are due to underlying damage to surrounding tissues (Table 1). Syndromes associated with cancer treatment may be related to surgery or other invasive procedures, chemotherapy, radiation therapy, hormonal therapy, or other antitumor or supportive treatment (Table 2). The underlying mechanisms of these pains vary

TABLE 1 Cancer Pain Syndromes Associated with Tumor Involvement (58–61)

Bone metastases
  Bone marrow expansion
  Base of skull involvement
  Local infiltration
  Vertebral syndrome
  Back pain and cord compression
Headache and facial pain
  Primary or metastatic brain tumors
  Trigeminal, facial nerve involvement
Muscle pain
  Cramping and pain usually due to skeletal tumors
Visceral pain
  Hepatic capsule distension
  Retroperitoneal syndrome
  Malignant bowel obstruction
  Ureteral obstruction
Neuropathies/plexopathies
  Mono or polyneuropathies
  Cauda equina syndrome
Paraneoplastic syndromes
  Osteoarthropathy
  Sensorimotor peripheral neuropathy

TABLE 2   Pain Syndromes Secondary to Cancer Treatment (11, 60–63)

Chemotherapy
   Avascular necrosis
   Mucositis
   Painful peripheral neuropathy
Aromatase inhibitors
   Arthralgias/myalgias
Hormonal therapy
   Bone pain flare
   Gynecomastia in men treated for prostate cancer
Procedure-related pain
   Bone marrow aspiration or biopsy
   Lumbar puncture
   Paracentesis
   Thoracentesis
   Venipuncture
Radiation
   Enteritis and proctitis
   Fibrosis
   Neuropathy (e.g., brachial or sacral plexus involvement)
   Osteoradionecrosis
   Radiopharmaceutical induced pain flare (e.g., Strontium-89)
Surgery
   Frozen shoulder
   Lymphedema
   Phantom limb pain
   Postsurgical syndromes
      Postmastectomy syndrome
      Postnephrectomy syndrome
      Postradical neck dissection
      Postthoracotomy syndrome

---

greatly. There are likely other factors, such as rapid weight loss or secondary infections, which can also lead to cancer pain.

Consideration of common cancer pain syndromes will inform the assessment, lead to more accurate diagnosis, and result in tailored treatment strategies. Cancer pain can be categorized by its duration (acute vs. chronic), the intensity (mild, moderate, or severe), the quality of the pain (neuropathic, nociceptive, or mixed), and its temporal pattern (continuous, breakthrough, or both). Another strategy for categorization is by etiology, including pain directly related to the tumor, pain related to treatment, or pain unrelated to these factors. Of particular importance is the evolving field of chemotherapy-induced painful peripheral neuropathies.

Chemotherapy-Induced Painful Peripheral Neuropathies

Chemotherapy-induced painful peripheral neuropathies are increasing in importance, in part, due to the increasing numbers of neurotoxic agents being used (Table 3). These sensory neuropathies are bilateral, affecting distal areas in a stocking–glove distribution. Patients experience significant paresthesias and dysesthesias, with cold sensitivity and, often, proprioceptive changes (9). Functional impairment occurs as sensory changes lead to difficulties with normal

TABLE 3 Chemotherapeutic Agents Most
Commonly Associated with Peripheral
Neuropathy (9,11)

Platinum-based agents
Carboplatin
Cisplatin
Oxaliplatin
Taxanes
Docetaxel
Paclitaxel
Nanoparticle albumin formation of paclitaxel
Immunomodulatory agents
Thalidomide
Lenalidomide
Vinca alkaloids
Vinblastine
Vincristine
Vinorelbine
Proteasome inhibitor
Bortezomib

tasks, particularly those requiring fine tactile sensation such as buttoning or picking up small items. Proprioceptive changes lead to safety concerns, as these individuals are at risk for falls and dropping items. They cannot sense the temperature of bath water, for example, leading to burns. For most, but not all chemotherapeutic agents, neuropathies occur in a dose-dependent fashion, and there is often a delay of approximately two weeks from administration to onset of pain (10). Little is known about the true prevalence, risk factors, time to resolution, and potential for persistent pain.

The consequences of chemotherapy-induced painful peripheral neuropathies can be profound. Reductions in potentially curative doses of drug, or even cessation of chemotherapy treatment can occur (11). Furthermore, for some patients, the neuropathies do not resolve, leaving them with severe, persistent chronic pain and impairments in activities of daily living.

Breakthrough Pain

Finally, although not unique to cancer pain, breakthrough pain is quite common in this population. Cancer patients experience breakthrough pains several times each day, with each episode lasting from a few moments to many minutes, often occurring without warning (12). Several types of breakthrough pain have been well categorized, including incident pain (pain associated with specific activities), spontaneous pain (no obvious etiology or trigger), and end-of-dose failure (pain that occurs toward the end of the usual dosing interval of a regularly scheduled analgesic). In one study of cancer patients near the end of life, 93% had breakthrough pain with 72% of the episodes related to movement or weight bearing.

TREATMENT

The management of cancer pain includes pharmacological interventions, antitumor therapies, along with nonpharmacological techniques. Because a significant percentage of people will progress and eventually die from their disease, awareness of care of those with advanced cancer is critical.

Pharmacological Therapies

Pharmacological therapies used to treat cancer pain include nonopioids, opioids, and adjuvant analgesics, discussed in depth in chapters 23, 24, 26 and 27. Specific cancer-related applications of each of these agents are addressed below. As with other complex pain syndromes, multimodal therapies are indicated. Combination therapies, such as opioids and anticonvulsant medications, have been shown to provide better relief than when given individually (13).

Nonopioids

Acetaminophen

Acetaminophen is analgesic and antipyretic but has limited anti-inflammatory effect, a common mechanism of bone pain in cancer. The maximum recommended dose is 4000 mg/day, although this does not take into account hepatic dysfunction, limited oral intake in the patient with anorexia, or other factors that may alter metabolism (14). Dose adjustment should be made for individuals with hepatic dysfunction, including those patients with liver metastases and individuals who use alcohol. Careful attention to over-the-counter drugs is indicated during the history as acetaminophen is common in these medications, leading to inadvertent overdose (15).

Nonsteroidal Anti-inflammatory Drugs

Nonsteroidal anti-inflammatory drugs (NSAIDs) are analgesic, antipyretic, and anti-inflammatory; thus, they can be effective agents in the treatment of cancer-related pain (16). The adverse effects associated with NSAIDS are of particular concern, including gastrointestinal bleeding, renal dysfunction, and clotting abnormalities (17). NSAIDs should be avoided in persons with multiple myeloma due to their high risk for renal dysfunction, as well as in patients receiving chemotherapeutic agents that can cause thrombocytopenia.

Opioids

The pharmacology of opioids has been thoroughly reviewed in chapter 24. Pure agonists are the primary opioids used in cancer pain management in the United States. There is no role for mixed agonist–antagonist agents in cancer pain control (18). Although partial agonists, such as transdermal buprenorphine, are used in Europe, the lack of an oral immediate-release formulation in the United States prohibits its use in cancer pain management.

Multiple routes of administration are warranted in cancer care. For example, mucositis or dysphagia due to irradiation of or tumor in the aerodigestive system can lead to inability to tolerate oral administration of opioids. Alternatives to oral opioid administration are described in Table 4. Additionally, long-acting (or sustained release) formulations are indicated in this population. Generally, the patient is first titrated using an immediate-release compound until an effective dose is determined and that dose is then converted to one of the available long-acting formulations. Selection is based upon efficacy of a particular opioid; the need for an oral, enteral, or transdermal delivery method; support

TABLE 4   Alternate Routes of Drug Administration Useful in Cancer Populations (64, 65)

Buccal, sublingual, and transmucosal

Buccal fentanyl is now commercially available, with a more rapid onset of effect when compared with immediate-release oral morphine.

Sublingual administration can be used with buccal tablets. Liquid morphine is often given sublingually to patients at the end of life or those who cannot swallow; however, due to the hydrophilic nature of morphine, the medication is not being absorbed by this route. Rather, the liquid is gradually trickling down the back of the throat and absorbed enterally. This is effective and acceptable as long as the volume is not so high as to lead to aspiration.

OTFC provides rapid onset for breakthrough pain.

Enteral

Opioids and other analgesics can be administered *via* feeding tube when compounded as a liquid or crushed and delivered in solution.

Medications can be placed rectally or in an ostomy, either in commercially available suppository preparations, or by placing the tablet directly into the orifice. Long-acting oral opioid preparations have been used in this manner when patients can no longer swallow.

Nasal

Currently, no opioids are commercially available for people with cancer (the only commercially produced product, butorphanol, is contraindicated as it is a mixed agonist–antagonist).

Studies are under way examining the use of intranasal fentanyl.

Parenteral

Intravenous and subcutaneous; intramuscular route is not recommended due to the lack of muscle mass in most cachectic patients, the variability in uptake of the drug, and the pain caused by this route of administration.

May incorporate intermittent injections, continuous infusions, or patient-controlled analgesia.

Spinal

Epidural or intrathecal.

Opioids may be given in combination with local anesthetics or other agents.

Delivery method, including external catheters or implanted ports or pumps, should be determined based upon projected life span of patient and the capacity of caregivers to manage the technique.

Transdermal

Fentanyl is commercially available for transdermal delivery in 12.5, 25, 50, 75 and 100 μg/hr formulations.

There is no evidence to support the use of topical morphine or other hydrophilic opioids applied to intact skin for pain control.

Abbreviation: OTFC, oral transmucosal fentanyl citrate.

in the home to adhere to a particular regimen; preference; and cost. Options are included in Table 5. Along with a long-acting opioid, short-acting opioids are indicated to manage breakthrough pain. Breakthrough dosing of oral opioids is generally 10% to 20% of the 24-hour oral dose. This can be administered as frequently as every hour.

Adverse Effects

Side effects of opioids are generally preventable or easily managed in most individuals with cancer (19). Nausea can occur when patients are first exposed to an opioid; providing an around-the-clock antiemetic for the first 24 to 48 hours in patients who have experienced this adverse effect of opioids in the past can manage this effect. Since many people with cancer have already been treated with an antiemetic during chemotherapy administration, select an antiemetic that has been well tolerated by the patient in the past, such as phenothiazines, including

TABLE 5 Long-Acting Opioid Formulations Used in Cancer Pain Management (66–68)

Long-acting morphine
  Tablets are administered every 12 hr, although some patients require 8-hr dosing.
  Capsules are administered daily, can be opened and sprinkled in applesauce for patients who can swallow soft items but not pills; these can also be placed in some enteral feeding tubes as long as the volume is low.
Long-acting oxycodone
  Tablets are administered every 12 hr, although 8-hr delivery is occasionally warranted.
Long-acting oxymorphone
  Tablets are administered every 12 hr.
Transdermal fentanyl
  Transdermal fentanyl is applied as a patch every 72 hr, although some patients require change in patch every 48 hr.
Methadone
  Advantages include low cost; efficacy in neuropathic pain (likely due to biding at mu opioid receptors and as an antagonist at the NMDA receptor); ability to be administered every 8 hr for pain relief; and availability in oral tablets, liquid, and parenteral formulations.
  Challenges include its long half-life (approximately 15–60 hr), thus necessitating very slow titration, numerous drug–drug interactions, prolonged QT interval, and complicated equianalgesic dosing.

Abbreviation: NMDA, *N*-methyl-D-aspartate.

prochlorperazine, or prokinetic agents such as metoclopramide. In more refractory cases, haloperidol or dexamethasone may be effective. Serotonin 5-HT3 receptor antagonists likely have limited utility in the management of prolonged opioid-induced nausea and vomiting. Other potential causes of nausea, such as malignant bowel obstruction, concomitant medications, or increased pressure from intracranial metastases, should be ruled out.

Constipation occurs in the majority of those requiring opioids for pain control, and prevention is usually effective using a combination stimulant laxative/softener, such as senna and docusate. As the dose of opioid is increased, the dose of laxative/softener generally needs to be titrated upward. If patients are unable to swallow or are too weak to generate the maneuvers necessary to evacuate the stool, laxative suppositories (such as bisacodyl) are indicated. Dietary changes, bulking agents such as methylcellulose, and increased fluid intake are rarely sufficient to counteract the constipating effects of opioid therapy in people with cancer. Methylnaltrexone is a peripherally acting opioid antagonist that has been shown to reliably reverse the effects of opioid-induced constipation when given subcutaneously at a dose of 0.15 mg/kg. The majority of patients respond within four hours (20).

Sedation is a common symptom in persons with cancer and may be related, in part, to opioid administration. It is generally managed by switching to an alternate opioid (opioid "rotation" or "switching") or adding a psychostimulant, such as methylphenidate. In one study that allowed doses up to 20 mg/day taken at any time (morning, afternoon, or evening), patients were found to have relief of sedation, reduced fatigue, improved appetite, as well as enhanced nighttime sleep (21). Doses as high as 60 mg or more have been described as safe and effective. Interestingly, a subsequent randomized trial failed to demonstrate any superiority of methylphenidate over placebo (22).

Myoclonus is a neurotoxicity of opioid administration and has been reported with all opioids. This syndrome is usually seen with higher doses of opioid, with concomitant renal dysfunction, and is more common in advanced malignancy (23–26). Treatment includes adding a benzodiazepine, such as clonazepam 0.5 mg orally twice daily, or midazolam if the parenteral route is warranted. Opioid rotation may be effective. In advanced cases that are refractory to treatment, where patients may have hours to days to live, palliative sedation may be indicated.

Adjuvant Analgesics

Adjuvant analgesics used in oncology include anticonvulsants, antidepressants, corticosteroids, and local anesthetics. These are key components of the multimodal therapy necessary to treat cancer pain, generally in combination with opioids. In more complicated pain syndromes, N-methyl-D-aspartate (NMDA) antagonists, such as ketamine, may be employed.

Antidepressants

Tricyclic antidepressants inhibit reuptake of norepinephrine and serotonin (27). Although not specific to cancer pain, a recent consensus panel listed this category as one of several first-line therapies for the management of neuropathic pains (28). Amitriptyline has significant adverse effects that are generally not well tolerated in the cancer population, yet other agents such as nortriptyline can be useful (29). Cardiac arrhythmias, conduction abnormalities, narrow-angle glaucoma, and clinically significant prostatic hyperplasia are relative contraindications to the tricyclic antidepressants (30). Their sleep-enhancing and mood-elevating effects may be of benefit in selected cancer patients. The delay in onset of pain relief of days to weeks may preclude the use of these agents for pain relief in patients with limited life expectancy.

Atypical antidepressants, including venlafaxine, has been shown to reduce neuropathy associated with chemotherapy-induced painful neuropathy and has the added advantage of treating hot flashes, a common phenomenon in oncology patients (31, 32). Duloxetine is a useful alternative.

Anticonvulsants

Older anticonvulsants, such as carbamazepine, are effective at relieving neuropathic pain, likely by blocking sodium channels. However, serious adverse effects associated with this agent, including aplastic anemia and hepatic dysfunction, limit its use in oncology. Newer agents are quite effective in cancer care (33). Gabapentin and pregabalin are generally well tolerated. The more common reasons for stopping the drug in this population are dizziness and fluid retention. Other anticonvulsants have been used with success in treating neuropathies, including lamotrigine, levetiracetam, tiagabine, topiramate, and zonisamide, yet no randomized controlled clinical trials in cancer are currently available (34).

Corticosteroids

Corticosteroids are particularly useful for relief of bone pain, neuropathic pain syndromes, including plexopathies, and visceral pain, including malignant bowel obstruction and pain associated with stretching of the liver capsule due to metastases (35). Dexamethasone produces the least amount of mineralocorticoid effect and is available in oral, intravenous, subcutaneous, and epidural formulations. The standard dose is 4 to 24 mg/day and can be administered once daily due to the long half-life of this drug. Intravenous bolus doses should be pushed slowly to prevent uncomfortable perineal burning and itching.

Local Anesthetics

Local anesthetics inhibit the movement of ions across the neural membrane and are useful for relieving neuropathic pain. Local anesthetics can be given orally, topically, intravenously, subcutaneously, or spinally. Gels have been used to prevent the pain associated with needle stick and other minor procedures. Lidocaine patches have been shown to reduce the pain of postherpetic neuropathy, a syndrome common in malignancy (36). Although historically used as a monthly infusion in chronic pain clinics, similar protocols using lidocaine have been adapted for use in patients with intractable pain at end of life. Intravenous lidocaine at 1 to 2 mg/kg administered over 30 to 60 minutes, followed by a continuous infusion of 1 to 2 mg/kg/hr has been reported to reduce intractable neuropathic pain in patients in inpatient palliative care and home hospice settings (37). Immediate signs of toxicity include numbness around the lips or a sensation of thickness of the tongue. These symptoms of toxicity are transient and easily reversible by lowering the infusion rate. Finally, epidural or intrathecal lidocaine or bupivacaine, usually delivered with an opioid, can reduce neuropathic pain (38).

NMDA Antagonists

Ketamine, a dissociative anesthetic, is thought to relieve severe neuropathic pain by blocking NMDA receptors. Routine use often is limited by cognitive changes and other adverse effects and a Cochrane review found insufficient trials conducted to determine safety and efficacy in cancer pain (39). However, in cases of intractable neuropathic pain, or in attempting to limit opioid doses due to adverse effects, ketamine can provide benefit (40). In a small ($n = 10$) study of cancer patients who reported pain unrelieved with morphine, a slow bolus of ketamine (0.25 or 0.50 mg/kg) was evaluated using a randomized, double-blind, crossover, double-dose design. Ketamine significantly reduced the pain intensity in almost all the patients at both doses, with the greatest effect being in those treated with higher doses. Adverse effects, including hallucinations and unpleasant cognitive sensations, responded to diazepam 1 mg intravenously (41). The investigators concluded that ketamine improved morphine analgesia in a variety of difficult pain syndromes, yet central adverse effects can limit the use of this therapy. Another study of young children and adolescents who were on high doses of opioids and had uncontrolled cancer pain, examined the effect of adding a low-dose ketamine infusion. In 8 of 11 patients, ketamine infusions used as an adjuvant to opioid analgesia provided improvement in pain and were associated with opioid-sparing effects. This resulted in reduction in opioid dose that ultimately improved social interaction (42).

Ketamine is given by a variety of routes: oral, intravenous, subcutaneous, intranasal, sublingual, epidural, intrathecal, and topical (43). The usual oral dose of ketamine is 10 to 15 mg every six hours. Because oral preparations are not commercially available in the United States, the solution used for injection is administered orally, usually mixed with juice or cola to hide the bitter taste.

Parenteral dosing is typically 0.04 mg/kg/hr with titration to a maximum of 0.3 mg/kg/hr. Onset of analgesia is 15 to 30 minutes with a duration of effect ranging between 15 minutes and 2 hours. A general recommendation is to reduce the opioid dose by approximately 25% to 50% when starting ketamine to avoid sedation. Severe side effects are generally associated with doses of parenteral ketamine above 0.5 mg/kg and include psychotomimetic phenomena such as dysphoria, nightmares, hallucinations, excessive salivation, and tachycardia (44).

Anticancer Therapies

Radiation Therapy and Radiopharmaceuticals
Radiotherapy is an essential treatment option in the relief of pain and is particularly beneficial in relieving pain due to bone metastases or other lesions (45). In many cases, single-fraction external-beam therapy can be used to facilitate treatment (46). Additionally, radiosurgery is being used with greater frequency for solitary lesions (47). Radiolabeled agents such as strontium-89 and samarium-153 have been shown to be highly effective at reducing widespread metastatic bone pain (48). Thrombocytopenia and leukopenia are relative contraindications since radionuclides can cause bone marrow suppression. Because there is a delayed onset of effect, radiopharmaceuticals should be considered only in those patients with a projected life span of greater than three months. A transitory pain flare is reported by as many as 10% of individuals receiving strontium-89; thus, patient education and additional analgesics are warranted.

Chemotherapy
Palliative chemotherapy has been shown to relieve pain when the underlying mechanism is related to the tumor (49). When considering this option, patient goals, their performance status, the sensitivity of the tumor to chemotherapy, and potential toxicities must be carefully weighed. Honest communication with the patient and family must include the goals of this therapy (palliate vs. cure) so that expectations are realistic.

Bisphosphonates
Bisphosphonates inhibit osteoclast-mediated bone resorption, thereby reducing pain related to metastatic bone disease. These agents are also used to prevent skeletal complications and to treat hypercalcemia (50, 51). Pamidronate disodium has been shown to reduce pain, hypercalcemia, and skeletal morbidity associated with breast cancer and multiple myeloma. The drug is administered as an intravenous infusion and dosing is generally repeated every four weeks, with an analgesic effect typically seen in two to four weeks. Zoledronic acid has been shown to relieve pain due to metastatic bone disease and is somewhat more convenient in that it can be infused over a shorter duration of time (50). Risedronate, alendronate, and ibandronate are oral formulations taken daily or weekly, weekly, and monthly, respectively. Therapy should be discontinued and parenteral delivery of other agents considered when patients are unable to sit up for at least 30 to 60 minutes after swallowing the tablets.

Concerns regarding osteonecrosis of the jaw in patients who have been given bisphosphonates have led to particular care in the use of these agents

(52). Dental evaluation prior to initiating therapy is crucial as poor dentition is thought to be a risk factor.

Interventional Therapies

Interventional therapies are of significant benefit in cancer pain relief, including nerve blocks, vertebroplasty, radiofrequency ablation of painful metastases, procedures to drain painful effusions, and other techniques. Nevertheless, few of these procedures have undergone controlled clinical studies, particularly in cancer pain. One technique, the celiac plexus block, has been shown to be superior to morphine in patients with pain due to unresectable pancreatic cancer (53). Selection of these techniques is dependent upon the availability of experts in this area who understand the special needs of cancer patients, the patient's ability to undergo the procedure, and the patient and family's goals of care.

Nonpharmacological Therapies

Nondrug therapies, including cognitive–behavioral techniques and physical measures, can serve as adjuncts to analgesic management in cancer pain management. These strategies are particularly useful to address periods of increased pain intensity, while waiting for the onset of the immediate-release analgesic. The patient's and caregivers' interest and ability to participate must be considered when selecting one of these therapies, including their fatigue level, belief in the use of these types of techniques, cognitive ability, and other factors.

Cognitive–Behavioral Therapies

Cognitive–behavioral therapy includes strategies that improve coping, reframe the meaning of pain and the disease experience, as well as enhance relaxation (54). Examples include art and music therapy, distraction, guided imagery, education, and prayer. One randomized clinical trial of patients undergoing bone marrow transplantation revealed a reduction in pain in those patients who received relaxation and imagery training and in those who received cognitive–behavioral skill development with relaxation and imagery (55). Patients who received treatment as usual or who were randomized to receive support from a therapist demonstrated no such benefit. These therapies may serve to relieve symptoms in addition to pain. For example, a prospective study of art therapy in an inpatient cancer unit revealed a significant reduction in pain, anxiety, fatigue, and other symptoms (56).

Physical measures, such as active or passive range of motion, massage, reflexology, heat, chiropractic, and other techniques, can relieve pain (57). In a study of male cancer patients, a 10-minute massage was found to relieve pain. These are simple, relatively inexpensive procedures that can incorporate family members and other caregivers, who are often seeking strategies to demonstrate support of their loved one.

REFERENCES

1. van den Beuken-van Everdingen MH, de Rijke JM, Kessels AG, et al. Prevalence of pain in patients with cancer: a systematic review of the past 40 years. Ann Oncol 2007; 18(9):1437–1449.

2. Halabi S, Vogelzang NJ, Kornblith AB, et al. Pain predicts overall survival in men with metastatic castration-refractory prostate cancer. J Clin Oncol 2008; 26(15):2544–2549.
3. Potter J, Hami F, Bryan T, et al. Symptoms in 400 patients referred to palliative care services: prevalence and patterns. Palliat Med 2003; 17(4):310–314.
4. Soares LG. Poor social conditions, criminality and urban violence: unmentioned barriers for effective cancer pain control at the end of life. J Pain Symptom Manage 2003; 26(2):693–695.
5. Miaskowski C, Cleary J, Burney R, et al. Guideline for the management of cancer pain in adults and children. APS Clinical Practice Guideline Series, No. 3. Glenview, IL: American Pain Society, 2005.
6. Chang VT, Hwang SS, Feuerman M, et al. The memorial symptom assessment scale short form (MSAS-SF). Cancer 2000; 89(5):1162–1171.
7. Cleeland CS, Mendoza TR, Wang XS, et al. Assessing symptom distress in cancer patients: the M.D. Anderson Symptom Inventory. Cancer 2000; 89(7):1634–1646.
8. Paice JA. Assessment of symptom clusters in people with cancer. J Natl Cancer Inst Monogr 2004; (32):98–102.
9. Hausheer FH, Schilsky RL, Bain S, et al. Diagnosis, management, and evaluation of chemotherapy-induced peripheral neuropathy. Semin Oncol 2006; 33(1):15–49.
10. Lee JJ, Swain SM. Peripheral neuropathy induced by microtubule-stabilizing agents. J Clin Oncol 2006; 24(10):1633–1642.
11. Windebank AJ, Grisold W. Chemotherapy-induced neuropathy. J Peripher Nerv Syst 2008; 13(1):27–46.
12. Caraceni A, Martini C, Zecca E, et al. Breakthrough pain characteristics and syndromes in patients with cancer pain. An international survey. Palliat Med 2004; 18(3):177–183.
13. Gilron I, Bailey JM, Tu D, et al. Morphine, gabapentin, or their combination for neuropathic pain. N Engl J Med 2005; 352(13):1324–1334.
14. Tanaka E, Yamazaki K, Misawa S. Update: the clinical importance of acetaminophen hepatotoxicity in non-alcoholic and alcoholic subjects. J Clin Pharm Ther 2000; 25(5):325–332.
15. Schiodt FV, Rochling FA, Casey DL, et al. Acetaminophen toxicity in an urban county hospital. N Engl J Med 1997; 337(16):1112–1117.
16. Mercadante S. The use of anti-inflammatory drugs in cancer pain. Can Treat Rev 2001; 27(1):51–61.
17. Wolfe MM, Lichtenstein DR, Singh G. Gastrointestinal toxicity of nonsteroidal antiinflammatory drugs. N Engl J Med 1999; 340(24):1888–1899.
18. Hanks GW, Conno F, Cherny N, et al. Morphine and alternative opioids in cancer pain: the EAPC recommendations. Br J Cancer 2001; 84(5):587–593.
19. Cherny N, Ripamonti C, Pereira J, et al. Strategies to manage the adverse effects of oral morphine: an evidence-based report. J Clin Oncol 2001; 19(9):2542–2554.
20. Thomas J, Karver S, Cooney GA, et al. Methylnaltrexone for opioid-induced constipation in advanced illness. N Engl J Med 2008; 358(22):2332–2343.
21. Bruera E, Driver L, Barnes EA, et al. Patient-controlled methylphenidate for the management of fatigue in patients with advanced cancer: a preliminary report. J Clin Oncol 2003; 21(23):4439–4443.
22. Bruera E, Valero V, Driver L, et al. Patient-controlled methylphenidate for cancer fatigue: a double-blind, randomized, placebo-controlled trial. J Clin Oncol 2006; 24(13):2073–2078.
23. Smith MT. Neuroexcitatory effects of morphine and hydromorphone: evidence implicating the 3-glucuronide metabolites. Clin Exp Pharmacol Physiol 2000; 27(7):524–528.
24. Sarhill N, Davis MP, Walsh D, et al. Methadone-induced myoclonus in advanced cancer. Am J Hosp Palliat Care 2001; 18(1):51–53.
25. Wright AW, Mather LE, Smith MT. Hydromorphone-3-glucuronide: a more potent neuro-excitant than its structural analogue, morphine-3-glucuronide. Life Sci 2001; 69(4):409–420.

26. Patel S, Roshan VR, Lee KC, et al. A myoclonic reaction with low-dose hydromorphone. Ann Pharmacother 2006; 40(11):2068–2070.

27. Hammack JE, Michalak JC, Loprinzi CL, et al. Phase III evaluation of nortriptyline for alleviation of symptoms of *cis*-platinum-induced peripheral neuropathy. Pain 2002; 98(1–2):195–203.

28. Dworkin RH, O'Connor AB, Backonja M, et al. Pharmacologic management of neuropathic pain: evidence-based recommendations. Pain 2007; 132(3):237–251.

29. Mercadante S, Arcuri E, Tirelli W, et al. Amitriptyline in neuropathic cancer pain in patients on morphine therapy: a randomized placebo-controlled, double-blind crossover study. Tumori 2002; 88(3):239–242.

30. Saarto T, Wiffen PJ. Antidepressants for neuropathic pain. Cochrane Database Syst Rev 2007; (4):CD005454.

31. Tasmuth T, Hartel B, Kalso E. Venlafaxine in neuropathic pain following treatment of breast cancer. Eur J Pain 2002; 6(1):17–24.

32. Durand JP, Goldwasser F. Dramatic recovery of paclitaxel-disabling neurosensory toxicity following treatment with venlafaxine. Anticancer Drugs 2002; 13(7):777–780.

33. Grothey A. Clinical management of oxaliplatin-associated neurotoxicity. Clin Colorectal Cancer 2005; 5(suppl 1):S38–S46.

34. Farrar JT, Portenoy RK. Neuropathic cancer pain: the role of adjuvant analgesics. Oncology (Huntington) 2001; 15(11):1435–1442.

35. Wooldridge JE, Anderson CM, Perry MC. Corticosteroids in advanced cancer. Oncology (Williston Park) 2001; 15(2):225–234.

36. Argoff CE, Galer BS, Jensen MP, et al. Effectiveness of the lidocaine patch 5% on pain qualities in three chronic pain states: assessment with the neuropathic pain scale. Curr Med Res Opin 2004; 20(suppl 2):S21–S28.

37. Ferrini R, Paice JA. How to initiate and monitor infusional lidocaine for severe and/or neuropathic pain. J Support Oncol 2004; 2(1):90–94.

38. Deer TR, Caraway DL, Kim CK, et al. Clinical experience with intrathecal bupivacaine in combination with opioid for the treatment of chronic pain related to failed back surgery syndrome and metastatic cancer pain of the spine. Spine J 2002; 2(4):274–278.

39. Bell R, Eccleston C, Kalso E. Ketamine as an adjuvant to opioids for cancer pain. Cochrane Database Syst Rev 2003; (1):CD003351.

40. Legge J, Ball N, Elliott DP. The potential role of ketamine in hospice analgesia: a literature review. Consult Pharm 2006; 21(1):51–57.

41. Mercadante S, Arcuri E, Tirelli W, et al. Analgesic effect of intravenous ketamine in cancer patients on morphine therapy: a randomized, controlled, double-blind, crossover, double-dose study. J Pain Symptom Manage 2000; 20(4):246–252.

42. Finkel JC, Pestieau SR, Quezado ZM. Ketamine as an adjuvant for treatment of cancer pain in children and adolescents. J Pain 2007; 8(6):515–521.

43. Lossignol DA, Obiols-Portis M, Body JJ. Successful use of ketamine for intractable cancer pain. Support Care Cancer 2005; 13(3):188–193.

44. Fitzgibbon EJ, Viola R. Parenteral ketamine as an analgesic adjuvant for severe pain: development and retrospective audit of a protocol for a palliative care unit. J Palliat Med 2005; 8(1):49–57.

45. Janjan N. Palliation and supportive care in radiation medicine. Hematol Oncol Clin North Am 2006; 20(1):187–211.

46. Jeremic B. Single fraction external beam radiation therapy in the treatment of localized metastatic bone pain. A review. J Pain Symptom Manage 2001; 22(6):1048–1058.

47. Ryu S, Jin R, Jin JY, et al. Pain control by image-guided radiosurgery for solitary spinal metastasis. J Pain Symptom Manage 2008; 35(3):292–298.

48. Maini CL, Sciuto R, Romano L, et al. Radionuclide therapy with bone seeking radionuclides in palliation of painful bone metastases. J Exp Clin Cancer Res 2003; 22(4 suppl):71–74.

49. Prommer E. Guidelines for the use of palliative chemotherapy. AAHPM Bull 2004; 5:1–4.

50. Berenson JR. Zoledronic acid in cancer patients with bone metastases: results of Phase I and II trials. Semin Oncol 2001; 28(2 suppl 6):25–34.
51. Walker K, Medhurst SJ, Kidd BL, et al. Disease modifying and anti-nociceptive effects of the bisphosphonate, zoledronic acid in a model of bone cancer pain. Pain 2002; 100(3):219–229.
52. Marx RE, Sawatari Y, Fortin M, et al. Bisphosphonate-induced exposed bone (osteonecrosis/osteopetrosis) of the jaws: risk factors, recognition, prevention, and treatment [see comment]. J Oral Maxillofac Surg 2005; 63(11):1567–1575.
53. Mercadante S, Fulfaro F, Casuccio A. Pain mechanisms involved and outcome in advanced cancer patients with possible indications for celiac plexus block and superior hypogastric plexus block. Tumori 2002; 88(3):243–245.
54. Robb KA, Williams JE, Duvivier V, et al. A pain management program for chronic cancer-treatment-related pain: a preliminary study. J Pain 2006; 7(2):82–90.
55. Syrjala KL, Donaldson GW, Davis MW, et al. Relaxation and imagery and cognitive–behavioral training reduce pain during cancer treatment: a controlled clinical trial. Pain 1995; 63(2):189–198.
56. Nainis N, Paice JA, Ratner J, et al. Relieving symptoms in cancer: innovative use of art therapy. J Pain Symptom Manage 2006; 31(2):162–169.
57. Ernst E. Manual therapies for pain control: chiropractic and massage. Clin J Pain 2004; 20(1):8–12.
58. Caraceni A, Weinstein SM. Classification of cancer pain syndromes. Oncology (Huntington) 2001; 15(12):1627–1640, 1642.
59. Katz N. Neuropathic pain in cancer and AIDS. Clin J Pain 2000; 16(2 suppl):S41–S48.
60. Chang VT, Janjan N, Jain S, et al. Regional cancer pain syndromes. J Palliat Med 2006; 9(6):1435–1453.
61. Chang VT, Janjan N, Jain S, et al. Update in cancer pain syndromes. J Palliat Med 2006; 9(6):1414–1434.
62. Quasthoff S, Hartung HP. Chemotherapy-induced peripheral neuropathy. J Neurol 2002; 249(1):9–17.
63. Leonard GD, Wright MA, Quinn MG, et al. Survey of oxaliplatin-associated neurotoxicity using an interview-based questionnaire in patients with metastatic colorectal cancer. BMC Cancer 2005; 5:116.
64. Paice JA, Von Roenn JH, Hudgins JC, et al. Morphine bioavailability from a topical gel formulation in volunteers. J Pain Symptom Manage 2008; 35(3):314–320.
65. Reisfield GM, Wilson GR. Rational use of sublingual opioids in palliative medicine. J Palliat Med 2007; 10(2):465–475.
66. Lauretti GR, Oliveira GM, Pereira NL. Comparison of sustained-release morphine with sustained-release oxycodone in advanced cancer patients [see comment]. Br J Cancer 2003; 89(11):2027–2030.
67. Dale O, Sheffels P, Kharasch ED. Bioavailabilities of rectal and oral methadone in healthy subjects. Br J Clin Pharmacol 2004; 58(2):156–162.
68. Centeno C, Vara F. Intermittent subcutaneous methadone administration in the management of cancer pain. J Pain Palliat Care Pharmacother 2005; 19(2):7–12.

19 Palliative Care Pain Management

Kathleen Broglio

New York University School of Medicine, Bellevue Pain Center, New York, New York, U.S.A.

PALLIATIVE CARE PAIN MANAGEMENT

Palliative care is an interdisciplinary approach for patients and families facing life-threatening illnesses. The palliative care team (physicians, nurses, social workers, pastoral counselors, psychologists, physical, occupational, music and art therapists) works to prevent and relieve suffering by participating in the management of the physical, psychological, social, and spiritual needs of patients and their families (1, 2).

Pain is one of many symptoms affecting people and their families with advanced disease. Pain management in advanced disease and at the end of life can be challenging due to multiple factors. As the disease state progresses, pain may worsen and be complicated by metabolic changes, weight loss, decreased function, psychological and existential distress. Dame Cicely Saunders, the founder of the hospice movement, uses the term "total pain" which encompasses physical, emotional, spiritual, and existential distress (3). An understanding of the physical, psychological, social, and spiritual issues important to the patient is fundamental for effective pain management through an interdisciplinary approach. Toward the end of life, goals of care may determine the setting for end of life, types of caregivers, and available modalities for pain management. Rather than winding down care at the end of life, for most people in their last weeks of life analgesic management includes analgesic rotation, dosing changes, changes in routes of administration to manage physical pain; and psychological, emotional, and spiritual support to manage "total" pain.

PREVALENCE OF PAIN AT THE END OF LIFE AND IN ADVANCED DISEASE

Pain is a significant symptom for at least 20% of the approximately 1 million people in the United States who die yearly in the hospital setting (4). Surveys indicate that the prevalence of pain ranges from 35% to 96% for hospice patients residing in nursing homes, adult cancer patients in hospice or palliative care settings, and people with terminal illness living at home (5–7).

The prevalence of pain related to cancer, which has been the most widely studied, is estimated to be 30% to 50% for people undergoing active treatment and up to 70% to 90% for those with advanced disease (8–10). Cardiovascular, renal, and pulmonary diseases account for significant end-of-life pain. For cardiovascular disease, the prevalence of pain is between 41% and 77% (11) with up to 75% of people in heart failure experiencing pain in the last six months of their lives (12). About 50% of the people with renal disease and between 34% and 77% people with chronic obstructive pulmonary disease experience pain (11). Many with these diseases have comorbidities such as osteoarthritis and diabetes, causing them even more daily pain. Pain is prevalent for people with neurological diseases such as multiple sclerosis, Parkinson's disease, and central pain related to cerebral vascular disease or spinal cord injury (13–15). The extent of pain experienced by those with dementia is unclear due to difficulty with assessment in advanced stages. However, at the end of life, functional decline, weight loss, development of skin breakdown, and contractures all are sources of pain. In a survey of caregivers of people with dementia, more than 50% reported patient pain at a moderate intensity or higher on average in the last two weeks of life (16). The prevalence of pain in people living with acquired immunodeficiency syndrome ranges from 63% to 88% (11, 17, 18), yet at the end of their lives this was observed to be 93% in an inpatient setting (19). On the basis of these statistics, it can be assumed that most people will have pain to some degree at the end of life.

CARE SETTING AND PAIN MANAGEMENT AT THE END OF LIFE
People die in a variety of settings in the United States and although surveys suggest that most people would prefer to die at home, only 25% do so. About 50% die in hospital settings and 25% in either nursing homes or other long-term care facilities (20).

Data from numerous sources suggest that rates of undertreatment of pain in advanced disease may be as high as 40% (21). Family members perceive that 40% of patients with cancer have distressing pain at the end of life, and that the setting of care (i.e., hospital, long-term care setting, home, or hospice) does not change the perception of pain experienced (22). With the advent of the hospice benefit in the 1980s, people have the opportunity to receive support for their pain and symptom management at the end of life, yet only 36% utilize this benefit, with a median length of stay of 20 days (23).

Pain management in the hospital setting should be easy to achieve, given the technological and nursing resources available. The undertreatment of cancer pain can be attributed to the combined effects of lack of knowledge, attitudes, fear of hastening death, patient underreporting, therapeutic nonadherence, and system-wide impediments to optimal analgesic therapy (24, 25). The inadequacy of pain management due to lack of staff education may be changing with the advent of more education in end-of-life care (26). More than 1200 hospitals in the United States (30%) have palliative care programs, thus have access to specialist knowledge (27). In the absence of palliative specialists, access to critical resources include end-of-life clinical pathways (28), simplified algorithms, and equianalgesic tables to improve pain management at the end of life.

Pain management in the long-term care setting is inadequate, and undertreatment of institutionalized elderly patients with cancer has been linked to being older than 85 years, minority race, impaired cognition, and requiring multiple medications (29). Barriers arise from fear of regulatory scrutiny, lack of acceptance of opioid use for nonmalignant pain, less physician involvement in daily care, lack of knowledge about pain assessment, and high ratios of patients to nursing staff (30). Suggestions for improving pain management include education for nurses and nursing assistants in end-of-life care (31), using scheduled medications versus as-needed medications for those with constant pain, minimizing use of simultaneous as-needed orders, and using scheduled medications for anticipated pain related to activity (e.g., 30 minutes prior to bath) (32).

Pain management at the end of life in the home can be challenging for the person in severe pain if trained professional support is not available. Health care provider and family fears of opioid use and knowledge deficits can hinder appropriate pain management (33). When home care is implemented, it is important for the nursing staff to be educated on end-of-life care and to teach patients and their families to manage pain at home (34). Regimens should be simplified when family members are primary caregivers; however, in communities where adequate nursing and infusion technology exists, people can be maintained at home on intravenous, subcutaneous, or neuraxial infusion until their end of life.

PAIN ASSESSMENT IN ADVANCED DISEASE

In the ideal setting, a thorough pain assessment includes location, duration, onset, characteristics, severity, alleviating and relieving factors, and associated symptoms. Identification of the pain etiology (nociceptive vs. neuropathic) is important for effective pain management. In advanced disease and at the end of life, the impact of pain on simple measures such as sitting up or even turning in bed must be assessed.

As the end of life nears and cognition decreases, it becomes increasingly important to utilize behavioral tools because it becomes difficult to obtain information or utilize the more widely used pain intensity scales. Behavioral tools such as the Pain Assessment in Advanced Dementia (PAINAID) rely on the use of behaviors, vocalization, breathing patterns, facial patterns, and consolability to assess pain (35). Validated tools are also available to assess pain for those in the intensive care unit, although their use is primarily limited to research settings (36, 37).

There has been reluctance to use surrogates (i.e., individuals who make medical decisions when patients cannot) to report patients' pain because of their emotional attachment to these patients and their potential for overestimating the pain. In a large study of seriously ill hospitalized patients, surrogates correctly identified the existence of pain 73% of the time and estimated its severity with 53% accuracy (38). Although surrogates may be less accurate about estimating pain severity, they may be able to provide essential information to assist clinicians managing pain.

In lieu of tools, if unable to adequately assess pain, clinicians should ask the following question: "Would I be in pain in this situation?" If the answer is "yes," or if the condition is known to cause pain, it is best to assume that pain is present and treat it. One can then determine the efficacy of treatment by changes in physiologic or behavioral signs.

PHARMACOTHERAPY IN ADVANCED DISEASE AND AT THE END OF LIFE

Pharmacotherapy is the mainstay of pain treatment at the end of life. Opioids are the principal analgesics used to treat moderate to severe pain associated with advanced illness and at the end of life and provide adequate pain relief to more than three-quarters of patients with cancer pain (39, 40). There is no uniformly preferred agent, and the selection of the opioids is based on the individual response, clinical judgment, access, and cost and/or availability of parenteral formulations.

Morphine, the most widely used analgesic for cancer pain, is considered a mainstay in end-of-life care and is the standard by which other opioids are compared. Morphine is primarily metabolized in the liver, and its active metabolites morphine-3-glucuronide and morphine-6-glucunoride are renally excreted. Actual accumulation and clinical effects of morphine's metabolites are still unclear due to lack of conclusive trials (41). However, it has been postulated that accumulation of morphine-6-glucuronide and morphine-3-glucuronide in those with renal insufficiency produces opioid toxicity and adverse effects such as nausea, sedation, delirium, and respiratory depression (42–46). From a clinical perspective, even with inconclusive evidence, morphine use should be avoided for patients with known renal insufficiency or failure unless no other opioid alternatives are available.

In home care or long-term care settings, morphine may be administered through concentrated solution (20 mg/mL) or suppositories for those unable to tolerate oral medication. Although morphine has been widely used sublingually in the hospice setting, it is poorly absorbed through this route. As cognition declines, for those who require around-the-clock opioid therapy, it may be necessary to change to a subcutaneous or intravenous route of administration or rotate to fentanyl transdermally.

Fentanyl is a high-potency, lipid-soluble, synthetic opioid with no active metabolites that is tolerated in older, more frail people. Available formulations include intravenous, neuraxial, transdermal, and oral transmucosal delivery systems, with nasal and sublingual sprays, buccal tablets, and inhaled aerosol spray formulations in development (47).

The fentanyl transdermal system may be more difficult to titrate at the end of life when pain escalates. It is never appropriate for acute pain, as onset of action can be delayed for 12 to 24 hours. The fentanyl patch may need to be changed every 48 hours versus every 72 hours especially in those with cachexia. Fever or application of heat can increase absorption and precipitate an overdose due to rapid distribution of the medication (47).

Breakthrough pain may be treated with oral transmucosal fentanyl, with the caveat that the two available formulations are not dose equivalent due to differences in their absorption. This route of delivery provides quicker onset for pain relief than immediate-release morphine (48).

Hydromorphone, a semisynthetic opioid, has an efficacy and side effect profile similar to those of other opioids (49). Hydromorphone's metabolites may account for neuroexcitatory effects, but there are conflicting reports of adverse effects and toxicities in clinical settings (50). Hydromorphone can easily be concentrated to 10 mg/mL, therefore, making it an ideal agent for subcutaneous administration when high doses are needed. In the nursing home or home care setting, hydromorphone in tablet, liquid, or suppository forms may be preferred to morphine due to its potency. At the present time, sustained-release hydromorphone, not available in the United States, is in clinical trials.

Methadone, an inexpensive, synthetic opioid with very high oral bioavailability, and no known active metabolites, used for decades for opioid addiction, has reemerged in the area of pain management and palliative care (51, 52). Clinically, people with significant pain have shown dramatic improvement when rotated to methadone (53). In vitro studies have shown methadone to be a relatively potent *N*-methyl-D-aspartate (NMDA) inhibitor; and it has been postulated that this could decrease development of tolerance and increase analgesia for painful neuropathies (54), but there have not been clinically relevant trials of applicability of NMDA antagonists in the treatment of neuropathic pain. Methadone has a rapid distribution phase, but a very slow elimination phase (ranges 15–190 hours). Its relative potency in comparison to other opioids and its slow elimination phase create the potential for oversedation occurring several days after initiation or titration. The complexities and potential toxicities of methadone pose challenges for the clinician.

There are several proposed methods for converting to methadone from other opioids (51, 55, 56). A simple guide is to take the total oral morphine dose and if it is less than 1000 mg daily, start methadone at 10% of that dose and start dosing it every eight hours, and if it is more than 1000 mg daily, start methadone at 5% of the daily dose every eight hours. Generally, it is not advisable to use methadone as the breakthrough medication. Methadone may be used intravenously, but there are conflicting reports about the successful use subcutaneously due to skin erythema, induration, and edema (57–59). However, a trial of subcutaneous infusion may be warranted if no other alternatives are available.

There is a rising concern about the use of methadone due to its potential to prolong the QTc interval, a phenomenon that predisposes one to a life-threatening cardiac arrhythmia, torsades de pointes (60). There are no established guidelines, but it is reasonable to consider an electrocardiogram prior to initiation of methadone therapy, and when titrating doses. One may need to weigh risks/benefits when considering methadone for people with underlying heart disease or who are utilizing other medications prolonging the QTc interval. Another concern is the cytochrome P450 metabolism of methadone with the possibility of level increases due to drug–drug interactions. In a recently published review, the authors conclude that the effects of potential interactions are still poorly understood, thereby making clinical judgment difficult when utilizing medications with potential interactions (61). For clinicians, it is important to recognize the possibility of interactions and changes in metabolism when initiating or discontinuing medications with potential interactions.

Oxycodone is a widely used, semisynthetic opioid available in extended-release and short-acting oral preparations. It has higher bioavailability than morphine, producing more consistent plasma concentrations. In some trials, there is less reported incidence of hallucinations and pruritis. As its elimination is primarily renal, dose reduction may be necessary for those with worsening renal function and for those with significant hepatic disease (62). Although used extensively for cancer-related pain, its use at the end of life may be limited for those no longer able to take oral medications.

Combination opioid analgesics with acetaminophen or nonsteroidal anti-inflammatory drugs (NSAIDs) are widely used for pain. However, their role is limited in the end-of-life setting except for those instances when pain is mild to moderate and occasional versus constant.

Meperidine use should be avoided for pain management in any setting because it is first metabolized to normeperidine in the liver (with a half-life of 15–20 hours) and then is renally excreted. Accumulation of normeperidine, which cannot be reversed with naloxone, has direct neurotoxic effects resulting in seizures, hallucinations, and delirium (63).

ROUTE OF ADMINISTRATION

Oral, sublingual, and buccal opioid administrations are ideal for those able to swallow and whose pain can be controlled by these routes. However, as the disease progresses and/or pain increases, rotation to transdermal, transmucosal, intravenous, subcutaneous, rectal, vaginal, and neuraxial opioid administration may be necessary. In a study of cancer patients at the end of life, less than 50% were able to use the oral route of analgesia in the last week of life and more than 50% required more than one route of medication (64).

When technology and resources are available, intravenous or subcutaneous administration of opioids via bolus dosing for moderate pain, continuous infusion for moderate or severe pain that is poorly controlled with boluses, or patient-controlled analgesia may provide the greatest benefit due to superior absorption and the ability to rapidly titrate doses. Neuraxial infusion may provide the most benefit for those with refractory pain and/or intolerable side effects. A variety of techniques for intraspinal opioid delivery (percutaneous or implanted epidural or intraspinal catheters) have been adapted to long-term treatment, and properly selected patients can benefit greatly (65).

DOSING AND TITRATION

The starting dose of an opioid for severe pain is usually equivalent to morphine sulfate 5 to 10 mg intravenously every four hours for patients with limited prior opioid exposure. There is no consensus on opioid dose titration, and at the present time, current practice is based on expert opinion and experience (66). Rate of titration may be either the total quantity of rescue drug consumed during the previous day, or 30% to 50% of the current total daily dose. The increment can be larger (75–100% of the total daily dose) if pain is severe, or smaller if the patient is already experiencing opioid toxicity or is predisposed to adverse effects because of advanced age or major organ failure. Rapid titration may be done in patients in hospital settings with severe pain. Parenteral dosing can be repeated every 30 minutes until pain is partially relieved with subsequent calculation of approximate maintenance doses. In outpatient settings, sustained-release formulations are generally titrated every three to five days, with the exception being methadone that is usually titrated weekly due to the long half-life (67). In the setting of renal and/or hepatic failure, dose and timing adjustments may be necessary (68, 69).

OPIOID ROTATION

Opioid rotation, trials of different opioid drugs, can be used to attain the most favorable balance between analgesia and side effects. According to a systematic review of data, clinical improvement is seen in more than 50% of patients after opioid rotation. Reasons to consider opioid rotation are adequate pain control, but adverse side effect profile; inadequate pain control with inability to escalate dose secondary to side effects; and rapid dose escalation without pain relief (70). Prediction of response to the new opioid is variable due to effects of cross-tolerance and the incomplete understanding of exact equianalgesic doses. A commonly used practice to rotate opioids is to calculate the sum of opioids given during the previous 24-hour period in units of oral morphine equivalents. From this calculation, the new agent can be dosed up to 50% to 80% of the new agent's equianalgesic dose except in the case of methadone.

CONTINUOUS VS. AS-NEEDED ANALGESIA

Patients at the end of life often need around-the-clock analgesia. As-needed (PRN) medication administration may lead to inadequate pain control unless pain is only incidental to a certain activity such as repositioning or performing wound care. Continuous intravenous or subcutaneous infusion is the preferred route of administration to provide consistent analgesia for dying patients in the hospital setting. However, a recent small study of continuous versus intermittent subcutaneous administration of opioids for cancer pain revealed no difference in efficacy of pain control, side effects, or patient preference (71), and decisions may be based on ease of administration and care setting. Sufficient breakthrough medication (at least 10% of the total daily dose of the basal medication) should be given on a PRN basis, especially during times when patients are stimulated or moved (e.g., bathing, turning, suctioning). Patient-controlled analgesia is optimal when patients are able to participate because it can provide a continuous infusion for those who need continuous opioids and/or can provide controlled bolus doses with short lockout periods for breakthrough or incidental pain.

BREAKTHROUGH MEDICATION

Breakthrough pain is a transitory increase in intensity when baseline pain is controlled on an analgesic regimen (72). Uncontrolled breakthrough pain results in poor overall pain control, decreased satisfaction with pain control, negative impact on quality of life, and increased economic burden. The incidence of breakthrough pain is 40% to 80% for those with cancer. The causes are multifactorial and include end-of-dose failure for those on sustained-release analgesics, incident pain related to activity, and spontaneous pain from unknown causes (73). In an observational study, the average number of episodes of breakthrough pain was four times daily with a duration of 35 minutes for each episode. In the same study, there was evidence of inadequate utilization of breakthrough medication with reported reasons for underutilization being lack of pain severity, adverse side effects, fear of pharmacologic dependence, and spontaneous resolution of pain (74). The general guiding principle for giving breakthrough medication is to utilize 10% to 15% of total daily dose opioids (75), with the European Association of Palliative Care recommending 17% of total daily dose (76). A confirmatory study of the use of intravenous morphine for breakthrough pain demonstrated that 20% total daily dose of opioids was tolerated without adverse side effects (77). Rapid-onset opioids (i.e., oral transmucosal fentanyl) may provide the quickest form of pain relief (78), but the range of dosing for breakthrough pain can be quite variable and may need to be individualized (79). In palliative pain management, rescue doses should be offered every one to two hours for oral medications and every 15 to 30 minutes for intravenous medications when pain is severe. The general practice is to use the same medication for breakthrough pain as the sustained-release agent, with the exception of methadone due to its long half-life, or when the use of rapid-onset opioids is a consideration.

SIDE EFFECT MANAGEMENT

Side effects from opioids such as nausea, vomiting, constipation, confusion, sleepiness, and dry mouth occur in 25% to 80% of people on opioid therapy (80). Patients may find side effects of nausea, vomiting, and confusion more distressing than other side effects (81). Most guidelines for treatment are based on consensus and expert opinion due to the lack of randomized controlled studies (82, 83).

Nausea and vomiting occur in about 10% to 30% of those with cancer on opioid therapy (84). There are multiple mechanisms including decreased gastrointestinal activity, stimulation of the chemoreceptive trigger zone, and enhanced vestibular sensitivity. Treatment options include the use of prokinetics, antipsychotics, serotonin antagonists, antihistamines, and corticosteroids. Optimally, choice should depend on the mechanism of action, patient characteristics, risk of adverse effects, and cost. Trials of antiemetics from different classes and combination use may be necessary to control nausea. If nausea persists despite the use of antiemetics of different classes and combination therapy, consider opioid rotation.

Constipation, the most common side effect of chronic opioid use, should be managed prophylactically even at the end of life when oral intake may be minimal due to the possibility of added abdominal discomfort. Most regimens are based on anecdotal evidence and current common practices such as the use of sennosides with docusate may not be as effective as the use of sennosides alone (85). The peripherally acting subcutaneously administered opioid antagonist, methylnaltrexone, for treatment of opioid-induced constipation may prove useful especially in advanced disease states when oral intake is limited (86, 87). There is evidence that the incidence of constipation may be less with the use of transdermal opiates versus extended-release morphine (88).

Pruritis is more commonly experienced with the use of intraspinal opioids. The underlying etiology is unclear and may involve the release of histamine and/or the involvement of spinal opioid receptors. Antihistamines are often used, but evidence from prospective studies is lacking (82). In some cases of refractory pruritis, the use of low-dose parenteral naloxone may be warranted. Consider opioid rotation if pruritis persists.

Sedation and cognitive adverse effects may occur with opioids especially at initiation and during significant titration. This symptom usually resolves after a few days. Since cognitive changes often occur at the end of life due to a variety of factors, these side effects may be difficult to assess. If the sedation or cognitive changes persist, the treatment of sedation may include reduced doses or rotation of opioids, neuraxial route analgesia, or adjuvant therapy such as methylphenidate.

Respiratory depression due to opioids can be a concern even at the end of life. This adverse effect can usually be avoided through careful monitoring and adjustment of opioid medications. If patients are not arousable with respiratory rates of less than 8 breaths per minute, naloxone should be given by diluting 0.4 mg in 10 mL of normal saline and administering 1-mL increments every two minutes until respiratory rate increases and patients are arousable (89).

NSAIDs IN ADVANCED DISEASE AND AT THE END OF LIFE

NSAIDs are generally not preferred analgesics in advanced disease and at the end of life. Gastrointestinal side effects and the risk of cardiovascular events may limit their usefulness in advanced disease states, especially in those with cardiovascular disease and prothrombotic states (90). One parenteral NSAID, ketorolac, has been used successfully as an adjunct therapy, with the addition of prophylactic gastrointestinal protection, for cancer-related pain in advanced disease (91), but again risks/benefits must be considered.

ADJUVANT ANALGESICS

Adjuvant analgesics are often used in pain management. Commonly used agents, corticosteroids, antidepressants, and anticonvulsants, may prove beneficial in painful syndromes in advanced disease such as bony metastases, neuropathies, and malignant bowel obstruction. However, many agents are not available as intravenous preparations, thus, limiting their use at the end of life.

Neuropathic pain in advanced disease may be related to the disease process itself, such as nerve compression from tumor burden; the effects of therapy, or comorbid conditions. Opioids may be utilized to treat neuropathic pain especially in advanced disease states where oral administration of medications is not optimal. Gabapentin has been shown to be effective for cancer-related neuropathic pain (92). Combinations of opioids and gabapentin are more effective than monotherapy in neuropathic pain related to diabetic neuropathy and cancer (93–96). If oral analgesics are tolerated, consider using opioids in combination with anticonvulsants (such as pregabalin and gabapentin), or serotonin-norepinephrine reuptake inhibitors (such as duloxetine, effexor or milnacipran), realizing that their use is off-label unless pain is related to diabetic peripheral neuropathic pain, fibromyalgia, or postherpetic neuralgia. For severe, refractory neuropathic pain, consideration may be given for the use of lidocaine or ketamine.

Bone pain related to malignancy is the most common cause of pain in persons with cancer. Pharmacotherapeutic options include corticosteroids, osteoclast inhibitors, and NSAIDs. Corticosteroids possess excellent anti-inflammatory and analgesic properties and may also control nausea and improve appetite (97, 98). Dexamethasone, which can be administered by oral, intravenous, and subcutaneous routes, is a preferred agent due to the longer duration of action and less mineralocorticoid effects and can be used at low doses (2–4 mg daily) in those with advanced cancer who have pain that is not optimally controlled with opioids. Although there is the long-term risk of side effects related to steroid use, this is usually not an issue at the end of life.

Pain related to bowel obstruction requires intensive palliative interventions for people who are not surgical candidates to reduce pain and other obstructive symptoms, including distention, nausea, and vomiting. The use of opioids, a corticosteroid, anticholinergic drugs, and the somatostatin analog, octreotide, can provide good symptom control and, for many, obviate the need for nasogastric tube drainage (99, 100).

A variety of anticholinergic drugs can be utilized with scopolamine (1.5 mg transdermal), often being the first trialed medication. Hyoscyamine (available in sublingual form) and glycopyrrolate have less blood–brain barrier penetration and, therefore, may be less likely to produce central nervous system toxicity. Octreotide inhibits the secretion of gastric, pancreatic, and intestinal secretions and reduces gastrointestinal motility; and its use in the symptomatic treatment of bowel obstruction is supported by favorable anecdotal experience (101).

PHARMACOTHERAPEUTIC APPROACHES FOR REFRACTORY PAIN

Lidocaine has been utilized for pain refractory to opioid therapy with reported favorable responses (102, 103). There have been different approaches to therapy including a one-time bolus therapy and continuous infusion (104). If technology and nursing support are available, lidocaine can be safely administered in the home and in a long-term care setting via intravenous or subcutaneous routes. Using 0.5 to 1 mg/kg/hr continuously or by short-term infusion in some cases produces excellent analgesia in combination with opioid therapy without cardiotoxicity.

Ketamine, an NMDA antagonist most commonly used as an anesthetic agent, has had a positive effect in the setting of severe, opioid refractory pain in far advanced disease, but this medication has a difficult side effect profile, including nightmares and delirium, and its long-term use is likely to be limited (105, 106). Ketamine can be started at 0.1 mg/kg/hr by continuous infusion and titrated slowly to 0.5 mg/kg/hr. Because of the psychotomimetic effects, it may be prudent to pretreat with a low-dose antipsychotic agent prior to initiation and as needed during the infusion.

INTERVENTIONAL STRATEGIES

Neural blockade with neurolytic solutions, usually alcohol, phenol, or glycerol, has been in use for many decades (107). The risks associated with the injection of neurolytic substances suggest that these techniques generally should be reserved for patients with refractory pain in the setting of advanced cancer or with an appropriate risk–benefit ratio. The commonly accepted exception is celiac plexus blockade in patients with pancreatic cancer, as the favorable response to this blockade warrants its use whenever the typical pancreatic pain syndrome occurs (108).

NONPHARMACOLOGIC APPROACHES TO PAIN MANAGEMENT

Pain in advanced disease is multifactorial, and the use of approaches such as massage, acupuncture, self-hypnosis, supportive group therapy, and transcutaneous electrical nerve stimulation may provide some pain relief when used as adjuncts to pharmacotherapy. There is minimal confirmatory literature in this area, but if the therapeutic approach is not harmful, then a trial is warranted (109). The comfort derived from human touch such as massage may be beneficial in ways that cannot be tangibly measured.

PALLIATIVE SEDATION

There are certain circumstances when pain and other symptoms, which may be complicated by psychological and existential suffering, cannot be controlled despite the best efforts of trained professionals. For a select group, the use of palliative sedation may be the only means to relieve suffering at the end of life. Sedation at the end of life may be controversial, especially if the ethical foundation is not adequately understood (110, 111). Although there continues to be considerable discussion among palliative care specialists about the role of and practical strategies for sedation in the imminently dying, the approach is widely accepted as a specific medical intervention to treat refractory pain and suffering in exceptional circumstances.

There is no consensus on the approach to palliative sedation and a variety of agents such as benzodiazepines, sedating antipsychotics, barbiturates, and general anesthetics are used to induce sedation. The goals of sedation (mild, deep, intermittent) and the patient's response will determine the agent and dose utilized (110). Sedation could potentially accelerate the dying process, but if the intention is to relieve suffering, it is ethical and should not be confused with euthanasia.

Palliative sedation should be implemented under the guidance of knowledgeable palliative care specialists only after the medical situation has been carefully assessed, a thorough discussion with the patient and family has taken place, consent has been obtained, and the goals of care have been clearly established. Once sedation has been activated, ongoing information should be provided to family and staff; and with prior approval by the patient or proxy, a plan for reducing sedation at times, to determine symptom burden and state of mind, may be put in place (112).

CONCLUSION

Clinicians will experience the deaths of many patients, loved ones, and ultimately themselves. There is an opportunity to provide expert pain and symptom management at the end of life, ultimately easing pain of loved ones surrounding the dying patient. It is a noble goal to leave them with a memory of a peaceful transition and not an agonizing end. Health care providers should attend to the management of patients at the end of life as they hope to be treated. As the end of life approaches, the philosophy "What else can I do to provide comfort?" replaces "There is nothing else that can be done."

REFERENCES

1. World Health Organization. WHO definition of palliative care, 2008. Available at: http://www.who.int/cancer/palliative/definition/en/. Accessed June 1, 2008.
2. National Consensus Project for Quality Palliative Care. Clinical practices guidelines for quality palliative care, 2004. Available at: http://www.nationalconsensusproject.org. Accessed June 1, 2008.
3. Saunders C. A personal therapeutic journey. BMJ 1996; 313:1599–1601.
4. von Gunten CF. Interventions to manage symptoms at end of life. J Palliat Med 2005; 8(suppl 1):S88–S94.
5. Buchanan RJ, Choi MA, Wang SJ, et al. Analyses of nursing home residents in hospice care using the minimum data set. J Palliat Med 2002; 16:465–480.
6. Higginson IJ, Hearn J. A multicenter evaluation of cancer pain control by palliative care teams. J Pain Symptom Manage 1997; 14:29–35.
7. Emanuel EJ, Fairclough DL, Slutsman J, et al. Understanding economic and other burdens of terminal illness; the experience of patients and their caregivers. Ann Intern Med 2000; 132(6):451–459.
8. Teunissen SC, Wesker W, Kruitwagen C, et al. Symptom prevalence in patients with incurable cancer: a systematic review. J Pain Symptom Manage 2007; 34(1):94–104.
9. Cherny NI. The assessment of cancer pain. In: McMahon SB, Koltzenburg M, eds. Wall and Melzack's Textbook of Pain. London, UK: Elsevier Limited, 2006:1099–1125.
10. Chang VT, Janjan N, Jain S, et al. Update in cancer pain syndromes. J Palliat Med 2006; 9:1414–1434.
11. Solano JP, Gomes B, Higginson IJ. A comparison of symptom prevalence in far advanced cancer, AIDS, heart disease, chronic obstructive pulmonary disease and renal disease. J Pain Symptom Manage 2006; 31(1):58–69.
12. Nordgren L, Sorensen S. Symptoms expressed in last six months of life in patients with end-stage heart failure. Eur J Cardiovasc Nurs 2003; 2:213–217.
13. Ehde DM, Gibbons LE, Chwastiak L, et al. Chronic pain in a large community sample of persons with multiple sclerosis. Mult Scler 2003; 9:605–611.

14. Svendsen KB, Jensen TS, Overvad K, et al. Pain in patients with multiple sclerosis: a population based study. Arch Neurol 2003; 60:1089–1094.
15. Kong KH, Woon VC, Yang SY. Prevalence of chronic pain and its impact on health-related quality of life in stroke survivors. Arch Phys Med Rehabil 2004; 85:35–40.
16. Shega JW, Hougham GW, Stocking CB, et al. Patients dying with dementia: experience at the end of life and impact of hospice care. J Pain Symptom Manage 2008; 35(5):499–507.
17. Frich LM, Borgbjerg FM. Pain and pain treatment in AIDS patients: a longitudinal study. J Pain Symptom Manage 2000; 19:339–347.
18. Karus D, Raveis VH, Alexander C, et al. Patient reports of symptoms and their treatment at three palliative care projects servicing individuals with HIV/AIDS. J Pain Symptom Manage 2005; 30(5):408–417.
19. Kimball LR, McCormick WC. The pharmacologic management of pain and discomfort in persons with AIDS near the end of life; use of opioid analgesia in the hospice setting. J Pain Symptom Manage 1996; 11:88–94.
20. Grunier A, Mor V, Weitzen S, et al. Where people die: a multilevel approach to understanding influences on site of death in America. Med Care Res Rev 2007; 64: 351–378.
21. Cleeland CS, Gonin R, Hatfield AK, et al. Pain and its treatment in outpatients with metastatic cancer. N Engl J Med 1994; 330:592–596.
22. Trask PC, Teno JM, Nash J. Transitions of care and changes in distressing pain. J Pain Symptom Manage 2006; 32:104–109.
23. National Hospice and Palliative Care Organization. NHPCO facts and figures: hospice care in America. November 2007 edition. Available at: http://www.nhpco.org/files/public/Statistics Research/NHPCO fact-and-figures Nov2007.pdf. Accessed July 20, 2008.
24. Pargeon KL, Hailey BJ. Barriers to effective cancer pain management: a review of the literature. J Pain Symptom Manage 1999; 18:358–368.
25. Fineberg IC, Wenger NS, Brown-Saltzman K. Unrestricted opiate use for pain and suffering at the end of life: knowledge and attitudes as barriers to care. J Palliat Med 2006; 9:873–883.
26. Sulmasy D, Cimino JE, He MK, et al. U.S. medical students' perceptions of their schools' curricular attention to care at the end of life: 1998–2006. J Palliat Med 2008; 11(5):707–716.
27. Center to Advance Palliative Care. New analysis shows hospitals continue to implement palliative care programs at rapid pace. Available at: http://www.capc.org/news-and-events/releases/news-release-4–14-08. Accessed July 20, 2008.
28. Bookbinder M, Blank AE, Arney E, et al. Improving end-of-life care: development and pilot-test of a clinical pathway. J Pain Symptom Manage 2005; 29:529–543.
29. Bernabei R, Gambassi G, Lapane K, et al. Management of pain in elderly patients with cancer. JAMA 1998; 279:1877–1882.
30. Weissman DE, Griffie J, Muchka S, et al. Improving pain management in long-term care facilities. J Palliat Med 2001; 4(4):567–573.
31. Roscoe LA, Hyer K. Quality of life at the end of life for nursing home residents: perceptions of hospice and nursing home staff members. J Pain Symptom Manage 2008; 35(1):1–9.
32. Liao S, Weissman DE. Pain management in nursing homes: analgesic prescribing tip #89. J Palliat Med 2006; 9(6):1475–1476.
33. Childress SB, Stromness AR. Improving pain management at the end of life in the home care environment. Home Health Care Manage Pract 2003; 15(3):203–206.
34. Ferrell BR, Virani R, Grant M. Improving end-of-life care education in home care. J Palliat Med 1998; 1(1):11–19.
35. Warden V, Hurley AD, Volicer L. Development and psychometric evaluation of the Pain Assessment in Advanced Dementia (PAINAID) scale. J Am Med Dir Assoc 2003; 4(1):9–15.

36. Aissaoui Y, Zeggwagh AA, Zekraoui A, et al. Validation of a behavioral pain scale in critically ill, sedated, and mechanically ventilated patients. Anesth Analg 2005; 101:1470–1476.

37. Gelinas C, Johnston C. Pain assessment in the critically ill ventilated adult: validation of the critical care pain observation tool and physiologic indicators. Clin J Pain 2007; 23:497–505.

38. Desbiens NA, Mueller-Rizner N. How well do surrogates assess the pain of seriously ill patients? Crit Care Med 2000; 28:1347–1352.

39. World Health Organization. Cancer Pain Relief with a Guide to Opioid Availability. 2nd ed. Geneva, Switzerland: World Health Organization, 1996.

40. Jacox A, Carr DB, Payne R, et al. Management of Cancer Pain. Clinical Practice Guideline No. 9. Rockville, MD: U.S. Department of Health and Human Services, Public Health Service, 1994. AHCPR publication 94-0592.

41. Skarke C, Geisslinger G, Lotsch J. Is morphine-3-gluconoride of therapeutic relevance? Pain 2005; 116:117–180.

42. D'Honneur G, Gilton A, Sandouk P, et al. Plasma and cerebrospinal fluid concentrations of morphine and morphine glucuronides after oral morphine. The influence of renal failure. Anesthesiology 1994; 81:87–93.

43. Faura CC, Moore RA, Horga JF, et al. Morphine and morphine-6-glucuronide plasma concentrations and effect in cancer pain. J Pain Symptom Manage 1996; 11:95–102.

44. Tiseo PJ, Thale HT, Lapin J, et al. Morphine-6-glucuronide concentrations and opioid-related side effects: a survey in cancer patients. Pain 1995; 61:47–54.

45. Morita T, Tei Y, Tsunoda J, et al. Increased plasma morphine metabolites in terminally ill cancer patients with delirium: an intra-individual comparison. J Pain Symptom Manage 2002; 23:107–113.

46. Sjogren P. Clinical implications of morphine metabolites. In: Portenoy RK, Bruera EB, eds. Topics in Palliative Care. Vol 1. New York, NY: Oxford University Press, 1997:163–177.

47. Fine P, Portenoy RK. Opioid Analgesia. 2nd ed. New York, NY: McGraw-Hill, 2007:26.

48. Coluzzia MH, Schwartzberg L, Conroy JD, et al. Breakthrough cancer pain: a randomized trial comparing oral transmucosal fentanyl citrate (OTFC) and morphine sulfate immediate release (MSIR). Pain 2001; 9(1/2):123–130.

49. Quigley C, Wiffen P. A systematic review of hydromorphone in acute and chronic pain. J Pain Symptom Manage 2003; 25(2):169–178.

50. Murray A, Hagen N. Hydromorphone. J Pain Symptom Manage 2005; 29:S57–S66.

51. Bruera E, Sweeney C. Methadone use in cancer patients with pain: a review. J Palliat Med 2002; 5(1):127–138.

52. Fishman SM, Wilsey B, Mahajan G, et al. Methadone reincarnated: novel clinical application with related concerns. Pain Med 2002; 3(4):339–348.

53. Bruera E, Neumann CM. Role of methadone in the management of pain in cancer patients. Oncology 1999; 13:1275–1284.

54. Ebert B, Andersen S, Krogsgaard-Larsen P. Ketobemidone, methadone and pethidine are non-competitive N-methyl-D-aspartate (NMDA) antagonists in the rat cortex and spinal cord. Neurosci Lett 1995; 187(3):165–168.

55. Manfredi PL, Houde RW. Prescribing methadone, a unique analgesic. J Support Oncol 2003; 1:216–220.

56. Gazelle G, Fine PG. Fast Facts and Concepts #75: Methadone for the Treatment of Pain. 2nd ed. July 2006. End-of-Life/Palliative Education Resource Center. Available at: http://www.eperc.mcw.edu. Accessed July 20, 2008.

57. Viel-Kerkmeer PE, van Mansom I. Re: Subcutaneous methadone—an issue revisited. J Pain Symptom Manage 2008; 35(6):572.

58. Hum A, Fainsinger RL, Bielech M. Subcutaneous methadone—an issue revisited. J Pain Symptom Manage 2007; 34(6):573–575.

59. Bruera E, Fainsinger R, Moore M, et al. Local toxicity with subcutaneous methadone. Experience of two centers. Pain 1991; 45:141–143.

60. Cruciani RA, Homel P, Yap Y, et al. QTc measurements in patients on methadone. J Pain Symptom Manage 2005; 29:385–391.
61. Weschules DJ, Bain KT, Richeimer S. Actual and potential drug interactions associated with methadone. Pain Med 2008; 9(3):315–344.
62. Kalso E. Oxycodone. J Pain Symptom Manage 2005; 29:S47–S56.
63. Max MB, Payne R, Edwards WT, et al. American Pain Society Principles of Analgesic Use in the Treatment of Acute Pain and Cancer Pain. 5th ed. Glenview, IL: American Pain Society, 2005:22.
64. Coyle N, Adelhardt J, Foley KM, et al. Character of terminal illness in the advanced cancer patient: pain and other symptoms during the last four weeks of life. J Pain Symptom Manage 1990; 5:83–93.
65. Du Pen SL, Du Pen AR. Intraspinal analgesic therapy in palliative care: evolving perspective. In: Portenoy RK, Bruera EB, eds. Topics in Palliative Care. Vol 4. New York, NY: Oxford University Press, 2000:217–235.
66. Davis MP, Weissman DE, Arnold RM. Opioid dose titration for severe cancer pain: a systematic evidence-based review. J Palliat Med 2004; 7(3):462–468.
67. Fine P, Portenoy RK. Opioid Analgesia. 2nd ed. New York, NY: McGraw-Hill, 2007:56.
68. Rhee C, Broadbent AM. Palliation and liver failure: palliative medications dosage guidelines. J Palliat Med 2007; 10(3):677–685.
69. Cohen LM, Moss AH, Weisbord SD, et al. Renal palliative care. J Palliat Med 2006; 9(4):977–992.
70. Mercadante S, Bruera E. Opioid switching: a systematic and critical review. Cancer Treat Rev 2006; 32:304–315.
71. Watanabe S, Pereira J, Tarumi Y, et al. A randomized double-blind crossover comparison of continuous and intermittent subcutaneous administration of opioid for cancer pain. J Palliat Med 2008; 11(4):570–574.
72. Portenoy RK, Hagen NA. Breakthrough pain: definition, prevalence and characteristics. Pain 1990; 41:273–281.
73. Mercadante S, Radbruch L, Caraceni A, et al. Episodic (breakthrough) pain. Consensus conference of an expert working group of the European Association for Palliative Care. Cancer 2002; 94:832–839.
74. Davies AN, Vriens J, Kennett A, et al. An observational study of oncology patients' utilization of breakthrough pain medication. J Pain Symptom Manage2008; 35(4):406–411.
75. Fine P, Portenoy RK. Opioid Analgesia. 2nd ed. New York, NY: McGraw-Hill, 2007:55.
76. Hanks GW, De Conno F, Cherny N, et al. Morphine and alternative opioids in cancer pain: the EAPC recommendations. Br J Cancer 2001; 84:587–593.
77. Mercadante S, Intravaia G, Villari P, et al. Intravenous morphine for breakthrough (episodic) pain in an acute palliative care unit: a confirmatory study. J Pain Symptom Manage 2008; 35:307–313.
78. Zeppetella G. Opioids for cancer breakthrough pain: a pilot study reporting patient assessment of time to meaningful pain relief. J Pain Symptom Manage 2008; 35(5):563–567.
79. Hagen NA, Fisher K, Victorino C, et al. A titration strategy is needed to manage breakthrough cancer pain effectively: observations from data pooled from three clinical trials. J Palliat Med 2007; 10(1):47–55.
80. Villars P, Dodd M, West C, et al. Differences in the prevalence and severity of side effects based on type of analgesic prescription in patients with chronic cancer pain. J Pain Symptom Manage 2007; 33(1):67–77.
81. Palos GR, Mendoza TR, Cantor SB, et al. Perceptions of analgesic use and side effects: what the public values in pain management. J Pain Symptom Manage 2004; 28(5):460–473.
82. McNicol E, Horowicz-Mehler N, Fisk RA, et al. Management of opioid side effects in cancer-related and chronic noncancer pain: a systematic review. J Pain 2003; 4(5):231–256.

83. Swegle JM, Logemann C. Management of common opioid-induced adverse effects. Am Fam Physician 2006; 74:1347–1354.
84. Holzer P. Treatment of opioid-induced gut dysfunction. Expert Opin Investig Drugs 2007; 16:181–94.
85. Hawley PH, Byeon JJ. A comparison of sennosides-based bowel protocols with and without docusate in hospitalized patients with cancer. J Palliat Med 2008; 11(4):575–581.
86. Thomas J, Karver S, Cooney GA, et al. Methylnaltrexone for opioid-induced constipation in advanced illness. N Engl J Med 2008; 358:2332–2343.
87. Becker G, Galandi D, Blum HE. Peripherally acting opioid antagonists in the treatment of opioid-related constipation: a systematic review. J Pain Symptom Manage 2007; 34(5):547–565.
88. Tassinari D, Sartori S, Tamburini E, et al. Adverse effects of transdermal opiates treating moderate-severe cancer pain in comparison to long-acting morphine: a meta-analysis and systematic review of the literature. J Palliat Med 2008; 11(3): 492–501.
89. Pasero C, Portenoy RK, McCaffery M. Opioid analgesics. In: McCaffery M, Pasero C, eds. Pain: Clinical Manual. 2nd ed. St. Louis, MO: Mosby, 1999:268–271.
90. Antman EM, Bennett JS, Daugherty A, et al. Use of nonsteroidal antiinflammatory drugs: an update for clinicians: a scientific statement from the American Heart Association. Circulation 2007; 115:1634–1643.
91. Joishy SK, Walsh D. The opioid-sparing effects of intravenous ketorolac as an adjuvant analgesic in cancer pain: application in bone metastases and the opioid bowel syndrome. J Pain Symptom Manage 1998; 16:334–339.
92. Ross JR, Goller K, Hardy J, et al. Gabapentin is effective in the treatment of cancer-related neuropathic pain: a prospective open-label study. J Palliat Med 2005; 8(6):1118–1126.
93. Hanna M, O'Brien C, Wilson MC. Prolonged-release oxycodone enhances the effects of existing gabapentin therapy in painful diabetic neuropathy patients. Eur J Pain 2008; 12:804–813.
94. Keskinbora K, Pekel AF, Aydinli I. Gabapentin and an opioid combination versus opioid alone for the management of neuropathic cancer pain: a randomized open trial. J Pain Symptom Manage 2007; 34(2):183–189.
95. Gilron I, Bailey JM, Tu D, et al. Morphine, gabapentin, or their combination for neuropathic pain. N Engl J Med 2005; 352(13):1324–1334.
96. Caraceni A, Zecca E, Martini C, et al. Gabapentin as an adjuvant to opioid analgesia for neuropathic cancer pain. J Pain Symptom Manage 1999; 17(6):441–445.
97. Bruera E, Roca E, Cedaro L, et al. Action of oral methylprednisolone in terminal cancer patients: a prospective randomized double-blind study. Cancer Treat Rep 1985; 69:751–754.
98. Tannock I, Gospodarowicz M, Meakin W, et al. Treatment of metastatic prostatic cancer with low-dose prednisone: evaluation of pain and quality of life as pragmatic indices of response. J Clin Oncol 1989; 7:590–597.
99. Ripamonti C, Twycross R, Baines M, et al. Clinical-practice recommendations for the management of bowel obstruction in patients with end-stage cancer. Support Care Cancer 2001; 9:223–233.
100. Mercadante S, Casuccio A, Mangione S. Medical treatment of inoperable malignant bowel obstruction: a qualitative systematic review. J Pain Symptom Manage 2007; 33:217–223.
101. Mystakidou K, Tsilika E, Kalaidopoulou O, et al. Comparison of octreotide administration vs conservative treatment in the management of inoperable bowel obstruction in patients with far advanced cancer: a randomized, double-blind, controlled clinical trial. Anticancer Res 2002; 22:1187–1192.
102. Thomas J, Kronenberg R, Cox MCC, et al. Intravenous lidocaine relieves severe pain: results of an inpatient hospice chart review. J Palliat Med 2004; 7(5):60–667.
103. McCLeane G. Intravenous lidocaine: an outdated or underutilized treatment for pain? J Palliat Med 2007; 10(3):798–804.

104. Ferrini R, Paice JA. How to initiate and monitor infusion lidocaine for severe and/or neuropathic pain. J Support Oncol 2004; 2:90–94.

105. Fitzgibbon EJ, Viola R. Parenteral ketamine as an analgesic adjuvant for severe pain: development and retrospective audit of a protocol for a palliative care unit. J Palliat Med 2005; 8:49–57.

106. Subramaniam K, Subramaniam B, Steinbrook RA. Ketamine as adjuvant analgesic to opioids: a quantitative and qualitative systematic review. Anesth Analg 2004; 99:482–495.

107. Patt RB, Cousins MJ. Techniques for neurolytic neural blockade. In: Cousins MJ, Bridenbaugh PO, eds. Neural Blockade in Clinical Anesthesia and Management of Pain. 3rd ed. Philadelphia, PA: Lippincott-Raven, 1998:1007–1064.

108. Yan BM, Myers RP. Neurolytic celiac plexus block for pain control in unresectable pancreatic cancer. Am J Gastroenterol 2007; 102:430–438.

109. Pan CX, Morrison RS, Ness J, et al. Complementary and alternative medicine in the management of pain, dyspnea, and nausea and vomiting near the end of life. A systematic review. J Pain Symptom Manage 2000; 20:374–387.

110. DeGraeff A, Dean M. Palliative sedation therapy in the last weeks of life: a literature review and recommendations for standards. J Palliat Med 2007; 10(1):67–85.

111. Chater S, Viola R, Paterson J, et al. Sedation for intractable distress in the dying—a survey of experts. J Palliat Med 1998; 12:255–269.

112. LoB, Rubenfeld G. Palliative sedation in dying patients: "We turn to it when everything else hasn't worked." JAMA 2005; 294(14):1810–1816.

20 Chronic Pain Following Electrical Injury

Elena N. Bodnar

Electrical Trauma Program, Department of Surgery, The University of Chicago, Chicago, Illinois, U.S.A.

THE DISORDER

Electrical injury is a serious and growing concern in today's medical community. According to the National Institute for Occupational Safety and Health, there were an estimated 46,598 nonfatal electrical injuries in the United States between 1992 and 2002 (1). With the increasing effectiveness of critical care services, the number of electrical injury survivors, who often experience long-term disabling conditions, will continue to increase. The primary consequences of electrical injury involve neuromuscular and neuropsychological problems, with chronic pain syndromes presenting as a nearly universal complaint (2, 3).

Electrical injury patients often experience loss of skeletal muscle and nerve function despite little or no evidence of thermal burn injury, as well as other cell damage localization and characteristics that are inconsistent with simple thermal effects. It has recently been established that, in addition to Joule heating, membrane electroporation and electroconformational denaturation of membrane proteins are significant mechanisms of electrical injury. Nonthermal mechanisms of electrical injury preferentially target nerve and skeletal muscle cells in the pathway of current flow. The direct action of electrical forces on tissues is caused by the buildup of electrical charge on the membrane surface of muscle and nerve cells which in turn is caused by the externally imposed electric field. The resulting supraphysiologic membrane potentials alter the structure and compromise the functional integrity of cell membranes. Whereas thermal injury mechanisms require electrical exposure for seconds or more, nonthermal effects can cause tissue damage within milliseconds (4–6).

Many survivors of electrical injury are unable to return to work or to resume their previous lives. The successful rehabilitation of these patients depends on an in-depth understanding of the complex biophysical mechanisms of electrical injury. Timely diagnosis and specific treatment regimes may prevent some of the long-term sequelae of electrical injury.

DIAGNOSIS

Patients who survive electric shock and lightning strikes are often misdiagnosed because they are infrequently seen in a medical practice. The overlooked diagnosis rate for lightning injury and electrical injury patients has been reported to be 93% and 98.2%, respectively (7). The diagnosis of electrical injury is usually made by history, and from the clinical perspective, it is important to recognize the pattern of damage. Determination of the patient's incidental electrical current exposure is fundamental to understanding the mechanism of injury (8).

Many electrical injury sequelae are not easily documented or quantified with standard medical tests. Diagnosis of pain in electrical injury patients is challenging because it is usually multifactorial and its impact often appears disproportionate to measurable neuropathology. Patients with pain symptoms and neuropsychological impairments frequently show no abnormalities on CT scans, MRIs, EEGs, or EMGs for various technical reasons (9).

Delayed and progressive pain symptoms are particularly difficult to diagnose because the link between the injury and the symptoms can often go unrecognized by the patients and their physicians. Neuropsychological problems in electrical injury also often begin after the patient is discharged from the hospital. Long-term follow-up is particularly critical with electrical injury patients. Health-care professionals who work in acute-care settings need to be cognizant of the chronic effects of electrical trauma so that referrals can be made for appropriate postacute diagnostic and treatment interventions (10–13).

When symptoms of neurological complaints exist, neurodiagnostic studies are required to determine the presence and extent of neuromuscular dysfunction. The clinical history and physical exam remain the most sensitive means of diagnosing neurological injury. It is important, however, to identify the presence and degree of peripheral nerve injury though multiple means. Electromyography and nerve conduction studies are often necessary to assess function and help to discern differences between unshocked and shocked peripheral nerves, as well as to follow recovery after electrical injury. Such diagnostic modalities are standard electrodiagnostic tests that are widely available and must be performed as early as possible (14, 15).

Comparing the postshock values of the amplitude of the action potential and compound nerve conduction velocity with the preshock values does not give any information about the nonhomogeneity of peripheral nerve damage. Because of the lack of sensitivity and specificity, such electrodiagnostic procedures may demonstrate results that are inconsistent with the sensory examination of the patient. Many electrical injury patients often have persistent symptoms despite nerve conduction patterns that look normal (14–18).

The velocity of a peripheral nerve action potential depends upon the diameter of the nerve fiber and upon the presence of a myelin sheath. The axons within the nerve trunk, which are of various sizes and types, have action potentials of varying amplitude and velocity. The compound action potential is an aggregate of the individual axonal action potentials (8, 14). Smith and Kimura have developed a technique based on the refractory period of transmission that can differentiate between the various types of fibers in peripheral nerves. In a spectral analysis of the peripheral nerve compound action potential, a sequence of stimuli is delivered to the nerve with increasing interstimulation intervals. As the interval between the stimuli increases, even more nerves are activated until finally the full signal is reestablished. The spectrum of refractory periods of a nerve can pinpoint the damage done by an electrical shock and determine which nerve fibers are functioning normally and which ones are not (19).

Many electrical injuries are occupationally related and often involve litigation, which can complicate the diagnosis of chronic pain (20). Diagnosable malingering has been noted to occur in electrical injury, particularly in patients who lack evidence of biologically significant exposure to electrical current. The Slick et al. criteria for Malingering Neurocognitive Dysfunctioning, which is a systematic, comprehensive, integrated, and research-based approach to the diagnosis of malingering, may be included as a part of evaluation when evidence of exaggeration is reported by neuropsychological testing (21).

PATHOPHYSIOLOGY

Electrical injury causes tissue damage by multiple biophysical mechanisms, including heat-mediated damage, cell membrane electroporation, electroconformational denaturation of membrane proteins, electrochemical interactions at the contact points, and blunt mechanical trauma due to thermoacoustic blast from a high-energy electrical arc. The cellular membranes of excitable cells, including nerves, skeletal muscles, and blood vessels, are particularly vulnerable to damage by electrical forces (22). Any disruption in the integrity of the plasma membrane of a cell causes metabolic stress that, if uncorrected, may eventually lead to cell death.

Electrical Energy Transport in Tissues

When an applied electrical potential drop is established across the human body, mobile charges will migrate and an electrical current is established between the points of contact. The current flow through the body is usually initiated by direct mechanical contact in the case of low voltage (less than 1000 V) and by an arc current in the case of high voltage. The passage of current at the interface requires the conversion of charge carriers from electrons to mobile ions. This conversion is mediated by electrochemical reactions at the skin surface that produce heat and toxic chemical by-products, which contribute to local tissue injury (2, 4).

The frequency of the electrical current is an important factor to the distribution of current density through the body. At frequencies below approximately 10 kHz, electrical current penetrates into the deeper tissues and the current distribution around cells along the current pathway is determined by the cell density, cell orientation relative to the direction of current flow, and cell size. Electrical currents at frequencies higher than 10 kHz, such as those produced by lightning strikes, do not readily penetrate the epidermis but pass along the surface of the skin (4, 5).

After penetrating the epidermis, which presents the largest resistive barrier to current flow through the body, the ionic current spreads out and distributes according to the relative conductance of the various tissues. Within tissues, the electrical current pathway is determined by the path of least resistance. Provided that the integrity of the plasma membrane of cells in the current pathway is not disrupted by thermal or electrical forces, the high resistivity of cellular membranes relative to the intra- and extracellular fluids causes the ionic current to flow around the cells. Because of the low relative electrical resistance of nerves and blood vessels, large arteries and nerves experience the largest current density. However, because of greater volumetric proportions, the majority of the current passes through skeletal muscles (4–6, 22, 23).

Thermal Injury

Thermal burn injury caused by Joule heating was once considered to be the only mechanism of tissue damage in electrical injury. Joule heating is caused by the movement of salt ions in response to an externally imposed electric field, which increases the average kinetic energy of surrounding molecules. In a typical industrial electrical shock scenario, the rate of Joule heating greatly exceeds the heat-dissipating mechanisms of tissue blood perfusion and skin surface-to-air convection. As a result, the temperature of tissues in the current path increases. The heat produced in the pathway of current may also spread to neighboring tissues by transfer. The thermally induced rise in temperature scales in time with the resistance of the conducting tissues and the square of the current density. Thermal burn injury is most likely to occur in tissues with the highest electrical resistance and current density, namely the current entry and exit points (5, 24).

Exposure of tissues to temperatures in excess of 43°C results in tissue damage at a temperature-dependent rate (25). Within a few seconds of electrical contact, resistive heating in the subcutaneous tissues along the current path produces temperatures sufficient to cause substantial damage. The thermally mediated damage to cells is caused by the denaturation of macromolecules, disruption of cell membranes, and other effects that are typically fatal to cells. Cellular membranes appear to be particularly susceptible to thermally induced disruption of the lipid bilayer, which renders the plasma membrane freely permeable to small ions (2, 5, 6). Depending on the amount of heat produced, demyelination and necrosis of neurons may occur (26).

Nonthermal Injury: Electroporation and Electroconformational Denaturation

The exposure of a cell to supraphysiologic electric fields can cause electroporation, or rupturing, of cell membranes (24, 27). Membrane electroporation, or electric field–induced permeabilization, is due to the reorganization of lipids in the lipid bilayer that occurs when electrical forces drive polar water molecules into cellular membrane molecular-scale defects (4, 28). The enlargement of molecular-scale defects in the lipid bilayer by electrical forces can increase the rate of free diffusion of ions through the membrane by several orders of magnitude, which may result in cell death due to metabolic exhaustion. As opposed to Joule heating, electroporation can cause slow cellular death that is consistent with the often-reported delayed neurological and neuropsychological symptoms of electrical injury (4, 24).

Elongated cells such as nerves and skeletal muscles for which the long axis is parallel to the direction of current flow are most vulnerable to membrane damage by electroporation (29). For example, electroporation of skeletal muscle tissue should be expected when more than 0.5 A of electrical current is passed through an extremity. Also, an electric field of 200 V/m in the direction of a 1-cm-long skeletal muscle cell should be sufficient to cause electroporation (24). Classical cable theory predicts that an externally imposed electric field will induce the greatest membrane potential in nerve cells with larger space constants and shorter charging times. It follows that large myelinated nerve cells, which have greater conduction velocities, are the most susceptible to electrical injury due to the higher probability of electroporation. Since peripheral nerves consist of nerve fibers with various diameters and degrees of myelination, it is important to recognize that the pattern of electrical injury is likely to be nonhomogenous, with greater damage to faster-conducting than to the slower-conducting fibers (2, 5, 19).

In addition to inducing the formation of pore-like structures in the lipid bilayer of cell membranes, electrical forces can also contribute to muscle and nerve dysfunction by impairing the structural integrity and function of membrane proteins. Upward of 30% of the plasma membrane is composed of proteins that perform essential cellular functions, such as ion channels, transporters, and signal receptors. Supraphysiologic electrical forces can stretch membrane proteins beyond their native conformations, resulting in protein damage that is distinct from thermal denaturation. Individual positively and negatively charged residues of proteins, as well as secondary protein structures such as α-helices, have a dipole moment. As a result, protein residues and secondary structures move and reorient in response to an externally imposed electric field, and supraphysiologic electric fields can have significant allosteric effects on membrane proteins (4, 5).

The voltage sensing and selectivity filter domains of ion channels are especially susceptible to the effects of supraphysiologic membrane potentials such as those experienced by nerve and muscle cells in electrical injury. In vitro experiments have shown that electrical shock can produce a reduction of channel conductance, ion channel selectivity, and the resting membrane potential of affected cells (30). Both Na and K channels have been shown to be affected by electroconformational damage, of which delayed rectifier K channels are the most vulnerable.

Electrical Injury Pattern
Because of the influence of many factors, including the multiple modes of frequency-dependent tissue–field interactions and variations in current density along the paths through the body, electrical shock trauma tends to produce a very complex pattern of injury that is far ranging in extent and highly variable in magnitude. The anatomical pattern, extent of tissue injury, and the relative contribution of Joule heating versus nonthermal tissue injury mechanisms are, in part, determined by multiple interacting variables, including the amount of current passed through the body, the voltage, frequency and current type of the electrical power source, the anatomical location of the pathway of electrical current, electrical contact duration, the body size and body position of the victim during electrical contact, the use of personal protective equipment, and the health history of the victim (2, 27, 31, 32). Personal protection equipment such as industrial garments and gloves, face shields, safety glasses, and arc enclosures usually moderate the intensity of the patient's incidental exposure (6). The magnitude of injury will vary whether the exposures involve direct mechanical contact with the energized surface by an unprotected body part or occur through electrical arc current flow. For example, electrical injury survivors who are shocked by direct physical contact with the electrical power source, as opposed to an electrical arc-mediated exposure, are significantly more likely to experience certain neurological and musculoskeletal symptoms, including chronic pain and headaches (33). Other factors such as barotraumas due to thermoacoustic blast forces generated by arc-mediated contact, especially if the victim is in an enclosed physical environment during the accident, and injuries associated with falls due to loss of consciousness may also add to the magnitude of electrical injury (34).

The duration of electrical contact is one of the main variables that determine the relative contribution of thermal versus nonthermal mechanisms of tissue damage, which is an important contributor to the extent of electrical injury. In the case of brief electrical contact, nonthermal mechanisms of cell damage will dominate. As the duration of electrical contact increases, the extent of thermal burn injuries also increases. In some cases, the contact duration can be influenced by whether the victim is shocked by a direct current or an alternating current power source. In addition to being associated with ventricular fibrillation, alternating currents can cause tetanic muscular contractions of the hand and forearm flexors. This phenomenon can cause the no-let-go response in which a victim's hand is unable to release the power source, prolonging the duration of electrical contact (5, 23, 35).

Compared to electrical injury by commercial power sources, survivors of lightning injury typically experience milder and shorter-term symptoms. Although the current and voltage of a lightning strike can be enormous, the duration of electrical exposure is usually between only 10 and 100 milliseconds (35–37). As a result, lightning injury survivors typically present with superficial burn injuries that may not require surgical intervention.

Chronic Pain in Electrical Injury Survivors

The clinical presentation of electrical trauma commonly involves physical, cognitive, and emotional complaints. Chronic pain syndromes are quite common following electrical and lightning injury and often serve as the basis of a patient's failure to return to work (19, 37, 38). Muscle aches, joint pain and stiffness, extreme physical sensitivity, headaches, paresthesia, burning skin, nerve compression symptoms such as carpel tunnel, and chronic general pain are among the most commonly reported physical symptoms, regardless of injury parameters (2, 24, 39, 40). A study by Pliskin et al. of 63 electrical injury patients evaluated by the University of Chicago Electrical Trauma Research Program found that paresthesias (49%), headaches (48%), muscle pain (40%), and burning skin pain (37%) had significantly high incidence in electrical injury survivors (41).

Persistent neurological complications exist in up to 85% of electrical injury patients who require hospitalization (5). A wide range of neurological impairments, including peripheral neuropathies, can occur immediately after shock or be delayed in onset. Permanent neurological sequelae of electrical injury have been correlated with demonstrable anatomical lesions, which can develop even when there is little evidence of damage to other tissues (4, 23, 26). The median nerve is most commonly affected by electrical injury, followed by the ulnar, radial, and peroneal nerves. These neurological complications can also be temporary, permanent, or get progressively worse with time. Symptoms can appear days, months, or even years after the injury and intensify over time (42–45). In fact, a higher incidence of neurological and neuropsychological symptoms is reported at 5.3 months than at 1.5 months postinjury (39). Headaches and pain are more commonly reported in postacute, or greater than three months postinjury, patients (41). Muscular pain, headaches, and other diverse neurological and neurobehavioral problems are the most prominent clinical features that usually persist.

Although high-voltage electrical injuries account for the largest fraction of major neurological complications, it has been established that the long-term impact of low-voltage electrical and lightning injuries is also significant (33). High incidence of persistent neurological, psychological, and musculoskeletal symptoms due to low-voltage electrical and lightning injury has been reported (24). It has also been reported that only 56.6% of low-voltage electrical injury patients are able to successfully return to work (33). A survey of Lightning Strike and Electric Shock Survivors, International members, a self-help group for electrical trauma survivors, has shown that both electrical and lightning injury survivors report a 75% decrease in their ability to return to work (37).

Intense pain associated with autonomic nervous system dysfunction is a serious complication of lightning and electrical trauma, of which complex regional pain syndrome (CRPS), both CRPS I (reflex sympathetic dystrophy) and CRPS II (causalgia), is of particular concern to electrical trauma patients (3, 37, 44). Typically, pain due to CRPS begins hours or days after electrical injury, but the onset can be delayed over a longer period such as a month. Electrical injury patients with CRPS experience severe burning pain, allodynia, and hyperalgesia, which are increased by physical and emotional stimulation. The pain is often out of proportion to the severity of the trauma, may eventually spread beyond the area of injury, and may be persistent (6, 42, 45). Although the spontaneous remission of CRPS is uncommon, the relapse of CRPS many months after electrical shock has been reported (44).

Electrical injury survivors commonly suffer from pain symptoms related to lingering effects of burn wounds, and subsequent fibrosis and scar formation. Electrical burn scars can often remain inflamed for a prolonged period of time, leading to painful, pruritic, and hypertrophic scaring (2). In addition to pain directly associated with the burn injury itself at the contact site and pain caused by tissue regeneration, electrical injured patients can experience intense, longer-lasting tingling and itching sensations that are almost equal in discomfort to the pain itself (35). Electrical burn scars can be stiff and often entrap nerves, leading to compression and decreased conductance. The time for the fibrosis to develop, progress, and cause a compressive neuropathy can explain the potential lack of a direct temporal relationship between the electrical injury and the peripheral neuropathy (43, 46).

Psychiatric Comorbidity

Electrical injury is associated with a high rate of psychiatric morbidity, including posttraumatic stress disorder, anxiety disorders, and major depressive disorders, which certainly have a significant role in pain perception (37, 38). These problems commonly occur, regardless of whether or not the head is a point of direct contact with the electrical current (47–50).

Multiple studies of lightning and electrical injuries have identified disabling neuropsychiatric changes for some electrical injury survivors, often persistent and occasionally progressive (37). Electrical injury patients diagnosed with comorbid psychiatric conditions exhibit poorer cognitive outcomes as compared to electrical injury patients with no psychiatric diagnosis (51–54). Patients with more psychological symptoms also tend to have a higher incidence of neurological symptoms (39).

Neuropsychological studies, including case reports, have indicated that electrical injury survivors experience a broad range of impaired neuropsychological functions, although there has been considerable variability (9–12). Pliskin et al. reported that in a carefully controlled study of neuropsychological tests in a series of 29 electrical injury patients treated at the University of Chicago Electrical Trauma Program and a carefully screened and matched group of 29 demographically similar, healthy electricians, electrically injured patients performed significantly worse on composite measures of attention/mental speed and motor skills (38). These significant differences in neuropsychological deficits could not be explained by demographic differences, injury parameters, litigation status, and mood disturbance.

The neural substrate of reported deficits in attention, learning, and working memory postelectrical injury remains poorly characterized. The first study to document task-dependent, system-level cortical and subcortical dysfunction in electrical injured by Ramati et al. demonstrated abnormal patterns of brain activation during working memory and procedural learning tasks in 14 electrical injured subjects compared to 15 demographically matched healthy control subjects performing a spatial working memory paradigm and a procedural learning paradigm during functional magnetic resonance studies (13).

TREATMENT

Management of chronic pain syndrome in electrical injury survivals presents many complexities and requires a detailed appreciation for the pathophysiology and clinical manifestations of electrical trauma. It requires a multidisciplinary team approach, with coordination of medications, physical and occupational therapies, behavioral strategies, and, if necessary, invasive remedies. Individual differences in injury symptom presentation, personality traits, and life circumstances should be considered in the planning of treatment and rehabilitation that is focused on managing pain symptoms, learning compensatory skills, providing psychosocial support, and preventing maladaptive behaviors (2, 4, 6, 37).

The treatment needs of electrical injury patients are usually not apparent at the initial evaluation. Aside from acute, physically obvious impairments, electrical shock survivors commonly develop persistent neurological problems and require significant ongoing interventions. Treatment of chronic pain related to neurological disorders after lightning and electrical injuries must borrow from the treatment paradigms and medical management strategies developed for the associated specific neurological and neurobehavioral syndromes, the details of which are described elsewhere. A treatment of choice for patients who wish to avoid the cognitive side effects of pain medications is hypnosis, which has been reported to be helpful for the pain problems of electrical injury survivors (37).

Rehabilitation therapy should include efforts to avoid chronic pain and causalgia-like complications. Reduction of pain and inflammation helps patient compliance with physical and occupational therapy, resulting in a better outcome. The clinical management of electrical burn scars should aim to reduce inflammation and mechanical tension to prevent the development of hypertrophic scaring. Cyclooxygenase inhibitors, such as ibuprofen, naproxen, and nambutone, may be useful in reducing pain and decreasing inflammation that leads to fibrosis. Vitamin antioxidants may also help reduce tissue inflammation. If the acute injury is not accompanied by significant wounds or deep tissue necrosis, the use of protective splinting and rest of the affected extremity may be helpful in reducing further neuromuscular pain and speeding the recovery process (6). Topical nonsteroidal anti-inflammatory agents with an occlusive barrier to increase scar moisture and temperature seem to be effective. Reconstructive surgery may be necessary to resurface a stiff, scarred, and painful skin surface (2).

Health-care professionals working with electrical injury patients at all phases of recovery should devote careful attention to evaluating the patients' psychiatric and cognitive status and initiate appropriate, timely interventions. The treating physician is unlikely to be successful in managing chronic pain related to electrical injury without successfully managing the psychiatric problems. While the literature suggests that many victims of electrical injury will not be satisfactorily relieved of chronic pain despite the methods used, it also suggests that improvement will be optimized by combining somatic and psychosocial therapies. This requires considerable coordination of efforts so that a scheduled dialog between treating physicians occurs (2, 36). The education of electrical injury patients is also very important. If patients are made aware of what to expect after electrical injury, they may be more vigilant about the timely reporting of outcomes to their physicians and, hence, will promptly receive necessary treatment interventions (12, 39).

Gradual reentry into previous life activities, especially work-related activities, is essential. Physical, cognitive, and work-related activities should be given to add responsibilities and demands as is comfortable to the patient. The goal of successful workforce reentry should be guided by consultation with the patient, coworkers, employer, and an experienced rehabilitation team.

CONCLUSION

Many survivors of electrical injury are unable to return to work or to resume their previous lives. The successful rehabilitation of these patients depends on an in-depth understanding of the complex biophysical mechanisms and clinical manifestations of electrical trauma. It requires a multidisciplinary team approach, with coordination of medications, physical and occupational therapies, behavioral strategies, and, if necessary, invasive remedies. The planning of treatment should focus on managing pain symptoms, learning compensatory skills, providing psychosocial support, and preventing maladaptive behaviors.

Although the management of acute pain in electrical injury patients is reasonably effective, the needs of chronic pain patients are still largely unmet, creating an enormous emotional and financial burden to sufferers, careers, and society. Improvements in the ability of the medical community to diagnose the causes of chronic pain, as well as development of new modalities for the treatment and prevention of long-term sequelae of electrical injury, are desperately needed.

REFERENCES

1. Cawley JC, Homce GT. Trends in Electrical Injury in the U.S., 1992–2002. EE Trans Ind Appl 2008; 44(4):962–972.
2. Lee RC, Bodnar EN, Rojahn KE. Diagnosis and management of electrical injury. In: Boswell MV, Cole BE, eds. Weiner's Pain Management: A Practical Guide for Clinicians. Boca Raton, FL: CRC Press, 2006:553–560.
3. Cooper MA. Disability, not death, is the main problem with lightning injury. Annual Meeting of the National Weather Association; October 1998; Oklahoma City, OK.
4. Bier M, Chen W, Bodnar E, et al. Biophysical injury mechanisms associated with lightning injury. NeuroRehabilitation 2005; 20:53–62.
5. Lee RC, Aarsvold JN, Chen W, et al. Biophysical mechanisms of cell membrane damage in electrical shock. Semin Neurobiol 1995; 15(4):367–374.

6. Danielson JR, Capelli-Schellpfeffer M, Lee RC. Upper extremity electrical injury. Thermal Injuries 2000; 16(2):225–234.

7. Hendler N. Overlooked diagnoses in chronic pain: analysis of survivors of electric shock and lightning strike. J Occup Environ Med 2005; 47(8):796–805.

8. Lee RC, Bodnar EN, Betala P, et al. Electric shock trauma. In: Barnes FS, Greenebaum B, eds. Biological and Medical Aspects of Electromagnetic Fields. Boca Raton, FL: CRC Press, 2007:333–349.

9. Pliskin NH, Fink J, Malina A, et al. The neuropsychological effects of electrical injury: new insights. Ann N Y Acad Sci 1999; 888:140–149.

10. Baily B, Gaudreault P, Thivierge RL. Neurologic and neuropsyhchological symptoms during the first year after an electric shock: results of a prospective multicenter study. Am J Emerg Med 2008; 26:413–418.

11. Heilbronner RL. Rehabilitation of the neuropsychological sequelae associated with electrical trauma. Ann N Y Acad Sci 1994; 720:224–229.

12. Martin TA, Salvatore NF, Johnstone B. Cognitive decline over time following electrical injury. Brain Injury 2003; 17(9):817–823.

13. Ramati A, Pliskin N, Keedy S, et al. Alteration in functional brain systems after electrical injury. J Neurotrauma, Online ahead of editing: March 26, 2009.

14. Mankani MH, Abramov GS, Boddie A, et al. Detection of peripheral nerve injury in electrical shock patients. Ann N Y Acad Sci 1994; 720(1):206–212.

15. Dendooven AM, Lissens M, Bruyninckx F, et al. Electrical injuries to peripheral nerves. Acta Belg Med Phys 1990; 13(4):161–165.

16. Christensen JA, Sherman RT, Balis GA, et al. Delayed neurologic injury secondary to high-voltage current with recovery. J Trauma 1980; 20(12):166–168.

17. Ratnayake B, Emmanuel ER, Walker CC. Neurological sequelae following high voltage electrical burns. Burns 1996; 22(7):574–577.

18. Gilyard CM, Morse MS, Mohr WJ, et al. The undetected trauma: low voltage electrical injury. J Burn Care Res 2008; 29(2): S151.

19. Abramov GS, Bier M, Capelli-Schellpfeffer M, et al. Alteration in sensory nerve function following electrical shock. Burns 1996; 22(8):602–606.

20. Andrews CJ, Cooper MA, Darveniza M, et al., eds. Lightning Injuries: Electrical, Medical, and Legal Aspects. Boca Raton, FL: CRC Press, 1991:163–186.

21. Bianchini K, Love JM, Greve KW, et al. Detection and diagnosis of malingering in electrical injury. Arch Clin Neuropsychol 2005; 20:365–373.

22. Tropea BI, Lee RC. Thermal injury kinetics in electrical trauma. J Biomech Eng 1992; 114:241–250.

23. Duff K, McCarrfrey RJ. Electrical and lightning injury: a review of their mechanisms and neuropsychological, psychiatric, and neurological sequelae. Neuropsychol Rev 2001; 11(2):101–116.

24. Morse MS, Berg JS, TenWolde RL. Diffuse electrical injury: a study of 89 subjects reporting long-term symptomatology that is remote to the theoretical current pathway. IEEE Trans Biomed Eng 2004; 51(8):1449–1459.

25. Lee RC, Capelli-Schellpfeffer M. Electrical and lightning injuries. In: Cameron JL, ed. Current Surgical Therapy. Baltimore, MD: Mosby, 1998:1021–1023.

26. Wilbourn AJ. Peripheral nerve disorders in electrical and lightning injuries. Semin Neurol 1995; 15(3):241–255.

27. Lee RC, Zhang D, Hannig J. Biophysical injury mechanisms in electrical shock trauma. Annu Rev Biomed Eng 2000; 2:477–509.

28. Block TA, Aarsvold JN, Matthews KL, et al. The 1995 lindberg award. Nonthermally mediated muscle injury and necrosis in electrical trauma. J Burn Care Rehabil 1995; 16(6):581–588.

29. Reilly JP. Scales of reaction to electric shock: thresholds and biophysical mechanisms. Ann N Y Acad Sci 1994; 720(1):21–37.

30. Chen W, Lee RC. Altered ion channel conductance and ion selectivity induced by large imposed membrane potential pulse. Biophys J 1994; 67:603–612.

31. Cherington M. Central nervous system complications of lightning and electrical injuries. Semin Neurol 1995; 15(3):233–240.
32. Solem L, Fischer RP, Strate RG. The natural history of electrical injury. J Trauma 1977; 17(7):487–492.
33. Theman K, Singerman J, Gomez M, et al. Return to work after low voltage electrical injury. J Burn Care Res 2008; 29(6):959–974.
34. Capelli-Schellpfeffer M, Toner M, Diller K, et al. Correlation between electrical accident parameters and injury. IEEE Trans Ind Appl 1998; 4(5):25–31.
35. Selvaggi G, Monstrey S, Van Landuyt K, et al. Rehabilitation of burn injured patients following lightning and electrical trauma. NeuroRehabilitation 2005; 20:35–42.
36. Primeau M, Engelstatter GH, Bares KK. Behavioral consequences of lightning and electrical injury. Semin Neurol 1995; 15(3):279–285.
37. Primeau M. Neurorehabilitation of behavioral disorders following lightning and electrical trauma. NeuroRehabilitation 2005; 20:25–33.
38. Pliskin NH, Ammar AN, Fink JW, et al. Neuropsychological changes following electrical injury. J Int Neuropsychol Soc 2006; 12:17–23.
39. Singerman J, Gomez M, Fish JS. Long-term sequelae of low-voltage electrical injury. J Burn Care Res 2008; 29(5):773–777.
40. Andrews CJ. Further documentation of remote effects of electrical injuries, with comments on the place of neuropsychological testing and functional scanning. IEEE Trans Biomed Eng 2006; 53(10):2102–2113.
41. Pliskin NH, Capelli-Schellpfeffer M, Law RT, et al. Neuropsychological symptom presentation after electrical injury. J Trauma 1998; 44(4):709–715.
42. Cohen JA. Autonomic nervous system disorders and reflex sympathetic dystrophy in lightning and electrical injuries. Semin Neurol 1995; 15(4):387–390.
43. Grube BJ, Heimbach DM, Engrav LH, et al. Neurologic consequences of electrical burns. J Trauma 1990; 30(3):254–258.
44. Jost WH, Schönrock LM, Cherington M. Autonomic nervous system dysfunction in lightning and electrical injuries. NeuroRehabilitation 2005; 20:19–23.
45. Ryan CM. Neurological manifestations of electrical trauma. In: Proceedings of the 26th Annual International Conference of the IEEE EMBS; September 1–5, 2004:5437–5439; San Francisco, CA.
46. Smith MA, Muehlberger T, Dellon AL. Peripheral nerve compression associated with low-voltage electrical injury without associated significant cutaneous burn. Plast Reconstr Surg 2002; 119(1):137–144.
47. Bodnar E, Variakojis R, Kelley K, et al. Pain and PTSD in survivals of electrical trauma. In: Proceedings of the 16th Charles Huggins Research Symposium. Chicago, IL: The University of Chicago, 2009:57.
48. Janus TJ, Barrash J. Neurologic and neurobehavioral effects of electric and lightning injuries. J Burn Care Rehabil 1996; 17(5):409–415.
49. Pliskin NH, Meyer GJ, Dolske MC, et al. Neuropsychiatric aspects of electrical injury: a review of neuropsychological research. Ann N Y Acad Sci 1994; 720:219–223.
50. Yarnell PR, Lammertse DP. Neurorehabilitation of lightning and electrical injuries. Semin Neurol 1995; 15(4):391–396.
51. Bodnar E, Ammar A, Fink J, et al. Assessment of the impact of post-traumatic stress disorder on brain function in electrical injured patients. In: Proceedings of the 29th Meeting of the Bioelectromagnetic Society; 2007:419; Japan.
52. Mancusi-Ungaro HR, Tarbox AR, Wainwright DJ. Posttraumatic stress disorder in electric burn patients. J Burn Care Rehabil 1986; 7(6):521–525.
53. Kelley KM, Tkachenko TA, Pliskin NH, et al. Life after electrical injury: risk factors for psychiatric sequelae. Ann N Y Acad Sci 1999; 888:356–363.
54. Ramati A, Rubin L, Wicklund A, et al. Prevalence and predictors of psychiatric morbidity following electrical injury and its effects on cognitive outcomes. 40th Meeting American Burn Association. J Burn Care Res 2008; 29(2):S152.

21 Neurogenic Thoracic Outlet Syndrome—A Biopsychosocial Approach

Allen J. Togut

The Commonwealth Medical College of Pennsylvania, Wilkes-Barre, Pennsylvania, U.S.A.

THE DISORDER

Neurogenic thoracic outlet syndrome (N-TOS) is a chronic illness that may involve part or all of the brachial plexus. It is predominantly a sensory disorder of pain and paresthesias, although it often includes motor dysfunction. It represents an entrapment neuropathy of a highly irritable brachial plexus. Maneuvers to test its ability to glide and its irritability will reproduce symptoms. N-TOS is often the result of repetitive trauma. Previous trauma(s) create the initial sensory injury (A-delta and C-fibers). More recent trauma(s) aggravate the previous injury and impact the central nervous system. Not only is motor function impacted, but the injuries may cause radiation of sensory symptoms beyond the original dermatomes and central sensitization (complex regional pain syndrome 2). The motor nerve injury usually results from compression by a cervical rib or incomplete cervical rib or other congenital abnormality.

Patients with N-TOS often present with nerve compression at more than one location—the so-called multiple crush syndrome. "Axoplasm flowing in ante grade fashion can be restricted at a number of locations" (1). The challenge for the physician is to determine the significance of each location.

The diagnosis of N-TOS is based on a detailed clinical evaluation. Laboratory findings and test results only apply in the context of the clinical findings. One needs to commit time to determine the nature of the problem. Often, the clinical situation is not adequately evaluated, the symptoms are discounted, and the diagnosis is not considered, resulting in ineffective management of the patient's distress. At other times, the diagnosis is based on a superficial understanding of the condition, and N-TOS is overdiagnosed, again, resulting in ineffective management.

The patient's odyssey through the health care system seeking the diagnosis and treatment amplifies the stress and adjustment problems caused by this debilitating condition.

Therefore, a biopsychosocial approach is crucial in assessing and treating the patient with N-TOS (2). The effective physician needs to know how the illness has impacted the individual's life and how effectively the individual has coped with it. The pain is unrelenting and grinds on the psyche, particularly when the patient hears or even senses that the physician thinks "it's all in your head." The subsequent dysfunction and disability of the extremity and hand frequently has a devastating impact on the patient's identity associated with multiple role loses, for example, wage earner, parent, and spouse. Happiness and self-image are seriously affected and frequently lead to a sense of uselessness, helplessness, hopelessness, and depression. Recommended therapies for this condition must be based on what is learned from a thorough psychosocial assessment as well as a clinical examination.

This chapter will concentrate on four areas—anatomy, etiology, and symptoms; physical and neurological examination; the role of testing; and management.

PATHOPHYSIOLOGY

Anatomy–Etiology

In N-TOS, anatomy defines the etiology. The brachial plexus is formed by the ventral rami of the spinal nerves C5 through T1. C5 and C6 (later forming the upper trunk) nerves pass through a myofascial compartment associated with the anterior scalene muscle and may be tethered to the muscle itself. Then, the middle trunk (C7) and the lower trunk (C8-T1) accompany the upper trunk through the interscalene triangle followed by the costoclavicular compartment and, finally, through the coracoid compartment in which the brachial plexus lies posterior to the pectoralis minor muscle as it enters the axilla.

The vertical sides of the interscalene triangle are formed by the anterior and middle scalene muscles, with the base being the first thoracic rib. Myofascial anomalies have been described by Roos, Brantigan (3,5) and others (6) and include bands from a long transverse process of C7, complete and incomplete cervical ribs, variations of Sibson fascia, anterior and middle scalene muscles, and the presence of a scalene minimus muscle. These anatomic anomalies predispose patients to suffer abnormal brachial plexus compression and irritation from trauma to the cervical region being the provocative factor. The costoclavicular compartment is bounded by the clavicle superiorly and the first rib inferiorly. The brachial plexus passes through this narrow space but may be scissored by scalene muscle spasm with elevation of the first rib, or by the presence of a cervical rib. In the coracoid compartment, the pectoralis minor tendon is anterior to the cords of the brachial plexus and may compress it as it makes a 90-degree bend with shoulder abduction.

The trapezius, levator scapula, and rhomboid muscles support the scapula on the posterior chest wall. When overused, as in cumulative trauma (assembly line worker) or as injured in a whiplash (motor vehicle accident), these muscles develop tonic spasm that increases shoulder traction of the brachial plexus. This process also creates contraction of the sternocleidomastoid and scalene muscles, causing the head to move into a partially flexed and tilted position with further constriction of the brachial plexus (7, 8).

Stretch injury of the brachial plexus, itself, must be differentiated from N-TOS. A stretch injury not only causes sensory symptoms but also motor dysfunction immediately after a specific trauma. N-TOS, on the other hand, is usually related to repetitive trauma or represents the later consequences of a specific trauma.

Symptoms

The pain usually radiates from the neck through the shoulder and through the supraclavicular area, and then down the upper extremity. Frequently, it will define the most involved part of the brachial plexus. Pain radiating down the inner brachium and forearm with tingling and numbness of the ring and small finger is consistent with the lower trunk–medial cord (C8/T1) and ulnar nerve involvement; whereas, pain radiating down the anterior brachium, lateral forearm with tingling, and numbness of the thumb, index, and long fingers is consistent with involvement of the upper trunk–lateral cord (C5, 6, and 7) of the brachial plexus and median nerve. In some cases, the two patterns coexist, suggesting that both the upper and the lower parts of the brachial plexus are involved.

Women are more often affected than men by a 3:1 ratio. Women with pendulous breasts may have their symptoms accentuated by the weight of the breasts, pulling the shoulders further forward adding to the work and dysfunction of the trapezii. By lifting up on the bra straps, thus, placing the breasts flush against the chest wall, there will be less distress. This suggests a role that these breasts are playing in accentuating their symptoms. A corset offering better support is indicated.

Coldness and sweating of the hand; changes in the quality and growth of hair and nails; static and mechanical allodynia, where touch and cool breeze crossing the skin surface are painful; and weakness and tremor of the extremity implicate sensitization of the central nervous system (complex regional pain syndrome 2).

Pain, paresthesias, limb fatigue, and weakness usually increase with activities of daily living with repetitive use and elevation of the arm in personal hygiene, cleaning house, writing, driving, and job requirements. These add to frustration, anguish, and feelings of hopelessness and helplessness. Unrelenting pain that is not being managed successfully and is always high on the visual analog scale results in the progression of symptoms, dysfunction, and further emotional distress.

DIAGNOSIS

Physical and Neurological Examination

The patient's symptoms are usually consistently reproducible by appropriate physical and neurological examination. Testing whether there are sensory and motor deficits or whether the brachial plexus glides and is irritated is the key to making the diagnosis.

The abnormal position of the shoulder—down and forward—and the tilt of the neck suggest the problem. The cervical and parascapular muscles may be tight and tender with identifiable trigger points.

Sensory assessment of the C2-T1 dermatomes should be carried out with a brush and a pin, two-point static discrimination of fingertips (normal range 2–3 mm), and vibration sense between the two forearms, testing ulnar and radial styloids, should be evaluated. Comparison should be made with the asymptomatic extremity.

Gliding and irritability of the brachial plexus are tested in the following fashion:

1. Nerve tension test is performed by having the patient tilt his/her head to one side. This puts a stretch on the contralateral brachial plexus. At that point,

ask what the patient is experiencing. The contralateral arm is then abducted to 90 degrees, or as much as the individual is able to do, further stretching that brachial plexus; then, ask what has changed. If the brachial plexus does not glide, the patient will often respond that he/she has more pain in the contralateral neck and shoulder muscles on the first maneuver. The pain on that side increases, going down the arm with tingling and numbness of certain fingers on the second maneuver, thus, reproducing symptoms.

2. In N-TOS, the brachial plexus above the clavicle at Erb's point, just lateral to the palpable anterior scalene muscle and in its infraclavicular position, is often quite sensitive. With gradual pressure, pain is experienced locally and radiates down the extremity with tingling and numbness of the fingers.

3. With the three-minute elevated arm stress test (EAST or Roos test), the patient raises his/her arms to the "surrender position," opens and closes the fingers slowly, and reports what is happening. The symptoms are recorded. Placing the forearms in full extension will reduce the tension on the ulna nerve if it is suspected to be part of the diagnosis. These symptoms are also recorded. The patient may abort the test earlier than three minutes due to increasing distress. Reproduction of the patient's usual symptoms strongly supports the diagnosis. The Adson test is commonly positive in normal people and does not have acceptable sensitivity or specificity for diagnosis of N-TOS.

Color, temperature, and sweating of the hands, and nail and hair quality are evaluated. Weakness of a particular muscle group is common, though atrophy is not. Presence of a tremor at rest or with use is also noted. With the reproduction of the patient's symptoms, along with sensory and motor deficits, the diagnosis is established.

Testing
Unfortunately, there are no laboratory tests with reliable sensitivity and specificity that confirm or deny the diagnosis. Cervical spine X rays should be obtained and may identify cervical anomalies such as a transverse process of C7 longer than that of T1, and incomplete or complete cervical rib. These are associated with congenital fibrous bands and muscle variations in the interscalene triangle (3). Cervical spine films may show cervical spine lesions, which could contribute to the patient's symptom complex. The typical Electromyographic/Nerve Conduction Study (EMG/NCS) has a sensitivity of only 30%. But when positive, it supports the diagnosis. N-TOS is predominantly a sensory illness and positive EMGs are unusual. The A-alpha fiber (motor neuron) is larger than and not as vulnerable to trauma as the A-delta and C-fibers, which are also found in the epineurium. Somatosensory evoked potentials or conduction velocities and latencies across the upper trunk–lateral cord and lower trunk–medial cord are better tests.

An MR neurograph, an MRI with special software and protocols, will better demonstrate changes in the brachial plexus, its relationship to surrounding structures, and variations in myofascial structures, and will serve as a guide if surgery is deemed appropriate (4). An MRI of the cervical spine should be obtained if symptoms and physical examination findings are suggestive of cervical disk disease or osteophytic encroachment on the neural foramina.

TREATMENT

Patients with N-TOS have commonly seen many doctors and have received many different diagnoses. Validation of the diagnosis is critical. Patients need to be educated about their illness and how they can take charge. Usually, they are pleased to learn that their problem is a medical reality and that it is not all in "their head," as they often have been told. They need to be an integral part of their therapy using the concepts of adapting, pacing, delegating, and assisting in developing positive coping skills. They need to learn how to avoid negative thinking and feelings, for those will accentuate their symptoms (cognitive behavior therapy) (9).

They have to avoid using their arms in a repetitive fashion and avoid elevated arm exercise. They must move from the time-honored way they learned to do a specific task to shorter time frames, better ergonomics, and sensitivity to messages from their bodies. Relaxation, distraction, biofeedback techniques, treating myofascial trigger points, and using a combination of narcotic and nonnarcotics will help.

The physician should realize that the patients' pain and their suffering is real and is associated with significant depression. This reality must be communicated to family members. Patients' symptoms have a major effect on their psyche and their ability to function. Too often the spouse does not want to change his attitude and impression, will not admit that his wife has a real problem, and so he does not want to participate in treatment. This lack of involvement becomes a barrier to treatment. Unfortunately, there are many dysfunctional families, and even though help is available, goal achievement may be limited. Many women have divorced or separated from their spouse because of the psychosocial stresses.

Surgery, decompression of part or the entire brachial plexus, is of value in some patients (10–12). A biopsychosocial approach is used to select patients for surgery. As with all therapies, the patient has to be honestly informed and participate in the discussion of the benefit–burden equation. Surgery is not a quick fix but is part of an overall treatment plan that requires the patient's active participation. Is there more to be gained or to be lost by recommending a surgical approach? The possible need for surgery and its urgency is determined by the total evaluation. With an established clinical diagnosis of N-TOS, the following factors suggest the need for surgery:

1. Positive EMG/NCS findings, a cervical rib complex, with or without muscle atrophy
2. Positive EMG/NCS findings, the presence of myofascial bands relating to the plexus seen on MR neurography, and a failure of appropriate physical therapy
3. No EMG/NCS changes, the presence of myofascial bands on MR neurography, and failure of or inability to do physical therapy
4. No MR neurography and severe symptoms that fail to respond to all forms of conservative management

The following clinical factors suggest that surgery is not indicated:

- Psychiatric illness
- Limited ability to understand the diagnosis and participate in postoperative and postdischarge care

- A member of a dysfunctional family with no or limited supports
- Comorbid conditions that would make surgery difficult or would complicate postoperative care
- Severe parascapular dysfunction with significant structural change
- Severe complex regional pain syndrome

Biopsychosocial assessment of patients with this illness will allow the physician to understand the illness, its impact on the patient's life, and to define appropriate management. Reasonable goal setting is important. It is critical to validate, educate, and guide them and to effectively treat their suffering. The patient has to play an integral role in the plan and with professional help must take charge of his/her illness and its nonoperative management.

This plan should include services identified through the diagnostic process. Surgery has an important role in a carefully selected subset of individuals, but there are some patients in whom the results of surgery will be poor, no matter how strong the indication because of the psychosocial problems.

REFERENCES

1. Mackinnon S, Dellon AL. Multiple crush syndrome. In: Mackinnon S, Dellon AL., eds. Surgery of the Peripheral Nerve. New York, NY: Thiem, 1988:347–392.
2. Gatchel RJ, Howard KJ. The biopsychosocial approach to pain. Pract Pain Manag 2008; 8:27–39.
3. Roos DB. Congenital anomalies associated outlet syndrome. Symptoms, diagnosis and treatment. Am J Surg 1976; 132:771–778.
4. Filler A, Kliot M. Application of magnetic resonance neurography and evaluation of patients with peripheral nerve pathology. J Neurosurg 1996; 85:299–309.
5. Brantigan CO, Roos DB. Etiology of neurogenic thoracic outlet syndrome. Hand Clin 2004; 20:17–22.
6. Gilliatt RW. Wasting of the hand associated with a cervical rib or band. J Neurol Neurosurg Psychiatry 1970; 33:615–624.
7. Mackinnon S, Novak C. Pathogenesis of cumulative trauma disorder. J Hand Surg 1994; 19A:873–883.
8. Leffert R. Thoracic outlet syndrome and the shoulder. Clin Sports Med 1983; 2:439–452.
9. Caudill M. Managing Pain Before It Manages You. New York, NY: Guilford Press, 2002:222.
10. Roos D. Essentials and safeguards of surgery for thoracic outlet syndrome. Angiology 1981; 32:187–193.
11. Mackinnon S, Paterson A, Novak C. Thoracic outlet syndrome: a current overview. Semin Thorac Cardiovasc Surg 1996; 8:176–182, 190–200.
12. Luoma A, Nelems B. Thoracic outlet syndrome—thoracic surgery perspective, surgical management of peripheral nerve injury and entrapment. Neurosurg Clin North Am 1991; 2:187–226.

22   Osteoarthritis

Thomas J. Romano

Private Practice, Martins Ferry, Ohio, U.S.A.

THE DISORDER

Arthritis can bring with it not only pain, suffering, and physical limitations, but also a negative impact on employability, and even financial hardship. Over 46 million American adults have self-reported, doctor-diagnosed arthritis (1). Over a third of these individuals have limitations due to arthritis (2). This problem is likely to rise considerably due to increasingly large numbers of senior citizens in the population among other factors (3). In addition to arthritis prevalence increasing with age, it is also higher among women in every age group in the United States (4).

In addition to the cost of patient treatment, there are significant indirect costs resulting from work absences, decreased productivity, and work disability (5). The ensuing economic problems encountered by many arthritis sufferers adversely affect quality of life and life satisfaction (6).

Of the many and varied types of arthritis, osteoarthritis (OA) is the most common. A recent epidemiological study reported that OA affects nearly 27 million Americans, an increase from 21 million in 1990 (7). As opposed to other types of arthritis such as rheumatoid arthritis that is a systemic inflammatory connective tissue disease, OA affects joints and surrounding structures and not the internal organs. It is typically a musculoskeletal problem that causes stiffness, loss of mobility, pain, and swelling in one or more joints. These symptoms are due to inflammation and degeneration in such joint structures as cartilage, bone, muscles, ligaments, and synovium. Any joint can be affected by OA but, typically, weight-bearing joints such as the hips, knees, low back, and ankles are prone to this disorder. Furthermore, injuries to joints may predispose those parts of the body to early development of OA such as might be found in relatively young individuals who have sustained sports or occupational injuries.

DIAGNOSIS

As with other medical conditions, establishing the diagnosis of OA entails taking a thorough medical history, performing a careful physical examination, and obtaining appropriate laboratory studies and radiographic tests. The importance of a careful clinical evaluation cannot be overemphasized. A large percentage of correct diagnosis can be made after a good history is taken, and an even larger percentage established when a thorough physical examination had been performed (8). This process is particularly important when OA is being considered since OA can be caused by other underlying medical conditions (9–11) and frequently coexists with others (12, 13). The typical patient with OA complains of pain on use of a joint associated with gelling and stiffness of the joint. Gelling and stiffness, if present, typically last less than 30 minutes, and often, patients will say once they start moving the joint, they will feel a grinding, clicking, or crunching of the joint in question. The physical examination often reveals bony enlargement of joints. This can be most readily appreciated by examination of the fingers. Often, Heberden's nodes, and Bouchard's nodes, bony enlargements of the distal and proximal interphalangeal joints, respectively, can be easily detected. Tactile and/or audible crepitus confirms the presence of roughening of the articular cartilage and effusions may be present. The most frequently involved joints are those of the hands (distal interphalangeal, proximal interphalangeal, and first carpometacarpal), hips, knees, acromioclavicular, and first metatarsophalangeal joints. Joint effusions, when present, tend to occur in weight-bearing joints, most often the knees. Other signs include the atrophy of the muscles surrounding the joint and, in the case of OA of weight-bearing joints, an altered gait would often be present. Instability of joints occurs in late stages of OA. X rays typically show marginal osteophytes, joint space narrowing, some bony sclerosis, and some cyst formation as well as malalignment (14, 15). As opposed to rheumatoid arthritis and systemic lupus erythematosus, blood tests are not particularly helpful in the diagnosis of OA, although negative tests will help to rule out other disorders. For example, the erythrocyte sedimentation rate, typically a very sensitive test for systemic inflammation, tends to be normal or only slightly elevated in patients with OA compared to the autoimmune-mediated rheumatologic diseases. Moreover, serology tends to be negative or weakly positive. Synovial fluid analysis may be helpful in that the joint fluid in OA demonstrates a relatively noninflammatory pattern. The typically clear, yellow or straw-colored fluid tends to be slightly viscous and has only a few thousand leukocytes compared to the more intensely inflammatory joint fluid seen in other arthropathies. There is evidence to suggest that inflammation of the synovial membrane augers poorly as it is often associated with a faster disease progression and ensuing impairment (16). Furthermore, frequent use of magnetic resonance imaging has also been helpful in determining the severity of OA. One study suggested that bone marrow lesions detected by magnetic resonance imaging correlated fairly well with higher levels of pain in OA patients. Also, those patients with knee OA and such lesions did have more rapidly progressing disease.

The pain experienced by OA sufferers tends to be multifactorial in its generation and perpetuation. Both peripheral and central mechanisms attribute to the misery experienced by many OA patients. The periphery-linked wear and tear and/or injury cause activation of inflammatory mediators such as interleukin-1 and prostaglandins, which can lead to disease progression (17). In particular, prostaglandin E_2 can contribute to the inflammatory process by sensitizing peripheral nociceptor terminals producing localized pain. This may be due to a direct effect or due to the increase in cyclooxygenase-2 (COX-2) (18, 19). The central nervous system gets involved after the A-delta fibers and C fibers transmit the nociceptor impulses through the peripheral nerve up to the dorsal root into the dorsal horn of the spinal cord and eventually to the central nervous system. The nociceptive impulses are interpreted via connections between the thalamus and cortex, resulting in a conscious awareness of the pain. The two main systems responsible for the perception of pain are the lateral and medial systems of the lateral spinal thalamic tract. The former system deals with activation of the thalamic nuclei and relays information to the cortex where the painful/noxious stimulus is analyzed for such properties as intensity, quality, duration, and location. The latter system has to do more with the affective response to pain (20). This affective response may be extremely important in the appreciation of pain, particularly in patients whose objectively variable pathology (e.g., damage seen by X ray of number of swollen joints) seems to be at odds with the patients' reported pain level. It is not an uncommon clinical occurrence for joint inflammation to be successfully treated with pharmacologic agents only to have the patient still complaining bitterly of pain despite an apparent (to the physician) adequate objective result. It is this author's experience that, for example, many patients with arthritis have concomitant fibromyalgia (21) and other comorbidities contributing to the global perception of pain. Merely addressing the adverse nociceptive stimuli from inflamed joints would be inadequate to help the patient in an optimal way, and other interventions may be needed to optimize the ability of the patient to function (22–24).

PATHOPHYSIOLOGY
As a rule, the pathology of OA follows a progression starting with the loss of cartilage matrix that predisposes the affected joint to further injury. As OA progresses, there tends to be alterations to underlying bone as well as associated wear and tear on the cartilage with the development of bony outgrowths called osteophytes at the periphery of the affected joint. Often debris, cartilage, and bone degradation products occupy the joint space, and eventually, more cartilage breakdown occurs when the synovium or joint lining becomes inflamed due to the release of inflammatory mediators such as cytokines and enzymes. Further cartilage damage and reactive bone formation occurs, and eventually, if unchecked, the affected joint may become totally dysfunctional leading to significant morbidity and impairment.

OA is the most common joint disorder not only in the United States but worldwide. Radiographic evidence of OA is present in most people aged 65 years or older and in over 80% of those older than 75 years. Furthermore, approximately 11% of people older than 64 years have knee OA that is causing pain, and/or stiffness and/or functional limitations (25). Knee OA has been cited frequently as a cause of impairment and disability (26, 27). There are many reasons for that. The knee is a weight-bearing joint, and often, it had been injured by work activities and/or sporting activities. Many patients often gain weight as they age. Being overweight or obese can be a risk factor in the development and/or exacerbation of knee OA (28–30). In addition to obesity, age is the most common identifiable risk factor for OA. Certainly genetics may also play a role. Bone abnormalities or inherited traits such as dysplasia or malalignment can subject joints to unusual stresses that could increase the likelihood of the development of OA. There is also a slight sex difference, particularly in the location of OA independent of age or physical activity. For example, hand OA is more prevalent in women while men are more prone to develop hip OA.

OA is an extremely costly disease. It is the most common cause of disability in the United States. One study measured both direct medical payments and lost productivity and came to the conclusion that the cost to the United States was $86 billion in 1997 (31). The costs are bound to rise. A subcommittee of the American College of Rheumatology (ACR) estimated that more than 20 million Americans will develop OA (32) as the population ages and as obesity becomes more prevalent.

TREATMENT

The treatment of OA must be individualized to fit the unique needs of each patient. To help clinicians achieve this goal, the ACR published guidelines for the treatment of hip and knee OA (32). These can be applied to address each patient's needs with the understanding that not every treatment is appropriate for all patients. At the outset, the patient must be informed of the nature and extent of his arthritic condition and how he can actively participate in his treatment. Each patient should be made aware of any aggravating factors peculiar to his situation and also of any comorbidities that may be causing or contributing to the pathological processes culminating in OA. The OA patient with thyroid problems or acromegaly must have these endocrinological problems controlled so that conventional OA treatment can be employed to maximum effect. Moreover, the "weekend warrior" who persists in doing strenuous, potentially damaging exercise, which includes impact loading on the joints, must be cautioned that these activities could result in a worsening of his OA. Exercises and activities that cause little impact loading on the joints are preferable. For example, swimming is an excellent exercise as well as aqua-aerobics and water walking. If the patient is overweight, a weight reduction regimen should be initiated. Other nonpharmacologic treatments include supplementation with chondroitin sulfate. This is available over the counter; it is relatively inexpensive and has been shown to be effective in OA (33). That study also showed that chondroitin sulfate not only helped while the patient was taking the supplement but that there was a carry-over effect. Even after the chondroitin sulfate therapy ended, good results were noted for up to six months. The optimal dose appears to be 800 to 1200 mg chondroitin sulfate daily (34). However, the mainstay of pharmacologic treatment for OA is the use of nonsteroidal anti-inflammatory drugs (NSAIDs). These medications tend to decrease pain, stiffness, and swelling, but have never been touted to stop the progression of OA. In fact, there is some evidence that certain NSAIDs may lead to progression of disease (35, 36). Commonly used NSAIDs and their respective daily dosage ranges include ibuprofen (2400–3200 mg), piroxicam (10–20 mg), naproxen (1000–1500 mg), diclofenac (50–150 mg), sulindac (200–400 mg), nabumetone (1000–2000 mg), etodolac (600–1000 mg), meloxicam (7.5–15 mg), indomethacin (50–150 mg), tolmetin (1200–1800 mg), and ketoprofen (100–200 mg). These nonselective NSAIDs all carry the risk of serious side effects. The most common problems seen with NSAIDs are those affecting the gastrointestinal tract. These side effects range from dyspepsia to severe peptic ulcer disease, occasionally resulting in fatal hemorrhage. In the United States, there are 16,500 deaths attributable to NSAIDs annually as well as 100,000 hospitalizations per year (37). Other NSAID-associated side effects include renal abnormalities (38), hepatotoxicity (39), and interference with platelet aggregation (40). To protect the stomach, the clinician has several options. One is to prescribe an H_2 antagonist or proton pump inhibitor along with the NSAID. Another is to prescribe a synthetic prostaglandin misoprostol 100 to 200 μg q.i.d. for the purpose of gastric cytoprotection. An alternative to the above NSAIDs is the use of nonacetylated salsalate or choline magnesium trisalicylate (2000–3000 mg daily). These preparations do not inhibit constitutive prostaglandins, thus, do not interfere with platelet function, renal plasma flow, or gastric cytoprotective mechanisms. A preparation combining diclofenac (50 or 75 mg b.i.d. to t.i.d.) with 200 μg misoprostol is also available commercially. More recently, a selective NSAID, inhibiting COX-2, celecoxib, has demonstrated efficacy in treating OA in doses of 200 to 400 mg daily while sparing the gastrointestinal tract (41). However, NSAIDs and COX-2 inhibitors have been shown to be associated with cardio-thrombotic events (37,42). Thus, these medications need to be used with caution. Acetaminophen, in doses not exceeding 4 g/day, has also been used successfully to treat the pain associated with mild OA, but this medication may be hepatotoxic and should be used with caution in patients with pre-existing liver disease and those who drink alcohol (43). For pure analgesia, tramadol in doses of 50 to 100 mg t.i.d. to q.i.d. can be used. It is a centrally acting analgesic available only by prescription. It is a weak opioid and not only does it bind to the mu opioid receptor but it also inhibits the uptake of serotonin and norepinephrine, thus acting on more than simply the nociceptive aspect of the pain. It has no anti-inflammatory properties and is generally well tolerated, but in some patients there is an increased risk of seizures (44). Patients in whom NSAIDs, acetaminophen, and tramadol have proven ineffective may require stronger analgesics such as opioids. Opioids act at the mu, kappa, and delta opioid receptors as well as peripherally (45). Many physicians are reluctant to use opioids for patients who do not have malignancies for a variety of reasons among which are fear of causing addiction, fears of possible oversight, and concerns about possible diversion. However, these medications can be of great benefit in certain patients and should be prescribed with caution but not withheld unnecessarily. Opioids are among the pharmacologic agents recommended for OA treatment by ACR (24). Best results are usually obtained by employing a long-acting oral opioid (morphine sulfate, oxycodone) or a fentanyl patch with short-acting opioids used for breakthrough pain (46).

If pharmacologic and nonpharmacologic treatments for OA fall short of the mark, other courses of action may be necessary. Acupuncture, while theoretically appealing, has not been shown to be very helpful in OA (47). Intra-articular injection with a corticosteroid local anesthetic mixture has been used for decades and can be quite affective in relieving pain in an affected joint. Dr. Joseph Lee Hollander (48) pioneered this technique and it has been used effectively to give temporary relief to countless patients. However, there is no proven benefit in terms of the halting of disease progression. Viscosupplementation is an alternative approach for patients who failed the above therapies. There are several products on the market, all of which have been termed "Hyaluronans." Because OA patients tend to have a decreased concentration or decreased molecular weight of hyaluronic acids in the joint space, those substances no longer provide necessary shock absorption and lubrication as they had done in the past. Hyaluronan supplementation has been used to help replenish and restore normal joint function by replacing the hyaluronic acid molecules that have been heretofore degraded and changed. The active ingredient in all of the five available Hyaluronans on the market to date have been extracted from chicken combs or made from bacterial cells. All of the products are indicated for knee OA, but in principle, they can be used for OA of any joint. They have a good safety profile and there is some evidence that preparations can promote normal cartilage growth (49). Clinical acumen must dictate how and when these agents should be used. In contrast to intra-articular corticosteroid injections, Hyaluronans do not raise blood sugar and have not been shown to have an adverse affect on cartilage or the surrounding structures.

When all else fails, surgery should be considered. Surgery can help relieve pain and improve joint mobility and can enhance the quality of life for many patients who otherwise would not be able to ambulate or perform even the most modest of activities of daily living. Arthroscopic surgery can be used to provide short-term relief in some cases but for most of the definitive results conventional surgery may be necessary. There are several operations that are available including osteotomy, hip resurfacing, partial joint replacement, and complete joint replacement. There is evidence that patients with knee OA, but not hip OA, develop worsening joint stiffness and physical function while waiting for joint replacement (50). There are more than 400,000 total knee replacements and more than 250,000 total hip arthroplasties in the United States annually, with a success rate of 80% to 90% (51). It has been estimated that the numbers of these procedures will rise to over 3 million and 572,000, respectively, yearly, by the year 2030 (48), with the bulk of these procedures performed on the elderly. Total joint arthroplasties are major surgical endeavors, and there are significant risks involved including deep venous thrombosis, infection, pulmonary embolism prosthesis fracture, and dislocation. Post surgery, the patients must participate in an extensive rehabilitation program that must be followed carefully in order to obtain optimal results.

In addition to a description of the pharmacologic, surgical, and other treatments aimed at the nociceptive component of medications, like antidepressants, targeting the affective component needs to be discussed. This is especially important since, often, depression and anxiety are overlooked in some OA patients (52). Comorbid depression may also contribute to noncompliance with OA treatment (53) and, thus, should be addressed when necessary. Depression may be a contributing factor in pain perpetuation, an increase in the number and severity of physical symptoms, and enhancing subjective assessments of pain-related disability (54, 55). In addition to pharmacologic interventions, cognitive–behavioral therapy (CBT) may be helpful in OA treatments. CBT focuses on coping strategies and belief systems that can adversely affect patients with arthritis (56). CBT has been shown to enhance both physical and psychological well-being in arthritis sufferers (57). However, patient involvement in CBT or any psychological intervention is extremely important. While no studies regarding compliance with CBT have been done in OA, reports of results in rheumatoid arthritis patients (58, 59) suggest that OA patients would be similarly affected. OA patients who suffer from chronic pain and who likely have higher levels of distress and dysfunctional behavioral and cognitive characteristics may be helped most by CBT (60). In addition to CBT, self-regulatory treatments may be employed to help mitigate the pain experienced by reducing psychological responses that pain tends to provoke. Techniques such as biofeedback, relaxation training, and guided imagery may help patients to reduce muscle tension and decrease mental distress. Often self-regulatory treatments are used in combination with CBT. To date, two randomized controlled trials showed that guided imagery with relaxation training resulted in improvement in both self-rated pain levels and quality-of-life measures among older women with OA (61, 62).

In summary, while OA is not a systemic inflammatory connective tissue disease and is not associated with extraarticular manifestations, it can cause tremendous pain and depression. OA can be extremely costly in terms of direct costs (i.e., treatment modalities) as well as indirect costs (e.g., lost wages, decreased productivity, disability, etc.). To obtain the best results, the clinician must consider all comorbidities as well as the pharmacologic and nonpharmacologic approaches to treatment.

REFERENCES

1. Hootman J, Bolen J, Helmick C, et al. Prevalence of doctor-diagnosed arthritis and arthritis-attributable activity limitation—United States, 2003–2005. MMWR Morb Mortal Wkly Rep 2006; 55(40):1089–1092.
2. Hootman JM, Helmick CG. Projections of U.S. prevalence of arthritis and associated activity limitations [abstract]. Arthritis Rheum 2006; 54(1):226–229.
3. Elders MJ. The increasing impact of arthritis on public health. J Rheumatol Suppl 2000; 60:6–8.
4. Theis KA, Helmick CG, Hootman JM. Arthritis burden and impact are greater among U.S. women than men: intervention opportunities. J Women's Health 2007; 16(4):441–453.
5. Li X, Gignac MA, Anis AH. The indirect costs of arthritis resulting from unemployment, reduced performance, and occupational changes while at work. Med Care 2006; 44:304–310.
6. Abell JE, Hootman JM, Zack MM, et al. Physical activity and health related quality of life among people with arthritis. J Epidemiol Community Health 2005; 59:380–385.
7. Helmick CG, Felson DT, Lawrence RC, et al.; National Arthritis. Estimates of the prevalence of arthritis and other rheumatic conditions in the United States: Part 1. Arthritis Rheum 2008; 58:15–25.
8. Sackett DL. The science of the art of the clinical examination. JAMA 1992; 267:2650–2652.
9. Holt PJL. Locomotor abnormalities in acromegaly. Clin Rheum Dis 1981; 7:689–709.
10. Adams PC, Speechly M. The effect of arthritis on the quality of life in hereditary hemochromatosis. J Rheumatol 1996; 23:707–710.
11. Gaines JJ, Tin GD, Kahn KN. The ultrastructural and light microscopic study of the synovium in ochronotic arthropathy. Hum Pathol 1987; 18:1160–1164.
12. Devecerski G, Tomasevi S, Teofilovski M, et al. The frequency of metabolic and endocrine diseases in patients with various types of osteoarthritis. Med Pregl 2006; 59(suppl 1):41–45.
13. Dahaghin S, Bierma-Zeinstr SM, Koes BW, et al. Do metabolic factors add to the effect of overweight on hand osteoarthritis? The Rotterdam Study. Ann Rheum Dis 2007; 66:916–920.
14. Altman R, Asch E, Bloch D, et al. The American College of Rheumatology criteria for the classification and reporting of osteoarthritis of the knee. Arthritis Rheum 1986; 29:1039–1049.
15. Altman RD, Hochberg M, Murphy WA, et al. Atlas of individual radiographic features in osteoarthritis. Osteoarthritis Cartilage. 1995; 3(suppl A):3–70.
16. Dougados M. Evaluation of disease progression during nonsteroidal anti-inflammatory drug treatment: imaging by arthroscopy. Osteoarthritis Cartilage 1999; 7:345–347.
17. Felson DT, Chaisson CE, Hill CL, et al. The association of bone marrow lesions with pain in knee osteoarthritis. Ann Intern Med 2001; 134:541–549.
18. Dougados M. The role of anti-inflammatory drugs in the treatment of osteoarthritis: a European viewpoint. Clin Exp Rheumatol 2001; 19(suppl 25):S9–S14.
19. Samad TA, Moore KA, Sapirstein A, et al. Interleukin-1 beta-mediated induction of COX-2 in the CNS contributes to inflammatory pain hypersensitivity. Nature 2001; 410:471–475.
20. de Brum-Fernandes AJ, Morisset S, Bkaily G, et al. Characterization of the PGE_2 receptor subtype in bovine chondrocytes in culture. Br J Dermatol 1996; 118:1597–1604.

21. Romano TJ. Fibromyalgia syndrome in other rheumatic conditions. Lyon Mediterranee Medical Medecine due Sud-est, 1996 Tome XXXII N5/6:2143–2146.
22. Vogt BA. Pain and emotion interactions in subregions of the cingulate gyrus. Nat Rev Neurosci 2005; 6:533–544.
23. Pariser D, O'Hanlon A. Effects of telephone intervention on arthritis self-efficacy, depression, pain and fatigue in older adults with arthritis. J Geriatr Phys Ther 2005; 28:67–73.
24. Calfas KJ, Kaplan RM, Ingram RE. One-year evaluation of cognitive–behavioral intervention in osteoarthritis. Arthritis Care Res 1992; 5:202–209.
25. Mjanek NJ, Lane NE. Osteoarthritis: current concepts in diagnosis and management. Am Fam Physician 2000; 61:1795–1804.
26. Centers for Disease Control and Prevention (CDC). Prevalence of disabilities and associated health conditions—United States, 1999. MMWR Morb Mortal Wkly Rep 2001; 50:120–125.
27. Leveille SG, Fried LP, McMullen W, et al. Advancing the taxonomy of disability in older adults. J Gerontol A Biol Sci Med Sci 2004; 59:86–93.
28. Anderson JJ, Felson DT. Factors associated with osteoarthritis of the knee in the first national Health and Nutrition Examination Survey (HANES I). Evidence for an association with overweight, race, and physical demands of work. Am J Epidemiol 1988; 128:179–185.
29. Ettinger WH, Davis MA, Neuhas JM, et al. Long-term physical functioning in persons with knee osteoarthritis from NHANES I: effects of comorbid conditions. J Clin Epidemiol 1994; 47:809–813.
30. Felson Dt, Anderson JJ, Naimark A, et al. Obesity and knee osteoarthritis. The Framingham study. Ann Intern Med 1988; 109:18–24.
31. Center for Disease Control. Update: direct and indirect costs of arthritis and other rheumatic conditions—United States, 1997. MMWR Morb Mortal Wkly Rep 2004; 53:388–389.
32. American College of Rheumatology Subcommittee on Osteoarthritis Guidelines. Recommendations for the medical management of osteoarthritis of the hip and knee: 2000 update. American College of Rheumatology Subcommittee on Osteoarthritis Guidelines. Arthritis Rheum 2000; 43:1905–1915.
33. Mazieres B, Combe B, Phan Van A, et al. Chondroitin sulfate in osteoarthritis of the knee: a prospective, double blind, placebo controlled multicenter clinical study. J Rheumatol 2001; 28:173–181.
34. Pavelka K, Manopulo R, Bucsi L. Double blind, dose-effect study of oral chondroitin 4 & 6 sulphate 1200 mg, 800 mg, 200 mg and placebo in the treatment of knee osteoarthritis. Litera Rheumatol 1999; 24:21–30.
35. Huskisson EC, Berry H, Gishen P, et al; on behalf of the LINK Study Group. Effects of anti-inflammatory drugs on the progression of osteoarthritis of the knee. J Rheumatol 1995; 22:1941–1946.
36. Reijman M, Bierma-Zeinstra SM, Pols HA, et al. Is there an association between the use of different types of nonsteroidal anti-inflammatory drugs and radiologic progression of osteoarthritis? The Rotterdam Study. Arthritis Rheum 2005; 52:3137–3142.
37. Wilcox CM, Allison J, Benzuly K, et al. Consensus development conference on the use of nonsteroidal anti-inflammatory agents, including cyclooygenase-2 enzyme inhibitors and aspirin. Clin Gastroenterol Hepatol 2006; 4:1082–1089.
38. House AA, Oliveira SS, Ronco C. Anti-inflammatory drugs and the kidney. Int J Artif Organs 2007; 30:1042–1046.
39. Rostom A, Goldkind L, Laine L. Nonsteroidal anti-inflammatory drugs and hepatic toxicity: a systematic review of randomized controlled trials in arthritis patients. Clin Gastroenterol Hepatol 2005; 3:489–498.
40. Kocsis JJ, Hernandovich J, Silver MJ, et al. Duration of inhibition of platelet prostaglandin aggregation by ingested aspirin or indomethacin. Prostaglandin 1973; 3:141–144.

41. Singh G, Fort JG, Goldstein JL, et al. Celecoxib versus naproxen and diclofenac in osteoarthritis patients. SUCCESS-I Study. Am J Med 2006; 119:255–266.
42. White WB, Faich G, Whelton A, et al. Comparison of thromboembolic events in patients treated with celecoxib, a cyclooxygenase-2 specified inhibitor, versus ibuprofen or diclofenac. Am J Cardiol 2002; 89:425–430.
43. Hepatitis C. Support Project Fact Sheet, January 2005. Available at: http://www.hcvadvocate.org. Accessed May 23, 2006.
44. Harati Y, Gooch C, Swenson M, et al. Double-blind randomized trial of Tramadol for the treatment of the pain of diabetic neuropathy. Neurology 1998; 50:1842–1846.
45. Stein C. The control of pain in peripheral tissue by opioids. N Engl J Med 1995; 332:1685–1690.
46. Portenoy RK, Hagen NA. Breakthrough pain: definition, prevalence and characteristics. Pain 1990; 41:273–281.
47. Manheimer E, Linde K, Laol L, et al. Meta Analysis: acupuncture for osteoarthritis of the knee. Ann Int Med 2007; 1416:868–877.
48. Hollander JL, Brown EM, Jessar RA, et al Hydrocortisone and cortisone injected into arthritic joints: comparative effects of and use of hydrocortisone as a local antiarthritic agent. JAMA 1951; 147:1629–1635.
49. Altman RD, Moskowiwtz R. Intraarticular sodium hyaluronate (Hyalgan) in the treatment of patients with osteoarthritis of the knee: a randomized clinical trial. J Rheumatol 1998; 25:2203–2212.
50. Kapstad H, Rustoen T, Hanestad BR, et al. Changes in pain, stiffness and physical function in patients with osteoarthritis waiting for hip or knee joint replacement surgery. Osteoarthritis Cartilage 2007; 15:837–843.
51. Kurtz S, Ong K, Law E, et al. Projections of primary and revision hip and knee arthroplasty in the United States from 2005 to 2030. J Bone Joint Surg Am 2007; 89:780–785.
52. Memel DS, Kirwan JR, Sharp DJ, et al. General practitioners miss disability and anxiety as well as depression in their patients with osteoarthritis. Br J Gen Pract 2000; 50:645–648.
53. DiMatteo MR, Lepper HS, Croghan TW. Depression is a risk factor for noncompliance with medical treatment: meta-analysis of the effects of anxiety and depression on patient adherence. Arch Intern Med 2000; 160:2101–2107.
54. Burns JW, Johnson BJ, Mahoney N, et al. Cognitive and physical capacity process variable predict long-term outcome after treatment of chronic pain. J Consult Clin Psychol 1998; 66:434–439.
55. Holzberg AD, Robinson ME, Geisser ME, et al. The effects of depression and chronic pain on psychosocial and physical functioning. Clin J Pain 1996; 12:118–125.
56. Keefe FJ, Caldwell DS. Cognitive behavioral control of arthritis pain. Med Clin North Am 1997; 81:277–290.
57. Mullen PD, Laville EA, Biddle AK, et al. Efficacy of psycho-educational interventions on pain depression and disability in people with arthritis. A meta-analysis. J. Rheumatol 1987; 14(suppl 15):33–39.
58. Sinclair VG, Wallston KA. Predictors of improvement in a cognitive–behavioral intervention for women with rheumatoid arthritis. Ann Behav Med 2001; 23:291–297.
59. Sinclair VG, Wallston KA, Dwyer KA, et al. Effects of a cognitive behavioral intervention for women with rheumatoid arthritis. Res Nurs Health 1998; 21:315–326.
60. Turk DC, Okifuji A. Directions in prescriptive chronic pain management based on diagnostic characteristics of the patient. Aust Prosthodont Soc Bull 1998; 8:5–11.
61. Baird CL, Sands L. A pilot study of the effectiveness of guided imagery with progressive muscle relaxation to reduce chronic pain and mobility of osteoarthritis. Pain Mang Nurs 2004; 5(3):97–104.
62. Baird CL, Sands LP. Effect of guided imagery with relaxation on health-related quality of life in older women with osteoarthritis. Res Nurs Health 2006; 29:442–451.

Nonopiate Analgesics and Adjuvants

Gary W. Jay

Clinical Disease Area Expert-Pain, Pfizer, Inc., New London, Connecticut, U.S.A.

The purpose of this, and the next several chapters, is to give the reader basic clinical information regarding the medications mentioned elsewhere in this textbook.

There is no one way to use medications. It really depends on the patients with chronic noncancer pain and what they need. As will be noted below, there are some better methods of providing pain medication for the chronic noncancer pain patient, with specific reasons for both how and why. The use of adjunctive medication is also extremely important and will be discussed.

When a patient is initially seen, most physicians will follow the World Health Organization's three-step ladder (1), which divides pain into mild, moderate, and severe categories.

It is felt that mild pain should be treated with aspirin, acetaminophen (APAP), and nonsteroidal anti-inflammatory medications (NSAIDs), with or without the use of adjuvant medication.

For moderate pain, the World Health Organization indicates the use of mild narcotics (for the most part). These include codeine, hydrocodone, oxycodone, dihydrocodeine, and tramadol, with or without adjuvant medications.

Severe pain would mandate the use of the traditional opioids: morphine, hydromorphone, methadone, levorphanol, fentanyl, and oxycodone, with or without adjuvant medication.

Adjuvant medications include anticonvulsants, membrane stabilizers, N-methyl-D-aspartate (NMDA) antagonists, α_2 agonists, GABAnergic medications, and other agents including the antidepressants and neuroleptics. Opioids, antidepressants, and anticonvulsants will be discussed in the following chapters.

When used with opioids, NSAIDs may also be considered adjuvant medications. An important concept is multimodal (or balanced) analgesia, which is beneficial to both acute and chronic pain. This entails a rational combination of several analgesics, which have differing mechanisms of action to obtain improved efficacy and/or tolerability and safety when compared to similar or equianalgesic doses of a single drug (2).

For many years, NSAIDs have been used for treatment or management of mild to moderate pain, frequently in combination with APAP, which acts centrally and inhibits brain cyclooxygenase (COX) and nitric oxide synthase. New information has determined that APAP dosages of 4 g/day or more can induce hepatic abnormalities in normal healthy patients (3). NSAIDs can cause gastrointestinal symptoms and can potentially induce gastric bleeding. The selective COX-2 inhibitors were developed to deal with this problem, but they are now known to have potentially serious cardiovascular problems. New guidelines or statements from both the American (FDA) and European (EMEA) agencies indicate that when using NSAIDs, the smallest effective dose should be used for the shortest period of time (4). These reasons, among others, show the advantages of combining drugs at decreased dosages to give a better risk–benefit ratio for pain management. Weak opioids combined with APAP may be more beneficial, as more than one mechanism of action (MOA) are utilized (4, 5).

Studies have shown that combinations of NSAIDs and patient-controlled morphine analgesia offer advantages over morphine alone, another example of multimodal analgesia (6).

Multimodal analgesia is also used for outpatient surgery. These regimens should include nonopioid analgesics (i.e., local anesthetics, NSAIDs, COX inhibitors, APAP, ketamine, and α_2 agonists, for example) to supplement opioid analgesics. As this procedure may give good opioid-sparing effects, this may lead to a reduction in nausea, vomiting, constipation, urinary retention, sedation, and respiratory depression (7).

NONOPIOID ANALGESICS

The simple analgesics are easily chosen by the patient, if not the physician. They are inexpensive and easy to obtain. They include aspirin and APAP. Aspirin appears to work by inhibiting the synthesis of prostaglandin by blocking the action of COX, an enzyme that enables the conversion of arachidonic acid to prostaglandin to occur. Prostaglandins are synthesized from cellular membrane phospholipids after activation or injury, and sensitize pain receptors.

Aspirin, the prototypical NSAID, has anti-inflammatory and antipyretic properties, along with its pain-relieving properties. The recommended adult dose for treatment is 650 mg every six hours. Taking the aspirin with milk or food may decrease gastric irritation. Aspirin can also double bleeding time for four to seven days after taking 65 g. Peak blood levels are found after 45 minutes. The plasma half-life is two to three hours.

Acetaminophen (called Paracetamol in the United Kingdom)

This medication is used fairly universally for mild to moderate pain of all forms, including musculoskeletal pain, neuropathic pain, and even osteoarthritis (OA). An aniline derivative (coal tar analgesic), it is an antipyretic (with possible effects in the hypothalamic thermoregulatory center) and is very commonly used in combination drugs for pain and many other uses including combination cold (URI) preparations. It was first used clinically by von Mering in 1887 (8).

Acetaminophen, or N-acetyl-para-amino-phenol (APAP) appears to work centrally; its MOA appears far more complex than initially thought. Oral APAP has efficacy in the prevention of the development of hyperalgesia induced via direct activation of algetic spinal receptors (9). It is able to penetrate into the brain enabling both antipyresis and analgesic properties (10). The MOA of APAP appears to involve several systems:

- The eicosanoid system: APAP inhibits the COX enzyme and interferes with the conversion of arachidonic acid to prostaglandins (11, 12); COX-3 may be at least one site of APAP action (13).
- The serotonergic system: Up to fivefold increase in serotonin levels in multiple areas of the central nervous system (CNS) has been detected after APAP treatment (14). APAP analgesia is inhibited by tropisetron, an antiemetic and serotonin (5-HT) type 3 antagonist (15).

- The cannabinoid system: In the human CNS, paracetamol is metabolized to P-aminophenol which, via fatty acid amide hydrolase is transformed into N-arachidonoyl-phenolamine (AM404) (16). AM404 is a ligand at selective cannabinoid subtype 1 (CB1) receptors, as well as an agonist of transient receptor potential vanilloid type 1 receptors (TRPV1) and an inhibitor of fatty acid amide hydrolase, which would inhibit the reuptake and metabolism of anandamide, an endocannabinoid with analgesic properties (14, 16–19). The cannabinoids as well as endocannabinoids induce antinociceptive effects that are secondary mainly to CB1 receptors (20, 21).
- The opioid system: Cannabinoid-induced antinociception does appear to be associated with the release of opioid peptides into the brain (22). Opioid mu receptors, like the CB1 receptors found on many of the same neurons, are both associated with G proteins. The APAP metabolite AM404 may activate, at least in part, both the opioid and cannabinoid systems. The secondary interaction between CB1 and opiate receptors may then modulate other neurotransmitters including 5-HT, gamma-aminobutyric acid, both antinociceptive, as well as glutamate (21, 23, 24).

Naloxone (an opiate receptor antagonist) can prevent APAP's activity; APAP may be involved with the dynorphin system, as dynorphins interact with kappa receptors, and if they are blocked, the APAP-induced antinociceptive effects are reversed (25).

APAP is used for mild to moderate pain. It is considered first-line treatment for OA (26). It has few adverse effects except for hepatic toxicity, even leading to death, most typically found at dosages of 4 g/day or more, especially in patients with hepatic problems secondary to chronic alcohol abuse. Newer research finds the same problem (elevations in aminotransferase) in healthy adults taking 4 g of APAP a day for 14 days (3).

It is important to take a very specific history from patients regarding their APAP intake as they may neglect to tell you about APAP found in combination with other medications, which the patients may not even be aware of.

Its recommended dosage is 325 to 650 mg every four hours or 325 to 500 mg every three hours, with a maximum of 4 g (4000 mg) a day. The author tries to limit his patients' APAP to 2500 to 3000 mg a day, maximum. For moderate pain, 1 g may need to be given for optimal effectiveness, three times a day.

APAP is not extensively bound to proteins (only 10–25%). It has a high bioavailability (85–98%), a two-hour plasma half-life, and easily crosses the blood–brain barrier (BBB) with a peak concentration in the CSF in two to three hours.

Nonsteroidal Anti-inflammatory Drugs

NSAIDs are anti-inflammatory, analgesic, and antipyretic agents. They decrease prostaglandin production by inhibiting COX-1 and COX-2 enzymes. They are the drugs of choice for use in OA and rheumatoid arthritis for pain.

In June 2005, the FDA recommended a black box warning, which received final approval in January 2006 for CV events for all NSAIDs, prescription and over-the-counter forms. This black box warning noted NSAIDs could cause an increased risk of serious cardiovascular thrombotic events, myocardial infarction, and stroke, which could be fatal. This risk could increase with duration of use. Patients with cardiovascular disease or risk factors for cardiovascular disease may be at greater risk (27). This black box warning was in addition to the gastrointestinal black box warning regarding bleeding, ulcerations, and perforation of the stomach or intestines.

Renal events have also been reported with non-COX-2–specific NSAIDs as well as coxibs, including increased BUN, dysuria, urinary micturition frequency, hematuria, increased creatinine, renal insufficiency including renal failure, interstitial nephritis, albuminuria, urinary casts, cystitis, azotemia, nocturia, glomerular nephritis, polyuria, and more (28).

There are two type of NSAIDs: nonselective and selective (COX-2 inhibitors—only celecoxib remains in this group). All nonselective NSAIDs and coxibs are given at dosages that inhibit COX-2. This inhibition provides their antipyretic, anti-inflammatory, and analgesic effects. COX-2-selective drugs (celecoxib) might also be known as COX-1-sparing drugs, compared to nonselective NSAIDs (29).

Both nonselective and selective NSAIDs are considered second-line treatment for OA, as well as showing good efficacy for the pain of surgical procedures and other conditions that have an inflammatory component, such as dental surgery (30).

There are over 20 different NSAIDs in the United States in 10 different chemical classes:

1. Propionic acids (ibuprofen, naproxen, ketoprofen, ketorolac)
2. Indoleacetic acids (indomethacin, sulindac, etodolac)
3. Salicylic acids (nonacetylated)—(sodium salsalate, choline magnesium trisalicylate)—aspirin is acetylated
4. Phenylacetic acid (diclofenac)
5. Naphthylalkanone (Nabumetone)
6. Oxicam (Piroxicam)
7. Anthranilic acid (enolic)—(mefenamic acid, meclofenamate)
8. Pyrroleacetic acid (tolmetin)
9. Pyrazolone (phenylbutazone)
10. COX-2 inhibitors (celecoxib—rofecoxib and valdecoxib have been withdrawn from the market secondary to cardiovascular concerns)

The most frequently prescribed NSAIDs include the following:

- Naproxen sodium (Anaprox), which reaches peak plasma levels in one to two hours, and has a mean half-life of 13 hours. It can be taken at 275 or 550 mg every six to eight hours, with a top dosage of 1375 mg/day.
- Ibuprofen (Motrin) is prescribed in dosages of 600 and 800 mg per tablet. The suggested dosage for mild to moderate pain is 400 mg every four to six hours as needed.
- Ketoprofen (Orudis) is a COX inhibitor but also stabilizes lysosomal membranes and possibly antagonizes the actions of bradykinin. Its peak plasma level is reached in one to two hours and has a two-hour plasma half-life. It is now over the counter (12.5-mg tablets) but is best used as 50- to 75-mg capsules. The recommended daily dosage is 150 to 300 mg a day in three or four

divided doses. GI side effects are generally mild. Care should be taken when given to a patient with impaired renal function.

- Ketorolac Tromethamine (Toradol) can be given orally or parentally for moderate to severe acute pain. Peak plasma levels occur after intramuscular injection in about 50 minutes. Its analgesic effect is considered to be roughly equivalent to a 10-mg dose of IM morphine. The typical injectable dose is 60 mg. Because of its potentially significant hepatic/renal side effects, the FDA has stated that Toradol should be given orally, after an IM injection of 60 mg, at 10 mg, every eight hours, for a maximum of five days.

The import of the different chemical classes is simple: not every NSAID will help every patient. If a patient does not receive relief from ibuprofen, the clinician should not try naproxen, which is in the same drug class, but another NSAID from another class should be utilized.

NSAIDs are extensively bound to serum albumin (95%). They are metabolized by the cytochrome P450 system (the CYP2C0 isoform) in the liver and excreted in the urine. Therefore, their use in patients with renal or hepatic dysfunction may be problematic. The half-lives of the NSAIDs vary greatly, ranging from an hour to longer than 55 hours.

NSAIDs may induce problems including constipation, confusion, headaches, and the aforementioned renal and hepatic toxicity, as well as GI ulcerations. They should be avoided in the elderly and those patients with congestive heart failure, coronary artery disease, hypertension, cirrhosis, and renal insufficiency. NSAIDs do have drug interactions, including ACE inhibitors, anticoagulants, beta-blockers, and loop diuretics.

The selective COX-2 inhibitor celecoxib has less risk of GI toxicity and has no reported effect on platelets/coagulation.

Risk factors for nonselective NSAID GI toxicity include combinations of NSAIDs; concomitant use of glucocorticoids and a past history of peptic ulcer disease, bleeding, or perforation. Again, their use in the older patient increases possible problems.

The idiosyncratic adverse effects of NSAIDs are also important to note and include the following:

- Rash
- Photosensitivity
- Tinnitus
- Aseptic meningitis
- Psychosis
- Cognitive dysfunction (especially in the elderly treated with indomethacin)
- Possible infertility
- Pulmonary infiltrates with eosinophilia
- Possible hypertension from naproxen and ibuprofen

Finally, long-term use of some NSAIDs appears to have accelerated cartilage damage in OA and some question the appropriateness of the use of NSAIDs in OA.

Some prescribing information:

- Ibuprofen (Motrin): Its half-life is 2 to 2.5 hours after multiple dosing. Typical adult dose is 1200 to 2400 mg/day.

- Naproxen: It is highly protein bound with a half-life of 12 to 15 hours. May use naproxen sodium 275- and 550-mg tablets twice a day.
- Ketoprofen (Orudis): It is 99% protein bound; its half-life is between 1.4 and 3.3 hours. It is available in 25, 50, and 75 mg and an extended-release 200-mg capsule. It can be taken three times a day.
- Oxaprozin (Daypro): Elimination half-life is between 50 and 60 hours after repeated doses—adult dose is 600 to 1200 mg/day. Patients can begin with a loading dose of 1800 mg.
- Etodolac (Lodine): The elimination half-life is six to seven hours. Maximum analgesia in one hour after oral dose. Doses range, in the adult, from 400 to 1200 mg/day.
- Indomethacin (Indocin): Elimination half-life is 2 to 11 hours. Adult dose is 75 to 150 mg/day.
- Diclofenac [Cataflam (potassium salt), Voltaren (enteric coated)]: It has a 75-minute half-life. The adult dose is 75 to 225 mg/day.
- Nabumetone (Relafen): A prodrug, metabolized to active metabolite with half-life of 24 hours. Adult dose is 1000 to 2000 mg/day.
- Ketorolac (Toradol): It is the only NSAID with parenteral usage; its half-life is four to six hours. Oral dosing is 10 mg three or four times a day. If given via IM or IV route, typically oral dosing is limited to four to five days.
- When using NSAIDs in the elderly, dosages should be decreased, in many cases, by 50%.
- Celecoxib (Celebrex): It has a half-life of 11 hours; adult dose is 100 to 400 mg a day.

Finally, it may be safe to give a COX-1 or COX-2 to patients with asthma and aspirin intolerance (31).

These medications are frequently sold in combination with other drugs such as caffeine, which exerts no specific analgesic effects, but may potentiate the analgesic effects of aspirin and APAP. There are aspirin–caffeine combination drugs (Anacin) and aspirin, APAP, and caffeine combinations (Excedrin Extra-Strength, Excedrin Migraine, and Vanquish). The recommended dosage is two tablets every six hours as needed.

MUSCLE RELAXANTS

Muscle relaxants are given for acute soft tissue spasm/pain by some clinicians. They are probably best utilized during the first one to three weeks post injury. They may be useful in patients with significant muscle spasm and pain. They are used appropriately after the development of muscle spasm after an injury such as a slip and fall, motor vehicle accident, work and athletic injuries, or over-stretching.

These medications work via the development of a therapeutic plasma level. Their exact MOA is unknown, but they do not directly affect striated muscle, the myoneural junction, or motor nerves. They produce relaxation by depressing the central pathways, possibly through their effects on higher CNS centers, which modifies the central perception of pain without effecting the peripheral pain reflexes or motor activity.

Carisoprodol (Soma) is a CNS depressant that metabolizes into a barbiturate, meprobamate, which makes it both addictive and particularly inappropriate to use for patients with pain from muscle spasm in addition to minor traumatic brain injury. It acts as a sedative and it is thought to depress polysynaptic transmission in interneuronal pools at the supraspinal level in the brain stem reticular formation. It is short lived, with peak plasma levels in one to two hours and a four to six hour half-life. Dosage is 350 mg every six to eight hours. It should not be mixed with other CNS depressants. It is also marketed in two other combined forms (with aspirin as Soma Compound) and with Codeine, for additional analgesic effects. It may be associated with postural hypotension, syncope, tachycardia, trembling, diplopia, blurred vision, and dyspnea, among other pharmacodynamic effects. Use caution in patients with hepatic and renal dysfunction.

Chlorzoxazone (Parafon Forte DSC) is a centrally acting muscle relaxant with fewer sedative properties. It is reported to inhibit the reflex arcs involved in producing and maintaining muscle spasm at the level of the spinal cord and subcortical areas of the brain. It reaches its peak plasma level in one to two hours, and duration of action is 6 to 12 hours. It is well tolerated, and side effects are uncommon. Dosage is 500 mg three times a day. Pharmacodynamic changes demonstrate a generally well-tolerated drug. Cautions include anaphylaxis.

Metaxalone (Skelaxin) is a centrally acting skeletal muscle relaxant which is chemically related to mephenoxalone, a mild tranquilizer. It is thought to induce muscle relaxation via CNS depression. Onset of action is about one hour, with peak blood levels in two hours, and duration of action is four to six hours. The recommended dose is 2400 to 3200 mg a day in divided doses (tablets are 400 mg each). It should be used carefully in patients with impaired liver function and should not be used at all in patients with significant renal or liver disease as well as a history of drug-induced anemias. Side effects include nausea, vomiting, GI upset, drowsiness, dizziness, headache, nervousness, and irritability as well as rash or pruritus. Jaundice and hemolytic anemia are rare. Use caution in patients with history of drug-induced anemias and with pre-existing liver damage. Serial liver function tests (LFTs) should be performed.

Methocarbamol (Robaxin) is a centrally acting skeletal muscle relaxant. It may inhibit nerve transmission in the internuncial neurons of the spinal cord. It has a 30- to 45-minute onset of action. Peak levels are found in about two hours, and its duration of action is four to six hours. It comes as 500- and 750-mg tablets. Tablets containing methocarbamol and aspirin (Robaxisal) are also available. The recommended dose of Robaxin is 750 mg three times a day. As with all of these medications, it should be taken for 7 to 10 days. It is well tolerated, with initial side effects which resolve over time, including lightheadedness, dizziness, vertigo, headache, rash, GI upset, nasal congestion, fever, blurred vision, urticaria, and mild muscular incoordination. In situations of severe, seemingly intractable muscle spasm, Robaxin may be given intravenously in doses of about 1 g every 8 to 12 hours.

Orphenadrine citrate (Norflex, Norgesic) is a centrally acting skeletal muscle relaxant with anticholinergic properties thought to work by blocking neuronal circuits, the hyperactivity of which may be implicated in hypertonia and spasm. It is available in injectable and oral formulations. The IM dose of Norflex is 2 mg, while the intravenous dosage is 60 mg in aqueous solution. The oral formulation (Norflex) is given in 100-mg tablets—one tablet every 12 hours. Norgesic is a combination form, including caffeine and aspirin and should be given one or two tablets every six to eight hours. Norgesic Forte, a stronger combination, is given one half to one tablet every six to eight hours. Because of its anticholinergic effects, it should be contraindicated in patients with glaucoma, prostatic enlargement, or bladder outlet obstruction. Its major side effects are also secondary to its anticholinergic properties and include tachycardia, palpitations, urinary retention, nausea, vomiting, dizziness, constipation, and drowsiness. It may also cause confusion, excitation, hallucinations, and syncope.

Many of these medications are given in combination with other drugs, including barbiturates (butalbital and meprobamate) and narcotics (codeine, oxycodone, propoxyphene, etc.) This is probably not a good idea, as the barbiturates and narcotics can easily help develop patient dependence.

A useful combination may include methocarbamol 750 mg three times a day for 10 days in patients with significant spasm, accompanied by ketoprofen, 75 mg, every six to eight hours as needed, with food as needed. For the acute posttraumatic soft tissue injury, one tablet of each taken together every six to eight hours for two to three doses works very well. These muscle relaxants are for acute cases of muscle spasm and pain. If there is no help within 10 days or so, they most probably won't work. In such cases, particularly in patients with painful muscle spasm lasting three weeks or longer, tizanidine would be the drug of choice.

Tizanidine has been used for painful conditions involving painful muscle spasm of three weeks' duration or longer, spasticity, myofascial pain, tension-type headache, acute low back pain, and fibromyalgia. This medication is very sedating, but it works well when given at h.s., rather than t.i.d. Peak effect is in one to two hours, with a duration of effect between three and six hours. Half-life is about 2.5 hours. It should be used with caution in patients with renal insufficiency. Adverse events may include hypertension, bradycardia, palpitations, prolonged QT interval, pruritus, and xerostomia. Dosages should be in the range of 12 to 16 mg given at night. Also, the generic forms of tizanidine are very frequently found to have side effects of hallucinations and vivid dreams, much more frequently than the nongeneric form (Zanaflex).

There are few high-quality, randomized controlled trials (RCTs) providing evidence of the effectiveness of muscle relaxants. It is felt that a combination of a skeletal muscle relaxant with an NSAID or with tramadol/APAP may be superior to single muscle relaxants (32).

OTHER ADJUNCTIVE MEDICATIONS

Other possible forms of adjunctive medications include NMDA receptor antagonists. There are no NMDA receptor antagonists approved for the treatment of pain; Memantine is approved for treatment of Alzheimer's disease. The NMDA receptor antagonists include ketamine, dextromethorphan, amantadine, magnesium, and methadone, an opiate which is considered to have a 10% NMDA receptor antagonism. These medications may, in the future, be very beneficial; particularly antagonists at the glycine-site NR2B sites, at which weak-binding channel blockers have shown an improved side effect profile in animal models of pain (33). Ketamine is used as an adjunctive therapy in the hospice setting when opioid therapy is not sufficient (34). Ketamine alone, or with midazolam, have long been used for sedating children undergoing minor operative procedures or painful procedures such as changing dressings for burn patients (35, 36).

Finally, subanesthetic dosages of ketamine used in analgesia appear to act largely as a dopamine D2 receptor agonist.

The α_2 agonists include clonidine and tizanidine. Clonidine is widely used, orally, transdermally, epidurally, and intrathecally, for the treatment of pain secondary to cancer, postoperative pain, neuropathies, postherpetic neuralgia, headaches, labor, and complex regional pain syndrome, restless leg syndrome, and orofacial pain.

Vistaril, an antihistamine, can also be used in combination with narcotics as an adjunctive medication to prolong and possibly amplify their effects.

Tramadol

Tramadol appears to be the most widely used analgesic for chronic noncancer pain of all types in the relatively (in parts) opiophobic European Union.

Tramadol is a centrally acting analgesic that is related structurally to codeine and morphine. It consists of two enantiomers, both of which are important in the drug's analgesic mechanisms. The (+)-tramadol and the metabolite (+)-O-desmethyl-tramadol (also called M1) are mu opioid receptor agonists. The (+)-tramadol also inhibits serotonin reuptake, while the (−)-tramadol enantiomers inhibit norepinephrine reuptake, enhancing inhibitory effects on spinal cord pain transmission (33).

Tramadol is rapidly absorbed after oral administration. It is rapidly distributed in the plasma, with about 20% plasma protein binding. It is metabolized by O- and N-demethylation and by conjugation forming glucuronides and sulfates. Tramadol and its metabolites are excreted mainly by the kidneys, with a mean elimination half-life of about six hours (33, 34). The O-demethylation of the drug to M1 is catalyzed by cytochrome P450 (CYP) 2D6 (35). The analgesic potency of tramadol is only 10% of that of morphine status post parenteral administration. Tramadol produces less constipation and problems with dependence than equianalgesic dosages of opioids (36). There are no respiratory or cardiovascular problems associated with the drug (37). M1 has a greater affinity to the mu receptor and is felt to be mainly responsible for tramadol opiate activity (36). It is felt that the dual activity (opioid and nonopioid) explains its effectiveness in pain that may not be responsive to opiates alone: neuropathic pain (38). Tramadol is felt to be one of the first-choice drugs for the treatment of neuropathic pain; it has been found to be effective in several placebo-controlled studies (39–45).

In a Cochrane evidence-based review, tramadol was found to be "an effective treatment for neuropathic pain" (46). The reviewers found five "eligible" RCTs, three comparing tramadol with placebo, one comparing tramadol with clomipramine, and one comparing tramadol with morphine. All three trials comparing tramadol to placebo were positive, with tramadol being superior to placebo. There was not enough evidence to develop a conclusion regarding tramadol versus morphine or clomipramine (47). It was determined that the NNT was 3.5 (NNT is the number needed to treat, to find one patient with a greater than 50% diminution of pain) (47).

Tramadol has been found to be useful in the treatment of fibromyalgia (48). It is also now thought to have antidepressant activity (49). For moderate to severe pain, start at 25 mg PO q.a.m., then increase by 25 mg/day every three days to 25 mg q.i.d., then increase by 50 mg/day every three days to 50 mg q.i.d.

Maximum dosage should not exceed 50 to 100 mg every four to six hours as needed. Typically, no more than 300 to 400 mg a day should be used. Large studies have found that tramadol abuse is statistically low, about 1 patient in 100,000 (49).

Antiarrhythmics

Antiarrhythmics block ectopic neuronal activity at central and peripheral sites (50). Lidocaine, mexiletine, and phenytoin—type I antiarrhythmics—stabilize neural membranes by sodium channel blockade. Lidocaine suppresses spontaneous impulse generation on injured nerve segments, dorsal root ganglia, and dorsal horn wide dynamic range neurons (51, 52). Lidocaine infusions have been used to predict the response of a given neuropathic pain disorder to antiarrhythmic therapy (53). Lidocaine may be effective at subanesthetic doses, and following nerve blocks analgesia may outlast conduction block for days or weeks (53–55). It has been reported that patients with peripheral nervous system (PNS) injury experience better pain relief than those with central pain syndromes (56). If a trial infusion of lidocaine is effective, a trial of oral mexiletine is worth considering.

Mexiletine and ketamine produced a moderate decrement of static but not dynamic allodynia associated with postherpetic neuralgia (57). Also, mexiletine was used to treat the peripheral neuropathy secondary to chemotherapy with taxol—a 50% improvement was seen (58).

Prior to starting mexiletine, a baseline electrocardiogram is recommended to determine if the patient has underlying ischemic heart disease. Dosages may be increased from 150 to 250 mg three times a day over several days. Taking the medication with food may minimize gastric side effects, which are common and a major reason for discontinuing the drug. Other side effects of mexiletine are nervous system effects such as tremor and diplopia. Once on a stable dose, a serum level should be obtained (the therapeutic range is between 0.5 and 2.0 mg/mL).

Topical Preparations of Local Anesthetics

Topical preparations of local anesthetics may be effective for neuropathic pain when there is localized allodynia or hypersensitivity. Topical blockade of small- and large-fiber nerve endings should reduce mechanical and thermal allodynia. A topical lidocaine patch (Lidoderm 5% lidocaine) has become available, which can be applied to painful areas in shingles (herpes zoster) and in more chronic forms of neuropathic pain such as diabetic neuropathy or the ischemic neuropathies created by prolonged peripheral vascular insufficiency. Up to three patches may be applied at one time to the painful area. The patches can be worn for up to 12 hours a day. However, the treating physician must ensure that the patient understands that chronic forms of neuropathic pain may require a longer therapeutic trial, for example, 30 days, before optimal symptomatic control can be determined. In patients with diabetic neuropathy, Rowbotham et al. (59) have found that the addition of topical lidocaine patches to exogenous GABAergic oral agents may provide further improvement of symptom control.

A topical cream, eutectic mixture of local anesthetic (EMLA cream), a mixture of lidocaine and prilocaine, may also be useful for cutaneous pain. The cream may be applied three or four times a day to the painful area.

Corticosteroids

Corticosteroids are clearly useful for neuropathic pain, particularly in stimulus-evoked pain such as lumbar radiculopathy. The anti-inflammatory effects of corticosteroids are well known, which may partly explain their efficacy for pain. When administered epidurally for treatment of discogenic radiculopathy, corticosteroids inhibit phospholipase A2 activity and suppress the perineural inflammatory response caused by leakage of disk material around the painful nerve root (60). However, corticosteroids also act as membrane stabilizers by suppressing ectopic neural discharges (61, 62). Therefore, some of the pain-relieving action of corticosteroids may be due to a lidocaine-like effect.

Depot forms of corticosteroids injected around injured nerves provide pain relief and reduce pain associated with entrapment syndromes. Corticosteroids are also effective if given orally or systemically. In cancer pain syndromes, steroids such as dexamethasone may be first-line therapy for neuropathic pain. The potential side effects of corticosteroids are well known and may be seen whether given orally, systemically, or epidurally.

As interventional treatment of pain becomes the most likely type of treatment a pain patient can receive, more steroids are being used than ever before, in spite of objective lack of level A or 1 evidence-based medicine. A number of $n = 1$ studies are published showing that "Corticosteroids cure pelvic pain" (63). Larger studies show that psychopathology/psychiatric comorbidity is associated with diminished pain relief after a medial branch nerve block with steroids (64), an issue that is most frequently ignored. Some RCTs are being done. In one, it was found that there were no differences in short-term outcomes found between local ultrasound guided corticosteroid injection and systemic corticosteroid injection in rotator cuff disease (65).

Finally, corticosteroid-induced psychosis was found in a patient following a cervical epidural, four medial branch blocks, four trigger point injections, and a tendon injection, all with corticosteroids, all performed in one treatment session. Seven days later, the patient developed psychotic episodes, with racing thoughts, anger, agitation, pressured hyperverbal speech, and paranoia. The symptoms resolved spontaneously within 7 to 10 days. This is possibly the first report of this known potential complication (66).

Baclofen

Baclofen is useful for trigeminal neuralgia and other types of neuropathic pain (67), particularly as an add-on drug. Baclofen is a GABA-B agonist and is presumed to hyperpolarize inhibitory neurons in the spinal cord (68), thereby reducing pain. This GABA effect appears to be similar to benzodiazepines, such as clonazepam. Side effects of baclofen can be significant and include sedation, confusion, nausea, vomiting, and weakness, especially in the elderly. A typical starting dose is 5 mg three times a day. Thereafter, the drug can be increased slowly to 20 mg four times a day. Abrupt cessation may precipitate withdrawal with hallucinations, anxiety, and tachycardia. The drug is excreted by the kidneys, and the dosage must be reduced in renal insufficiency.

Baclofen is more commonly being used intrathecally via an implanted pump for pain as well as spasticity. It is also being used for refractory cancer pain, neuropathic pain, and visceral pain (69–72).

Capsaicin

Capsaicin is a C fiber–specific neurotoxin and is one of the components of hot peppers that produces a burning sensation on contact with mucous membranes. Topical preparations are available over the counter and are widely used for chronic pain syndromes. Capsaicin is a vanilloid receptor (TRPV1) agonist and activates ion channels on C fibers that are thermotransducers of noxious heat (>43°C) (73). With repeated application in sufficient quantities, capsaicin can inactivate primary afferent nociceptors via desensitization. For patients with pain due to sensitized nociceptors, capsaicin may be effective, if they can tolerate the pain induced by the medication. The drug causes intense burning, which may abate with repeated applications and gradual inactivation of the nociceptors. However, in patients with tactile allodynia, which is probably mediated by large fibers, capsaicin may not be as effective. Capsaicin extracts are available commercially as topical preparations, containing 0.025% and 0.075% and should be applied to the painful area three to five times a day. The preparation may be better tolerated if it is used after application of a topical local anesthetic cream.

TRPVI (vanilloid) receptors have become a major research target for both agonists and antagonists, with multiple treatment indications including postsurgical pain, postherpetic neuralgia, diabetic neuropathic pain, OA, and others, including cancer (74). Further research has found evidence that TRPVI receptors on the central branches of dorsal root ganglion (DRG) neurons in the spinal cord may play an important role in pain modulation and nociceptive transmission (75). It has also been noted that capsaicin-induced calcium desensitizes the TRPVI channels and contributes to capsaicin-induced analgesia (76).

TRPV1 receptors, as neuronally expressed, are nonselective Ca(2+) preferring cation channels. Other than capsaicin, this channel is activated by different stimuli including heat, acid, certain arachidonic acid derivatives, and direct phosphorylation via protein kinase C (PKC—see below) (77).

Protein Kinase C (PKC) Inhibitors

Activation of PKC has been implicated in noted changes in pain perception. When activated by phorbol esters, PKC enhances thermal hyperalgesia in diabetic mice. Activated PKC also leads to enhancement of excitatory amino acids (EAAs) in dorsal horn neurons as well as trigeminal neurons. It is therefore possible that PKC may induce neuronal sensitization that produces hyperalgesia in diabetic neuropathy. Ruboxistaurin, a PKC inhibitor, may be a valid treatment for diabetic neuropathic pain (78–80).

TRPV1 and TRPV4 channels are coexpressed in certain DRG neurons and TRPV4 can be sensitized by PKC in the DRG neuronal cell bodies as well as in the central sensory and nonsensory nerve terminals. This PKC-induced sensitization may play a synergistic role in nociception (81).

REFERENCES

1. World Health Organization. Cancer Pain Relief with a Guide to Opioid Availability; World Health Organization; 1996.
2. Schug SA. Combination analgesia in 2005—a rational approach: focus on paracetamol-tramadol. Clin Rheumatol 2006; 25(suppl 1):S16–S21.

3. Watkins PB, Kaplowitz N, Slattery JT, et al. Aminotransferase elevations in healthy adults receiving 4 grams of acetaminophen daily: a randomized, controlled trial. JAMA 2006; 296(1):87–93.

4. Langford RM. Pain management today—what have we learned? Clin Rheumatol 2006; 25(suppl 7):2–8.

5. Schnitzer TJ. Update on guidelines for the treatment of chronic musculoskeletal pain. Clin Rheumatol 2006; 25(suppl 7):22–29.

6. Elia N, Lysakowski C, Tramer MR. Does multimodal analgesia with acetaminophen, nonsteroidal antiinflammatory drugs or selective cyclooxygenase-2 inhibitors and patient-controlled analgesia morphine offer advantages over morphine alone? Meta-analysis of randomized trials. Anesthesiology 2005; 103(6):1296–1304.

7. White PF. The changing role of non-opioid analgesic techniques in the management of postoperative pain. Anesth Analg 2005; 101(5 suppl):S5–S22.

8. von Mering J. Beitrage zur Kenntniss der Antipyretica. Ther Monatscyh 1983; 7:577–587.

9. Crawley B, Saito O, Malkmus S, et al. Acetaminophen prevents hyperalgesia in central pain cascade. Neurosci Lett 2008; 442:50–53.

10. Courad JP, Besse D, Delchambre C, et al. Acetaminophen distribution in the rat central nervous system. Life Sci 2001; 69:1455–1464.

11. Rowlinson SW, Kiefer JR, Prusakiewicz JJ, et al. A novel mechanism of cyclooxygenase-2 inhibition involving interactions with Ser-530 and Tyr-385. J Biol Chem 2003; 278:45763–45769.

12. Anderson BJ. Paracetamol (acetaminophen): mechanisms of action. Paediatr Anaesth 2008; 18:915–921.

13. Warner TD, Mitchell JA. Cyclooxygenase-3 (COX-3): filling in the gaps toward a COX continuum? Proc Natl Acad Sci U S A 2002; 99:13371–13373.

14. Smith HS. Potential analgesic mechanisms of acetaminophen. Pain Physician 2009; 12:269–280.

15. Picering G, Loriot MA, Libert F, et al. Analgesic effect of acetaminophen in humans: first evidence of a central serotonergic mechanism. Clin Pharm Ther 2006; 79(4):371–378.

16. Bertolini A, Ferrara A, Ottani A, et al. Paracetamol: new vistas of an old drug. CNS Drug Rev 2006; 12(3/4):250–275.

17. Sinning C, Bernhard W, Coste O, et al. New analgesics synthetically derived from the paracetamol metabolite N-(4-hydroxyphenyl)-(5Z,8Z,11Z,14Z)-icosatetra-5,8,11,14-enamide. J Med Chem 2008; 51(24):7800–7805.

18. Di Marzo V, Deutsch DG. Biochemistry of the endogenous ligands of cannabinoid receptors. Neurobiol Dis 1998; 5:386–404.

19. Hogestatt ED, Jonsson BA, Ermund A, et al. Conversion of acetaminophen to bioactive N-acylphenolamine AM404 via fatty acid amide hydrolase-dependent arachidonic acid conjugation in the nervous system. J Biol Chem 2005; 280:31405–31412.

20. Manzanares J, Julian MD, Carrascosa A. Role of the cannabinoid system in pain control and therapeutic implications for the management of acute and chronic pain episodes. Curr Neuropharmacol 2006; 4:239–257.

21. Rice ASC, Farquhar-Smith WP, Nagy I. Endocannabinoids and pain: spinal and peripheral analgesia in inflammation and neuropathy. Prostaglandins Leukot Essent Fatty Acids 2002; 66(2/3):243–256.

22. Palazzo E, de Novellis V, Petrosino S, et al. Neuropathic pain and the endocannabinoid system in the dorsal raphe: pharmacological treatment and interactions with the serotonergic systems. Eur J Neurosci 2006; 24:2011–2020.

23. Schoffelmeer ANM, Hogenboom F, Wardeh G, et al. Interaction between CB1 and μ opioid receptors mediating inhibition of neurotransmitter release in rat nucleus accumbens core. Neuropharmacology 2006; 51:773–781.

24. Ruggieri V, Vitale G, Pini LA, et al. Differential involvement of opioidergic and serotonergic systems in the antinociceptive activity of N-arachidonoyl-phenolamine

(AM404) in the rat: comparison with paracetamol. Naunyn Schmiedebergs Arch Pharmacol 2008; 337:219–229.

25. Sandrini M, Romualdi P, Capobianco A. The effect of paracetamol on nociception and dynorphin A levels in the rat brain. Neuropeptides 2001; 35:110–116.
26. American College of Rheumatology Subcommittee on Osteoarthritis Guidelines. Recommendations for the medical management of osteoarthritis of the hip and knee: 2000 update. Arthritis Rheum 2000; 43:1905–1915.
27. World Health Organization (WHO) Pharmaceuticals Newsletter 2005; 3:8.
28. Barkin RL, Buvanendran A. Focus on the COX-1 and COX-2 agents: renal events of nonsteroidal and anti-inflammatory drugs-NSAIDs. Am J Ther 2004; 11:124–129.
29. Warner TD, Mitchell JA. COX-2 selectivity alone does not define the cardiovascular risks associated with non-steroidal anti-inflammatory drugs. Lancet 2008: 371(9608):270–273.
30. Barkin RL, Romano RJ. Nonopioid drugs for pain management. Patient Care 2004: 41–51.
31. Szczeklik A, Murray JJ; Celecoxib in Aspirin-Intolerant Asthma Study Group. Celecoxib in patients with asthma and aspirin intolerance. The Celecoxib in Aspirin-Intolerant Asthma Study Group. N Engl J Med 2001; 344(2):142.
32. Beebe FA, Barkin RL, Barkin S. A clinical and pharmacologic review of skeletal muscle relaxants for musculoskeletal conditions. Am J Ther 2005; 12:151–171.
33. Brown DG, Krupp JJ. N-methyl-D-aspartate Receptor (NMDA) antagonists as potential pain therapeutics. Curr Top Med Chem 2006; 6(8):749–770.
34. Legge J, Ball N, Elliott DP. The potential role of ketamine in hospice analgesia: a literature review. Consult Pharm 2006; 21(1):51–57.
35. Owens VF, Palmieri TL, Comroe CM, et al. Ketamine: a safe and effective agent for painful procedures in the pediatric burn patient. J Burn Care Res 2006; 27(2): 211–216.
36. Cheuk DK, Wong WH, Ma E, et al. Use of midazolam and ketamine as sedation for children undergoing minor operative procedures. Support Care Cancer 2005; 13(12):1001–1009.
37. Grond S, Sablotzki A. Clinical pharmacology of tramadol. Clin Pharmacokinet 2004; 43(13):879–923.
38. Desmeules JA. The tramadol option. Eur J Pain 2000; 4(suppl A):15–21.
39. Dworkin RH, Backonja M, Rowbotham MC, et al. Advances in neuropathic pain. Arch Neurol 2003; 60:1524–1534.
40. Stacey BR. Management of peripheral neuropathic pain. Am J Phys Med Rehabil 2005; 84(suppl 3):S4–S16.
41. Marchettini P, Teloni L, Formaglio Lacerenza M. Pain in diabetic neuropathy case study: whole patient management. Eur J Neurol 2004; (suppl 1):12–21.
42. Mullins CR, Wild TL. Pain management in a long-term care facility: compliance with JCAHO standards. J Pain Palliat Care Pharmacother 2003; 17(2):63–70.
43. Sindrup SH, Andersen G, Madsen C, et al. Tramadol relieves pain and allodynia in polineurpathy: a randomised, double-blind, controlled trial. Pain 1999; 83:85–90.
44. Waikakul S, Waikakul W. Penkitti P, et al. Comparison of analgesics for pain after brachial plexus injury: tramadol vs. paracetamol with codeine. Pain Clinic 1998; 11:119–124.
45. Harati Y, Gooch C, Sweenson M, et al. Double-blind randomized trial of tramadol for the treatment of the pain of diabetic neuropathy. Neurology 1998; 50:1842–1846.
46. Duhmke RM, Cornblath DD, Hollingshead JR. Tramadol for neuropathic pain. Cochrane Database Syst Rev 2004; 2:CD003726.
47. Cook RJ, Sackett DL. The number needed to treat: a clinically useful measure of treatment effect. BMJ 1995; 310:452–454.
48. Sumpton JE, Moulin DE. Fibromyalgia: presentation and management with a focus on pharmacological treatment. Pain Res Manage 2009; 13(6):477–483.
49. Reeves RR, Burke RS. Tramadol: basic pharmacology and emerging concepts. Drugs Today (Barc) 2008; 44(11):827–836.

50. Chabal C, Jacobson L, Mariano A, et al. The use of oral mexiletine for the treatment of pain after peripheral nerve injury. Anesthesiology 1992; 76:513–517.
51. Abram SE, Yaksh TL. Systemic lidocaine blocks nerve injury-induced hyperalgesia and nociceptor-driven spinal sensitization in the rat. Anesthesiology 1994; 80:383–391.
52. Swerdlow M. Anticonvulsant drugs and chronic pain. Clin Neuropharmacol 1984; 7:51–82.
53. Burchiel KJ, Chabal C. A role for systemic lidocaine challenge in the classification of neuropathic pains. Pain Forum 1995; 4:81–82.
54. Chaplan SR, Flemming BW, Shafer SL, et al. Prolonged alleviation of tactile allodynia by intravenous lidocaine in neuropathic rats. Anesthesiology 1995; 83:775–785.
55. Jaffe RA, Rowe MA. Subanesthetic concentrations of lidocaine selectively inhibit a nociceptive response in the isolated rat spinal cord. Pain 1995; 60:167–174.
56. Galer BS, Miller KV, Rowbotham MC. Response to intravenous lidocaine infusion differs based on clinical diagnosis and site of nervous system injury. Neurology 1993; 43:1233–1235.
57. Sasaki A, Serizawa K, Andoh T, et al. Pharmacological differences between static and dynamic allodynia in mice with herpetic or postherpetic pain. J Pharmacol Sci 2008; 108(3):266–273.
58. Yano T, Yamane H, Fukuoka R, et al. Evaluation of efficacy and safety of adjuvant analgesics for peripheral neuropathy induced by cancer chemotherapy in digestive cancer patients—a pilot study. Gan To Kagaku Ryoho 2009; 36(1):83–87.
59. Rowbotham MC, Davies PS, Verkernpinck C, et al. Lidocaine patch: double-blind, controlled study of a new treatment method for post-herpetic neuralgia. Pain 1996; 65:39–44.
60. Saal JS, Franson RC, Dobrow R, et al. High levels of inflammatory phospholipase A2 activity in lumbar disc herniations. Spine 1990; 15:674–678.
61. Castillo J, Curley J, Hotz J, et al. Glucocorticoids prolong rat sciatic nerve blockade in vivo from bupivacaine microspheres. Anesthesiology 1996; 85:1157–1166.
62. Devor M, Govrin-Lippmann R, Raber P. Corticosteroids suppress ectopic neural discharge originating in experimental neuromas. Pain 1985; 22:127–137.
63. Antolak SJ Jr, Antolak CM. Therapeutic pudendal nerve blocks using corticosteroids cure pelvic pain after failure of sacral neuromodulation. Pain Med 2009; 10(1):186–189.
64. Wasan AD, Jamison RN, Pham L, et al. Psychopathology predicts the outcome of medical branch blocks with corticosteroids for chronic axial low back or cervical pain: a prospective cohort study. BMC Musculoskelet Disord 2009; 10(1):22.
65. Ekeberg OM, Bautz-Holter E, Tveita EK, et al. Subacromial ultrasound guided or systemic steroid injection for rotator cuff disease: a randomized double blind study. BMJ 2009; 338:a3112.
66. Benyamin RM, Valleho R, Kramer J, et al. Corticosteroid induced psychosis in the pain management setting. Pain Physician 2008; 11(6):917–920.
67. Fromm GH, Terrence CF, Chattha AS. Baclofen in the treatment of trigeminal neuralgia: double-blind study and long-term follow-up. Ann Neurol 1984; 15:240–244.
68. Yaksh TL, Malmberg AB. Central pharmacology of nociceptive transmission. In: Wall PD, Melzack R, eds. Textbook of Pain. 3rd ed. Edinburgh, UK: Churchill Livingstone, 1994:165–200.
69. Newsome S, Frawley BJ, Argoff CE. Intrathecal analgesia for refractory cancer pain. Curr Pain Headache Rep 2008; 12(4):249–256.
70. Brennan PM, Whittle IR. Intrathecal baclofen therapy for neurological disorders: a sound knowledge base but many challenges remain. Br J Neurosurg 2008; 22(4):508–519.
71. Gronseth G, Cruccu G, Alksne J, et al. Practice parameter: the diagnostic evaluation and treatment of trigeminal neuralgia (an evidence based review): report of the Quality Standards Subcommittee of the American Academy of Neurology and the European Federation of Neurological Societies. Neurology 2008; 71(125):1183–1190.

72. Brusberg M, Ravnefjord A, Martinsson R, et al. The GABA(B) receptor agonist baclofen and the positive allosteric modulator CGP7930, inhibit visceral pain-related responses to colorectal distension in rats. Neuropharmacology 2009; 56(2):362–367.
73. Caternia MJ, Schumacher MA, Tominga M, et al. The capsaicin receptor: a heat-activated ion channel in the pain pathway. Nature 1997; 389:816–824.
74. Wong GY, Gavva NR. Therapeutic potential of vanilloid receptor TRPVI agonists and antagonists as analgesics: recent advances and setbacks. Brain Res Rev 2009; doi:10.1016/j.brainresrev.2008.12.006.
75. Spicarova D, Palecek J. The role of spinal cord vanilloid (TRPV1) receptors in pain modulation. Physiol Res 2008; 57(suppl 3):S69–S77.
76. Vyklicky L, Novakova-Tousova K, Benedikt J, et al. Calcium-dependent desensitization of vanilloid receptor TRPV1: a mechanism possibly involved in analgesia induced by topical application of capsaicin. Physiol Res 2008; 57(suppl 3):S59–S68.
77. Adcock JJ. TRPV1 receptors in sensitization of cough and pain reflexes. Pulm Pharmacol Ther 2009, doi:10.1016/j.pupt.2008.12.014.
78. Kamel J, Mizoguchi H, Narita M, et al. Therapeutic potential of PKC inhibitors in painful diabetic neuropathy. Exp Opin Invest Drugs 2001; 10(9):1653–1664.
79. Haslbeck M. New options in the treatment of various forms of diabetic neuropathy. MMW Fortschr Med 2004; 146(21):47–50.
80. Vinik AI, Bril V, Kempler P, et al. Treatment of symptomatic diabetic peripheral neuropathy with the protein kinase C beta-inhibitor ruboxistaurin mesylate during a 1-year, randomized, placebo controlled, double-blind clinical trial. Clin Ther 2005; 27(8):1164.
81. Cao DS, Yu SQ, Premkumar LS. Modulation of transient receptor potential vanilloid 4-mediated membrane currents and synaptic transmission by protein kinase C. Mol Pain 2009; 5:5.

24 Opioid Medications and Correct Medical Usage—An Update

Gary W. Jay

Clinical Disease Area Expert-Pain, Pfizer, Inc., New London, Connecticut, U.S.A.

The antinociceptive pain pathways have been described in detail in *Chronic Pain* (1). The descending pathways are opioid and monoaminergic based. The opioid analgesics appear to produce analgesia by inhibiting the ascending pain pathways (which carry nociceptive information to the brain), and activate the descending pain control pathways, which go from the CNS down the ventro-medial medulla and down to the spinal cord dorsal horn. Opioids act in the periaqueductal gray (via μ receptors) to decrease GABAergic inhibition of the descending pathways.

The basic mode of opioid action is to inhibit the release of excitatory amino acids such as glutamate from peripheral nociceptors and postsynaptic neurons in the spinal cord dorsal horn.

After acute pain, algetic or pain-inducing chemicals are released from the nociceptors' terminals, including substance P, glutamate, calcitonin gene–related peptide (CGRP), neurokinins, and more. These chemicals will enable nociceptive information to reach the dorsal horn (via the substantia gelatinosa) and move rostrally via the ascending pain pathways. Locally, these algetic chemicals induce a neurogenic or sterile inflammation, the presence of which continues to feed nociceptive information centrally.

Glutamate will anneal to the N-methyl-D-aspartate (NMDA) receptor as well as the AMPA (alpha-amino-3-hydroxy-5-methyl-4-isoxazole propionic acid) receptor.

The AMPA receptor has a low threshold and quickly fluxes sodium and potassium through it. The NMDA receptor has a voltage-gated magnesium "plug." Typically, in acute pain this is not dislodged and the NMDA receptor provides only minimal stimulation.

As a consequence of the pathophysiology of chronic pain, the magnesium is forced out of the NMDA receptor (secondary to continuous stimulation, in part) and calcium fluxes through the receptor and into the cell, where it reacts with protein kinase C and nitric oxide synthase, which enables the formation of nitric oxide. The nitric oxide leaves the cell and reacts with guanyl synthase, which closes the sodium channel. This enables the development of pain that will not respond to opioids, as opioids can only work on the terminal if the sodium channel is open. A major goal is to prevent this from occurring by treating pain earlier rather than later.

Continued nociceptive stimulation will produce other phenomena, including "wind-up" secondary to continuous C-fiber stimulation to the dorsal horn which will enable the wide-dynamic range neurons, which are essentially "on–off" cells, to turn on and not go off, producing, with the help of the NMDA receptors, central sensitization with changes in perception inducing hyperalgesia, mechanical hypersensitivity, and allodynia. When this occurs, simple analgesics and even strong opioids may not be able to diminish the pain.

As noted, the NMDA receptors contribute significantly to these problems. They help effectuate wind-up; they stimulate apoptosis (along with increases of excitatory amino acids such as glutamate); and one can see the induction of cell death by "hyperstimulation" by the excitatory amino acids.

Neuronal plasticity occurs—new neuronal connections are made in the dorsal root ganglia (DRG) as well as the spinal cord dorsal horn. One example is the formation of new sympathetic neurons sprouting in the DRG. The sympathetic nervous system responds to pain only during pathological conditions. This enables greater hypersensitivity in the DRG and the corresponding areas of the dorsal horn.

CNS plasticity is the focus of a major research initiative.

When the sympathetic nerves sprout into the DRG's somatic nerves, this interaction makes the pain more difficult to treat.

Does all chronic noncancer pain (CNCP) involve sympathetic nervous system input? Probably yes, but to a lesser degree.

The use of opioids becomes important, as the majority of CNCP may not involve significant degrees of central sensitization. This is important in that the more significant the degree of central sensitization that exists, the less likely the opioids will be very effective in stopping the pain.

Opioids are used for moderate to severe pain. They are agonists of opioid receptors (μ, the most common; κ, dealing with spinal cord and supraspinal information and may contribute to nociception; and δ).

Genetic variations of the μ receptor exist. Patients respond differently to μ-opioid receptor agonists (2). When the μ receptor is genetically changed in mice, they may be insensitive to one opioid but remain sensitive to other opiates (3). This may also explain the phenomenon of incomplete opiate cross-tolerance in humans. The μ-opioid receptor gene is called *MOR1*, and genetic differences may explain differences in opiate effectiveness (4).

Evaluation of studies of long-term use of opioids on the quality of life of patients with CNCP identified both moderate/high-quality and low-quality evidence, indicating long-term treatment with opioids can lead to significant improvements in functional outcomes, including quality of life in patients with CNCP (5).

There are no randomized controlled trials of opiates that are longer than 12 weeks. There are, however, open-label trials lasting 6 to 24 months (6). Average pain relief was found to be 30% in 11 reviewed studies. The studies reviewed also found that the most common adverse events were constipation, nausea, and somnolence. Further, only 44% of 344 patients in the open-label trials remained on opiates between 7 and 24 months (6).

Other studies reviewed opiate use in neuropathic pain and general persistent noncancer pain in both very short (<24 hours) to intermediate-length studies (8–56 days). All these studies found opiates to be first-line drugs for pain treatment, as they separated well from placebo (7–10). When number needed to harm (NNH) was evaluated, the range for the common adverse events of nausea (3.6), constipation (4.6), drowsiness (5.3), vomiting (6.2), and dizziness (6.7) were determined (9).

Opioids are considered safe drugs in that they have been used for centuries and we know a fair bit about them. The most common adverse events include constipation, dizziness, nausea, vomiting, somnolence, and confusion. The serious adverse events include respiratory depression and death.

Addiction, a nonphysiological reaction, is also considered a serious adverse event.

Opioid medications have multiple routes of administration, including oral, IV, IM, SQ, sublingual, intranasal, inhaled, transdermal, vaginal, rectal, intrathecal, and epidural.

Opioids are either hydrophilic (propoxyphene, codeine, morphine, hydrocodone and oxycodone, hydromorphone and methadone) (which also has NMDA antagonistic properties) or lipophilic (fentanyl and sufentanil). The lipophilic drugs are more lipid soluble and have greater μ receptor affinity.

Another way of evaluating opiates is looking at them as weak or strong. Going along with the WHO three-step process, this may make more sense.

Weak Opiates:

- Codeine has a weak affinity to μ-opioid receptors; it is about 15% as potent as morphine (the opiate "gold standard"). It has a 2.5- to 3-hour half-life; major side effects include constipation and nausea; dosages greater than 65 mg every four to six hours are not appropriate. Most analgesic activity requires biotransformation to morphine by CYP2D6. Therefore, patients taking a CYP2D6 inhibitor may obviate the effectiveness of the drug.
- Hydrocodone (Vicodin, Vicoprofen, Lorcet, Lortab)—considered to be the most abused analgesic, per DAWN studies (Drug Abuse Warning Network); analgesic and antitussive; has active metabolites (hydromorphone, dihydrocodeine; renal dysfunction will be problematic; same half-life as codeine; typically found in combination with acetaminophen or an NSAID; use 1 to 2 q4–6 hours as needed. As with all PRN analgesics, limit use to 7 or 10 days. Its analgesic efficacy may depend on CYP2D6 activity. Available only as combination tablets with ibuprofen or acetaminophen or ASA. Watch for maximal acetaminophen intake >4 g/day.
- Oxycodone (Percodan, Percocet, Roxicet, Tylox)—elimination half-life of 3 to 3.5 hours; no active metabolites; effectiveness is 7.7 times the potency of codeine; typically found in combination with acetaminophen; has fewer side effects than morphine when given orally; no ceiling effect for analgesia; typically given 1 to 2 orally every four to six hours. The combination tablets have different strengths of oxycodone (2.5/325, 5/325, 7.5/325 and 500, 10/325 and 650), which should be monitored with appropriate dose escalation.
  - OxyContin, extended-release oxycodone, has many good characteristics: short half-life, long duration of action; no clinically active metabolites; easy titration, with a steady state found in 24 to 36 hours; no ceiling dose; minimal adverse effects; low first-pass effect; 60% to 87% bioavailability; no crushing/chewing. Comes in 10-, 20-, 40-, 60-, and 80-mg tablets. At least one review of studies on the use of controlled-release oxycodone has found it to be a good alternative in the treatment of CNCP (11). Unfortunately, this drug is subject to multiple misconceptions and has been given the appellation "hillbilly heroin" by the news. It was considered a major drug of diversion. Of interest is a recent note that OxyContin on the street is so

expensive that addicts are going back to heroin (11). It is second on the DAWN list of medications associated with overdoses.

- Meperidine (Demerol)—has 10% of the efficacy of morphine; has significant anticholinergic properties; has been associated with tachycardia, mydriasis; the half-life is three hours; its metabolite normeperidine (half-life of 15–30 minutes) is considered neurotoxic, with the ability to induce seizures and myoclonus. It is rarely used at this time.
- Propoxyphene (Darvon)—related to methadone; efficacy similar to that of codeine; half-life is 6 to 12 hours, but duration of effect is three to five hours; its demethylated metabolite norpropoxyphene has a very long half-life of 30 to 60 hours and can induce cardiotoxicity; it can induce seizures; it is also a weak competitive NMDA receptor antagonist. It should be used with care in the elderly if it should be used at all in this patient population. At the time this is being written, there is a movement for the FDA to withdraw this drug.
- Tramadol (Ultram) (also see chap. 23)—a synthetic analog of codeine, with oral potency equal to that of codeine; it inhibits norepinephrine and serotonin (5-HT$_3$) reuptake and has weak central opioid receptor activity (about 30%); half-life is 6.7 hours; peak plasma level in 2.3 hours; has active metabolite; analgesia from tramadol and its metabolite; typically used at 50 to 100 mg every six hours, maximum dose of 400 mg/day.
  - Possible seizure risk with concurrent tricyclic antidepressant, selective serotonin reuptake inhibitor (SSRI), monoamine oxidase inhibitor (MAOI), and opioid use
  - Serotonin syndrome has been reported with the combined use of tramadol and other serotonergic agents including tricyclic antidepressants, MAOIs, bupropion, SSRIs, buspirone, venlafaxine, etc.
  - Ultracet is tramadol (37 mg) in combination with acetaminophen. The combination of these two drugs has been found to have a possibly significant role in multimodal analgesia (12).
  - Tramadol can induce delirium in healthy elder patients (13).

Strong Opiates:

- Morphine—the prototypical opiate; half-life of two hours, but an analgesic effect lasting four to five hours; 50% of oral morphine reaches the central compartment within 30 minutes; it has active metabolites morphine-6-glucuronide (M6G) and morphine-3-glucuronide (M3G). M6G is found to be more potent than morphine when given intrathecally as well as less potent than morphine when comparing central effects; M3G has no affinity for the μ- and δ-opioid receptors and appears to have no analgesic potency; it can induce allodynia and hyperalgesia and, with higher dosages, myoclonus and seizures—this appears to induce antinociceptive activity. It can also bring on a syndrome similar to opioid withdrawal. Renal impairment will enhance the buildup of M3G and M6G. When given anally, M6G is found in much higher concentrations than M3G.
  - Has extended-release formulations: Kadian and MS-Contin, given every 8 to 12 hours, and Avinza, given once daily
  - MS-Contin—50% of oral dose reaches the central compartment within 1.5 hours and peaks at 2.5 to 4 hours; steady state is reached in 24 hours; no chewing/crushing

○ Kadian—peak level in 9 to 10 hours, lasts six to seven hours; typical use is q 12 hours; consider q.d. use in the elderly; no crushing or chewing
○ Avinza—once a day; no crushing or chewing; equal milligram doses over a 24-hour period with one Avinza and a six times a day immediate-release morphine (MSIR)
- Hydromorphone (Dilaudid)—an analog of morphine; given IV, 1.5 mg of hydromorphone is equivalent to 10 mg of morphine; duration of action is three to four hours; it is metabolized primarily to hydromorphone-3-glucuronide and accumulation of the hydromorphone-3-glucuronide, which is also not analgesically active, can induce neuroexcitatory side effects including allodynia, myoclonus, and seizures.
○ Palladone, an extended-release formulation, was withdrawn secondary to overdosages when mixed with alcohol.
- Methadone—a synthetic μ-opioid agonist with approximately 10% NMDA antagonistic activity; considered equipotent to morphine when given parenterally; terminal elimination half-life is 50 to 120 hours; 90% protein bound; undergoes N-demethylation in liver and is excreted in urine; duration of analgesia is four hours; given chronically every six to eight hours; given in 5- and 10-mg tablets.
○ Major problem is the half-life—clinically, one should wait at least five to seven days (longer is better) before adjusting methadone dose—if increased too soon, as steady state is not reached quickly, patient may develop significant sedation and/or overdosage—discordance between analgesic duration and half-life.
  - If patient develops respiratory depression, long half-life necessitates at least a 36- to 48-hour observation period; multiple dosages of opiate antagonist may be necessary.
○ Cipro inhibits CYP1A2 and 3A4 (of the P450 system in the liver), thus increasing plasma levels of methadone.

The Federal Drug Administration (FDA) issued an alert/warning in November of 2006 regarding death, narcotic overdose, and serious cardiac arrhythmias secondary to methadone use. It noted that the duration of analgesic action (four to eight hours) was much shorter than its elimination half-life (8–59 hours) and suggested that physicians using the drug needed to be more knowledgeable about it.

Therapeutic levels of methadone were found to cause sudden death secondary to cardiac arrest. It is known that QTc prolongation and arrhythmogenesis can be induced by methadone (14–16). Methadone should not be a first-line opiate used for moderate to severe pain patients who are opiate naïve.

Methadone is well tolerated and effective in both cancer and noncancer chronic pain patients (17, 18).

- Fentanyl—oldest synthetic phenylpiperidine opioid agonist; 80 times more potent than morphine; it is very lipophilic; used IV for perioperative pain control; can be used epidurally or intrathecally. A buccal formulation has recently been approved.
○ Duragesic transdermal therapeutic system—four dosages used for 72 hours per patch (25-, 50-, 75-, and 100-μg patches); reaches steady state within 12 to 24 hours; can have end-of-dose failure; after the generic

formulation of the patch, the Drug Enforcement Agency (DEA) gave notice of increased overdosage.
- ○ Actiq—given orally for transmucosal absorption; swallowed fentanyl has significant first-pass (hepatic and intestinal) metabolism; fentanyl does have good buccal mucosal absorption—what is not absorbed here is swallowed; high lipid solubility means rapid transit to CNS.
- ○ Fentora, an effervescent buccal tablet, has been used in the treatment of breakthrough pain. Dosages range from 100 to 800 μg.

A black box warning exists indicating that the use of fentanyl of any type is only for patients with cancer pain who are opioid tolerant; it is contraindicated in acute and postoperative pain. Actiq cannot be converted microgram per microgram. Actiq is still used for migraine in some emergency departments. It is dangerous to use any form of fentanyl on patients who are opiate naïve.

- • Oxymorphone (Opana)—Dosages should be in the range of 5 to 20 mg q 4–6 hours, PRN. Peak action is in 30 minutes, with an average six-hour duration. Half-life is 7.2 to 9.4 hours. A relatively significant food effect on absorption exists.

USING NARCOTICS APPROPRIATELY

State and federal clinical practice guidelines do indicate that it is appropriate to ameliorate pain, and that the use of pain medications to do so is not illegal (19, 20). A set of "Frequently Asked Questions" was released by the DEA along with pain specialists from the University of Wisconsin in August 2004, the purpose of which was to indicate that physicians "cannot be arrested for properly prescribing narcotic pain killers that are the best treatment for millions of suffering patients" (21, 22). Unfortunately, the FAQ was withdrawn by the DEA and many statements retracted. This is discussed in greater detail below.

The Joint Commission for Accreditation of Health Care Organizations has determined that pain is the "Fifth Vital Sign" and mandated significant changes in hospital facilities to deal with this problem (23).

Undertreatment with opioid pain medication is becoming all too common for an estimated 40% to 70% of patients with chronic, intractable noncancer pain (24).

Medically, there are significant adverse effects of undertreatment of pain:

- • Physical
  - ○ Increased pulse, blood pressure, and respiration
  - ○ Increased risk of cardiac event in patients so predisposed
  - ○ Increased risk of atelectasis, pneumonia
  - ○ Decreased tissue oxygenation, leading to muscle breakdown, poor healing, weakness
  - ○ Decreased activity and mobility leading to decreased recovery secondary to limited ambulation
  - ○ Increased risk of thromboembolic events
- • Psychological
  - ○ Depression, anxiety disorders
  - ○ Sleep deprivation
  - ○ Anorexia
- • Immunological

- Decreased immune response secondary to decreased nature killer cells
- Socioeconomic
  - Decreased productivity, loss of work
  - Increased use of health care resources
  - Familial breakdown

The treatment of the CNCP patient with only narcotics is problematic and most often leads to failure. The most appropriate treatment is within an interdisciplinary pain management program (25–29). An important issue here is that part of the typical interdisciplinary program is the use and then weaning off of chronic opioid medications, as tolerated by the patient, and reflected by their continued and improved functionality.

Kalso et al. (6) note recommendations for the use of opioids in the CNCP patient. They indicate that the management of the patients' pain should be directed by the underlying cause of the pain. The prescribing physician should be aware of the patient's psychosocial status. Finally, they note that opioid treatment should not be considered a lifelong treatment.

The use of opioids in the CNCP patient does not have a routine, non-individualized answer. Clinically, many patients with CNCP with a very poor quality of life can improve their function with the use of time-release (around-the-clock, ATC) opioid pain medications. On the other hand, some patients may develop decreased functionality with chronic opioids. Therefore, *function* is the most important issue when dealing with pain patients and chronic opioid medications. If these patients are not showing an improved functionality on these medications, they may need to be stopped.

Most importantly, prior to the use of chronic opioid medications, the CNCP patients must have received all conservative and/or appropriate surgical treatment and failed it—meaning, their pain was not ameliorated and their functionality continued to be poor or show further decline.

For patients who have had and failed all appropriate treatment, the use of chronic narcotics may certainly be appropriate on an individualized basis. There are several tenets that should be followed. First, these patients should receive long-acting opioids on an ATC basis to maintain an acceptable level of comfort. These medications provide a relatively flat dose–response curve, which engenders effective levels of analgesia without the peaks and valleys seen with short-acting pain medications, and therefore provide less risk for potential drug abuse.

There are four basic time-release medications:

- Duragesic patches (Janssen) (percutaneous Fentanyl)—used on the skin for, most typically, 72 hours at a time. This medication also enables the patient to stop taking pain pills multiple times a day, helping to extinguish a medication-related behavior. A generic patch with a different mechanism is now being used.
- Morphine sulfate—different time-release formulations: MS-Contin (Purdue Pharma Stamford, CT) and Kadian (King Pharmaceuticals, Bristol, TN); both formulations to be given, most typically every 12 hours; Avinza (King Pharmaceuticals), a once a day preparation. There are generic forms of MS-Contin.
- OxyContin (Purdue Pharma, Stamford, CT)—time-release oxycodone, typically taken every 12 hours. It was this medication along with its nickname hillbilly heroin and multiple stories of drug abuse and drug diversion and

addiction that brought the current crises regarding the use of these medications to a head.

- Methadone (generic)—a very old medication, developed in the mid-20th century. This medication has a long half-life: it is not a "time-release" medication. It may be given every 8 to 12 hours. The difficulty in its use is twofold: poor understanding of its clinical attributes and use by many physicians and the fact that it is also used in specific government-approved heroin/opioid detoxification programs. Some pharmacies insist on having the words "for pain" on the prescription, or they would not fill it; another institutional problem for these patients—the stigma.

Many pharmacy formularies would not pay for the more expensive Oxy-Contin or Duragesic patches, leaving the morphine-derived time-release medications as well as methadone to be used. The problem here is natural selection. One of the breakdown products of morphine, M3G is pronociceptive and can induce significant side effects in the elderly as well as (less frequently) the young, including increased pain.

Even with a time-release medication, the CNCP patients on occasion need to be given a "breakthrough pain" medication, typically a short-acting, immediate-release opioid, which may be needed to lower nociceptive pain brought about by an acute exacerbation of pain secondary to any number of factors such as overactivity.

There are three types of breakthrough pain: incident or episodic—patients know what can cause the pain and take a pre-emptive, fast-acting pain medication. Next is idiopathic or spontaneous breakthrough pain, which comes on suddenly and not infrequently for no obvious reason. Lastly is end-of-dose failure, which is not as unusual as one would expect. Some patients will need to take MS-Contin or even OxyContin two or three times a day (q8h). Some patients use transdermal fentanyl patches, which are labeled to last 72 hours, but in some patients they may last only 48 hours. The physician can see the end-of-dose failure by the marked increase in breakthrough pain that occurs when the time-release medication has been metabolized and the blood level is dropping.

Breakthrough pain can be of moderate to severe intensity. It comes on quickly, typically in less than two to three minutes to maximal intensity. It can last, on average, 13 to 30 minutes, or longer, especially in cancer patients. For these reasons, the goal of treatment would be to use a pain medication with fast onset, such as transmucosal fentanyl.

The typical immediate-release medications used for breakthrough pain include the following:

- Ultram, Ultracet (Tramadol, with or without acetaminophen)—a medication which stimulates the μ-opioid receptors as well as affects serotonin and norepinephrine reuptake.
- Vicodin (Abbott Pharmaceutical, Abbott Park, IL)—hydrocodone and acetaminophen, given every four to six hours for breakthrough pain.
- Lorcet (Forest Pharmaceuticals, New York, NY), Lortab (UCB Pharma, Inc., Belgium), Norco (Watson Pharmaceuticals, Corona, CA)—hydrocodone and acetaminophen, to be used every four to six hours for breakthrough pain. Norco has the smallest dosages of acetaminophen, making the acetaminophen load lowest, and is therefore the least hepatotoxic, depending on the number utilized each day.

- Percocet (Endo Pharmaceuticals, Chadds Ford, PA)—oxycodone and acetaminophen, given every four to six hours for breakthrough pain.
- Roxicodone (Roxane Pharmaceuticals—a member of the Boehringer Ingelheim group of Pharmaceutical Companies (Ridgefield, CT)—oxycodone without acetaminophen, given every four to six hours for breakthrough pain.
- Actiq (Cephalon, Inc., Frazer, PA)—fentanyl oral transmucosal, an oralette or "lollypop" on a stick; allowed to dissolve in the mouth, with medication entering the system transmucosally; to be used every four to six hours for severe breakthrough pain. While labeled for breakthrough pain in cancer patients, it is now being used by many clinicians for moderate to severe breakthrough pain in the CNCP patients.

The use of immediate-release narcotics with acetaminophen and/or a nonsteroidal anti-inflammatory medication must be looked at carefully secondary to possible hepatotoxicity and nephrotoxicity.

In medical practice, physicians should use an extended-release (ATC) pain medication for the CNCP patient, with attention being focused on analgesia and improved function, as well as the number of breakthrough pain episodes. The extended-relief opioid typically enables an increased function, which may be responsible for the episodes of breakthrough pain that were not seen when the patient was bed/chair bound.

If the patient has more than three or four episodes of breakthrough pain, the ATC medications should be slowly increased, keeping an eye on continued improvement in function and the onset of drug-related problems such as sedation or poor cognitive function. If this occurs, the ATC medication should be decreased. Consideration of opioid rotation should be performed in such cases, as well as generally every four to six months as needed.

The use of breakthrough, instant/immediate-release pain medication for breakthrough pain should be limited to three to five times a typical day for a patient.

The science is important. There is no one perfect opioid that will work for all patients. Typical side effects, such as constipation, should be treated at the same time an opioid is started.

Individual responses to opioids may vary, possibly secondary to genetic factors, but this must be recognized. If one opioid does not give good analgesia with a small number of side effects, it should be changed. The use of an adjuvant to help with pain management and possibly allow a smaller dosage of opiate should always be considered.

When prescribing an opiate, always follow established principles and the guidelines and laws applicable from the state and the federal levels; follow both, but particularly whichever is most strict.

Pain management physicians must always document (while monitoring) the four A's: Analgesia; Activities of daily living; Adverse effects; and Aberrant drug-taking behaviors (30). By default, the pain management physician is responsible for identifying the rare drug abuser or drug diverter. When concerned, get a consult from an addictionologist and even cotreat with this clinician.

The use of chronic opioids alone should only be done after the patient has had, if needed, narcotic medication to help enable them to undergo appropriate rehabilitation. The initial use of chronic opioids is medically not indicated,

However, there is a very common caveat to this: a patient's insurance company may not pay for rehabilitation. Many will pay for interventional pain medicine, where a patient may receive a series of epidural steroid medications, for example, and be placed on pain medications simultaneously, but all will pay for pain medications (sometimes only specific pain medications, for extended and immediate release).

The new reality is that the pain management physician must provide care while preventing misuse and drug diversion. Physicians are being turned into police, creating a significant problem in the older established patient/physician relationship. Physicians feel that they cannot always/just cannot trust a pain patient who may divert a pain medication and get the physician into trouble. Patients are afraid, possibly with good reason, that even in the presence of real pain, their pain management needs may not be met.

DEFINITIONS

There are several definitions that must be kept in mind. They are presented with only a little variation, as the concepts and definitions are very important:

- *Physical dependence*: seen when the body has adapted to an opiate and there is a class-specific withdrawal syndrome that can be produced by the abrupt cessation, rapid dose reduction, and/or administration of an opiate antagonist. This is not addiction. It is associated with the following:
- *Tolerance*: a state of adaptation in which exposure to a drug can induce changes that cause the body to enable a diminution of one or more of the drug's effects over time, with all other conditions/aspects of disease being the same. If the physical disorder is getting worse, or progressing, it may cause a need for more medication. If a patient's functional activity is continuing to progress, he/she may need more medication to make up for the tolerance induced, and an increase in breakthrough pain secondary to activity.
- *Pseudoaddiction*: this is seen in pain patients who are seeking more pain medication, even doctor shopping to obtain these medications, secondary to the patient's real pain syndrome being undertreated. When the treatment enables the patient to achieve appropriate relief, all inappropriate behavior ends.
- *Addiction*: a primary, chronic, neurobiologic disease associated with genetic, psychosocial, and environmental factors which significantly influence its development and how it manifests. It is specifically characterized by behaviors that are typified by impaired control over drug use, compulsive use, craving the drug, and compulsive use in spite of self-induced harm.

A consensus document regarding these definitions was published in 2001 as a joint effort of the American Academy of Pain Medicine, The American Pain Society and the American Society of Addiction Medicine (31).

An important question is the risk of addiction and aberrant behavior. Portenoy and Savage (32) stated that addiction to opioids in the context of pain treatment is rare in those with no history of addictive behavior.

The Boston Collaborative Drug Surveillance Project looked at 11,882 inpatients who received an opioid while hospitalized; subsequently, only four cases of addiction could be identified (33).

Passik and Portenoy (34, 35) worked to develop a model of aberrant drug-taking behaviors. They felt that predictive behaviors included: selling prescription drugs; prescription forgery; stealing or borrowing another patient's drugs; injecting oral formulations; obtaining prescription drugs from nonmedical sources; concurrent abuse of related illicit drugs; multiple unsanctioned dose escalations; recurrent prescription losses. Behaviors felt to be less predictive included: aggressive complaining about a need for higher medication doses; drug hoarding during periods of reduced symptoms; requesting specific drugs; acquisition of similar drugs from other medical sources; unsanctioned medication dose escalation one to two times; unapproved use of the drug to treat another symptom; and reporting psychic effects not intended by the clinician.

TREATMENT PROCEDURES
CNCP patients should be seen monthly, at least for the first six months or more. If an escalation of the amount of breakthrough pain medication is seen, this may indicate a need to increase the time-release chronic narcotics.

In routine practice, the CNCP patients should be given a pain medication agreement, which indicates the possible side effects of narcotic usage (including sedation, nausea, vomiting, itching, loss of sexual function, and immunological problems, among others). Also, the patient must agree that only one physician will provide his/her narcotic pain medications, and the prescriptions will be taken to one (listed) pharmacy. Urine or blood tests may be performed at any time, and if an untoward substance (i.e., cocaine or narcotics not prescribed the pain specialist) is found in patients' urine or blood, or if their blood/urine level of the prescribed pain medication is very inappropriate, the physician may wean the patient off of their opioid medications and treat them without further use of narcotics or discharge them. Other reasons for tapering and ending opioid maintenance include evidence of opioid hoarding; obtaining pain medications from other prescribers; obtaining drugs from others (diversion); and uncontrolled dose escalation or other aberrant behaviors (frequent loss of one's medication—"my dog ate it"; reports of stolen medications without a proper police report; frequently calling in requesting medications earlier than should be indicated after being given a one-month drug prescription). A past history of substance abuse may be considered a relative contraindication for the use of chronic opioids. However, it is not felt that it is infeasible to treat a chronic pain patient with a history of drug abuse. These patients, as noted above, may need to be treated while they are being seen by an addictionologist.

In some practices, urine testing is felt to be an important part of managing a chronic pain patient safely. Appropriate urine testing can help the prescriber determine if the patient is taking the prescribed medication, if he/she is taking the correct dosages, and if there is any other untoward drug in his/her system. Some clinicians do this routinely; some do not do it at all. Some clinicians will have consenting patients observed, to be certain that the urine is theirs. Rare practices may frisk patients to be certain that they do not have a urine receptacle that they have used to transport "clean" urine. Both general class-specific urine testing should be done in combination with gas chromatography/mass spectrometry to find the identity of, or confirm the presence or absence of, a specific drug and/or its metabolites (36).

Another very useful tool is serial testing using drug-related questionnaires, such as the CAGE questionnaire (37), or the Pain Outcome Profile (POP+) developed by the American Academy of Pain Management (38).

The Web site www.legalsideofpain by former federal prosecutor Jennifer Bolen is an excellent resource for all physicians in pain management. Ms. Bolen has excellent examples of patient opioid medication agreements and informed consents for the use of opioids, as well as much more that is useful and should be mandatorily used, in one form or another by all pain management physicians (see chap. 25).

So-called "Universal Precautions" in pain medicine need to be remembered (39):

1. Diagnosis with appropriate differential
2. Psychological assessment
3. Informed consent for the use of opiates
4. Treatment agreements
5. Pain and function assessments
6. Trial of opiate therapy
7. Reassessment of pain and function
8. Regular assessment of the "4 A's"—Analgesia; Activities of daily living; Adverse events; Aberrant drug-taking behavior
9. Periodic review of diagnosis and comorbidities
10. Documentation (and lots of it!)

Chronic Opioid Use in Patients with CNCP

Two interesting studies from Canada note important facts which would most likely be replicated if done in the United States.

A report in 2001 by Moulin et al. (40) found that 340 Canadian pain patients with an average pain intensity of 6.3 (on a 1–10 scale) were taking medication for pain. Eighty percent complained of moderate to severe pain. Their average pain history was 10.7 years. Only 22% of these patients were taking opioid medications and two-thirds of these patients were only taking codeine preparations.

A more recent report (2003) found that a cohort of 154 Canadian pain patients had a mean pain score of 7.7 on a Likert scale (0–10), with a mean duration of pain being 4.7 years. Over 40% of these patients had not used opioids and about 25% had not used any other antineuropathic pain medication in spite of these high levels of pain (41).

A number of authors feel that while the use of opioids may be helpful to treat the CNCP patient, there are no specific guidelines and therefore a greater degree of hesitancy and fear exists (6,42–49). The "correct" way to use opiates as noted in these various studies is described above. The most basic points being: make certain the patient is examined and documentation is excellent; symptom control leading to improved function and quality of life is primary; chronic opioid therapy should be considered for both continuous nociceptive and neuropathic pain if all other appropriate therapies have been tried and failed, utilizing the proper time frame for the medications to work; know the psychosocial status of the patient; use ATC medications, with instant-release opioids for breakthrough pain; monitor treatment including re-examinations, functional assessments, and urine testing; the physician and the patient should have an appropriate opioid agreement which spells out the patient's rights and responsibilities.

Opioid therapy can be enhanced via the use of adjunctive medications (see chap. 23). These may include NMDA antagonists, clonidine, calcium channel blockers, alpha-2-adrenergic agonists, NSAIDs, gabapentinoids and neurokinin-1 (NK-1) receptor antagonists (50, 51).

The number of published opioid trials lasting longer than 6 to 12 weeks is very small. This leads to the concern regarding the safety of chronic narcotic usage. Reports show that there were 11 studies with 1025 patients that compared oral opioids with placebo and lasted for four days to eight weeks. Six trials had an open label follow-up of 6 to 24 months (7). The adverse events noted included constipation, nausea, and somnolence being the most common adverse events noted (at least one of the three) in 80% of patients. Also of interest is that only 44% of 388 patients placed in the open-label trails were still taking opioids after therapy for between 7 and 24 months, showing a relatively small group of patients continuing with long-term opioid treatment (7).

Another study looked at the impact of opioid use on CNCP patients. The authors found 11 studies which evaluated long-term opioid treatment for CNCP and also looked at quality of life and included 2877 patients. Six were randomized controlled trials and five were observational studies. The authors concluded that there was both moderate/high- and low-quality evidence indicating that long-term treatment with opiates can help CNCP patients develop an increased quality of life and significant improvements in function (5).

Maier et al. (52) looked at 121 patients with a three-year history of opioid use and found that the patients with long-term opioid use had significantly lower pain intensity and good improvements in quality of life, global assessments, and physical status. During the five years of this study, 33% had no change in opioid dosage, 16% had their dosages decreased, and 27% had a slight overall increase and 19% had significant dose increases (secondary to loss of opioid efficacy). It was concluded that there was a very low frequency of withdrawal in CNCP patients taking long-term opiates, and there was no evidence for tolerance development, especially if the treatment was performed in a pain center.

Several controlled studies of opioids in CNCP have shown pain relief of 30% to 50% with chronic dosing, but no development of significant tolerance, except for side effects such as nausea and sedation (53).

A more recent meta-analysis of the effectiveness and side effects of opioids when used for CNCP found that both weak and strong opioids outperformed placebo for both pain and function in all types of CNCP (54). The authors of this review also noted that better functional outcomes were found with other drugs which were, for pain relief, only outperformed by strong opioids (54). They also found that in spite of the typically short time for opioid trials, more than one-third of participants withdrew from the treatment (54).

The most common side effect/adverse event stemming from the use of opioids is constipation. Typically, when a patient is started on an opiate, a stimulant and stool-softening agent is stated at the same time. There are many patients who continue to have problems with significant constipation. A peripheral opioid receptor antagonist, methylnaltrexone, for the treatment of severe constipation has been found to be useful in managing opioid-induced constipation without significant adverse events including opiate withdrawal (55, 56). This drug, which is still in clinical development, can reverse morphine-induced gastrointestinal hypomotility (57–59).

It is also interesting to note that opioids have been ascribed anti-inflammatory properties (60).

Tolerance and Opioid-Induced Pain

Over time, continued opiate usage will induce "tolerance," a known effect, to the opioid analgesic effect (see above). It has been felt that most commonly, dose escalation is secondary to increasing pain, as a result of increasing nociception from ongoing disease processes. However, studies and additional clinical activity indicate that tolerance to different opioid effects can develop at different rates (selective tolerance); for example, one can rapidly develop tolerance to nausea and vomiting, sedation, and respiratory depression, but little if any tolerance to constipation and miosis (61). Patient dose variability (genetic polymorphism) can occur as differences in opioid receptor synthesis and differences in various opioid affinities of ligands causing a wide margin of dose variability in patients (61). It is felt that once tolerance to analgesic effects of a specific opiate has developed, simultaneous use of analgesics, which are mediated by different receptors, may help avoid further tolerance; this concept, known as multimodal analgesia, is growing more common and involves techniques such as opioid switching/rotation and the use of adjuvant medications.

Two possible mechanisms have also been postulated regarding the development of drug tolerance. First, a within-system mechanism, which involves opioid receptors downregulating at the highest affinity sites and uncoupling from G-proteins. The between-systems mechanism is proposed, with the opiate-activated opponent systems—the pain facility systems may be involved with the development of opioid tolerance (62). The first mechanism (within system) is the mechanism most often considered; other mechanisms indicate that chronic opiate treatment may also activate the pain facilitatory systems (NMDA receptors, nitric oxide production, and COX activation) during the development of opiate tolerance (62).

Data shows that opioids can increase pain through activation of the bulbospinal facilitation from the rostral ventromedial medulla (RVM); increased pain can decrease spinal opioid antinociceptive potency and finally blockade of pain restores the antinociceptive potency (63).

Tolerance can also be induced by a state of hyperalgesia that results from opioid exposure. The paradoxical or abnormal pain secondary to opiate therapy may also be secondary to neuroplastic changes in the brain and spinal cord, including the activation of the descending pain facilitation mechanism from the RVM. This may be developed, at least in part, by the increased activity of cholecystokinin (CCK) in the RVM. This may induce more pronociceptive events including the upregulation of spinal dynorphin levels and increased CGRP and substance P expression in the DRG. It then appears that opioids can initiate pain due to descending facilitation, upregulation of spinal dynorphin, and increased evoked release of excitatory neurotransmitters from primary afferents (64, 65). The neuroplastic changes secondary to chronic opioid utilization may be secondary to adaptive changes needed to promote increased pain transmission and induced tolerance (decreased antinociception) (66).

It has also been noted that chronic opioid use may be associated with the development of hyperalgesia (67). The use of chronic opiates does appear to induce the development of antinociceptive tolerance, which would necessitate increasing the doses of the opiate to maintain adequate analgesia. "Analgesic tolerance" has been associated with paradoxical pain in regions previously not affected by pain, as a result of sustained morphine utilization (67). Many neuropeptides and neurotransmitters (antagonists of algetic chemicals) have been able to block or reverse the antinociceptive tolerance (see below).

Chronic opioid use does upregulate substance P and calcitonin gene–related peptide, which in turn increases the release of algetic, or pain-inducing substances from primary afferent nerve fibers after stimulation. This is correlated with the onset of the abnormal pain states and the opioid antinociceptive tolerance (67).

The descending pain modulatory pathway from the brain stem RVM occurs via the dorsolateral funiculus (DLF) and maintains changes in the spinal cord secondary to abnormal pain states, paradoxical pain, and antinociceptive tolerance. Lesioning the DLF in animals prevented increased evoked algetic neuropeptide release and the development of antinociceptive tolerance and abnormal pain secondary to chronic opiate exposure (67).

Microinjecting lidocaine or a CCK antagonist into the RVM blocks both thermal and touch hypersensitivity and antinociceptive tolerance. It is concluded that chronic opioid exposure will enhance a descending pain facilitatory pathway from the RVM that is mediated by CCK, among other neuropeptides, and is essential for the maintenance of antinociceptive tolerance (67, 68). "Nociceptin," also called "orphanin FQ," or OFQ, is a ligand for the "opioid receptor–like 1" receptor. When injected into the RVM, OFQ suppresses firing of all types of neurons and blocks opioid-induced cell activation. In the medulla, OFQ can produce an antiopioid effect. It appears that depending upon in which region OFQ is placed, it may be able to produce either hyperalgesia or hypalgesia (69).

Chronic opioid administration induces increased expression of spinal dynorphin, which causes increased sensitivity to nonnoxious and noxious stimuli: a decrease in spinal antinociceptive properties (70, 71). Experimental use of a cannabinoid CB1 agonist to the spinal cord will also induce paradoxical/abnormal pain, inducing increased spinal dynorphin (71). Continuous morphine use induces neuroplasticity in primary afferents and the spinal cord and induces increased levels of CGRP and dynorphin (72). Dynorphin antiserum can block increased release of CGRP from rats given chronic morphine; so can lesions of the DLF (72).

NMDA receptor antagonists do decrease or prevent the development of tolerance to the antinociceptive effects of opioids (73, 74). It is thought that a range of NMDA receptor antagonists potentiate morphine-induced antinociception (73).

Another study found that the mechanism of tolerance to receptor-selective μ- and δ-opioids may be different compared to that associated with morphine tolerance (74). This would indicate that studies looking at paradoxical pain from chronic morphine utilization may not be generalizable to all opiates.

Specific neurons in the RVM include "off-cells," which are felt to inhibit nociceptive transmission, and "on-cells," which facilitate nociception. When these cells are tested with an NMDA antagonist, several things are noted: systemic morphine produces analgesia in part by involving an NMDA-mediated excitatory process to activate off-cells in the RVM. Secondly, activation of on-cells is mediated by a non-NMDA receptor, and this activation does not appear to be significant in regulating reflex responses to acute, noxious stimuli. Excitatory amino acid–induced excitation appears to work several ways in the RVM, activating off-cells and on-cells under different conditions (75).

Algetic or pain-inducing neuropeptides are involved in both the development of tolerance and paradoxical/abnormal pain. Sustained morphine use increases substance P and NK-1 receptor expression in the spinal cord dorsal horn. It also increases capsaicin-evoked substance P release and internalization of NK-1 receptors in the presence of noxious stimuli. It appears that NK-1 receptors have an important role in the expression of chronic morphine-induced hyperalgesia. It may also indicate that chronic opiate usage can induce changes that are similar to those found in inflammatory pain (76).

As noted earlier, CGRP has been found to be increased in the spinal cord dorsal horn during morphine tolerance. The opiate receptors appear to be involved in upregulation of CGRP and substance P following exposure to chronic opiates; protein kinase C appears to have a role in this upregulation (77). Prostaglandins are also upregulated (78). Both CGRP and substance P, which are colocalized and coreleased, are involved in the development of tolerance to spinal antinociceptive effects of μ- and δ-related agonists. CGRP antagonists may be helpful in the prevention and reversal of opioid tolerance (79–81).

CCK, which is enhanced in the RVM during chronic opiate exposure, may also decrease spinal morphine antinociception by causing a descending pain facilitatory mechanism to exacerbate spinal nociceptive activity. A CCK receptor antagonist may also be a useful tool in the prevention of paradoxical pain and analgesic tolerance (82).

Via the use of a 5-HT$_1$ A receptor agonist, it was determined that, as opioids produce bidirectional hypo- and proanalgesic activity, the 5-HT$_1$ A receptor activation counteracts the various aspects of opioid-induced pain. An interesting point is made by the authors of this study that opioid addiction may be self-therapy of opioid-induced pathological pain (83).

Another very important research target is CNS microglia. Spinal cord glia are important contributors to the creation of enhanced pain states secondary to the release of neuroexcitatory substances. Glia (microglia and astrocytes) also release neuroexcitatory substances in response to morphine, opposing its effects (84). After activation of microglial cells under neuropathic pain conditions induces proinflammatory cytokines including interleukin-1 beta, interleukin-6, tumor necrosis factor, complement components (C1q, C3, C4, C5, C5a), and multiple other substances that facilitate pain transmission (85).

Glia create and maintain enhanced pain states such as neuropathic pain and also compromise the efficacy of morphine and other opiates for pain control. Glia have essentially no role in pain under basal conditions, but pain is amplified when the glia become activated and induce the release of the proinflammatory products, those noted above and especially proinflammatory cytokines (86).

Glia are activated via multiple neuron-to-glia signals including neuronal chemokines, neurotransmitters, and substances released by damaged, dying, and dead neurons (86).

Glia become increasingly activated in response to repeated administration of opiates, which induces neuronal excitability via numerous mechanisms, including direct receptor-mediated actions, upregulation of excitatory amino acid receptor function, downregulation of GABA receptor function, as well as others (85, 86). These effects of glial activation amplify pain, decrease efficacy of opioid analgesia, contribute to the loss of opioid analgesia after repeated opioid administration (tolerance), and contribute to the development of opioid dependence (86, 87).

Toll-like receptors (TLR; a family of receptors that provide needed links between immune stimulants produced by microorganisms and the initiation of host defenses) are seemingly important players in this multifaceted problem. Activation of TLR4 induces the release of antimicrobial peptides, inflammatory cytokines, and chemokines, among other activities. TLR4-mediated glial activation is central to neuropathic pain, compromised acute opioid analgesia, and unwanted opioid side effects including tolerance, dependence, and reward. Selective antagonism of TLR4 has been shown to reverse neuropathic pain and potentiate opioid analgesia (88).

The p38 mitogen-activated protein kinases (p38 MAPK) are signaling molecules, part of a family of serine/threonine protein kinases, which play a role in cellular responses to external stress signals. Inhibitors of two members of the p38 family have anti-inflammatory effects via inhibiting the expression of inflammatory mediators (89). Activation of p38 MAPK in spinal microglia mediates morphine antinociceptive tolerance. Minocycline, a selective inhibitor of microglia activation, has been reported to attenuate peripheral inflammation-induced hyperalgesia by inhibiting p38 MAPK in the spinal microglia. These authors demonstrated that minocycline antagonizes morphine antinociceptive tolerance, possibly due to the inhibition of p38 activation in spinal microglia (90).

It was found that inhibiting neuronal nitric oxide synthase diminished morphine antinociceptive tolerance by reducing p38 MAPK activation in the spinal microglia (91). Another group provided evidence that p38 activation in spinal microglia played an important role in the development of tolerance to morphine analgesia (92).

Neuroglia

It has been found that glial activation contributes to a state of opioid analgesic tolerance, and the induced neuroglial communication is possibly responsible, at least in part, for the altered functional competence in δ-opioid receptor–mediated effects following morphine treatment; chronic morphine treatment has been found to involve the activation and hypertrophy of spinal glia cells (93).

Finally, a study notes that activity of endocannabinoids, mediated via CB1 receptors, contributes to both the development and maintenance of opioid tolerance by influencing the opioid-induced increase in spinal CGRP (94).

Sexual Dimorphism

More evidence is being found that indicates anatomical and neuropsychological differences exist between the nociceptive systems of males and females (95). Differences appear to exist between male and female perception of and response to pain (96). Women have been found to experience more severe and longer lasting pain than men (97).

Woman experience greater clinical pain, suffer greater pain-related distress, and show increased sensitivity to experimentally induced pain when compared to men. Some of the multifactorial issues helping to explain the sex differences include psychosocial factors (pain-related catastrophizing). Gonadal hormone levels in cycling women are also responsible for a substantial impact on pain perception and analgesic response. Women perceive more pain during their luteal phase, and estrogen antagonists provide long-term pain relief in certain situations (98).

Dyspnea exerts an inhibitory effect on pain; one study shows the inhibitory effect of dyspnea on pain sensation is less in females than in males, but the sex difference may not be explained by the female reproductive hormones alone (99). Another group looked at sexually dimorphic recruitment of spinal opioid analgesic pathways by the spinal application of morphine in rats, and found that in females, but not males, activation by intrathecal (IT) morphine of spinal κ-opioid receptors is a prerequisite for spinal morphine antinociception. Also, in females, but not males, IT application of antidynorphin antibodies substantially attenuates the antinociception produced by IT morphine. It was felt that the female-specific recruitment by IT morphine of a spinal dynorphin/κ-opioid receptor pathway results from organizational consequences of ovarian sex steroids and not the absence of testicular hormones (100).

Differences in analgesic responses to μ-opioid agonists have been seen, but the findings have varied. One study found women to have more a more robust response to morphine than men, in contrast to prior studies (101). Typically, the μ-opioid antinociceptive response is greater in male rats than in female rats (102). A recent study found sexual dimorphism in the opioid effects was related to the opioid receptors on which a particular opioid predominately acts (102).

Studies have found that the analgesic effect of kappa partial agonists (pentazocine, butorphanol, nalbuphine) is much greater in women than in men. This may be secondary to a naloxone-sensitive antinociceptive effect of these agonist/antagonists inducing decreased analgesia or increased pain (103, 104).

Other studies suggest that it is estrogen receptors in trigeminal neurons which modulate nociceptive responses via serotonin and other neuropeptides. It was thought that the variation in estrogen receptor signaling and neuropeptide plasticity in the trigeminal neurons may have an inducing effect on mensuration-related migraine (95).

Finally, inflammation and inflammatory disorders are thought to be sexually dimorphic, via neuroimmune mechanisms underlying sexual dimorphism in three possible aspects of the inflammatory process: plasma extravasation, neutrophil function, and inflammatory hyperalgesia (105).

Barriers to the Use of Opioids

There are patient and physician barriers to appropriate use of opioids: fears of addiction, medication dependence, and drug tolerance, with frequent lack of understanding of the differences between these issues.

Physicians are frequently afraid to prescribe opioids secondary to

- an inadequate understanding of pain management principles;
- inability to appropriately assess a patient's pain;
- fear/concern about regulation of controlled substances;
- fear that giving pain medication to one patient would make the physician a target of the DEA as well as other patients wanting/needing pain medications;
- fears of patient addiction and other problems leading to liability;
- concern about patients becoming tolerant to opioids, needing higher dosages, and needing them for extended periods of time (years);
- concern about side effects of opioids.

Patient barriers to appropriate opioid use include

- fear that pain means a disease is worse;
- concern that talking about pain would prevent a physician from dealing with a significant underlying disease;
- wanting to be a good patient and not alienate the physician by reporting pain;
- concerns about developing tolerance or addiction to pain medications;
- fear of showing "weakness";
- embarrassment to go to the pharmacy for these medications; further embarrassment that they may be construed a "drug addict," even though they have no aberrant drug-related behavior and a physiological reason for their pain.

Systemic/institutional barriers include

- restrictive regulation of controlled substances;
- poor access to treatment;
- poor access to pain management specialists;
- poor insurance.
  - The most appropriate treatment would not be reimbursed.
  - The most appropriate treatment is too costly for the patient.
  - Lack of rehabilitation benefits—"Bad Insurance."
    - Inability to obtain any rehabilitation or even just physical therapy or psychological care, as they are far more expensive than pain medications (an hour of physical therapy may bill at US $150 to $200, while a single generic Tylenol #4 tablet—one grain of codeine—costs only pennies).

Other barriers to pain relief:

- Pharmacies do not stock adequate and/or appropriate opioids.
- No continuity in patient care.

SUMMARY

The complexity of this subject is great, even though the medical aspects are fairly straightforward. It is the multitudes of other problems and barriers to appropriate pain management and opioid usage that make this problem so complex.

When one considers that the clinical definition of pain is simple—whatever the patient says it is—it is then up to the clinician to determine exactly what the patient means, utilizing a history, examination, and any necessary tests. Then appropriate treatment should be rendered. The utilization of chronic opioid analgesics is one very important treatment modality, which, when used appropriately, may help improve patients' function and ameliorate their pain.

In February 2009, the FDA issued a call for tightened regulations of extended-release oral medications, methadone, and patch opioid medications as well as for reducing diversion, overdoses, and inappropriate use of schedule II opioid medications (106). This may place more difficulty on physicians who utilize opioids in the treatment of CNCP patients and make continued treatment of these patients more onerous. While they are requesting more thorough risk management plans from the makers of these medications, the ramifications to the physician are not yet clear.

REFERENCES

1. Jay GW. Chronic Pain. New York: Informa Healthcare, 2007.
2. Pasternak GW. The pharmacology of mu analgesics: from patients to genes. Neuroscientist 2001; 7(3):220–231.
3. Rossi GC, Brown GP, Leventhal, et al. Novel receptor mechanisms for heroin and morphine-6 beta glucuronide analgesia. Neurosci Lett 1996; 216(1):1–4.
4. Pasternak GW. Molecular biology of opioid analgesia. J Pain Symptom Manage 2005; 29(5 suppl):S2–S9.
5. Devulder J, Richarz U, Nataraja S. Impact of long-term use of opioids on quality of life in patients with chronic, non-malignant pain. Curr Med Res Opin 2005; 21(10):1555–1568.
6. Kalso E, Allan L, Dellemijn PLI, et al. Recommendations for using opioids in chronic non-cancer pain. Eur J Pain 2003; 7(5):381–386.
7. Kalso E, Edwards JE, Moore RA, et al. Opioids in chronic non-cancer pain: a systemic review of efficacy and safety. Pain 2004; 112:372–380.
8. Watson CP, Watt-Watson JH, Chaipman ML. Chronic non-cancer pain and the long term utility of opioids. Pain Res Manage 2004; 9:19–24.
9. Eisenberg E, McNicol ED, Carr DB. Efficacy and safety of opioid agonists in the treatment of neuropathic pain of nonmalignant origin: systemic review and meta-analysis trials. JAMA 2005; 293:3043–3052.
10. Dworkin RH, Backonja M, Rowbotham MB, et al. Advances in neuropathic pain: diagnosis, mechanisms, and treatment recommendations. Arch Neurol 2003; 60:1524–1534.
11. Stiehl M. Controlled release oxycodone—a new option in the treatment of severe and very severe pain. Review of studies on neuropathic, physical activity-related and postoperative pain. NNW Fortschr Med 2004; 145(suppl 2):61–69.
12. Schug SA. Combination analgesia in 2005—a rational approach: focus on paracetamol–tramadol. Clin Rheumatol 2006; 25(suppl 1):S16–S21.
13. Kunig G, Datwyler S, Eschen A, et al. Unrecognized long-lasting tramadol-induced delirium in two elderly patients. Pharmacopsychiatry 2006; 39(5):194–199.
14. Chugh SS, Socoteanu C, Reinier K, et al. A community-based evaluation of sudden death associated with therapeutic levels of methadone. Am J Med 2008; 121(1):66–71.
15. Burgess FW, Pawasauskas J. Methadone analgesia: balancing the risks and benefits. Pain Medicine News Special Edition. December 2008:53–58.
16. Burgas FW, KRantz MJ, Barkin RL. Methadone: unintended mortality due to overdose and arrhythmia. Pain Medicine News. May/June 2007:1–6.
17. Fredheim OM, Kaasa S, Dale O, et al. Opioid switching from slow release morphine to oral methadone may improve pain control in chronic non-malignant pain: a nine-month follow-up study. Palliat Med 2006; 20(1):35–41.
18. Fredheim OM, Borchgrevink PC, Klepstad P, et al. Long term methadone for chronic pain: a pilot study of pharmacokinetic aspects. Eur J Pain 2007; 11(6):599–604.
19. Florida Administrative Code. Title 64, Department of Health, Board of Medicine, Chapter 64B8–9 Standards of Practice for Medical Doctors. 64B8–9.013 Standards for the Use of Controlled Substances for Treatment of Pain. Available at: http://www.medsch.wisc.edu/painpolicy/domestic/fllaw.htm. Accessed February 14, 2009.
20. Federation of State Medical Boards of the United States: Model policy for the use of controlled substances for the treatment of pain. May 2004. Available at: http://www.fsmb.org. Accessed February 14, 2009.
21. DEA issues new guidelines on pain drugs. Associated Press, August 11, 2004. Available at: http://www.msnbc.msn.com/id/5673456. Accessed February 14, 2009.
22. U.S. Department of Justice, Drug Enforcement Administration, with Pain & Policy Studies Group, University of Wisconsin. Frequently asked questions and answers for Health Care Professionals and Law Enforcement Personnel. Available at: http://www.deadiversion.usdoj.gov/. Accessed February 14, 2009.

23. Joint Commission on Accreditation of Healthcare Organizations. Pain Assessment and Management: An Organizational Approach. Oakbrook Terrace, Illinois: JCAHO, 2000:3.
24. Furrow BR. Pain management and provider liability: no more excuses. J Law Med Ethics 2001; 29(1):29–51.
25. Rosomoff HL, Rosomoff RS. Comprehensive multidisciplinary pain center approach to the treatment of low back pain. Neurosurg Clin N Am 1991; 2(4):877–890.
26. Cutler RB, Fishbain DA, Abdel-Moty E, et al. Does nonsurgical pain center treatment of chronic pain return patients to work? A review and meta-analysis of the literature. Spine 1994; 19:643–652.
27. Flor H, Fydrich T, Turk DC. Efficacy of multidisciplinary pain treatment centers: a meta-analytic review. Pain 1992; 49:22–30.
28. Chapman SL, Brena SF, Bradford LA. Treatment outcomes in a chronic pain rehabilitation program. Pain 1981; 11:255–268.
29. Turk DC, Loeser JD, Monarch ES. Chronic pain: purposes and costs of interdisciplinary pain rehabilitation programs. TEN 2002; 4(2):64–69.
30. www.fda.gov/ohrms/dockets/ac/02/slides/3820s2_05_passik.ppt. Accessed February 14, 2009.
31. Consensus document from the American Academy of Pain Medicine, The American Pain Society and the American Society of Addiction Medicine. Definitions related to the use of opioids for the treatment of pain. 2001.
32. Portenoy RK, Savage SR. Clinical realities and economic considerations: special therapeutic issues in intrathecal therapy—tolerance and addiction. J Pain Symptom Manage 1997; 14(3 suppl):S27–S35.
33. Porter J, Jick H. Addiction rare in patients treated with narcotics. N Engl J Med 1980; 302(2):123.
34. Passik SD, Portenoy RK, Ricketts PL. Substance abuse issues in cancer patients. Part 1: Prevalence and diagnosis. Oncology 1998; 12(4):517–521.
35. Passik SD, Portenoy RK, Ricketts PL. Substance abuse issues in cancer patients. Part 2: Evaluation and treatment. Oncology. 1998; 12(5):729–734.
36. Heit HA, Gourlay D. Urine drug testing in pain medicine. J Pain Symptom Manage 2004; 27(3):260–267.
37. Fiellin DA, Reid MC, O'Connor PG. Outpatient management of patients with alcohol problems. Ann Intern Med 2000; 133(10):815–827.
38. Federal Register 2004; 69(220):67170–67172.
39. Gourlay DL, Heit HA, Almahrezi A. Universal precautions in pain medicine: a rational approach to the treatment of chronic pain. Pain Med 2005; 6(2):107–112.
40. Moulin DE, Clark AJ, Speechley M, et al. Chronic pain in Canada. A patient survey. In: Proceedings of the 10th World Congress on Pain. San Diego, CA; 2002:93. Abstract.
41. Gilron I, Bailey JM. Trends in opioid use for chronic neuropathic pain: a survey of patients pursuing enrollment in clinical trials. Can J Anesth 2003; 50:42–47.
42. Nicholson B. Responsible prescribing of opioids for the management of chronic pain. Drugs 2003; 63(1):17–32.
43. Portenoy RK, Foley KM. Chronic use of opioid analgesics in non-malignant pain: report of 38 cases. Pain 1986; 25:171–186.
44. Portenoy RK. Opioid therapy for chronic nonmalignant pain: a review of critical issues. J Pain Symptom Manage 1996; 11(4):203–217.
45. Cowan DT, Allan L, Griffiths P. A pilot study into the problematic use of opioid analgesics in chronic non-cancer pain patients. Int J Nurs Stud 2002; 39(1):59–69.
46. Portenoy RK. Appropriate use of opioids for persistent non-cancer pain. Lancet 2004; 364(9436):739–740.
47. Breivik H. Opioids in chronic non-cancer pain, indications and controversies. Eur J Pain 2005; 9(2):127–130.
48. Reder RF. Opioid formulations: tailoring to the needs in chronic pain. Eur J Pain 2001; 5(suppl A):109–111.

49. Chou R, Clark E, Helfand M. Comparative efficacy and safety of long-acting oral opioids for chronic non-cancer pain: a systematic review. J Pain Symptom Manage 2003; 26(5):1026–1048.

50. Kalso E. Improving opioid effectiveness: from ideas to evidence. Eur J Pain 2005; 9(2):131–135.

51. Christo PJ, Grabow TS, Raja SN. Opioid effectiveness, addiction, and depression in chronic pain. Adv Psychosom Med 2004; 25:123–137.

52. Maier C, Schaub C, Willweber-Strumpf A, et al. Long-term efficiency of opioid medication in patients with chronic non-cancer-associated pain. Results of a survey 5 years after onset of medical treatment [abstract]. Schmerz 2005; 19(5):410–417.

53. Jovey JD, Ennis J, Gardner-Nix, et al. Use of opioid analgesics for the treatment of chronic noncancer pain—a consensus statement and guidelines from the Canadian Pain Society. Pain Res Manage 1998; 3:197–222.

54. Furlan AD, Sandoval JA, Mailis-Gagnon A, et al. Opioids for chronic noncancer pain: a meta-analysis of effectiveness and side effects. CMAJ 2006; 174(11):1589–1594.

55. Yuan CS, Foss JF, O'Connor M, et al. Methylnaltrexone for reversal of constipation due to chronic methadone use: a randomized controlled trial. JAMA 2000; 283(3):367–372.

56. Yuan CS, Foss JF. Oral methylnaltrexone for opioid-induced constipation. JAMA 2000; 284(11):1383–1384.

57. Yuan CS. Clinical status of methylnaltrexone, a new agent to prevent and manage opioid-induced side effects. J Support Oncol 2004; 2(2):111–117.

58. Greenwood-Van MB, Gardner CJ, Little PJ, et al. Preclinical studies of opioids and opioid antagonists on gastrointestinal function. Neurogastroenterol Motil 2004; 16(suppl 2):46–53.

59. Yuan CS, Doshan H, Charney MR, et al. Tolerability, gut effects, and pharmacokinetics of methylnaltrexone following repeated intravenous administration in humans. J Clin Pharm 2005; 45(5):538–546.

60. Walker JS. Anti-inflammatory effects of opioids. Adv Exp Med Biol 2003; 521:148–160.

61. Freye E, Latasch L. Development of opioid tolerance—molecular mechanisms and clinical consequences [abstract]. Anasthesiol Intensivmed Notfallmed Schmerzther 2003; 38(1):14–26.

62. Hsu MM, Wong CS. The roles of pain facilitatory systems in opioid tolerance. Acta Anaesthesiol Sin 2000; 38(3):155–166.

63. Vanderah TW, Suenaga NM, Ossipov MH, et al. Tonic descending facilitation from the rostral ventromedial medulla mediates opioid-induced abnormal pain and antinociceptive tolerance. J Neurosci 2001; 21(1):279–286.

64. Ossipov MH, Lai J, King T, et al. Underlying mechanisms of pronociceptive consequences of prolonged morphine exposure. Biopolymers 2005; 80(2/3):319–324.

65. Ossipov MH, Lai J, King T, et al. Antinociceptive and nociceptive actions of opioids. J Neurobiol 2004; 61(1):126–148.

66. Mao J, Price DD, Mayer DJ. Mechanisms of hyperalgesia and opiate tolerance: a current view of their possible interactions. Pain 1995; 62:259–274.

67. King T, Ossipov MH, Vanderah TW, et al. Is paradoxical pain induced by sustained opioid exposure an underlying mechanism of opioid antinociceptive tolerance? Neurosignals 2005; 14(4):194–205.

68. Ossipov MH, Lai J, Vanderah TW, et al. Induction of pain faciliatation by sustained opioid exposure: relationship to opioid antinociceptive tolerance. Life Sci 2003; 73(6):783–800.

69. Heinricher MM, McGaraughty S, Grandy DK. Circuitry underlying antiopioid actions of orphanin FQ in the rostral ventromedial medulla. J Neurophysiol 1997; 78(6):3351–3358.

70. Vanderah TW, Gardell LR, Burgess SE, et al. Dynorphin promotes abnormal pain and spinal opioid antinociceptive tolerance. J Neurosci 2000; 20(18):7074–7079.

71. Gardell LR, Burgess SE, Dogrul A, et al. Pronociceptive effects of spinal dynorphin promote cannabinoid-induced pain and antinociceptive tolerance. Pain 2002; 98(1/2):79–88.

72. Gardel LR, Wang R, Burgess SE, et al. Sustained morphine exposure induces a spinal dynorphin-dependent enhancement of excitatory transmitter release from primary afferent fibers. J Neurosci 2002; 22(15):6747–6755.

73. Fischer BD, Carrigan KA, Dykstra LA. Effects of N-methyl-D-aspartate receptor antagonists on acute morphine-induced and l-methadone-induced antinociception in mice. J Pain 2005; 6(7):425–433.

74. Bilsky EJ, Inturrisi CE, Sadee W, et al. Competitive and non-competitive NMDA antagonists block the development of antinociceptive tolerance to morphine, but not to selective mu or delta opioid agonists in mice. Pain 1996; 68(2/3):229–237.

75. Heinricher MM, Schouten JC, Jobst EE. Activation of brainstem N-methyl-D-aspartate receptors is required for the analgesic actions of morphine given systemically. Pain 2001; 92(1/2):129–138.

76. King T, Gardell LR, Wang R, et al. Role of NK-1 neurotransmission in opioid-induced hyperalgesia. Pain 2005; 116(3):276–288.

77. Belanger S, Ma W, Chabot JG, et al. Expression of calcitonin gene-related peptide, substance P and protein kinase C in cultured dorsal root ganglion neurons following chronic exposure to mu, delta and kappa opiates. Neuroscience 2002; 115(2):441–453.

78. Powel KJ, Quirion R, Jhamandas K. Inhibition of neurokinin-1-substance P receptor and protanoid activity prevents and reverses the development of morphine tolerance in vivo and the morphine-induced increase in CGRP expression in cultured dorsal root ganglion neurons. Eur J Neurosci 2003; 18(6):1572–1583.

79. Menard DP, van Rossum D, Kar S, et al. A calcitonin gene-related peptide receptor antagonist prevents the development of tolerance to spinal morphine analgesia. J Neurosci 1996; 16(7):2342–2351.

80. Powell KJ, Ma W, Sutak M, et al. Blockade and reversal of spinal morphine tolerance by peptide and non-peptide calcitonin gene-related peptide receptor antagonists. Br J Pharmacol 2000; 131(5):875–884.

81. Menard DP, van Rossum D, Kar S, et al. Alteration of calcitonin gene-related peptide and its receptor binding sites during the development of tolerance to mu and delta opioids. Can J Physiol Pharmacol 1995; 73(7):1089–1095.

82. Xie JY, Herman DS, Stiller CO, et al. Cholecystokinin in the rostral ventromedial medulla mediates opioid-induced hyperalgesia and antinociceptive tolerance. J Neurosci 2005; 25(2):409–416.

83. Colpaert FC, Deseure KR, Stinus L, et al. High-efficacy 5-HT1 A receptor activation counteracts opioid hyperallodynia and affective conditioning. J Pharmacol Exp Ther 2006; 316(2):892–899.

84. Watkins LR, Hutchinson MR, Johnson IN, et al. Glia: novel counter-regulators of opioid analgesia. Trends Neurosci 2005; 28(12):661–669.

85. Mika J. Modulation of microglia can attenuate neuropathic pain symptoms and enhance morphine effectiveness. Pharmacol Rep 2008; 60(3):297–307.

86. Watkins LR, Hutchinson MR, Ledeboer A, et al. Norman Cousins Lecture: Glia as the "bad guys": implications for improving clinical pain control and the clinical utility of opioids. Brain Behav Immun 2007; 21(2):131–146.

87. DeLeo JA, Tanga FY, Tawfik VL. Neuroimmune activation and neuroinflammation in chronic pain and opioid tolerance/hyperalgesia. Neuroscientist 2004; 10(1):40–52.

88. Hutchinson MR, Bland ST, Johnson KW, et al. Opioid-induced glial activation: mechanisms of activation and implications for opioid analgesia, dependence and reward. Scientific World Journal 2007; 7:98–111.

89. Kumar S, Boehm J, Lee JC. p38 MAP kinases: key signaling molecules as therapeutic targets for inflammatory disease. Nat Rev Drug Discov 2003; 2(9):717–726.

90. Cui Y, Liao XX, Liu W, et al. A novel role of minicycline: attenuating morphine antinociceptive tolerance by inhibition of p38 MAPK in the activated spinal microglia. Brain Behave Immun 2008; 22(1):114–123.

91. Liu W, Wang CH, Cui Y, et al. Inhibition of neuronal nitric oxide synthase antago-
     nizes morphine antinociceptive tolerance by decreasing activation of p38 MAPK in
     the spinal microglia. Neurosci Lett 2006; 410(3):174–177.
92. Cui Y, Chen Y, Zhi JL, et al. Activation of p38 mitogen-activated protein kinase
     in spinal microglia mediates morphine antinociceptive tolerance. Brain Res 2006;
     1069(1):235–243.
93. Holdridge SV, Armstrong SA, Taylor AM, et al. Behavioral and morphological evi-
     dence for the involvement of glial cell activation in delta opioid receptor function:
     implications for the development of opioid tolerance. Mol Pain 2007; 3:7.
94. Trang T, Sutak M, Jhamandas K. Involvement of cannabinoid (CB1)-receptors in the
     development and maintenance of opioid tolerance. Neuroscience 2007; 146(3):1275–
     1288.
95. Lipozencic J. The 1st world congress on gender-specific medicine men, women and
     medicine in a new view of the biology of sex/gender differences and aging. Acta
     Dermatovenerol Croat 2006; 14(2):132–134.
96. Schwarz JB. Gender differences in response to drugs: pain medications. J Gend Specif
     Med 1999; 2(5):28–30.
97. Sun LS. Gender differences in pain sensitivity and responses to analgesia. J Gend
     Specif Med 1998; 1(1):28–30.
98. Paller CJ, Campbell CM, Edwards RR, et al. Sex-based differences in pain perception
     and treatment. Pain Med. 2009; 10(2):289–299.
99. Nishino T, Isono S, Ishikawa T, et al. Sex differences in the effect of dyspnea on
     thermal pain threshold in young healthy subjects. Anesthesiology 2008; 109(6):1100–
     1106.
100. Liu NJ, von Gizycki H, Gintzler AR. Sexually dimorphic recruitment of spinal opioid
     analgesic pathways by the spinal application of morphine. J Pharmacol Exp Ther
     2007; 322(2):654–660.
101. Fillingim RB, Ness TJ, Glover TL, et al. Morphine responses and experimental pain:
     sex differences in side effects and cardiovascular responses but not analgesia. J Pain
     2005; 6(2):116–124.
102. Holtman JR Jr, Wala EP. Characterization of the antinociceptive effect of oxycodone
     in male and female rats. Pharmacol Biochem Behav 2006; 83(1):100–108.
103. Gear RW, Gordon NC, Miaskowski, et al. Sexual dimorphism in very low dose nal-
     buphine postoperative analgesia. Neurosci Lett 2003; 339(1):1–4.
104. Gear RW, Gordon NC, Miaskowski C, et al. Dose ratio is important in maximiz-
     ing naloxone enhancement of nalbuphine analgesia in humans. Neurosci Lett 2003;
     351(1):5–8.
105. Levine JD, Khasar SG, Green PG. Neurogenic inflammation and arthritis. Ann N Y
     Acad Sci 2006; 1069:155–167.
106. Pain management: FDA to tighten regulations of extended-release and patch meds.
     Drug War Chronicle 2009; (572). Available at http://www.stopthedrugwars.org.
     Accessed February 15, 2009.

Legal Issues in Pain Management

Jennifer Bolen

The Legal Side of Pain®, The J. Bolen Group, LLC, Knoxville, Tennessee, U.S.A.

Chronic opioid therapy (COT) is but one of many possible treatments to help people living with chronic pain conditions, and for some the only treatment. Because opioids are controlled substances, clinicians who prescribe them must be aware of the clinical and legal guidelines surrounding their use and strive to balance patient access to these medications with the obligation to prevent abuse and diversion. This chapter contains a basic discussion of federal and state laws governing the use of controlled medications for pain management. Clinicians should become familiar with these materials and use the brief question guide at the end of this chapter to open a dialogue with legal counsel concerning regulatory compliance and risk management needs for the medical practice. In addition to the question guide, clinicians will find a short resource list from which to compile a basic handbook on legal/regulatory materials.

BACKGROUND

On October 23, 2001, the U.S. Drug Enforcement Administration (DEA), together with 21 health care organizations issued a joint statement promoting pain relief and the prevention of abuse and diversion (1). The joint statement acknowledged that the undertreatment of pain is serious health problem in the United States, and encourages the aggressive treatment of pain (1). At the same time, and to encourage clinicians to guard against the nonmedical use of controlled medications, the joint statement recognized that the abuse and diversion of these medications is a real problem requiring clinicians to adopt reasonable measures as part of routine daily practice to undertake a benefit-to-risk analysis when considering these medications as part of a treatment plan.

Nearly eight years have passed since the issuance of the joint statement and the challenges for the pain clinician remain the same: addressing undertreated pain and preventing abuse and diversion. In May 2009, the nation's Director of National Drug Control Policy issued his report on the nonmedical use of prescription drugs, citing a serious threat to public health and safety because of the growing number of unintentional deaths involving prescription opioids (increasing 114% from 2001 to 2005) and treatment admissions (increasing 74% in a similar four-year period) (2).

Despite the strict requirements of federal and state Controlled Substances Acts and corresponding federal regulations, controlled prescribed medications (CPMs) are diverted from legitimate sources for illicit distribution and/or abuse (3). Typically, CPM diversion "involves individuals who doctor-shop and forge prescriptions, unscrupulous physicians who sell prescriptions to drug dealers or abusers, unscrupulous pharmacists who falsify records and subsequently sell the drugs, employees who steal from inventory, executives who falsify orders to cover illicit sales, individuals who commit burglaries or robberies of pharmacies, and individuals who purchase CPDs from rogue Internet pharmacies" (3). Another avenue of CPM diversion is "the sharing or purchasing of drugs between family and friends or individual theft from family and friends" (3).

In response to the growing problem of CPM diversion, the federal government has empowered the U.S. Food and Drug Administration (FDA) with authority to place additional requirements on pharmaceutical companies in connection with medications in the opioid class (4). The problem of nonmedical use of prescribed controlled substances is so bad that the DEA, FDA, and several professional pain organizations have labeled it a "public health crisis" (5). In early 2009, in an unprecedented attempt to better deal with the public health aspects of opioid abuse and diversion, the FDA began a series of meetings with industry members and other stakeholders in the pain community to address the nature and substance of one such control measure known as an Opioid REMS (Risk Evaluation and Mitigation Strategy). At the same time, the American Pain Society (APS) and the American Academy of Pain Medicine (AAPM) published clinical guidelines for the use of COT in the treatment of chronic noncancer pain (CNCP). These guidelines, published in the *Journal of Pain* (6), contain approximately 37 recommendations broken down into sections that closely parallel regulatory guidelines and rules on prescribing controlled medications to treat pain. The APS-AAPM guidelines present challenges to the pain clinician because many of the recommendations are based on weak evidence and clinicians may find themselves without the ability to fulfill these recommendations because of the structure of the current health care system—it does not always provide for risk management tools such as urine drug testing, specialist referrals, and combination therapies for the management of patients with CNCP.

Legal and medical professionals recognize that controlled medications are important to the treatment of pain and often may be the only treatment available for some patients. All stakeholders in the pain community share a responsibility for ensuring that prescription pain medications remain available to patients who need them and are subject to "safe use" and "safe handling" measures to prevent abuse and diversion. While there is no question that preventing prescription drug abuse and diversion is an important societal goal, the October 2001 Joint Statement makes clear that abuse prevention methods should not "hinder patients' ability to receive the care they need and deserve" (1). Pain clinicians should not fear prescribing controlled medications to their patients, so long as their prescribing is for a legitimate medical purpose and in the usual course of professional practice. Over time, the efforts of federal and state agencies, together with professional pain organizations, will bridge the gap between undertreating pain and inappropriate prescribing and achieve the balance described above. Risk management will always be a critical component of pain medicine, and the pain practitioner must develop a daily practice routine that balances the tasks of treating pain and minimizing risk.

INTEGRATION OF LAW AND MEDICINE

Law and medicine are closely integrated when treatment involves controlled medications. Pain clinicians should strive to understand federal and state legal standards relating to controlled substances, and to use these legal standards as the framework for regulatory compliance policies. It is equally important for the pain clinician to evaluate current and relevant clinical guidelines, such as those issued in 2009 by APS-AAPM, and to follow them in good faith. The pain clinician's medical record documentation will play a crucial role in determining liability—administrative, civil, or criminal. The remainder of this chapter examines legal standards and parallel clinical guideline recommendations and offers the pain clinician suggestions on documentation and basic risk management protocols.

FEDERAL LEGAL/REGULATORY MATERIALS

Clinicians rarely receive formal training in legal and regulatory issues related to the prescribing of controlled substances. There are two basic levels of legal authorities for controlled substance prescribing: federal and state, with their own associated agencies. At the federal level (see Figure 1), there are three basic types of legal/regulatory materials: laws, regulations, and policy statements, the last of which includes the DEA's September 2006 *Final Policy Statement for the Dispensing of Controlled Substances for the Treatment of Pain* (the "Final Policy Statement") (7). Figure 1 contains a diagram of the three levels of federal legal materials and cites an example at each level.

The Controlled Substances Act of 1970

The federal Controlled Substances Act of 1970 (CSA) is the primary body of federal law governing the administration, dispensing, manufacturing, and prescribing of controlled medications. The CSA contains five (5) different "schedules" classifying the various substances under DEA's control. Federal law classifies each controlled substance into one of the five schedules based on

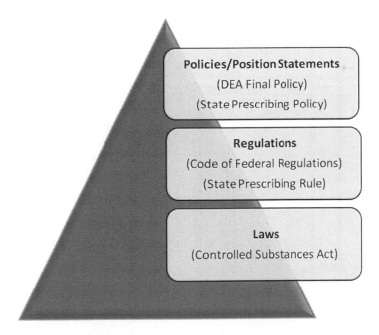

FIGURE 1 Federal Legal/Regulatory Materials.

medicinal value, potential harmfulness, and the potential for abuse (8). Each state has its own controlled substance act, usually referred to as a Uniform Controlled Substances Act. States must use the federal CSA as the platform for their own CSAs, but a state may be more restrictive depending on its individual abuse and diversion problems. Thus, some states schedule medications that are not currently scheduled under federal law. Two examples include (*i*) tramadol and (*ii*) carisoprodol. As with the federal law, state CSAs prohibit the nonmedical use of controlled substances.

The Code of Federal Regulations

The Code of Federal Regulations explains individual aspects of the federal CSA. Title 21, Code of Federal Regulations, Part 1300, contains several sections directly relating to the prescribing of controlled substances. This section is limited to a discussion of three of the key federal regulations governing the prescribing of controlled substances. Pain clinicians should use online resources, such as the DEA Office of Diversion Control's website (9), to review relevant federal pre-scribing regulations. In addition, pain clinicians should review the DEA's *Practitioner's Manual* (10), published in September 2006.

21. CFR 1306.04—Purpose of Issue of Prescription

Section 1306.04 of Title 21, Code of Federal Regulations, sets forth the fundamental federal legal standard for a valid controlled substance prescription, regardless of the prescribed drug's schedule. A controlled substance prescription is effective or valid only if it is (*i*) issued for a legitimate medical purpose by an individual practitioner, who is (*ii*) acting in the usual course of his professional practice (11). While the prescribing clinician is primarily responsible for the "proper prescribing and dispensing of controlled substances," "a corresponding responsibility rests with the pharmacist who fills the prescription" (11). If the prescribing clinician or dispensing pharmacist knowingly prescribes or fills a controlled substance prescription outside the usual course of professional practice (or outside the usual course of legitimate and authorized research), then the individual practitioner may be "prosecuted" (12) under federal law. Section 1306.04 also *prohibits* prescribing clinicians from issuing a prescription order:

1. "to obtain controlled substances for supplying the individual practitioner for the purpose of general dispensing to patients" (13); and
2. "for the dispensing of narcotic drugs listed in any schedule for 'detoxification treatment' or 'maintenance treatment'" (14).

21. CFR 1306.05—Manner of Issuance of Prescriptions

Section 1306.05 of Title 21, Code of Federal Regulations, governs the technical aspects of issuing a controlled substance prescription. Section 1306.05(a) requires that "all prescriptions for controlled substances *shall be dated as of, and signed on, the day when issued*" (15). In addition, this section requires that the patient's full name and address be on the prescription and that the body of the prescription contain the "drug name, strength, dosage form, quantity prescribed, directions for use, and the name, address, and registration number of the practitioner" (16). Section 1306.05(a) also contains a requirement that Schedule II controlled substance prescriptions *must* be "written with ink or indelible pencil or typewriter and *shall* be manually signed by the practitioner." While a clinician's agent or secretary may prepare the body of the prescription, the prescribing clinician (DEA registrant) must be the one to sign the prescription form and will be held accountable by DEA if the prescription itself "does not conform in all essential respects to the law and regulations" (16). Once again, pharmacists have a "corresponding liability" if they dispense a controlled substance prescription that does not conform to the federal requirements. There are some important exceptions to the requirements of Section 1306.05(a), which apply to those individual practitioners who are exempt from registration, such as a hospitalist who uses the hospital's registration number (17). Section 1306.05(c) also contains directions for individual practitioners employed by one of the armed forces or the public health service.

21. CFR 1306.12—Refilling Prescriptions
Section 1306.12 prohibits the refilling of a prescription for a Schedule II controlled substance, subject to the "multiple prescriptions" exception created in 2007 by DEA pursuant to its rule-making authority. As of December 19, 2007, federal law permits an individual practitioner to issue "multiple prescriptions authorizing the patient to receive *a total of up to a 90-day supply of a Schedule II controlled substance, but only if the practitioner meets the following conditions*:

a. Each separate prescription is issued for a legitimate medical purpose by an individual practitioner acting in the usual course of professional practice;
b. The individual practitioner provides written instructions on each prescription (other than the first prescription, if the prescribing practitioner intends for that prescription to be filled immediately) indicating the earliest date on which a pharmacy may fill each prescription;
c. The individual practitioner _concludes_ that providing the patient with multiple prescriptions in this manner does not create an undue risk of diversion or abuse;
d. The issuance of multiple prescriptions as described in this section is permissible under the applicable state laws; and
e. The individual practitioner complies fully with all other applicable requirements under the Act and these regulations as well as any additional requirements under state law" (18).

Of critical importance here is the fact that federal law *does not require* an individual practitioner to issue Schedule II prescriptions in this format, meaning that patients *do not have a legal right* to receive prescriptions in this format. Likewise, federal law *does not encourage* this practice, meaning the use of the multiple Schedule II prescriptions format is completely within the individual practitioner's discretion, and subject to the federal legal conditions set forth above, any additional state law conditions, and clinical guidelines and standards of care.

An equally important aspect of Section 1306.12 (the Final Rule) is the fact that DEA does not encourage individual practitioners to see their patients only once every 90 days when prescribing Schedule II controlled substances (19). Instead, DEA's position is that section 1306.12 requires individual practitioners to "determine on their own, based on sound medical judgment, and in accordance with established medical standards, whether it is appropriate to issue multiple prescriptions and how often to see their patients when doing so" (18). *This is a significant statement and one often disregarded by nonlawyer educators during lectures at pain conferences.* Quite simply, pain clinicians should remember that federal law *does not* encourage the "multiple Schedule II prescriptions" format. Thus, pain clinicians should carefully evaluate their use of this prescribing format and ensure that state law permits this practice and that each patient has been carefully evaluated—using a benefit-to-risk analysis—and document the rationale and safety measures for monitoring the patient during follow-up evaluations to prevent abuse and diversion.

DEA Policy Statements
Over almost a two-year period, beginning in November 2004 and ending in September 2006, DEA issued three policy statements relating to the use of controlled substances to treat pain (20). The *Interim Policy Statement* (November 2004) and the *Clarification Statement* (August 2005) both contain insight into DEA's position on prescribing of Schedule II controlled substances, and both ultimately give rise to the *Final Policy Statement* (September 2006) and the *Final Rule on Issuance of Multiple Prescriptions for Schedule II Controlled Substances* (November 2007) (discussed above). These three policy statements contain insight into DEA's position on registrant obligations. These statements are summarized below.

The DEA Interim Policy Statement—November 2004
In November 2004, following its October 2004, retraction of the FAQ and to explain its rationale or doing so, DEA published its Interim Policy Statement on Dispensing Controlled Substances to Treat Pain (the "Interim Policy Statement"). DEA said that "each of the [FAQ] factors—though not necessarily determinative—may indeed be indicative of diversion." Those factors, not viewed individually by the courts as indicative of criminal behavior (although prosecution on certain individual behaviors is possible), but in concomitant and recurrent patterns, included the following:

a. prescribing of an inordinately large quantity of controlled substances;
b. issuing large numbers of controlled substance prescriptions;
c. prescribing controlled substances without performing a physical examination;
d. the physician warned the patient to fill the controlled substance prescriptions at different drug stores;
e. the physician issued controlled substance prescriptions to a patient known to be delivering the drugs to others;
f. the physician prescribed controlled substances at intervals inconsistent with legitimate medical treatment;
g. the physician used street slang with patients rather than medical terminology to describe the controlled substances prescribed;
h. there was no logical relationship between the controlled substances prescribed and the treatment of the condition allegedly existing; and
i. the physician wrote more than one controlled substance prescription on occasions in order to spread them out.

These factors remain relevant today. However, it is important to note that DEA has stated that this does not mean that "the existence of any of [these] factors will automatically lead to the conclusion that the physician acted improperly" (21).

The DEA's Clarification Statement—August 2005

On August 26, 2005, DEA published a Clarification of Existing Requirements under the Controlled Substances Act for Prescribing Schedule II Controlled Substances, which DEA intended as a follow-up to its Interim Policy (November 2004) comments on prescriptions for Schedule II controlled substances. While not formally characterized as a "policy statement," this document provides insight into DEA's position on the use of Schedule II controlled substances to treat pain. "Schedule II controlled substances, by definition, have the highest potential for abuse, and are the most likely to cause dependence, of all the controlled substances that have an approved medical use" (22). "Physicians must use the utmost care in determining whether

a. their patients for whom they are prescribing schedule II controlled substances should be seen in person each time a prescription is issued; or
b. seeing the patient in person at somewhat less frequent intervals is consistent with sound medical practice and appropriate safeguards against diversion and misuse" (22).

"Physicians must also abide by any requirements imposed by their state medical boards with respect to proper prescribing practices and what constitutes a bona fide physician–patient relationship" (22). Subject to state laws which may prohibit prescribing in the absence of a face-to-face office visit, federal law permits physicians who regularly see each patient to issue a prescription for a Schedule II controlled substance for a legitimate medical purpose without seeing the patient in person, and may mail the prescription to the patient or pharmacy. DEA regulations state: "A prescription for a schedule II controlled substance may be transmitted by the practitioner or the practitioner's agent to a pharmacy via facsimile equipment, provided that the original written, signed prescription is presented to the pharmacist for review prior to the actual dispensing of the controlled substance, except as noted [elsewhere in this section of the regulations]" (23). Thus, as this provision of the regulations provides, faxing may be used to facilitate the filling of a Schedule II prescription, but only if the pharmacy receives the original written, signed prescription prior to dispensing the drug to the patient *and* only if state law permits it. Moreover, federal law *does not* set a specific limit on the number of days' worth of a Schedule II controlled substance that a physician may authorize per prescription. Some states, however, do impose specific limits on the amount of a Schedule II controlled substance that may be prescribed. Any limitations imposed by state law apply in addition to the corresponding requirements under federal law, so long as the state requirements do not conflict with or contravene federal requirements.

Remember, the essential federal legal standard is that a "prescription for a controlled substance be issued for a legitimate medical purpose in the usual course of professional practice." Both physicians and pharmacists "have a duty as DEA registrants to ensure that their prescribing and dispensing of controlled substances occur in a manner consistent with effective controls against diversion and misuse, taking into account the nature of the drug being prescribed." It took DEA a little more than a year after its Clarification Statement to publish a Final

Statement on Dispensing Controlled Substances to Treat Pain. Despite the large gap in time, DEA finally presented registrants with written materials containing regulatory boundaries on controlled substance prescribing.

DEA Final Policy Statement—September 2006

Federal case law makes clear: there is no "one size fits all" definition of legitimate medical purpose and usual course of professional practice. In administrative cases, the law is also clear: DEA evaluates each case on its own merits in view of the totality of the circumstances and individual facts tied to physician–patient relationships. DEA expects registrants to accept their responsibility and to put practices into place, as part of routine medical practice, to prevent abuse and diversion (24). According to a 2009 DEA administrative case involving the suspension and ultimate reinstatement of a physician's registration, DEA has the authority to suspend or revoke a registration if the registrant's behavior presents a threat to public health and safety (24). "A practitioner who ignores the warning signs that her patients are either personally abusing or diverting controlled substances commits 'acts inconsistent with the public interest,' 21 U.S.C. 824(a)(4), even if she is merely gullible or naive" (24).

The DEA Final Policy Statement contains the following critical language explaining DEA's position on DEA registrant responsibilities to prevent abuse and diversion when prescribing controlled medications to treat pain:

> *What are the general legal responsibilities of a physician to prevent diversion and abuse when prescribing controlled substances?*
>
> In each instance where a physician issues a prescription for a controlled substance, the physician must properly determine there is a legitimate medical purpose for the patient to be prescribed that controlled substance and the physician must be acting in the usual course of professional practice [internal citation omitted]. This is the basic legal requirement discussed above, which has been part of American law for decades. Moreover, as a condition of being a DEA registrant, a physician who prescribes controlled substances *has an obligation to take reasonable measures to prevent diversion* [internal citation omitted]. *The overwhelming majority of physicians in the United States who prescribe controlled substances do, in fact, exercise the appropriate degree of medical supervision—as part of their routine practice during office visits—to minimize the likelihood of diversion or abuse.* Again, each patient's situation is unique and the nature and degree of physician oversight should be tailored accordingly, based on the physician's sound medical judgment and consistent with established medical standards.
>
> *What additional precaution should be taken when a patient has a history of drug abuse?*
>
> As a DEA registrant, *a physician has a responsibility to exercise a much greater degree of oversight to prevent diversion and abuse in the case of a known or suspected addict than in the case of a patient for whom there are no indicators of drug abuse.* **Under no circumstances** may a physician dispense controlled substances with the knowledge they will be used for a nonmedical purpose or that they will be resold by the patient. Some physicians who treat patients having a history of drug abuse require each patient to sign a contract agreeing to certain terms designed to prevent diversion and abuse, *such as periodic urinalysis.* While such measures are not mandated by the CSA or DEA regulations, they can be very useful.
>
> *Can a physician be investigated solely on the basis of the number of tablets prescribed for an individual patient?*

The Supreme Court has long recognized that an administrative agency responsible for enforcing the law has broad investigative authority [internal citation omitted], and courts have recognized that prescribing an "inordinately large quantity of controlled substances" can be evidence of a violation of the CSA [internal citation omitted]. DEA therefore, as the agency responsible for administering the CSA, has the legal authority to investigate a suspicious prescription of any quantity. Nonetheless, the amount of dosage units per prescription will never be a basis for investigation for the overwhelming majority of physicians. As with every other profession, however, among the hundreds of thousands of physicians who practice medicine in this country in a manner that warrants no government scrutiny are a handful who engage in criminal behavior. In rare cases, it is possible that an aberrant physician could prescribe such an enormous quantity of controlled substances to a given patient that this alone will be a valid basis for investigation. For example, if a physician were to prescribe 1,600 (sixteen hundred) tablets per day of a schedule II opioid to a single patient, this would certainly warrant investigation as there is no conceivable medical basis for anyone to ingest that quantity of such a powerful narcotic in a single day. Again, however, such cases are extremely rare. The overwhelming majority of physicians who conclude that use of a particular controlled substance is medically appropriate for a given patient should prescribe the amount of that controlled substance which is consistent with their sound medical judgment and accepted medical standards without concern that doing so will subject them to DEA scrutiny (7).

Summary of Key Federal Legal Standards (Substantive Only)

By way of summary, the federal law sets forth the below-listed *substantive* legal standards that DEA registrants must follow when treatment involves controlled substances. For a more complete discussion of both substantive and technical requirements for controlled substance prescriptions, review the DEA Diversion website and the DEA's September 2006 *Practitioner's Manual*, which may also be found on the website.

1. Provides DEA authority to oversee the flow of controlled substances in the United States and gives DEA authority to register and oversee registrant activity through its administrative and enforcement arms.
2. Requires registrants to prescribe controlled substances for a legitimate medical purpose while acting in the usual course of professional practice.
3. Requires registrants to use reasonable measures, as part of routine daily medical practice, to prevent abuse and diversion.
4. Imposes a corresponding responsibility on pharmacists to ensure a legitimate medical purpose prior to dispensing a controlled substance prescription, and requires them to do so in the usual course of professional practice.
5. Provides for specific handling of controlled substances in Schedule II, and identifies certain exceptions to the federal rules requiring a written prescription for these medications, including a provision for faxing and emergency supply. Prohibits refills of Schedule II controlled substance prescriptions, unless the registrant is acting under the "multiple issuance" or "do not fill" rule of 21 CFR 1306.12 (described above). Registrants may not issue multiple prescriptions for Schedule II controlled substances unless state law authorizes them to do so.

6. Provides for specific handling of controlled substances in Schedule III, and includes a provision for oral prescribing and refills, subject to the legitimate medical purpose/usual course of professional practice rule.
7. Does not limit the quantity of any drug prescribed or dispensed, but does limit the number of refills permitted for each prescription for a Schedule III controlled substance.
8. With the exception of the Schedule II "multiple issuance" or "do not fill" rule, does not specify a quantity or duration to determine the clinician's ongoing use of a Schedule II controlled substance.
9. Does not establish a minimum or maximum dose for controlled substance prescriptions in Schedules II through V (some states DO set maximum doses for some controlled substances, so registrants should take care to review state law before prescribing).
10. Does not establish a "life" or period of validity for a Schedule II controlled substance prescription (some states DO set a "life" or period of validity, such as 7 days, 14 days, or 21 days, and registrants should take care to review state law before prescribing).
11. Does not limit the overall number of refills for Schedule III, IV, and V controlled substances, but does establish a rule of not more than five refills in six months (some states set more restrictions so registrants should check state law).
12. Permits the mailing of controlled substance prescriptions, subject to registrant discretion and policy suggestions.

State Legal/Regulatory Materials
State legal/regulatory materials in many ways parallel the federal framework, but there are differences in state policy–level material relating to the use of controlled medications to treat pain. While a state-by-state analysis of legal/regulatory materials is beyond the scope of this chapter, pain clinicians will find that the basic framework for state controlled substances acts, medical practice act regulations, and pain policy have many similarities and the same basic platform for critical elements. To date, all but three states (25) have regulations and/or policy or position statements specifically relating to prescribing controlled substances to treat pain.

There are three basic levels of state legal/regulatory materials:

1. *Laws,* such as a state's Uniform Controlled Substances Act; Medical, Nursing, and Pharmacy Practice Acts; and in some states an Intractable Pain Treatment Act;
2. *Regulations,* including professional licensing board rules outlining standards of professional conduct and often rules on prescribing controlled medications to treat pain; and
3. *Policy or Position Statements,* including state policies on the use of controlled medications to treat pain and the office-based treatment of opioid addiction.

Federation of State Medical Boards' Model Policy
Of critical relevance to many state licensing boards' position on prescribing controlled substances for the treatment of pain is the body of policy materials created by the Federation of State Medical Boards, located in Dallas, Texas (the FSMB).

The FSMB's mission is "to continuously improve the quality, safety, and integrity of health care through developing and promoting high standards for physician licensure and practice" (26). In 1997, and again in 2004, the FSMB published a *Model Policy for the Prescribing of Controlled Substances for the Treatment of Pain* (the *Model Policy*) (27). This document contains many helpful statements on the need for pain policy to achieve balance in patient care—access to pain management, including controlled medications, and measures to prevent abuse and diversion of those medications.

As with most state regulations and/or policy statements on prescribing controlled substances to treat pain, the FSMB's *Model Policy* contains seven (7) basic elements:

1. Patient Evaluation (History and Physical Examination);
2. Treatment Plan;
3. Informed Consent;
4. Treatment Agreements;
5. Periodic Review (Patient Follow-up Evaluation);
6. Consultations and Referrals; and
7. Medical Record and Regulatory Compliance.

Pain clinicians have an "ethical and professional responsibility" to assess patients' pain (27). When pain clinicians believe it is appropriate to prescribe controlled medications to treat pain, they must document their clinical rationale for doing so (the legitimate medical purpose requirement) and take those steps outlined in currently accepted standards of care or, in the absence of a directly applicable statement of such a standard, clinical guidelines, such as the APS-AAPM 2009 clinical guideline (usual course of professional practice requirement) (6). Failure to adhere to state rules and, without a documented reason, state policy or position statements may result in administrative and legal sanctions.

One of the easiest ways to signal the intent to comply with state legal/regulatory requirements on the use of controlled substances to treat pain is to incorporate key phrases from state prescribing rules and policies into the medical record. For example, if a state prescribing rule requires a risk–benefit analysis prior to prescribing a controlled substance, then the prescribing clinician should enter a note in the patient chart integrating or referring to the legal/regulatory language, as illustrated in Figure 2. This format is easily transferred into electronic medical record systems or templates.

"The anticipated benefits for this patient's use of DRUG A are as follows:

The potential risks related to the use of DRUG A are as follows:

I have discussed these matters with the patient in detail, and based on all of the information in my possession at this time, including statements made to me by the patient, I believe the benefits of using DRUG A outweigh the risks associated with use, and I am going to prescribe a trial of DRUG A to the patient as follows . . . ."

FIGURE 2 Example of patient chart note.

There is no legal requirement requiring clinicians to incorporate legal/regulatory language into the medical record, but pain clinicians should realize that licensing board investigators and law enforcement agents speak a different language when it comes to pain management and occasional references to the materials these individuals use on a daily basis may help prevent misunderstandings and, more importantly, provide the prescribing clinician with a reference point should there be a challenge to one's prescribing patterns. Once again, there is no magic formula for avoiding legal scrutiny. However, pain clinicians must do what they can to ensure evidence of good faith prescribing and patient care as part of routine medical practice. The remainder of this section contains a discussion of each of the key elements of the FSMB's *Model Policy*, providing a framework for state licensing board materials. Pain clinicians should also consult parallel recommendations contained in the APS-AAPM Clinical Guidelines on the Use of COT to Treat CNCP to ensure practice in compliance with generally accepted clinical standards of care (28).

Patient Evaluation and Risk Assessment

Both the *Model Policy* and the APS-AAPM COT guideline require pain clinicians to engage in a careful evaluation of the patient prior to prescribing COT. The evaluation process has many components, most of which are also referred to by state licensing boards in prescribing regulations and policies. Language in the APS-AAPM COT guideline and many state regulations and policy statements suggest that the evaluation and risk assessment process should take place *prior to prescribing controlled substances to the patient* (6). The difficulty with such a requirement is obvious: many patients present already using controlled substances to treat pain and the timing of many patient visits is such that patients are almost out of their medications, requiring a prescription to avoid the discomforts of acute withdrawal. Common sense tells us that pain clinicians must balance their role as health care providers with their legal and professional obligation to prevent abuse and diversion. Thus, early in any relationship between a pain clinician and a patient, prescribing should be done in a controlled and trial fashion to ensure pain management and minimize risk.

In the patient evaluation phase, legal/regulatory materials recommend that clinicians:

1. obtain information about the patient's past medical history;
2. evaluate a recent physical examination or perform a new, condition-specific physical examination and document the results in the medical record;
3. document the nature and intensity of the patient's pain, current and past treatments for pain, any underlying or coexisting diseases or conditions, the effect of pain on the patient's physical and psychological function; and
4. ascertain the patient's history of substance abuse (alcohol and drug) (29).

The APS-AAPM COT guideline (6) expands upon the "risk assessment" portion of patient evaluation, making the following very important recommendations that directly correlate with the legal/regulatory recommendations:

1.1 *Before initiating COT*, clinicians *should* conduct a history, physical examination, and appropriate testing, including an assessment of risk of substance abuse, misuse, or addiction (*strong recommendation, low-quality evidence*).

1.2 Clinicians *may* consider a trial of COT as an option if CNCP is moderate or severe, pain is having an adverse impact on function or quality of life, and potential therapeutic benefits outweigh or are likely to outweigh potential harms (*strong recommendation, low-quality evidence*).

1.3 A benefit-to-harm evaluation, including a history, physical examination, and appropriate diagnostic testing, *should* be performed and documented before and on an ongoing basis during COT (*strong recommendation, low-quality evidence*) (6).

"Proper patient selection is critical and requires a comprehensive benefit-to-harm evaluation that weighs the potential positive effects of opioids on pain and function against potential risks." "*Thorough risk assessment and stratification is appropriate in every case*" (30).

In 2009, risk assessment requires all pain management clinicians to be familiar with the various risk factors for opioid abuse and the methods for assessing risk and evaluating the potential for opioid-associated adverse effects. "A thorough history and physical examination, including an assessment of psychosocial factors and family history, is essential for adequate risk stratification. Implicit in the recommendation to conduct a comprehensive benefit-to-harm analysis is the recognition that an opioid trial may not be appropriate. Clinicians should obtain appropriate diagnostic tests to evaluate the underlying pain condition, and should consider whether the pain condition may be treated more effectively with nonopioid therapy rather than with COT" (6).

Newer risk assessment measures include screening tools that assess the potential risks associated with COT based on patient characteristics, such as environmental factors, experience with medications, experience with lawsuits, emotions and feelings, and several others (6). The APS-AAPM COT guideline states these tools "are likely to be helpful for risk stratification, though more validation and prospective outcome studies are needed to understand how their use predicts and affects clinical outcomes" (6). Unfortunately, however, the current health care system does not provide focused reimbursement methods for the use of these tools, making it just one more thing pain clinicians are told they "should" do prior to prescribing controlled substances. In addition, many clinicians have yet to review these tools (31) and decide whether and how to incorporate their use into the medical practice.

In summary, pain clinicians should consider the following measures in connection with patient evaluation:

1. verify the patient's self-report of medication usage with prior providers or through a state prescription drug monitoring program or pharmacy profile;
2. discuss medication options with the patient and determine whether patient has had a trial of nonopioids and document patient's response to same or reason why the trial was inappropriate or did not work;
3. review documentation from prior providers;
4. consider overall risk assessment issues and whether a urine drug test would support your prescribing rationale.

The pain clinician's rationale for the use of controlled substances is a critical documentation topic. Overall, the clinician should document their rationale for using controlled substances, medication quantity, the duration of use and, where applicable, medication combinations, and document one or more currently accepted clinical indications for the use of controlled substances. Doing so will go a long way to establishing a legitimate medical purpose.

Treatment Plan

After deciding whether to prescribe controlled substances to the patient, legal/regulatory materials require/suggest the use of a *written* treatment plan documenting the patient's diagnosis (or working diagnosis) and a summary of treatment goals and the time frame for reevaluating the patient's progress toward the same. The plan does not have to be elaborate, but it should clearly document the legitimate medical purpose for which controlled substances are prescribed and provide enough information to demonstrate that the clinician is acting within the usual course of professional practice. Most state licensing board rules/policies require some version of the following in connection with the treatment plan:

> The medical record should include (A) how the medication relates to the chief presenting complaint of chronic pain; (B) dosage and frequency of prescribed, (C) further testing and diagnostic evaluations to be ordered, (D) other treatments that are planned or considered, (E) periodic reviews planned, and (F) objectives that will be used to determine treatment success, such as pain relief and improved physical and psychosocial function (32).

Most states require clinicians to periodically review the treatment plan to ensure that the benefit-to-risk analysis remains the focus and to evaluate the necessary level of medical supervision to prevent abuse and diversion in the patient's individual case.

Informed Consent and Treatment Agreement

Informed consent and the agreement for treatment are critical components of most state rules/policies on prescribing controlled substances to treat pain. It is important to remember, however, that informed consent is a separate legal concept from a treatment agreement and one that is grounded in medical ethics. While it is possible to address informed consent and treatment agreement issues with the patient during a single visit, the better practice is to address these matters separately, using separate forms designed to reinforce the relevant subject matter with the patient. A full-blown discussion of the informed consent and treatment agreement is beyond the scope of this chapter.

Informed consent is the process by which the clinician fulfills the ethical responsibility to give the patient information from which he/she can make informed decisions about health care (33). It involves a process and a discussion with the patient about

1. the risks of the recommended treatment, including any medications prescribed;
2. the anticipated benefits of the recommended treatment;
3. any alternative or complimentary therapies; and
4. special issues related to the recommended treatment, such as treatment safety, driving, and decision-making (33).

Some states require a separate form documenting the informed consent process, while others permit the clinician to use a contemporaneous note describing it in the medical record. Be sure to check state licensing board requirements to ensure compliance. Also, a clinician's failure to provide the patient with adequate information may give rise to a claim of negligence. Check with legal counsel to ensure informed consent forms are current and written in conformance with state case law in mind. In summary, informed consent process and related documentation focuses on the patient's mindset and whether he/she has sufficient information to provide his/her consent to the recommended treatment. If the patient withholds information from a clinician about a material component of informed consent, such as withholding personal history of substance abuse, then any claim of negligence against the treating clinician may be mitigated by the patient's actions. These matters require careful legal analysis and are best left to the clinician's local legal counsel.

By contrast, a treatment agreement (often inappropriately referred to as a "narcotic contract") involves a form and a conversation between the patient and the clinician about the clinician's expectations of patient behaviors—what the patient must or must not do during the treatment period involving controlled substances. In fact, the treatment agreement is a unique tool arising out of state rules/policies on prescribing controlled substances to treat pain; informed consent is not and applies to any recommended medical treatment within the clinician–patient relationship. While both processes involve efforts designed to improve patient care and prevent abuse and diversion, the **informed consent** favors the patient's need for information *prior to making health care decisions* and the **treatment agreement** favors the clinician's need to set *behavioral boundaries* designed to protect the individual patient and the public's health and safety and to enforce them based on the individual patient's case.

The FSMB's *Model Policy* contains the following basic suggestions regarding the use of treatment agreements:

1. A written treatment agreement should be considered if the patient has a history of substance abuse (34).
2. The agreement should explain the purpose and terms of its use and should seek the patient's agreement to:
   a. use a single clinician for the prescribing of controlled substances;
   b. select a single pharmacy to use for filling controlled substance prescriptions (35);
   c. produce a blood/urine sample as requested for compliance and therapeutic testing; and
   d. bring with them to each office visit original medication bottles containing all remaining medication.
3. The agreement should clearly state the reasons for which controlled substance therapy or treatment overall may be discontinued (36).

It is vital that the pain clinician draft the treatment agreement using clear and simple language and even consider translating it into other languages to serve the entirety of the clinician's patient population. It is also important to remember that treatment agreements are part of the medical record and may be used in administrative hearings and court to address the clinician's prescribing habits. Often, treatment agreements and other practice forms are shown to hearing officers and jurors and provide an impression of the clinician's attention to detail and professionalism and tone toward patients. Thus, great care should be given to the drafting and review of treatment agreements and other office forms.

PERIODIC REVIEW AND RISK MONITORING

Periodic review involves patient follow-up care and medical supervision commensurate with the individual patient needs and the scope of the clinician's medical practice. Clinical standards of care require the clinician to evaluate the patient's progress (or lack thereof) toward the treatment plan goals and the patient's compliance with medication instructions—safe use and handling, etc. The timing of follow-up visits should be individualized to each patient, taking into consideration the patient's history, overall risk potential, and developing facts of patient care. Some state rules/policies require the clinician to see the patient at least every 12 weeks (37). Most states, however, do not suggest a specific follow-up period and leave the decision to the clinician, thereby requiring the clinician to exercise medical decision-making consistent with current standards of care and evolving patient needs. The language of the DEA's *Clarification Statement* (August 2005) and *Final Policy Statement* (September 2006), and its administrative opinion *in the matter of Jayam Krishna-Iyer* (January 2009), indicates growing regulatory emphasis on individualized treatment plans, follow-up periods, and patient risk monitoring. In many ways, periodic review emphasizes both sides of the balance issue—ensuring the patient's continued access to quality pain management, including where appropriate controlled medications, and routine measures as part of daily medical practice to prevent abuse and diversion. Pain clinicians may face regulatory scrutiny if patient follow-up does not include reasonable and regular means designed to prevent abuse and diversion, such as periodic urinalysis (38), medication counts (39) or attention to the amount of medication a patient has on hand and determining whether there is a need for the safe disposal of expired or unused medications, and other measures designed to address these concerns.

The APS-AAPM COT guideline provides the following recommendations in connection with patient monitoring:

> 5.1 Clinicians should reassess patients on COT periodically and as warranted by changing circumstances. Monitoring should include documentation of pain intensity and level of functioning, assessments of progress toward achieving therapeutic goals, presence of adverse events, and adherence to prescribed therapies (*strong recommendation, low-quality evidence*).
> 5.2 In patients on COT who are at high risk or who have engaged in aberrant drug-related behaviors, clinicians should periodically obtain urine drug screens or other information to confirm adherence to the COT plan of care (*strong recommendation, low-quality evidence*).
> 5.3 In patients on COT not at high risk and not known to have engaged in aberrant drug-related behaviors, clinicians should consider periodically obtaining urine drug screens or other information to confirm adherence to the COT plan of care (*weak recommendation, low-quality evidence*) (6).

According to a panel of experts who authored the APS-AAPM clinical guidelines on COT to treat CNCP:

> Clinicians should periodically reassess all patients on COT. Regular monitoring of patients once COT is initiated is critical because therapeutic risks and benefits do not remain static and can be affected by changes in

the underlying pain condition, presence of coexisting disease, or changes in psychological or social circumstances. Monitoring is essential to identify patients who are benefiting from COT, those who might benefit more with restructuring of treatment or receiving additional services such as treatment for addiction, and those whose benefits from treatment are outweighed by harms (6).

These guidelines state that the evidence is insufficient to guide precise recommendations on appropriate monitoring intervals. From a regulatory perspective, if this is the case with a patient, then the clinician should document this fact in the medical record.

Likewise, the APS-AAPM clinical guideline states:

Risk stratification is useful for guiding the approach to monitoring. In patients at low risk for adverse outcomes and on stable doses of opioids, monitoring at least once every three to six months may be sufficient. Patients who may need more frequent or intense monitoring, at least for a period of time after initiation of therapy or changes in opioid doses, include those with a prior history of an addictive disorder, those in an occupation demanding mental acuity, older adults, patients with an unstable or dysfunctional social environment, and those with comorbid psychiatric or medical conditions. For patients at very high risk for adverse outcomes, monitoring on a weekly basis may be a reasonable strategy (6).

It is important to note that the language of this clinical guideline may actually conflict with specific regulatory requirements in some states, such as Louisiana and New Jersey, both of which mandate that patients on chronic controlled substance therapy be seen at least every 12 weeks and, more frequently, depending on the patient's individual circumstances. Pain clinicians should document the interval for periodic review and supply a statement of the rationale for the period selected.

"There is general agreement that monitoring should routinely include assessment and documentation of pain severity and functional ability, progress toward achieving therapeutic goals, and presence of adverse effects" (6). Monitoring also include a complete and routine "clinical assessment for presence of aberrant drug-related behaviors, substance use, and psychological issues" (40).

Clinical and regulatory guidelines acknowledge that periodic urine drug screening can be a helpful tool to monitor patients using controlled medications (41). A detailed discussion of urine drug testing is beyond the scope of this chapter. However, several federal cases address the lack of urine drug testing and the failure to address the results of a urine drug test with the patient, indicating that the defendant-clinician's failure to use urine drug testing or the results of such toxicology tests as evidence of a lack of legitimate medical purpose and a provider acting outside the usual course of professional practice (42).

Overall, the pain clinician is responsible for determining whether the patient's response to controlled substance therapy is satisfactory and that ongoing use remains indicated. Many states suggest clinicians indicate a satisfactory response to controlled substance therapy by documenting facts associated with "the patient's decreased pain, increased level of function, or improved quality of life" (27). Many clinicians find themselves in hot water with licensing boards if they merely document the above-quoted phrase instead of making the effort to document facts demonstrating decreased pain, that is, the patient reports a decrease in pain from level 7 to level 4. Or, the patient reports "she is now working part time and doing house hold chores and engaging in social activities with her family—she states she went to the movies with her husband and children and sat through most of the movie without too much discomfort." In essence, clinicians should monitor the patient for "[o]bjective evidence of improved or diminished function ... and [consider] information from family members or other caregivers in determining the patient's response to treatment" (27). State legal/regulatory and clinical guidelines make very clear: "[i]f the patient's progress is unsatisfactory, the clinician should asses the appropriateness of continued use of the current treatment plan [especially one involving controlled substances] and consider the use of other therapeutic modalities" (27).

It is important to note that both clinical guidelines and legal/regulatory materials distinguish initial and ongoing treatment for "high-risk" patients. Pain clinicians should carefully review clinical and regulatory resources to ensure compliance. As questions arise, check with clinical colleagues and confirm practice policies with legal counsel.

CONSULTATIONS AND REFERRALS

The use of consultations and referrals is contemplated on an "as necessary" basis by both current clinical standards of care and state pain rules/policies. Some patients may need to see behavioral health specialists; others may need professionals qualified in addiction medicine or other specialty area. Unfortunately, the current health care system does not always support the use of necessary consultations and referrals, often making it difficult for both the clinician and the patient to address specific treatment concerns.

MEDICAL RECORDS

Pain clinicians are required to keep accurate and careful documentation of their interaction with patients and treatment recommendations. Like state regulations and policy statements, the *Model Policy* contains a list of medical records that pain clinicians should keep. Remember, state licensing boards and state laws may

---

The following list of Medical Records is quoted from the FSMB's Model Policy Statement on the Use of Controlled Substances for the Treatment of Pain (April 2004) (27). Similar lists appear in many state prescribing guidelines and regulations.
  "Medical Records—The physician should keep accurate and complete records to include

1. the medical history and physical examination,
2. diagnostic, therapeutic and laboratory results,
3. evaluations and consultations,
4. treatment objectives,
5. discussion of risks and benefits,
6. informed consent,
7. treatments,
8. medications (including date, type, dosage and quantity prescribed),
9. instructions and agreements and
10. periodic reviews.

Records should remain current and be maintained in an accessible manner and readily available for review.

FIGURE 3 List of medical records.

TABLE 1 Key Legal/Regulatory Compliance Recommendations and Documentation Steps in the Treatment of Pain with Controlled Substances

Legal/Regulatory Component	Documentation Checklist
Patient Evaluation (History, Physical Examination, Risk Assessment)	*General patient history *Specific pain history *Past treatments for pain (including medication/procedures) and records from prior provider *Family and Patient history of chemical/substance abuse *Current report of pain (nature, intensity) *Condition-appropriate physical examination *Risk Assessment Questionnaire if Chronic Opioid Therapy is contemplated *Urine Drug Testing (point of care and laboratory confirmation), for illegal drugs and other controlled prescribed drugs *Electronic prescription drug monitoring program or patient pharmacy profile
Treatment Plan and Medication Trial	*Written treatment plan *Set goals for treatment and reasonable trial period *Discuss methods used to measure patient's progress and next steps outline *Set time for return visits using patient risk level (L, M, H) to guide decision making *Order additional testing (diagnostic and laboratory) *Use consultations and referrals as necessary *Take reasonable steps to prevent abuse and diversion via medication trial and safety steps
Informed Consent	*Informed consent is a process whereby the clinician discusses the (1) risks, including adverse effects, known side-effects, potential for addiction, (2) benefits, (3) alternatives to using controlled substances (if any), and (4) special issues, such as medication safety, driving, operating heavy machinery, making important decisions, caring for others, and carrying weapon. Clinicians should give patients a chance to ask questions. *Consider documenting informed consent SEPARATE from a Treatment Agreement. The two processes are not the same, and some state licensing boards make this point very clear. *The American Academy of Pain Medicine has a sample Informed Consent document on its website. Some states require a written, signed form; others allow a contemporaneous note in the patient's medical record. *Applies to both medications and treatments. Informed consent process is not unique to opioids, although the actual document usually is. *You should review your informed consent practices with your legal counsel.
Treatment Agreement	*Addresses practice boundaries and rules relating to obtaining, filling, and safe handling and usage of controlled substances. *Usually a written document discussing treatment accountability and drug boundary issues. *Should NOT be limited to opioids; Most state materials apply it to controlled substances rather than just opioids. *Should NOT be titled a Contract or a Narcotic Contract.

TABLE 1   (Continued)

Legal/Regulatory Component	Documentation Checklist
	*You should review this document with your legal counsel. *Most state licensing board rules/policies provide sample language for a treatment agreement; use this language and tailor it as appropriate to your practice. *The American Academy of Pain Medicine has a sample Treatment Agreement, but make sure you change the language to cover all controlled substances instead of leaving it as limited to opioids – especially for those who are in states that take this approach. *Remember, a Treatment Agreement is also a process and the pain clinician should address patient violations with balance in mind – access to pain care with obligation to prevent abuse and diversion. Failure to address aberrant patient behaviors may increase legal exposure.
Periodic Review	*Assess the patient periodically, based on the individual circumstances of each patient's case and according to the standard of care and state rules/guidelines. Some states require follow-up review at least every 12 weeks. Others require more frequent visits. *Standard of care may dictate more frequent visits due to the patient's risk level. *Remember to demonstrate reasonable measures to prevent abuse and diversion, such as periodic urine drug testing, medication counts, and referrals. *State rules/policies contain a checklist for follow-up care. *The APS-AAPM COT guideline contains additional suggestions.
Consultations and Referrals	*Use as necessary. *If patient's insurance does not cover, then document as much and advocate for coverage or alternatives. *Most state rules/policies suggest that consultations and referrals "are necessary" when a patient has a history of substance abuse and a pain condition necessitating controlled substances. Be sure to review these state materials.
Documentation	*Consult state rules/policies for a specific list of required documents.

require additional documentation, so pain clinicians should check with appropriate state agencies and their legal counsel to ensure compliance (Table 1). Medical record documentation often serves as a deciding factor in the outcome of legal challenges. While there can be no guarantee that having all of the items listed in Figure 3 will prevent a lawsuit, the better the pain clinician's documentation, the easier it is to explain the clinician's treatment rationale and the patient's consent to the same. In fact, solid documentation of the patient's informed consent to current and generally accepted treatments can mitigate risk and improve legal outcomes.

SUMMARY
The law is not designed to prevent the use of controlled substances to treat pain. Instead, federal and state legal/regulatory materials set boundaries within which

pain clinicians must operate to maintain their medical license and DEA registration. Familiarity with legal/regulatory boundaries enables pain clinicians to achieve balance in the treatment of chronic pain with controlled substances—treating pain while taking reasonable steps to prevent abuse and diversion. By integrating legal/regulatory principles with clinical guidelines through the creation and implementation of compliance and risk management policies, the pain clinician can minimize the potential for legal exposure. A good faith effort to comply with legal/regulatory directives and policies, together with clinical guidelines, may not stop a lawsuit but can certainly help determine its outcome and, most importantly, preserve patient access to quality medical care.

REFERENCES

1. Promoting Pain Relief and Preventing Abuse of Pain Medications: A Critical Balancing Act, A Joint Statement from 21 Health Organizations and the Drug Enforcement Administration, October 23, 2001. Available at: http://www.painpolicy.wisc.edu/dea01.htm.
2. National Prescription Drug Threat Assessment 2009, National Drug Intelligence Center, Drug Enforcement Administration. Available at: http://www.usdoj.gov/ndic/pubs33/33775/33775p.pdf. "Among the general population, nonmedical use of controlled prescription drugs was stable from 2003–2007, with 7 million Americans, aged 12 and older, reporting past month nonmedical use of prescription drugs. Pain relievers are the most widely diverted and abused, with one in five new drug abusers initiating with potent narcotics. Diversion and abuse of controlled prescription drugs cost public and private medical insurers an estimated $72.5 billion per year."
3. National Prescription Drug Threat Assessment 2009, National Drug Intelligence Center, Drug Enforcement Administration. Available at: http://www.usdoj.gov/ndic/pubs33/33775/33775p.pdf.<CE: Ref. 4, Duplicate Refs. 5 and 6.>
4. The Food and Drug Administration Amendments Act of 2007 (FDAAA), Public Law 110-85, 110th Congress. Available at: http://frwebgate.access.gpo.gov/cgi-bin/getdoc.cgi?dbname = 110_cong_public_laws&docid = f:publ085.110.
5. See, for example, Jayam Krishna-Iyer, MD. Suspension of Registration; Granting of Renewal Application Subject to Condition, 2009; 74(3):459–464 (DEA); and Chou R, et al. Clinical guidelines for the use of chronic opioid therapy in chronic noncancer pain. J Pain 2009; 10(2):113–130. Available at: www.sciencedirect.com.
6. Chou R, et al. Clinical guidelines for the use of chronic opioid therapy in chronic noncancer pain. J Pain 2009; 10(2):113–130. Available at: www.sciencedirect.com.
7. U.S. Drug Enforcement Administration, Final Policy Statement on Dispensing Controlled Substances for the Treatment of Pain. Federal Register 2006; 71(172):52716–52723. Available at: http://wais.access.gpo.gov (DOCID:fr fr06se06–139).
8. U.S. Drug Enforcement Administration, Codified Controlled Substances Act of 1970. Available at: http://www.deadiversion.usdoj.gov/21cfr/21usc/21ibusct.htm.
9. www.deadiversion.usdoj.gov.
10. U.S. Drug Enforcement Administration, Practitioner's Manual: An Informational Outline of the Controlled Substances Act 2006 Edition. Available at: http://www.deadiversion.usdoj.gov/pubs/manuals/pract/index.html. Clinicians should keep a copy of this manual in their office and review it periodically to ensure compliance with federal legal requirements for registration and prescribing.
11. 21 CFR 1306.04.
12. Here, prosecuted means both administrative and criminal actions. The ultimate direction of any investigation and prosecution is subject to a careful analysis of facts and legal authority of the regulatory agency, in this case the U.S. Department of Justice (DOJ) through DEA, who has authority to pursue administrative and criminal actions against registrants. When criminal actions are pursued, federal prosecutors

evaluate the investigative value of the case and decide whether to present the matter for prosecution. DEA often works with other law enforcement agencies on criminal cases involving prescribing clinicians and dispensing pharmacists. In administrative matters, DEA uses its own attorneys and its diversion investigators to initiate enforcement actions against DEA registrants. To learn more about these matters, use the DEA Diversion website at www.deadiversion.usdoj.gov.

13. 21 CFR 1306.04(b). The rationale for this rule is tied to the federal requirement of a separate registration for each dispensing location, because dispensing of controlled substances requires a great deal more paperwork and security that the act of prescribing. Pain clinicians should review the federal and state laws relating to dispensing controlled substances out of the medical practice and discuss these matters with legal counsel. While it may be that dispensing controlled substances provides an additional income stream to the clinician and the convenience of on-sight medications for patients, many clinicians find themselves unprepared to handle the significant increase of paperwork and DEA scrutiny.

14. 21 CFR 1306.04(c). Once again, narcotic treatment centers involve a separate registration and additional regulatory hurdles for clinicians who work in them. It is important to note, however, that the Drug Abuse Treatment Act of 2000 (DATA 2000) provides for special registration of qualified clinicians to prescribe controlled substances in Schedules III, IV, and V for the treatment of opioid addiction (commonly known as X-Registration for the prescribing of buprenorphine for detoxification within the privacy of the medical practice). To read more about these matters, consult the DEA Diversion website www.deadiversion.usdoj.gov.

15. "Issued" means the date the controlled substance prescription is released to the ultimate user, whether by hand delivery or posting via U.S. mail. *Citation*: Section 1306.05(a) makes clear "[a] practitioner may sign a prescription in the same manner as he would sign a check or legal document (e.g., J.H. Smith or John H. Smith)." In other words, pre- or postdating a controlled substance prescription is prohibited. *Important note*: While the act of pre- or postdating a prescription is prohibited under federal law, the act of providing fill date instructions, including a delayed fill date for a Schedule II controlled substance, *is not prohibited*. See the comments for 21 CFR 1306.12, concerning the issuance of multiple prescriptions for Schedule II controlled substances. Remember too that clinicians should consult individual state laws on multiple Schedule II prescriptions, because some states prohibit this prescribing format.

16. 21 CFR 1306.05(a).

17. 21 CFR 1306.05(b). Here, the individual practitioner must use the special registration number provided to the hospital and ensure that the following information is contained on the controlled substance prescription: the physician stamped, typed, or hand-printed on it, as well as the signature of the physician.

18. 21 CFR 1306.12 and U.S. Drug Enforcement Administration, Final Rule on Issuance of Multiple Prescriptions for Schedule II Controlled Substances, November 17, 2007 (effective December 17, 2007). Federal Register 2007; 72(222):64921–64930. Available at: http://wais.access.gpo.gov (DOCID:fr19no07–2).

19. U.S. Drug Enforcement Administration, Final Rule on Issuance of Multiple Prescriptions for Schedule II Controlled Substances, November 17, 2007 (effective December 17, 2007). Federal Register 2007; 72(222):64921–64930. Available at: http://wais.access.gpo.gov (DOCID:fr19no07–2).

20. Prior to the DEA's publication of its Final Policy Statement, DEA published two preliminary statements in the Federal Register: (1) U.S. Drug Enforcement Administration, Interim Policy Statement on Dispensing Controlled Substances for the Treatment of Pain. Federal Register 2004; 69(220):67170–67172. Available at: http://wais.access.gpo.gov (DOCID:fr16no04–82); and (2) the U.S. Drug Enforcement Administration, Clarification of Existing Requirements Under the Controlled Substances Act for Prescribing Schedule II Controlled Substances. Federal Register 2005; 70(165):50408–50409. Available at: http://wais.access.gpo.gov (DOCID:fr26au05–139).

21. U.S. Drug Enforcement Administration, Interim Policy Statement on Dispensing Controlled Substances for the Treatment of Pain. Federal Register 2004; 69(220):67170–67172. Available at: http://wais.access.gpo.gov (DOCID:fr16no04–82).
22. U.S. Drug Enforcement Administration, Clarification of Existing Requirements Under the Controlled Substances Act for Prescribing Schedule II Controlled Substances. Federal Register 2005; 70(165):50408–50409. Available at: http://wais.access.gpo.gov (DOCID:fr26au05–139).
23. 21 CFR 1306.11.
24. Jayam Krishna-Iyer, MD. Suspension of Registration; Granting of Renewal Application Subject to Condition, 2009; 74(3):459–464 (DEA).
25. To date, those three states include DE, IL, and IN. There is a great deal of pressure on these states to adopt some form of pain policy to ensure basic guidance to clinicians practicing in DE, IL, and IN.
26. www.fsmb.org (home page).
27. Federation of State Medical Boards, Model Policy for the Use of Controlled Substances for the Treatment of Pain (May 2004). Available at: http://www.fsmb.org/pdf/2004_grpol_Controlled_Substances.pdf.
28. The APS-AAPM document acknowledges that many of its recommendations are based on "weak evidence," because of the lack of data and evidence-based medicine studies on the treatment of chronic pain with opioids. Unfortunately, however, because these professional organizations published these clinical guidelines and structured them as "clinical recommendations," every attorney involved in any level of litigation (administrative, civil, or criminal) will work through hired medical experts and use the directives and specific language of the APS-AAPM guideline to measure the propriety of a defendant-clinician's prescribing habits. Thus, it is critical that pain clinicians attempt to follow these recommendations in good faith, and document reasons for varying from them—especially when the health care system inhibits or prevents compliance as is often the case with specific measures such as urine drug testing, behavioral medicine referrals, and even alternative means of treatment.
29. Federation of State Medical Boards, Model Policy for the Use of Controlled Substances for the Treatment of Pain (May 2004). Available at: http://www.fsmb.org/pdf/2004_grpol_Controlled_Substances.pdf; Texas Medical Board Rules [chap 170]. Available at: http://www.tmb.state.tx.us/rules/rules/bdrules.php.
30. Chou R, et al. Clinical guidelines for the use of chronic opioid therapy in chronic non-cancer pain. J Pain 2009; 10(2):113–130. Available at: www.sciencedirect.com. According to the guideline, "[t]his approach is justified by estimates of aberrant drug-related behaviors (see Appendix B, Glossary), drug abuse, or misuse in patients with CNCP, which range from 0% to 50%, depending on the population evaluated and methods used to define and identify these outcomes [internal citation omitted]. Risk stratification pertaining to outcomes associated with the abuse liability of opioids—misuse, abuse, addiction and diversion—is a vital but relatively undeveloped skill for many clinicians [internal citation omitted]."
31. There are several tools, several of which are referenced by the APS-AAPM COT guideline: "Tools that appear to have good content, face, and construct validity include the Screener and Opioid Assessment for Patients with Pain (SOAPP) Version 1 (Appendix 3), the revised SOAPP (SOAPP-R), the Opioid Risk Tool (ORT) (Appendix 4), and the Diagnosis, Intractability, Risk, Efficacy (DIRE) instrument (Appendix 5). DIRE is clinician-administered and is designed to assess potential efficacy as well as harms. The SOAPP Version 1, SOAPP-R and ORT are patient self-report questionnaires that assess risk of aberrant drug-related behaviors." Chou R, et al. Clinical guidelines for the use of chronic opioid therapy in chronic noncancer pain. J Pain 2009; 10(2):113–130. Available at: www.sciencedirect.com.
32. State example comes from Texas Medical Board Rules, Texas Admin. Code, Title 22, Part 9, chap 170. Available at: http://www.tmb.state.tx.us/rules/rules/bdrules.php.

33. American Medical Association, Informed Consent. Available at: http://www.ama-assn.org/ama/pub/physician-resources/legal-topics/patient-physician-relationship-topics/informed-consent.shtml.
34. It is very important for pain clinicians to check state pain rules/policies for guidance on the use of treatment agreements. Many states recommend/suggest the use of treatment agreements if there is to be long-term prescribing of controlled substances. Thus, while the FSMB's Model Policy ties the use of a treatment agreement to the patient's known risk of substance abuse, many state rules/policies tie the use of a treatment agreement to all patients who are placed on long-term controlled substance therapy (not just opioid therapy). This distinction may be critical in any legal evaluation of the pain clinician's prescribing practices.
35. From a risk management perspective, pain clinicians should encourage patients to fill all of their prescriptions—controlled or not—at a single pharmacy to better enable the pharmacist to evaluate potential drug–drug interactions, provide additional patient education, and communicate possible drug conflicts to the pain clinician. While this may prove difficult in today's health care system largely due to the popularity or even required use of mail order pharmacies, the pain clinician may validly argue that such a control measure minimizes risk to not only the individual patient, but also to other stakeholders involved in patient's health care, including the health plan.
36. The American Academy of Pain Medicine publishes a sample treatment agreement on its website www.painmed.org. While this agreement is written for long-term opioid therapy, it can easily be tailored to meet the requirements of most state rules/policies by changing opioid therapy to controlled substance therapy. Pain clinicians should check with local legal counsel to ensure compliance with state licensing board expectations and current standards of care.
37. Louisiana and New Jersey are two states with such requirements. Readers should contact their medical board for more information.
38. Periodic urinalysis is cited as a term in a treatment agreement that is designed to prevent abuse and diversion, as stated in the DEA's Final Policy Statement (September 2006). In addition, periodic urinalysis (in one fashion or another) has been cited as an important risk management tool in several federal criminal case opinions (along with supporting trial transcripts). See, for example, US v. Williams, 445 F.3d 1302 (11th Cir. 2006); US v. Merrill, No. 06–14076 (11th Cir. 1/17/2008) (11th Cir. 2008).
39. Medication counts are often referred to as "pill counts" and are not always an accurate measure of a patient's compliance because it is relatively easy for a patient to save enough medication to remain consistent with expected medication usage. Some "patients" will go as far as borrowing or purchasing enough medication to meet count expectations. In many ways, counting medication may seem silly, but it can prove helpful especially when a patient is using a controlled substance for "breakthrough" pain management. Check with your state licensing board to determine its position on the value of medication counts in pain management.
40. The APS-AAPM clinical guidelines state: "Because patient self-report may be unreliable for determining amount of opioid use, functionality, or aberrant drug-related behaviors (internal citations omitted), pill counts, urine drug screening, family member or caregiver interviews, and use of prescription monitoring program data can be useful supplements. Although evidence is lacking on the accuracy and effects on clinical outcomes of formal screening instruments for identification of aberrant drug-related behaviors, use of tools with strong content, face, and construct validity, such as the PADT (Appendix 8 and 9) (internal citations omitted), is recommended as an efficient method of assessment and documentation."
41. Chou R, et al. Clinical guidelines for the use of chronic opioid therapy in chronic noncancer pain. J Pain 2009; 10(2):113–130. Available at: www.sciencedirect.com; U.S. Drug Enforcement Administration, Final Policy Statement on Dispensing Controlled Substances for the Treatment of Pain. Federal Register 2006; 71(172):52716–52723. Available at: http://wais.access.gpo.gov (DOCID:fr fr06se06–139).
42. US v. Williams, 445 F.3d 1302 (11th Cir. 2006); US v. Merrill, No. 06–14076 (11th Cir. 1/17/2008) (11th Cir. 2008).

26 Antidepressant Medications

Gary W. Jay

Clinical Disease Area Expert-Pain, Pfizer, Inc., New London, Connecticut, U.S.A.

The purpose of this chapter is to discuss the use of antidepressant medications (ADMs) in terms of their use for pain/analgesia.

TRICYCLIC ANTIDEPRESSANTS

Tricyclic antidepressants (TCAs) include amitriptyline, nortriptyline, desipramine, imipramine, and doxepin (which are used most frequently). Their starting dose is between 10 and 50 mg at night. It is best to start low and increase slowly. Dosages with effectiveness for pain are typically between 25 and 150 mg at night (q.h.s.). The most typical indications include neuropathic pain, fibromyalgia, and, in general, any type of chronic pain.

These medications work via a blockade of the reuptake of both serotonin and norepinephrine. They should be used with caution in the elderly and in patients with cardiovascular disorders, urinary hesitancy, or history of seizures. TCAs are contraindicated in patients with a history of recent myocardial infarction, narrow angle glaucoma, or within 14 days of the use of a monoamine oxidase inhibitor (MAOI).

TCAs should be used with caution with selective serotonin reuptake inhibitors (SSRIs) (as they increase the risk of serotonin syndrome), anticholinergic medications, antiarrhythmics, clonidine, lithium, and tramadol (which has the same reuptake inhibition). These medications should not be used in combination with drugs that prolong the QTc interval, as this may increase the risk for cardiac arrhythmia.

The major adverse effects of TCAs are secondary to cholinergic/muscarinic receptor blockade, histaminergic blockade (H1, H2), as well as blockade of the dopaminergic system. The anticholinergic side effects predominate and can include blurred vision, xerostomia, sinus tachycardia, constipation, urinary retention, confusion, and memory dysfunction. Histaminergic blockade can induce sedation, weight gain, dizziness, and hypotension. It also potentiates the effects of other CNS depressants. Alpha-1 adrenergic blockade can be associated with postural hypotension and dizziness. Blockade of dopaminergic receptors can induce extrapyramidal syndrome, dystonia, akinesia, neuroleptic malignant syndrome, tardive dyskinesia, and endocrine changes. Tachycardia and prolonged PR and QRS intervals with membrane stabilization can occur. The QT interval can become prolonged (1, 2).

An electrocardiogram is recommended if there is a history of cardiac disease. Electrocardiogram changes such as QRS widening, PR and QT prolongation, and T wave flattening can be induced by these agents as noted. TCAs may have quinidine-like actions, consistent with their sodium channel–blocking effects, particularly in patients with underlying ischemic cardiac disease or arrhythmias (3). Because abrupt discontinuation of antidepressants may precipitate withdrawal symptoms, such as insomnia, restlessness, and vivid dreams, a gradual taper over 5 to 10 days is recommended. Occasional blood levels as well as complete blood count (CBC) and hepatic studies are recommended to monitor for organ toxicity.

The TCA medication of choice is amitriptyline, a sedating TCA. Like all of the tricyclics, it works in the synapse to decrease reuptake of serotonin and, depending on the individual medication, norepinephrine. Amitriptyline, unlike the other TCAs, also works to repair the damage in stage 4 sleep architecture. It is the most sedating tricyclic. The typical dosage is between 10 and 50 mg at night. The author has found it rare to need more than 20 or 30 mg at night.

Doxepin is also a frequently used tricyclic. Anticholinergic side effects such as sedation are reduced (but not by much) when compared to amitriptyline. It does not work on the sleep architecture. It is used at the same dosage levels as amitriptyline.

Notice that the tricyclics are not used in their antidepressant dosages, anywhere from 100 to 350 mg a day. Even though the doses are low, their effectiveness in the treatment of pain is there.

Amitriptyline is indicated for use in neuropathic pain, while nortriptyline is more often used with fibromyalgia (4, 5). However, the increased sedation of amitriptyline may be useful in the treatment of fibromyalgia patients, although it is not FDA approved for this indication.

TCAs such as amitriptyline, desipramine, and imipramine, for example, block the induction of long-term potentiation by inhibiting actions on n-methyl-D-aspartate (NMDA) receptors (6).

TCAs have been used for years for the management of neuropathic pain syndromes, including diabetic peripheral neuropathy, postherpetic neuralgia, and migraine headache (6–8). However, pain relief is often modest and accompanied by side effects. Controlled studies indicate that approximately one-third of patients will obtain more than 50% pain relief, one-third will have minor adverse reactions, and 4% will discontinue the antidepressant because of major side effects (9). Fortunately, some patients obtain excellent pain relief.

Because comparisons between TCAs have not shown great differences in efficacy (8, 9), the choice of which antidepressant to use often depends on the side effect profile of a given drug. For example, when a patient is having difficulty in sleeping because of pain, a more sedating drug, such as amitriptyline, may be indicated. On the other hand, desipramine, which is less sedating, may be better tolerated in elderly patients.

TCAs have the lowest number needed to treat (NNT—the number of patients that need to be treated to achieve a 50% decrement in pain in one patient). The NNT for TCAs is 2.4 versus 6.7 for the SSRIs.

SELECTIVE SEROTONIN REUPTAKE INHIBITORS

The SSRIs include fluoxetine, paroxetine, and citalopram, escitalopram and sertraline, among others. These medications are not typically sedating, although for some patients they may be, and with the exclusion of those patients, they are energizing. They should be given in the morning. Fluoxetine and paroxetine should start at 10 to 20 mg a day and the dose can be increased to 60 to 80 mg. Sertraline should be given at 25 to 50 mg in the morning, up to 150 mg in divided doses. The doses should be divided, giving one when the patient gets up in the morning (around 7:00 AM) and one at noon. Patients should understand that taking these medications later than noon can, in many cases, give them problems sleeping.

The clinician can also safely combine 10 to 40 mg of fluoxetine or paroxetine, or 50 mg of sertraline given in the morning with a small dose of amitriptyline or doxepin (10–30 mg) at night. Inappropriate dosages of these two forms of medications can, rarely, induce the serotonin syndrome.

Compared with tricyclic agents, SSRIs for neuropathic pain have been relatively disappointing. In addition, they are more expensive than the older generic agents. Nonetheless, at relatively high doses (e.g., 60 mg), paroxetine is effective for diabetic neuropathy (10). Fluoxetine may also be useful in the treatment of rheumatic pain conditions, many of which have neuropathic components (11). SSRIs are better tolerated than TCAs and should be considered as first-line drugs in patients with concomitant depression. In this group, they may serve double duty.

SSRIs specifically blockade serotonin reuptake. They should be used cautiously in patients with a history of seizures. They should not be used in conjunction with MAOIs, as death has been reported (12).

There is an increased risk of the serotonin syndrome when SSRIs are combined with MAOIs, triptans, TCAs, bupropion, other SSRIs, buspirone, tramadol, and venlafaxine. Increased bleeding can be seen when used with warfarin (12).

The major side effects include nausea, diarrhea, anxiety, dyspepsia, diaphoresis, headache, insomnia, dizziness, tremor, nervousness, sedation, and sexual dysfunction.

SSRIs inhibit the CYP450 enzyme system and can cause delayed clearance of some medications, particularly those that use the CYP450 1A2 and 2D6 and 3A4 enzymes as metabolic substrates (1).

Norepinephrine–Serotonin Reuptake Inhibitors

These drugs include venlafaxine, duloxetine, and milnacipran. Venlafaxine can be started at 37.5 mg/day or b.i.d. and effective dosages are 150 to 300 mg/day. Duloxetine should be started at 20 mg b.i.d. and its effective dose is 60 mg/day. Milnacipran is used at dosages of 100 to 200 mg/day.

Venlafaxine is a novel phenylethylamine antidepressant that is chemically distinct from the older TCAs and the SSRIs. Although venlafaxine blocks serotonin and norepinephrine reuptake, its analgesic actions may be mediated by both an opioid mechanism and adrenergic effects (13). It appears to block serotonin reuptake at low dosages, and norepinephrine reuptake at high dosages, and dopamine at very high dosages (1). The drug may be at least as well tolerated as tricyclic agents and more effective for pain than standard doses of serotonin-selective drugs. Indeed, an initial report suggests that venlafaxine is effective for neuropathic pain (14). Venlafaxine should be started at one-half of a 37.5 mg tablet twice daily and titrated weekly to a maximum of 75 mg, taken twice a day. Nausea appears to be the most common side effect. An extended-release formulation of the drug was effective in relieving the pain associated with diabetic neuropathy. The NNT values for the higher dose of venlafaxine ER are comparable with those of the TCAs and gabapentin (15).

Venlafaxine has been used for the treatment of neuropathic pain (but is not FDA approved for this indication) (4).

It should be used with caution in hypertensive patients or patients with a history of seizures. It should be withdrawn slowly.

Venlafaxine has increased risk of serotonin syndrome when used with MAOIs, TCAs, SSRIs, tramadol, bupropion, and buspirone.

The most common adverse events include nausea, headache, nervousness, tremor, dry mouth somnolence, diaphoresis, constipation, and sexual dysfunction.

Duloxetine is a serotonergic and noradrenergic reuptake inhibitor with low affinity for other neurotransmitter systems. The most common adverse events are referable to the gastrointestinal and nervous systems. Duloxetine is primarily eliminated via the urine after significant hepatic metabolism via multiple oxidative pathways, methylation, and conjugation. The half-life is 12.1 hours. Duloxetine does cause inhibition of CYP 2D6. It should not be used in combination with nonselective MAOIs or CYP 1A2 inhibitors (16). It is effective for major depressive disorders as well as for the treatment of diabetic peripheral neuropathic pain (17–19).

Several double-blind, randomized, multicenter trails comparing duloxetine with placebo for the treatment of diabetic peripheral neuropathy have been done. In one, patients received duloxetine 60 mg daily, twice a day, or placebo. Duloxetine was superior to placebo in both dosages; discontinuations secondary to adverse events were more frequent in the duloxetine 60 mg/b.i.d. group (20).

In the second, a 12-week double-blind, placebo-controlled study in types 1 and 2 diabetics with peripheral diabetic neuropathy (PDN), both 60 and 120 mg/day dosages demonstrated statistically significant improvement in pain compared to placebo (21).

Duloxetine has also been found to be an effective and safe treatment for many symptoms associated with fibromyalgia in subjects with or without a major depressive disorder, particularly for women, who had the best outcomes, with significant improvement over most outcome measures (18, 22, 23).

Duloxetine is FDA approved for the treatment of neuropathic pain, fibromyalgia, and diabetic neuropathic pain.

Milnacipran, a new norepinephrine serotonin reuptake inhibitor, was approved in January 2009 for the treatment of fibromyalgia. This norepinephrine serotonin reuptake inhibitor preferentially blocks the reuptake of norepinephrine with higher potency than serotonin. Other than published studies, there is no clinical experience with this drug in the United States. The drug has been used in Europe, Asia, and Australia under the name Ixel. Milnacipran is said to block both serotonin and norepinephrine equally. Side effects include itching, sweating and chills, vertigo, headache, gastrointestinal complaints, orthostatic dizziness, depression, lethargy, hot flashes, and difficulty urinating. An exacerbation of hypertension can be seen at higher dosages (24, 25).

Norepinephrine–Dopamine Reuptake Inhibitor

Bupropion can be used as an antidepressant or for nicotine withdrawal. Dosages range, initially, from 75 to 150 mg/day to a maximum of 300 mg/day. It has been noted to help with neuropathic pain, but is not approved by the FDA for this indication (26).

The drug works by blockading the reuptake of norepinephrine and dopamine. It should not be used in patients with seizure disorders, anorexia, bulimia, or within 14 days of the use of MAOIs. Its toxicity is increased by levodopa and amantadine; there is an increased risk of seizure with agents that lower the seizure threshold. Common side effects include agitation, tremor, insomnia, nausea, headache, xerostomia, somnolence, hypertension, and tachycardia (12).

Atypical Antidepressants

Mirtazapine is an atypical ADM, described as a noradrenergic serotonin-specific antagonist. The drug facilitates enhanced noradrenergic and serotonergic output, which induces analgesia (1).

There are no reported problems with sexual dysfunction with this drug, and there is also a decrease in migraine headache as well as anxiety, agitation, depression, and insomnia (27–29).

BLACK BOX WARNING

Starting in 2004 the FDA requested a black box warning that children and adolescents taking antidepressants had an increased risk of suicide. In 2007, this warning was increased to include older patients and it reads, in part, "Antidepressants increased the risk compared to placebo of suicidal thinking and behavior (suicidality) in children, adolescents and young adults in short-term studies of major depressive disorder (MDD) and other psychiatric disorders." There did not appear to be a reported risk of suicide in adults over the age of 24.

This information should be kept in mind when prescribing antidepressants for pain or depression in the noted age groups, men and women up to the age of 24.

REFERENCES

1. Barkin RL, Barkin D. Pharmacologic management of acute and chronic pain: focus on drug interactions and patient-specific pharmacotherapeutic selection. South Med J 2001; 94(8):756–770.
2. Barkin RL, Fawcett J, Barkin S. Chronic pain management with a focus on the roll of newer antidepressants and centrally acting agents. In: Weiner RS, ed. Pain Management: A Practical Guide for Clinicians. 6th ed. New York, NY: CRC Press, 2002:415–434.
3. Glassman A, Roose S, Bigger J. The safety of tricyclic antidepressants in cardiac patients. Risk–benefit reconsidered. JAMA 1993; 269:2673–2677.
4. Sindrup SH, Otto M, Finnerup NB, et al. Antidepressants in the treatment of neuropathic pain. Basic Clin Pharmacol Toxicol 2005; 96(6):399–409.
5. Goldenberg DL, Burckhardt C, Crofford L. Management of fibromyalgia syndrome. JAMA 2004; 292(19):2388–2395.
6. Mico JA, Ardid D, Berrocoso E, et al. Antidepressants and pain. Trends Pharmacol Sci 2006; 27(7):348–354.
7. McQuay HJ, Tramer M, Nye BA, et al. A systematic review of antidepressants in neuropathic pain. Pain 1996; 68:217–227.
8. Max M. Antidepressants as analgesics. In: Fields HL, Liebskind JC, eds. Pharmacological Approaches to the Treatment of Chronic Pain: New Concepts and Critical Issues. Progress in Pain Research and Management. Vol 1. Seattle, WA: IASP Press, 1994:229–246.
9. Onghena P, van Houdenhove B. Antidepressant-induced analgesia in chronic nonmalignant pain: a meta-analysis of 39 placebo controlled studies. Pain 1992; 49:205–220.

10. Sobotka JL, Alexander B, Cook BL. A review of carbamazepine's hematologic reactions and monitoring recommendations. DICP 1990; 24:1214–1219.
11. Rani PU, Naidu MUR, Prasad VBN, et al. An evaluation of antidepressants in rheumatic pain conditions. Anesth Analg 1996; 83:371–375.
12. Lussier D, Beaulieu P, Fishbain D, et al. 2009 Overview of analgesic agents. Pain Medicine News Special Edition. December 2008:27–50.
13. Siegfried J. Long term results of electrical stimulation in the treatment of pain my means of implanted electrodes. In: Rizzi C, Visentin TA, eds. Pain Therapy. Amsterdam, The Netherlands: Elsevier, 1983:463–475.
14. Galer BS. Neuropathic pain of peripheral origin: advances in pharmacologic treatment. Neurology 1995; 45(suppl 9):S17–S25.
15. Rowbotham MC, Goli V, Kunz NR,et al. Venlafaxine extended release in the treatment of painful diabetic neuropathy: a double-blind, placebo controlled study. Pain 2004; 110(3):697–706.
16. Wernicke JF, Gahimer J, Yalcin I, et al. Safety and adverse event profile of duloxetine. Expert Opin Drug Saf 2005; 4(6):987–993.
17. Kirwin JL, Goren JL. Duloxetine: a dual serotonin–norepinephrine reuptake inhibitor for treatment of major depressive disorder. Pharmacotherapy 2005; 25(3):396–410.
18. Maizels M, McCarberg B. Antidepressants and antiepileptic drugs for chronic noncancer pain. Am Fam Physician 2005; 71(3):483–490.
19. Duloxetine (Cymbalta) for diabetic neuropathic pain. Med Lett Drugs Ther 2005; 47(1215/1216):67–68.
20. Raskin J, Pritchett YL, Wang F, et al. A double-blind, randomized multicenter trial comparing duloxetine with placebo in the management of diabetic peripheral neuropathic pain. Pain Med 2005; 6(5):346–356.
21. Goldstein DJ, Lu Y, Detke MJ, et al. Duloxetine vs. placebo in patients with painful diabetic neuropathy. Pain 2005; 116(1/2):109–118.
22. Arnold LM, Lu Y, Crofford LJ, et al. A double-blind, multicenter trial comparing duloxetine with placebo in the treatment of fibromyalgia patients with or without major depressive disorder. Arthritis Rheum 2004; 50(9):2974–2984.
23. Offenbaecher M, Ackenheil M. Current trends in neuropathic pain treatments with special reference to fibromyalgia. CNS Spectr 2005; 10(4):285–297.
24. Development of milnacipran for fibromyalgia hits a snag. Medscape Medical News. October 2005. Available at: medscape.com/viewarticle/538358. Accessed February 22, 2009.
25. Gendreau RM, Thorn MD, Gendreau JF, et al. Efficacy of milnacipran in patients with fibromyalgia. J Rheumatol 2005; 32:1975–1985.
26. Semenchuk MR, Sherman S, Davis B. Double-blind, randomized trial of bupropion SR for the treatment of neuropathic pain. Neurology 2001; 57(9):1583–1588.
27. Barkin RL, Chor PN, Braun BG, et al. A trilogy case review highlighting the clinical and pharmacologic applications of mirtazapine in reducing polypharmacy for anxiety, agitation, insomnia, depression and sexual dysfunction. J Clin Psychiatry 1999; 1:172–175.
28. Fawcett J, Barkin RL. Review of the results from clinical studies on the efficacy, safety and tolerability of mirtazapine for the treatment of patients with major depression. J Affect Disord 1998; 51:267–285.
29. Braverman B, O'Connor C, Barkin RL. Pharmacology, physiology and anesthetic management of antidepressants. In: Pharmacology and Physiology in Anesthesia. Philadelphia, PA: Lippincott Health Care Publications, 1993:1–15.

27 Anticonvulsant Medications

Gary W. Jay

Clinical Disease Area Expert-Pain, Pfizer, Inc., New London, Connecticut, U.S.A.

While the most common treatments for nociceptive pain include anti-inflammatory and opioid medications, anticonvulsant medications (ACMs) are first-line drugs for neuropathic pain. Both older (conventional) and newer ACMs may be used in patients with neuropathic pain, migraine, essential tremor, spasticity, restless legs syndrome, and several psychiatric disorders including bipolar disorder and schizophrenia (1, 2).

Food and Drug Administration (FDA)-approved ACMs and ADMs and a patch for neuropathic pain and fibromyalgia include the following:

- Carbamazepine: trigeminal neuralgia
- Duloxetine
  - peripheral diabetic neuropathy
  - fibromyalgia
- Gabapentin: postherpetic neuralgia
- Lidocaine Patch 5%: postherpetic neuralgia
- Pregabalin
  - peripheral diabetic neuropathy
  - postherpetic neuralgia
  - fibromyalgia
- Milnacipran: fibromyalgia

There is not a great deal of knowledge regarding the mechanism of action of most ACMs. Of note here are the multiple proposed mechanisms of action of multiple drugs, indicative of the uncertainty of the MOA (3).

- Sodium current blockade: carbamazepine, oxcarbazepine, lamotrigine, valproic acid, phenytoin, topiramate, zonisamide
- Calcium current blockade: gabapentin, pregabalin, carbamazepine, oxcarbazepine, zonisamide
- Increased GABA: topiramate, valproic acid, clonazepam, tiagabine
- Gabapentinoids: gabapentin, pregabalin—bind to the $\alpha_2\delta$ subunit of calcium channel; block calcium influx, prevent presynaptic release of neurotransmitters
- Reduced excitatory amino acids (i.e., glutamate): topiramate, lamotrigine, phenytoin, pregabalin, gabapentin
- Unknown: levetiracetam

397

When using ACMs, there are some clinical actions which may maximize their effectiveness, or appropriate patient use:

1. Always start low and go slow when titrating an ACM.
2. Understand the pharmacokinetics as well as the mechanistic differences between the ACMs.
3. In treatment-resistant patients (poor effectiveness), it is useful to combine two ACMs, if necessary, but be certain to use drugs with different modes of action.
4. All too frequently a patient will state that he or she has tried and failed an ACM, or many of them. Be certain to find out exactly what happened. Most commonly, a patient took a very low dose of an ACM for a very short period of time (less than that would be necessary to develop a steady state with clinical efficacy) and claimed lack of effectiveness, at which point, instead of insisting that the titration be continued appropriately, a different ACM is used, and the same problems persist. If an ACM is not titrated appropriately, the drug was really not used, as clinically there would not have been any effectiveness. Stopping a drug secondary to adverse effects is absolutely appropriate.
5. Push the ACM dosages until you see clinical effectiveness or you have to stop it secondary to side effects.
6. In many patients, maximal effectiveness (in the treatment of neuropathic pain) is found with ACMs given at 50% to 100% of their antiepileptic dosages. This does not hold true for the FDA-approved ACMs, which were approved at specific dosages for the treatment of neuropathic pain.

As a form of multimodal analgesia, oral gabapentin as well as pregabalin has been used perioperatively for adjunctive management of postoperative pain, as a supplement to opioids and other analgesics (4, 5).

The most commonly used ACMs and their typical doses include the following:

Name	Half-life (hr)	Dosing (mg/day)/regimen
Carbamazepine (Tegretol)	10–20	400–1200 mg/t.i.d.
Gabapentin (Neurontin)	5–9	1200–3600 mg/t.i.d.
Phenytoin (Dilantin)	12–36	300–600 mg/t.i.d. (q.h.s-nongeneric)
Oxcarbazepine (Trileptal)	8–10	300–1800 mg/b.i.d.
Topiramate (Topamax)	18–30	50–400 mg/b.i.d. or q.h.s
Lamotrigine (Lamictal)	15–30	50–300 mg/b.i.d.
Valproate (Depakote)	6–16	500–1500 mg/t.i.d.
Clonazepam (Klonopin)	18–50	0.5–6.0 mg/q.h.s.
Levetiracetam (Keppra)	6–8	1000–2000 mg/b.i.d.
Zonisamide (Zonegran)	25–60	100–400 mg/q.h.s
Tiagabine	5–10	12–44 mg/t.i.d.
Pregabalin (Lyrica)	5–6.5	75–300 mg/day

Anticonvulsants are useful for trigeminal neuralgia, postherpetic neuralgia, diabetic neuropathy, as well as central pain (6, 7). Although anticonvulsants have traditionally been thought of as most useful for lancinating pain, they may also relieve burning dysesthesias. Chemically, anticonvulsants are a diverse group of drugs, are typically highly protein bound, and undergo extensive hepatic metabolism.

Carbamazepine has a long history of use for neuropathic pain, particularly trigeminal neuralgia. Carbamazepine is chemically related to the tricyclic antidepressant imipramine, has a slow and erratic absorption, and may produce numerous side effects, including sedation, nausea, vomiting, and hepatic enzyme induction. In 10% of patients, transient leukopenia and thrombocytopenia may occur, and in 2% of patients hematologic changes can be persistent, requiring stopping the drug (8–10). Aplastic anemia is the most severe complication associated with carbamazepine, which may occur in 1:200,000 patients. Although requirements for hematologic monitoring remain debatable, a complete blood cell count, hepatic enzymes, blood urea nitrogen (BUN), and creatinine are recommended at baseline; and these are checked again at 2, 4, and 6 weeks, and every 6 months thereafter. Carbamazepine levels should be drawn every 6 months and after changing the dose to monitor for toxic levels and verify that the drug is within the therapeutic range (4–12 mg/cc). Patients with low pretreatment white blood cell counts are at increased risk of developing leukopenia (WBC < 3000/mm^3). Because toxicity is entirely unpredictable, it is important to instruct patients to recognize clinical signs and symptoms of hematologic toxicity, such as infections, fatigue, ecchymosis, and abnormal bleeding, and to notify the physician if they develop. Check hepatic enzymes and CBC routinely to rule out (possibly aplastic) anemia and hepatic dysfunction. Also, check the patient's ECG, if one has not been done recently; do one to look for arrhythmias and evaluate the QT interval. To improve compliance, carbamazepine should be started at a low dose (e.g., 50 mg twice daily) and increased over several weeks to a therapeutic level (200–300 mg typically three times a day).

Oxcarbazepine is an analog of carbamazepine, but typically is not associated with blood dyscrasias, nor hepatic insult.

Phenytoin also has well-known sodium channel-blocking effects and is useful for neuropathic pain (11). However, it is less effective than carbamazepine for trigeminal neuralgia (12). We have also noted that neuropathic pain caused by structural lesions causing nerve or root compression can paradoxically increase when phenytoin is administered. Phenytoin has a slow and variable oral absorption, some of which is dependent upon GI motility and transit time. Toxicity includes CNS effects and cardiac conduction abnormalities. Side effects are common and include hirsutism, gastrointestinal and hematologic effects, and gingival hyperplasia (13). Allergies to phenytoin are common, and may involve skin, liver, and bone marrow. Phenytoin doses in the range of 100 mg twice or three times a day may be helpful for neuropathic pain; therapeutic blood levels are in the range of 10 to 20 mg/ml. There are numerous potential drug interactions, including induction of cytochrome P450 enzymes, which may accelerate the metabolism of other drugs. Because of side effects and toxicity, phenytoin is not a first-line drug for neuropathic pain.

Valproic acid appears to interact with sodium channels but may also increase GABA metabolism. The principal nonantiepileptic, FDA-approved, use of valproic acid is for the prophylaxis of migraine headache (14). Potential toxicity includes hepatic injury and thrombocytopenia, particularly in children on multiple antiepileptic medications, although valproic acid is generally considered safe for adults.

Divalproex sodium is better tolerated than valproic acid. The recommended starting dose is 250 mg twice daily, although some patients may benefit from doses up to 1000 mg/day. As a prophylactic drug, valproic acid can reduce the frequency of migraine attacks by about 50% (14). Although there is little published information on the efficacy of valproic acid for neuropathic pain syndromes, based on its mechanism of action it may be useful alone or in combination with other adjuvant drugs. The drug may be associated with weight gain, pancreatitis, and hepatic injury as well as hair loss. A "fetal valproate syndrome" exists, so it should not be used in pregnant women.

Clonazepam may be useful for radiculopathic pain and neuropathic pain of a lancinating character. Clonazepam enhances dorsal horn inhibition by a GABAergic mechanism. The drug has a long half-life (18–50 hours), which reduces the risk of inducing an abstinence syndrome on abrupt withdrawal. The major side effects of clonazepam include sedation and cognitive dysfunction, especially in the elderly. Although the risk of organ toxicity is minimal, some clinicians recommend periodic complete blood count (CBC) and liver function tests for monitoring. Starting doses of 0.5 to 1.0 mg at bedtime are appropriate to reduce the incidence of daytime sedation.

Topiramate was found to be identical to placebo in three placebo controlled trials for painful diabetic neuropathy, while a fourth, independent placebo-controlled trial used different methods to assess topiramate efficacy and tolerability. It was found that in this one study, topiramate monotherapy reduced pain and body weight more effectively than placebo (15). The drug may be associated with weight loss and cognitive dysfunction. Topiramate was approved for migraine prophylaxis by the FDA in 2004.

Gabapentin is a popular anticonvulsant for neuropathic pain. Gabapentin was approved for use in the United States in 1993, as an adjunctive treatment of adults with partial epilepsy. Almost immediately after its release, physicians began to use gabapentin for various neuropathic pain disorders, such as diabetic peripheral neuropathy and postherpetic neuralgia. The structural similarity of gabapentin to GABA suggested that the drug might be useful for neuropathic pain. Although tricyclic antidepressants have been proven clinically effective for neuropathic pain for years, they often fail to provide adequate pain relief or cause unacceptable side effects. Therefore, when gabapentin became available, its benign side effect profile quickly made it very popular among physicians. Although initial enthusiasm for the drug was based largely on word of mouth, anecdotal published reports, discussions at clinical meetings and animal studies have substantiated the efficacy of gabapentin in various types of neuropathic pain. Over time, a growing consensus concerning the usefulness of gabapentin has emerged supported by well-controlled clinical trials.

It is clear that gabapentin is not a direct GABA agonist, although indirect effects on GABA metabolism or action may occur. A leading hypothesis suggested that gabapentin interacts with a novel receptor on a voltage-activated calcium channel (16). Research has shown that it interacts with the $\alpha2\delta$ subunit on the voltage-gated calcium channel (17). The inhibition of voltage-gated sodium channel activity (such as that occurs with classical anticonvulsants, e.g., phenytoin and carbamazepine) and amino acid transport, which alters neurotransmitter synthesis, may also occur. Although gabapentin is not an NMDA antagonist, there is evidence that gabapentin interacts with the glycine site on the NMDA receptor (18).

Ligation of rat spinal nerves L5 and L6 (the Chung model) produces characteristic pain behaviors, including allodynia, which are typical of neuropathic pain. Chapman et al. (19) demonstrated that gabapentin reduces pain in the Chung model. Gabapentin appears to act primarily in the CNS, in contrast to amitriptyline, which seems to act centrally and peripherally (20). Gabapentin also is effective in reducing pain behavior in phase 2 of the formalin test, a model of central sensitization and neuropathic pain (21). Gabapentin reduces spinally mediated hyperalgesia seen after sustained nociceptive afferent input caused by peripheral tissue injury. Gabapentin also enhances spinal morphine analgesia in the rat tail-flick test, a laboratory model of nociceptive pain (21).

Gabapentin is effective in reducing painful dysesthesias and improving quality-of-life scores in patients with painful diabetic peripheral neuropathy (23). Of patients randomized to receive gabapentin, 56% achieved a daily dosage of 3600 mg divided into three doses per day. The average magnitude of the analgesic response was modest, with a 24% reduction in intensity at the completion of the study compared with controls. Side effects were common. Dizziness and somnolence occurred in about 25% of patients, and confusion occurred in 8% of patients.

Morello et al. (24) compared gabapentin with amitriptyline for diabetic neuropathy and found both equally effective. However, the number needed to treat (NNT) for the tricyclic antidepressants is 2.5 and 4.2 for gabapentin (25–27).

Postherpetic neuralgia (PHN) is another difficult neuropathic syndrome. PHN affects approximately 10% to 15% of patients who develop herpes zoster, and is a particularly painful syndrome associated with lancinating pain and burning dysesthesias. The incidence of PHN is age related, with up to 50% of patients older than 60 years developing persistent pain after a bout of herpes zoster. Pain relief usually requires pharmacological therapy. Unfortunately, most medications are not very effective. For example, only about one-half of patients obtain adequate relief with antidepressants.

Rowbotham et al. (28) evaluated the efficacy of gabapentin for the treatment of PHN. Of patients taking gabapentin, 65% achieved a daily dosage of 3600 mg. Although the average magnitude of pain reduction with gabapentin was modest, with approximately a 30% reduction in pain compared with controls, statistically pain reduction was highly significant. In addition, gabapentin improved sleep parameters and quality-of-life scores. Adverse effects that occurred more commonly in the gabapentin group included somnolence (27%), dizziness (24%), ataxia, peripheral edema, and infection (7–10%). Based on the data of Rowbotham and colleagues, it was reasonable to consider gabapentin as first-line therapy for postherpetic neuralgia.

The FDA approved gabapentin for use in postherpetic neuralgia in 2002.

Gabapentin probably is at least as effective as antidepressants, with fewer contraindications. Gabapentin may be used as monotherapy or add-on/adjunctive treatment. Other possible adverse reactions include confusion, dizziness, and possible weight gain.

Gabapentin is generally well tolerated, even in the geriatric population, and has a safer side effect profile than tricyclic antidepressants. In the PHN study, the majority of patients were titrated to 3600 mg/day, and the median patient age was 73 years. The kidneys excrete gabapentin, and the dosage must be reduced for patients with renal insufficiency (29).

Pregabalin is also a GABA analog, with a similar structure and function to gabapentin. A new class of anticonvulsants was named the "Gabapentinoids" of which these two drugs are the first known for inclusion. Pregabalin (Lyrica) is indicated/approved for the treatment of neuropathic pain associated with both diabetic peripheral neuropathy and postherpetic neuralgia, adjunctive treatment of partial seizures, as well as fibromyalgia (see chap. 12) (30).

Pregabalin has negligible hepatic metabolism; it is not protein bound and has a plasma half-life of about six hours. Most of the oral dose (95%) is found unchanged in the urine. Peak plasma levels are found in about one hour post oral doses; oral bioavailability is greater than 90% (31).

The time to peak concentration is 1.5 hours, while a food effect increased this to 3 hours. A steady state is reached in one to two days. Pregabalin does not bind to plasma proteins. Mean half-life is 6.3 hours. It should be used in lesser dosages in patients with renal insufficiency, as it is metabolized renally (31, 32).

The most common adverse events seen in >10% of patients include dizziness, somnolence, peripheral edema, infection, and dry mouth (31, 32).

Pregabalin binds to the $\alpha 2\delta$ subunit protein of the voltage-gated calcium channels, like gabapentin, and reduces the release of excitatory neurotransmitters (e.g., glutamate, norepinephrine, serotonin, dopamine, and substance P) (33, 34).

Several randomized clinical trials show pregabalin to be superior to placebo in the treatment of neuropathic pain (PHN and DPN) at doses of 300 to 600 mg/day. Sleep was improved. Common adverse events included dizziness, peripheral edema, weight gain, and somnolence (35).

Randomized controlled studies of pregabalin in painful diabetic peripheral neuropathy were also done and showed the drug to be superior to placebo in doses of 300 to 600 mg/day. Improvements in sleep were also seen (36–38).

While many countries in the European Union have approved pregabalin, it was also evaluated for use in Canada for the treatment of peripheral neuropathic pain. The past treatment was reviewed. It was noted that the number of subjects with >50% reduction in pain increased when pregabalin was compared to placebo. Withdrawal due to adverse events was more frequent with pregabalin than placebo. The authors concluded that while pregabalin appeared effective in the treatment of peripheral neuropathic pain, no evidence was found that it offered advantages over the treatments currently being used in Canada (39).

Pregabalin was the first drug approved for use in fibromyalgia, based on two RCTs of approximately 1800 patients (40). The initial two studies considered of a 14-week study, with some patients showing reductions in pain during the first week. Approximately 70% of patients on a total daily dose of 300 mg/day of pregabalin, and 78% of those on a total daily dose of 450 mg/day experienced improvement on the patient global impression of change scale compared to 48% of those on placebo. The 600 mg/day dose was no more effective than the lower doses, and there was evidence of dose-related side effects (40).

The second trial, a six-month randomized withdrawal study, found that at the end of the double-blind phase, 61% of placebo patients had loss of therapeutic response to pregabalin, *versus* 90 (32%) of the pregabalin group, demonstrating the durability of effect for relieving FMS pain (41).

Other clinical cautions for other ADMs include the following:

- Lamotrigine—can be associated with Stevens–Johnson syndrome/toxic epidermal necrolysis; visual blurring with long-term use.
- Levetiracetam—caution if used with carbamazepine; may have typical GI and CNS side effects (nausea, ataxia, headache, dizziness, and sedation).
- Zonisamide—contraindicated in patients with sulfonamide hypersensitivity, can be associated with renal calculi.

SUICIDALITY AND ACMs

In July of 2008, the FDA had an advisory board which recommended against a black box warning regarding an increased risk of suicidal thoughts and behaviors. In December of 2008, the FDA announced that it would require makers of ACMs to add a warning to their drug labels, but not a black box warning, regarding this problem.

The FDA based their actions on the agency's meta-analysis of 199 clinical trials, with 43,000 subjects, of 11 ACMs being taken for multiple indications, which showed that patients taking antiepileptics had almost twice the suicidal behavior or thoughts when compared to a placebo group (0.37% vs. 0.22%) (42).

The Advisory Board did not dispute the FDA's findings.

The FDA stated that "all patients who are currently taking or starting on any antiepileptic drug for any indication should be monitored for notable changes in behavior that could indicate the emergence or worsening of suicidal thoughts or behavior or depression" (43).

REFERENCES

1. White PF. The changing role of non-opioid analgesic techniques in the management of postoperative pain. Anesth Analg 2005; 101(5 Suppl):S5–S22.
2. Mico JA, Ardid D, Berrocoso E, et al. Antidepressants and pain. Trends Pharmacol Sci 2006; 27(7):348–354.
3. Lussier D, Beaulieu P, Huskey A, et al. 2009 Overview of Analgesic Agents. Pain Medicine News Special Edition, December 2008:27–50.
4. Hurley RW, Cohen SP, Williams KA, et al. The analgesic effects of perioperative gabapentin on postoperative pain: a meta-analysis. Reg Anesth Pain Med 2006; 31(3):237–247.
5. Agarwal A, Gautam S, Gupta D, et al. Evaluation of a single preoperative dose of pregabalin for attenuation of postoperative pain after laparoscopic cholecystectomy. Br J Aneasth 2008; 101(5):700–704.
6. Swerdlow M. Anticonvulsants in the therapy of neuralgic pain. Pain Clin 1986; 1:9–19.
7. Hegarty A, Portenoy RK. Pharmacotherapy of neuropathic pain. Semin Neurol 1994; 14:213–224.
8. Hart RG, Easton JD. Carbamazepine and hematological monitoring. Ann Neurol 1982; 11:309–312.
9. Sotgiu ML, Lacerenza M, Marchettini P. Effect of systemic lidocaine on dorsal horn neuron hyperactivity following chronic peripheral nerve injury in rats. Somatosens Mot Res 1992; 9:227–233.

10. Vanderah TW, Gardell LR, Burgess SH, et al. Dynorphin promotes abnormal pain and spinal opioid antinociceptive tolerance. J Neurosci 2000; 20:7074–7079.

11. McCleane GJ. Intravenous infusion of phenytoin relieves neuropathic pain: a randomized double-blinded, placebo controlled, crossover study. Anesth Analg 1999; 89:985.

12. Blom S. Trigeminal neuralgia: its treatment with a new anticonvulsant drug G-32883. Lancet 1962; 1:839–840.

13. Brodie MJ, Dichter MA. Antiepileptic drugs. N Engl J Med 1996; 334:168–175.

14. Matthew NT, Saper JR, Silberstein SD, et al. Migraine prophylaxis with divalproex. Arch Neurol 1995; 52:281–286.

15. Raskin P, Donofrio PD, Rosenthal NR, et al. Topiramate vs. placebo in painful diabetic neuropathy: analgesic and metabolic effects. Neurology 2004; 63:865–873.

16. Chaplan SR. Neuropathic pain: role of voltage-dependent calcium channels. Reg Anesth Pain Med 2000; 25:283–285.

17. Gee NS, Brown JP, Dissanayake VU, et al. The novel anticonvulsant drug, gabapentin (Neurontin) binds to the alpha2delta subunit of a calcium channel. J Biol Chem 1996; 271:5768–5776.

18. Jun JH, Yaksh TL. The effect of intrathecal gabapentin and 3-isobutyl gamma-aminobutyric acid on the hyperalgesia observed after thermal injury in the rat. Anesth Analg 1998; 86:348–354.

19. Chapman V, Suzuki R, Chamarette HLC,et al. Effects of systemic carbamazepine and gabapentin on spinal neuronal responses in spinal nerve ligated rats. Pain 1998; 75:261–272.

20. Abdi S, Lee DH, Chung JM. The anti-allodynic effects of amitriptyline, gabapentin, and lidocaine in a rat model of neuropathic pain. Anesth Analg 1998; 87:1360–1366.

21. Shimoyama M, Shimoyama N, Inturrisi CE, et al. Gabapentin enhances the antinociceptive effects of spinal morphine in the rat tail-flick test. Pain 1997; 72:375–382.

22. Sindrup SH, Gram LF, Brosen K, et al. The selective serotonin reuptake inhibitor paroxetine is effective in the treatment of diabetic neuropathy symptoms. Pain 1990; 42:135–144.

23. Backonja MM, Beydoun A, Edwards KR, et al. Gabapentin for the symptomatic treatment of painful neuropathy in patients with diabetes mellitus. A randomized controlled trial. JAMA 1998; 280:1831–1836.

24. Morello CM, Leckband SG, Stoner CP, et al. Randomized double-blind study comparing the efficacy of gabapentin with amitriptyline on diabetic peripheral neuropathy. Arch Int Med 1999; 159:1931–1937.

25. Mattia C, Coluzzi F. Tramadol: focus on musculoskeletal and neuropathic pain. Minerva Anestesiol 2005; 71:565–584.

26. Sindrup SH, Jensen TS. Efficacy of pharmacological treatments of neuropathic pain: an update and effect related to mechanism of drug action. Pain 1999; 83:389–400.

27. Sindrup SH, Jensen TS. Pharmacological treatment of pain in polyneuropathy. Neurology 2000; 55:915–920.

28. Rowbotham M, Harden N, Stacey B, et al. Gabapentin for the treatment of postherpetic neuralgia. A randomized controlled trial. JAMA 280:1837–1842.

29. Beydoun A, Uthman BM, Sackellares JC. Gabapentin: pharmacokinetics, efficacy, and safety. Clin Neuropharmacol 1995; 18:469–481.

30. Zareba G. Pregabalin: a new agent for the treatment of neuropathic pain. Drugs Today Barc 2005; 41(8):509–516.

31. Pfizer Inc. Pregabalin (Lyrica) package insert. New York: Pfizer, 2006.

32. Pregabalin Monograph. National PBM Drug Monograph. May, 2007. VHA Pharmacy Benefits Management Strategic Healthcare Group and the Medical Advisory Panel. www.phm.va.gov/monograph/Pregabalin.pdf. Accessed February 27, 2009.

33. Dooley DJ, Taylor CP, Donevan S, et al. Ca^{2+} channel $\alpha 2\delta$ ligands: novel modulators of neurotransmission. Trends Phramacol Sci 2007; 28:75–82.

34. Freynhagen R, Stojek K, Griesing T, et al. Efficacy of pregabalin in neuropathic pain evaluated in a 12-week, randomized, double-blind, multicenter, placebo-controlled trial of flexible- and fixed-dose regimens. Pain 2005; 115(3):254–263.
35. Lesser H, Sharma U, LaMoreaux L, et al. Pregabalin relieves symptoms of painful diabetic neuropathy: a randomized controlled trial. Neurology 2004; 63(11):2104–2110.
36. Richter RW, Portenoy R, Sharma U, et al. Relief of painful diabetic peripheral neuropathy with pregabalin: a randomized, placebo-controlled trial. J Pain 2005; 6(4):253–260.
37. Frampton JE, Scott LJ. Pregabalin: in the treatment of painful diabetic peripheral neuropathy. Drugs 2004; 64(24):2813–2820.
38. Rosenstock J, Tuchman M, LaMoreaux L, et al. Pregabalin for the treatment of painful diabetic peripheral neuropathy: a double-blind, placebo controlled trial. Pain 2004; 110(3):628–638.
39. Hadj Tahar A. Pregabalin for peripheral neuropathic pain. Issues Emerg Health Technol 2005; 67:1–4.
40. Mechcatie, E. Pregabalin is first drug approved for fibromyalgia. Pain Medicine (Lyrica from Pfizer Inc.). Clinical Psychiatry News. International Medical News Group. 2007. *HighBeam Research.* http://www.highbeam.com. Accessed July 10, 2009.
41. Crofford JL, MEase PJ, Simpson SL, et al. Fibromyalgia relapse evaluation and efficacy for durability of meaningful relief (FREEDOM): a 6-month, double-blind, placebo-controlled trial with pregabalin. Pain 2008; 136(3):419–431.
42. Food and Drug Administration. Statistical review and evaluation: antiepileptic drugs and suicidality. www.fda.gov/ohrms/dockets/ac/o8/briefing/2008-4372b1-01-FDA.pdf. Accessed May 23, 2008.
43. Food and Drug Administration. Suicidal behavior and ideation and antiepileptic drugs. FDA Alert, Information for Healthcare Professionals, updated December 16, 2008. www.fda.gov/cder/drug/infopage/antiepileptics/default.htm. Accessed January 31, 2008.

Index

Abductor pollicis brevis (APB), 89
ACE inhibitors, 6
Acetaminophen, 18, 253, 275, 322, 328–329
  FMS, 155
Acetaminophen and caffeine combinations,
  130
Acetylcholine-esterase (AChE), 126
Acetyl-L-carnitine (ALC), 6, 20
Achilles tendonitis, 93
Acromegaly, 85
Actiq, 348, 351
Active loci, 123
Active MTRP, 124
Acupuncture, 5, 19
  compression neuropathies, 99
  FMS, 162
  for neuropathic pain, 224
  osteoarthritis, 322
  PHN, 44
  PLP, 57
Acute bacterial prostatitis, 242
Acyclovir, 35
Addiction, 352
Adjuvant medications, 327
ALADIN III (Alpha-Lipoic Acid in Diabetic
  Neuropathy) study, 7
Alcoholism, 85
Aldose reductase inhibitors, 6–7
Allodynia, 24, 31, 53, 104, 155
  compression neuropathies, 85
  CRPS, 65, 72
  tremor of, 71
α-Adrenergic blockers, 252
Amitriptyline, 7, 20, 25, 392
  cancer pain, 278
  IC, 233
  MPS, 131–132
  phantom limb pain (PLP), 55–56
  PHN, 35, 38

AMPA (alpha-amino-3-hydroxy-5-methyl-4-
  isoxazole propionic acid) receptor,
  343
Amputations, 50
Amyloidosis, 85
Anaprox, 130
Anesthetic/steroid injections, 92
Annular tears, 215
Anorexia, 31
Anterior interosseous nerve (AIN) syndrome,
  90–91
Anthranilic acid, 330
Antiarrhythmics, 336
Anticancer therapies. *See* Cancer pain
Anticonvulsant medications (ACMs)
  clinical actions promoting, 398
  commonly used, 398
  Food and Drug Administration
    (FDA)-approved, 397
  mechanism of action, 397
  and suicidality, 403
Antidepressant medications (ADMs), 131
  FMS, 156
Antiepileptic drugs (AEDs), 8–9, 194
Antiretroviral toxic neuropathy (ATN), 15
  treatment, 20
Antiviral medications
  PHN, 34
Anxiety, 10
APAP, 327–328
Aplastic anemia, 399
Arsenic poisoning, 88
Arthritis, 318
Aspirin, 130, 253, 328
Aspirin, acetaminophen (APAP), 327
Aspirin-caffeine combination drugs (Anacin),
  130
Aspirin/diethyl ether, 41
ATC medications, 351

Attachment TRP, 125
Axillary radial nerve palsy, 91

Bacillus Calmette-Guerin (BCG), 235
Baclofen, 337
Barotraumas, 305
Benzodiazepines, 194
Bicycle-related injuries, 87
Biofeedback-assisted relaxation training, for
       PLP, 58
Biopsies, 96
Bisphosphonates, 280–281
Black box warning, 395
BoNT/A, 235
Brachial plexus, 314–315
   gliding and irritability of, 313
Breakthrough medication, 291
Breakthrough pain, 274, 288, 291
Brivudine, 35
Bupropion, 394

Calcitonin-gene–related peptide (CGRP), 65,
       125
Cancer pain
   consequences of inadequate relief, 271
   constipation problem, 277
   pathophysiology, 272–274
   screening, 271
      assessment tools, 272
   sedation, 277
   treatment
      adjuvant analgesics, 278–280
      anticancer therapies, 280–281
      interventional therapies, 281
      nonopioids, 275
      nonpharmacological therapies, 281
      opioids, 275–278
      pharmacological, 275
      routes of drug administration useful in,
         276
Cannabinoid system, 329
Cannabis, 19
Capsaicin patch, 19
Capsaicin (trans-8-methyl-N-vanillyl-6-
       nonenamide), 20, 40–41,
       338
Carbamazepine, 194, 278, 399
Carisoprodol, 131, 194, 332–333
Carpal tunnel syndrome (CTS), 85, 90
Cauda equina syndrome, 92
Causalgia, 105

Celecoxib, 131, 332
Central poststroke pain (CPSP) syndrome
   diagnosis, 23–24
   disinhibition hypothesis of, 24
   epileptiform discharges, 25
   evaluation of, 23–24
   imaging studies, 24
   incidence of, 23
   lesions, 24
   pain, 23–24
   pathophysiology, 24–25
   sensory abnormalities, 23
   treatment, 25–26
Central sensitivity, 153
Central sensitization, 127
C fibers
   and activation of NMDA receptors,
      152–153
   and capsaicin, 338
   CRPS, 65
   IC, 230–231
   loss in low back pain, 208
   N-TOS, 312, 314, 319
   unmyelinated, 4, 127, 189, 214
Charcot arthropathy, 2
Chemotherapy-induced painful peripheral
       neuropathies, 273–274
Chiropractics, 162
Chlorzoxazone, 131, 194, 333
Chronic bacterial prostatitis, 242
Chronic LBP (cLBP), 181, 190
Chronic noncancer pain (CNCP), treatment
   and neuroglial communications, 359
   and p38 MAPK activation, 359
   sexual dimorphism, 359–360
   "Universal Precautions" in pain medicine,
      354
   urine or blood tests, 353
   use of opioids, 344
      barriers, 360–361
      chronic, 354–355
      and tolerance, 356–359
Chronic opioid therapy (COT), 367
Chronic pain syndromes
   autonomic dysfunction in neuropathic
      pain, 105
   clinical assessment of neuropathic pain,
      102–104
   quantitative sensory testing (QST), 104–105
   quantitative sympathetic sudomotor
      testing, 106

selective tissue conductance (STC)
  technology, 106–107
  peripheral quantitative STC
    measurement, 107–108
  staging system, 108–111
Chronic pelvic pain (CPP), female
  causes of pain, 261
  diagnosis, 262–263
    laboratory studies, 262–263
    pelvic laparoscopic evaluation, 263
    physical examination, 262–263
    previous accidents or surgeries, role of,
      262
  pathophysiology
    causes, 264–265
    pelvic pain, 263
  psychosocial ramifications of, 261–262
  symptoms, 263
  treatment, 265–268
    algorithm, 266
Chronic pelvic pain syndrome (CPPS). *See*
      Chronic prostatitis (CP)
Chronic prostatitis (CP)
  definition, 242
  diagnosis
    anal sphincter electromyography and/or
      sphincter function profiles, 248
    cystoscopy, 248
    diagnostic office procedures, 246–248
    differential, 244
    digital rectal examination, 243
    evaluation of CCPS/CP, 244–245
    formal flow rate studies, 248
    impact of symptoms, 243
    laboratory evaluation, 245
    pain symptoms, 243
    physical findings, 243–244
    prostatic massage, 246–247
    quality of life, 243
    radiographic studies, 245
    third voided midstream urine specimen,
      247
    urinary symptoms, 243
    videourodynamic evaluation, 247–248
  diet for, 254–255
  outpatient care, 255
  pain management, 253
  pathophysiology
    cytokine activity, 248
    E. coli infection, 250
    occult bacteria, 249

propionibacterium acnes, 249–250
    role for fastidious bacteria, 249
  sexual dysfunctions, 244–245
  specialist consultation for
    andrology, 253–254
    pain, 253
    physical medicine, 254
    psychiatry, 253
  treatment
    antibiotics, 251–252
    challenges, 257–258
    evidence-based, 256–258
    muscle relaxants, 252
    prostatic massage (therapeutic), 250
    psychotropic medications, 253
    sitz baths, 251
    surgery, 252–253
    therapeutic ejaculation, 250
Chronic Prostatitis Symptom Index, 243
Cimetidine, 234
Ciprofloxacin, 251
Clomipramine, 7
Clonazepam, 131, 194, 400
Clonidine, 335
CNS plasticity, 344
Codeine, 327, 345
Cognitive behavioral therapy, 162
  cancer pain, 281
Cognitive dysfunction, 160
Cold Intolerance, 160
Combination therapy, PHN, 41
Compensatory pain, related to phantom
      sensations, 50
Complex regional pain syndrome (CRPS) I
      and II, 307
  autonomic dysregulation and edema, 68
  cortical reorganization, 71–72
  IASP criteria of, 62
  laboratory tests
    peripheral vasoconstrictor reflex, 63
    radiographic manifestations, 63
    skin temperature, 63
    sudomotor function tests, 64
    triple-phase bone scan technique, 64
  movement disorder of, 70–71
  neurogenic edema, 68–69
  pathophysiology, 64–66
  role of sympathetic nervous system in the
      pain, 67–68
  sickness response, 66–67
  signs and symptoms, 62–63

Complex regional pain syndrome (CRPS) I
  and II (*Cont.*)
  sympathetically maintained pain, 69–70
  treatment, 72
Compression neuropathies
  axonal degeneration, 96
  diagnosis
    autonomic studies, 95
    cardiovascular testing, 95
    cervical and spinal roots, 88
    cervical roots, 88–89
    cranial nerves, 88
    electrodiagnosis, 95
    laboratory studies, 95
    lumbosacral plexus compressive
      neuropathies, 92–94
    median nerve entrapment syndromes,
      90–91
    nerve biopsy, 96
    past medical history, 87
    physical examination, 88
    polyneuropathies, 95
    radial nerve entrapment syndromes,
      91–92
    radiculopathies, 95
    radiologic studies, 96
    thermography, 96
    thoracic outlet syndrome, 89
    ulnar nerve entrapment syndromes, 91
  epidemiology, 85–86
  etiology, 86–87
  healing process from peripheral nerve
    trauma, 97
  pathophysiology, 96–97
  symptoms, 85
  treatment, 97–99
  vascularity in, 85
Conductance, 107
Constipation, 94
Contraction knots, 123, 125
Convergence-facilitation, 127
Convergence-projection, 127
Corneal confocal microscopy, 3
Corticosteroids, 278–279, 337
  PHN, 35
COX-2 inhibitors, 327, 330
C-peptide deficiencies, 4
Cryotherapy, 142
C8–T1 innervated muscles, 89
Cyclic pelvic pain, 267
Cyclobenzaprine, 157, 194

Cyclooxygenase (COX), 327
Cyclooxygenase-2 inhibitors (Cox-2)
  FMS, 155
Cystometrography, 248
Cytochrome P450 system, 331

D3 agonist, 159
DdC (zalcitabine), 16
DdI (didanosine), 16
"D" drugs, 16
Deep brain stimulation (DBS), 26
Deep peroneal nerve entrapment (anterior
    tibial nerve), 93–94
Depression, 10
Desensitization techniques, PLP, 57
Desipramine, 7, 38, 392
Dexamethasone, 278
DEXA scanning, 96
Dextromethorphan, 56–57
DHEA (dehydroepiandrosterone), 159
DH neurons, 64–65
Diabetes, 1
Diabetes mellitus, 85
Diabetic peripheral neuropathy (DPN), 1, 108
  diagnosis of
    corneal confocal microscopy, 3
    general examination of feet, 2
    nerve conduction velocity (NCV) tests, 3
    neuropathic pain scales, 2–3
    testing methods, 2
    thermal thresholds, 3
  pain, 1
  pathophysiology of
    hyperglycemia, 3–4
    metabolic abnormalities, 4
    progression of disease, 4
  sensory abnormalities in feet or hands, 2
  sweating, 2
  treatment
    nonpharmacological, 5
    pharmacological, 6–10
    prevention of progression, 4–5
    surgery, 11
Diabetic peripheral sensory polyneuropathy,
  1
Diazepam, 253
Diclofenac, 332
Diclofenac/diethyl ether mixtures, 41
Diffuse hyperhidrosis (STC stage II), 109
Diffuse hypohidrosis (STC stage IV), 110–111
Dihydrocodeine, 327

Dimethylsulfoxide (DMSO), 234
Discography, 189
Disk prolapse, 215–216
Distal hyperhidrosis (STC stage I), 108
Distal hypohidrosis (STC stage III), 109–110
Distal reference peak (DRP), 108
Distal sensory polyneuropathy (DSP), 15
  antiretroviral-related, 17
  biopsies for, 17
  epidermal nerve fiber density in, 17
  and glycoprotein gp120, 17
  knee jerks in, 16
  laboratory evaluation in, 16
  mitochondrial abnormalities, 17
  neuropathologic changes of the dorsal root
    ganglia, 17
  pathogenesis of, 17
Distal symmetrical polyneuropathy, 17–20
Divalproex sodium, 400
Dorsal forefoot nerve entrapment, 93
Dorsal root ganglion blocks treatment, of
    PHN, 43
Doxepin, 392
D4T (stavudine), 16
Dualism theory, 51
Duloxetine, 8, 39, 131, 195, 278, 394
Duragesic transdermal therapeutic system,
    347–348
Dysautonomia, 160
Dysesthesia, 85
Dyspnea, 360

Eicosanoid system, 328
Electrical injury
  diagnosis, 301–303
  nonthermal mechanisms of, 301
  pathophysiology
    chronic pain in survivors, 306–308
    electrical energy transport in tissues, 303
    electrical injury pattern, 305–306
    electroconformational denaturation,
      304–305
    membrane electroporation, 304–305
    thermal burn injury, 303–304
  treatment, 308–309
Electrical stimulation (E-Stim), for MPS, 133
Electroacupuncture, 20
Electroconformational denaturation, 304–305
Electromyography, 95, 302
Electroporation, of skeletal muscle tissue, 304
Endoneural edema, 189

Enthesitis, 125
Enthesopathy, 125
Entrapment neuropathy, 211–213
Environmental impact record, 255
Epidural adhesions, 217
Ergonomics, for compression neuropathies,
    98
Etodolac, 332
Eutectic mixture of local anesthetic (EMLA
    cream), 336
Evidence based treatment
  chronic prostatitis (CP), 256–258
  fibromyalgia syndrome (FMS), 154–163
  myofascial pain syndrome (MPS), 134–135
Excitatory amino acids (EAAs), 338

Facet joint injections, 198–199
False L5-S1 pain syndrome. *See* Piriformis
    syndrome
Famciclovir, 35
Fatigue, 31, 88, 160
Fentanyl, 288, 327
Fentanyl patch, 288
Fentanyl percutaneous patches (Duragesic),
    155
Fentora, 348
Fibromyalgia, 154
Fibromyalgia fog, 146
Fibromyalgia Impact Questionnaire (FIQ),
    158
Fibromyalgia syndrome (FMS)
  ACR's classification criteria, 147
  activation of NMDA receptors, 152
  autonomic nervous system abnormalities,
    149
  brain imaging techniques, 148
  central pain processing abnormalities, 149
  central sensitization, 151–153
  clinical changes, 149
  definition, 144
  diagnosis of, 145–148
  functional cerebral abnormalities, 150
  hormonal differences, 148
  juvenile forms, 145
  and MPS, 153–154
  neurochemical abnormalities, 150
  neuroendocrine abnormalities, 150
  pathophysiology of, 148–154
  prevalence, 145
  psychological abnormalities, 149
  psychological distress, 146

Fibromyalgia syndrome (FMS) (*Cont.*)
  psychophysiological evidence of
      hyperalgesia, 148
  significant gender difference, 147
  symptoms associated, 146
  treatment, 154–163
    nonpharmacological management,
        160–163
    nonsteroidal anti-inflammatory drugs
        (NSAIDs), 155
Foot care advice, 5
Foot ulcers, 1
Foraminal stenosis, 216
Foscarnet, 35

Gabapentin, 9, 18, 20, 25
  as anticonvulsant for neuropathic pain,
      400
  as antidepressants, 401
  cancer pain, 278
  Chung model, 401
  IC, 234
  LFCN, 84
  phantom limb pain (PLP), 56
  PHN, 35–36, 38
  spinal pain, 194
  tolerance, 401
Gene regulatory abnormalities, 4
Genetic predisposition, to CP/CPPS, 249
Glucose metabolization, in hyperglycemia,
      3–4
Glutamate, 343
Glycosylation of tissue and plasma proteins, 3
Gonadotropin-releasing hormone agonist
      therapy, 267
Gray rami communicantes, 106
Guillain–Barré syndrome, 87

Healing touch, 19
Hereditary neuropathy with liability to
      pressure palsies (HNPP), 86
Herpes zoster vaccine, 34
Highly active antiretroviral therapy
      (HAART), 15
Hindlimb ischemia, 67
HIV/AIDS neuropathy
  diagnosis, 15–17
  forms, 15
  middle and late stages of, 15
  pathophysiology, 17
  treatment, 17–20

HMG-CoA reductase inhibitors (statins),
      6
Hydrocodone, 327, 345
Hydrodistention, 236
Hydromorphone, 288, 327
Hydroxyzine, 233–234
Hyperalgesia, 31, 66, 127
Hyperesthesia, 85, 104
Hyperglycemia, 3–4
Hypertriglyceridemia, 6
Hypothyroidism, 87

Ibuprofen, 130, 253, 330–331
Imipramine, 7, 392
Indoleacetic acids, 330
Indomethacin, 41, 332
Insomnia, 31
Insulin deficiencies, 4
Interleukin 1 and 6, 125
Interleukin-8 concentration
  PHN, 42
Interstitial cystitis (IC)
  ATP levels, 231
  bladder's mucosal lining in, 232
  classification, 228–229
  diagnosis of, 229–230
    bladder hydrodistention, 230
    cystoscopy, 230
    evaluation of the bladder as a "pain
        generator," 230–231
    potassium sensitivity test, 230
    urinary markers, 231
  neural inflammation/upregulation,
      231–232
  pathogenesis, 231–232
  symptoms, 231
  treatment
    conservative therapy, 232–233
    intravesical therapy, 234–235
    management strategies, 232
    medical therapy, 233–234
    role of urinary diversion, 237
    surgery, 235–237
Intrathecal (IT) morphine, 360
Intrathecal steroid injections, 42
Invasive interventions, for PHN, 35–36
Iontophoresis, for MPS, 133
Ipsilateral Achilles reflex, 142
Irritable bowel syndrome, 265
Ischemic nerve injury, 83
Isosorbide dinitrate, 9

Japanese acupuncture, 133
Joule heating, 303–304

Kadian, 347
K channels, 305
Ketamine, 56, 279–280, 294, 334–336
Ketamine coma, 72
Ketoprofen, 130, 330–332
Ketorolac, 131, 332
Ketorolac Tromethamine, 331
Key MTRP, 125

Lamotrigine, 18, 25, 278
Latent MTRP, 124
Lateral femoral cutaneous nerve (LFCN),
    92–93
  anatomy, 81–82
  pathophysiology, 83
  symptoms, 81–83
  treatment, 83–84
Laws governing, medications for pain
    management
  background, 367–368
  federal level
    Code of Federal Regulations, 370–372
    Controlled Substances Act of 1970 (CSA),
      369–370
    DEA Policy Statements, 372–375
    substantive legal standards, 375–376
  Federation of State Medical Boards' Model
    policy, 376–378
  informed consent and the agreement for
    treatment, 380–382
  integration of law and medicine, 368–369
  medical records, 384–386
  patient evaluation and risk assessment,
    378–380
  periodic review and risk monitoring,
    382–384
  state level, 376
  treatment plan, 380
  use of consultations and referrals, 384
Leeds Assessment of Neuropathic Symptoms
    and Signs (LANSS) Pain Scale, 2
Leprosy, 85
Leukopenia, 280
Levetiracetam, 278
Levofloxacin, 251
Levorphanol, 327
Lidocaine, 9, 20, 293–294, 336
  gel, 19

injection, 26, 156
  patch, 336
Lidoderm patch, 40
Linear gradient method, 108
Lipid-lowering agents, 6
A-lipoic acid, 7
Long-term depression (LTD), 65–66
Long-term potentiation (LTP), 65–66
Lorcet, 350
Low back pain (LBP). *See also* Spinal pain
  definition, 181
  neuropathic
    diagnosis, 208
    drug treatment of neuropathic low back
      pain, 222–223
    Dworkin's recommendations, 221
    pathophysiology, 209–218
    treatment, 218–224
Lower limb amputation, risk of, 1
L-tryptophan, 159
Lumbar epidural spinal injections (LESIs),
    199–201
Lumbar facet arthropathy, 217
Lumbosacral plexus compressive
    neuropathies, 92–94
Lyme disease, 87

Massage therapy, 99
McGill Pain Questionnaire, 103–104
McKenzie approach, for neuropathic pain,
    224
Medial branch blocks, 199
Mees' nail lines, 88
Memantine, 18–19, 56–57, 334
Membrane electroporation, 304–305
Meperidine, 289, 346
Meralgia paresthetica, 81, 92–93
  symptoms of, 81
Metaxalone, 131, 194, 333
Methadone, 56, 221, 288–289, 327
Methocarbamol, 131, 194, 333
Methylnaltrexone, 277
Mexiletine, 20, 336
Milnacipran, 158, 394
Mirror therapy, PLP, 57–58
Mirtazapine, 158, 395
  phantom limb pain (PLP), 55
Mononeuritis multiplex, 85
Morphine, 287–288, 346
Morphine-3-glucuronide, 288
Morphine-6-glucunoride, 288

Morton's neuroma, 85, 94
Motor abnormalities, in PHN, 31
Movement disorder, of CRPS, 70–71
Multiple crush syndrome, 312
Muscle compartment syndromes, 87
Muscle relaxants, 131, 332–334
Muscle spasmolytics, 193–194
Muscular biopsy, 94
Musculoskeletal anatomy, 209
Myelography, 187
Myoclonus, 71, 278
Myofascial pain syndrome (MPS), 215
    definition, 115
    diagnosis, 117–122
        cervical range of motion (ROM), 117
        correct, 117
        differential, 119–120
        endocrine problems associated with
            myofascial pain, 120–121
        perpetuating factors, 121–122
        TRP examination, 118–119
        vs fibromyalgia syndrome (FMS), 117
    due to trigger points, 116
    onset, 116
    pain, 116
    pathophysiology
        analysis of LTR, 123
        clinical diagnostic criteria of an MTRP,
            123–125
        packets of ACh, 122
        sympathetically maintained pain,
            127–128
        sympathetic aspects, 127
        trigger point (TRP) hypothesis, 125–126
    treatment
        conservative care, 129–130
        evidence-based, 134–135
        medications, 130–132
        physical therapy, 133–134
        psychological therapy, 134
        TPI therapy and interventional
            treatment, 132–133
Myofascial trigger points (MTRPs), 115–116,
    147
Myogelosis, 122
Myoinositol, 4
Myxedema, 85

Nabumetone, 332
N-acetyl-para-amino-phenol (APAP), 328
Na channels, 305

Na^+/K^+-ATPase, 4
Naloxone, 329
Naloxone injection, 26
Naphthylalkanone, 330
Naproxen, 332
Naproxen sodium, 330
Narcotics, 348–352
Needle electromyography, 16
Nerve biopsy, 17
Nerve conduction latency, 95
Nerve conduction velocity (NCV) tests, 3
Nerve entrapment syndromes, 87
Neural anatomy, 210–211
Neuraxial blocks treatment, of PHN, 42–43
Neurogenic thoracic outlet syndrome
        (N-TOS)
    biopsychosocial approach for, 312
    definition, 312
    diagnosis of, 312
        physical and neurological examination,
            313–314
        tests, 314
    EMG/NCS findings, 316
    pathophysiology
        anatomy-etiology, 314–315
        symptoms, 315
    treatment, 316–317
Neuromas, 52
Neuromuscular disease, 125
Neuromuscular Junction, 122
Neuronal plasticity, 344
Neuropathic discogenic pain, 213
Neuropathic medications, 220–221
Neuropathic pain (NP), 184, 293
    autonomic dysfunction in, 105
    7 clinical assessment of, 102–104
    definition, 206
    syndromes, 105
Neuropathic Pain Scale, 2
Neuropathy, 1
NIH prostatitis type III, 242
NMDA antagonists
    PHN, 41
N-methyl-d-aspartate (NMDA) inhibitor, 288,
    327
N-methyl-d-aspartate (NMDA) receptor, 343
Noninvasive, quantitative neurophysiological
        method, 106–107
Norepinephrine–dopamine reuptake
        inhibitor, 394–395
Norepinephrine (NEP), 125

Norepinephrine/serotonin reuptake inhibitors (NSRIs), 131, 393–394
Normal result (stage N), 108
Nortriptyline, 7, 38
NSAIDs, 18, 130–131
  cancer pain, 275
  combinations with analgesia, 328
  FMS, 155
  frequently prescribed, 330–331
  low back pain, 220
  OA, 331–332
  osteoarthritis, 321–322
  palliative care, 292–293
  and risk of GI toxicity, 331
  side effects, 327–328, 331
  spinal pain, 193
  types of, 330
Nucleoside reverse transcriptase inhibitors (NRTIs), 15
Number needed to harm (NNH), 344

Obesity, 10
Opioid medications
  spinal pain, 195
Opioid rotation, 289
Opioids, 9, 221, 322, 344
  phantom limb pain (PLP), 56
  PHN, 39–40
  strong, 346–348
  weak, 345–346
Opioid system, 329
Orphenadrine, 131
Orphenadrine citrate, 333–334
Osteoarthritis (OA), 146
  definition, 318
  diagnosis, 318–320
  pathophysiology, 320
  treatment, 321–324
Ovarian cysts, 264
Oxaprozin, 332
Oxcarbazepine, 399
Oxicam, 330
Oxidative stress, 4
Oxycodone, 39, 289, 327, 345–346
OxyContin, 155, 345
Oxymorphone, 348

Paget's disease, 87
Pain. *See also specific pain*
  bone, 293
  chronic spine-related, 190, 214–215
  generalized musculoskeletal, 145
  lumbosacral radicular, 189
  management. *See* Palliative care
  myofascial pain syndrome (MPS), 116
  myofascial trigger points (MTRPs), 116
  related to bowel obstruction, 293
  spatial characteristics of, 102
  sympathetically maintained, 127–128
    and the MPS, 128–129
Pain drawing, 103
Pain region, 103
Pain transmission neurons (PTNs), 64
Palliative care
  adjuvant analgesics, 293
  breakthrough medication, 291
  care setting, 286–287
  continuous *vs* as-needed analgesia, 291
  dosing and titration, 290
  interventional strategies, 294
  nonpharmacologic approaches to pain management, 294
  NSAIDs, 292–293
  opioid rotation, 290
  pain assessment in advanced disease, 287
  pain management, 285
  palliative sedation, 294–295
  pharmacotherapeutic approaches for refractory pain, 293–294
  pharmacotherapy, 287–289
  prevalence of pain related to cancer, 285–286
  route of administration, 290
  side effects management, 291–292
Palliative chemotherapy, 280
Palliative sedation, 294–295
Paresthesia, 85
Patient Global Impression of Change (PGIC), 158
Paxil, 131
Pelvic floor pain dysfunction, 265
Pelvic inflammatory disease, 264
Pelvic pain syndrome, 94
Pelvic varicosities, 265
Pentosan polysulfate sodium (PPS), 233
Percocet, 350
Perineal pain syndromes, 264–265
Peripheral nerve blocks treatment, of PHN, 43
Peripheral nervous system, 213–214
Peripheral neuropathy syndrome, in HIV-infected patients, 15–16
Peripheral vasoconstrictor reflex, 63

Peroneal neuropathy, 93
Phantom limb pain (PLP)
  cortical reorganization, 54
  definitions, 51–52
  history, 51
  incidence of, 50–51
  pathophysiology, 53–54
  peripheral and central changes, 53–54
  residual limb pain (RLP), 52–53
  treatment
    nonpharmacologic approaches, 57–58
    pharmacologic approaches, 55–57
Phantom pain, 51
Phantom sensation, 51
Phenylacetic acid, 330
Phenytoin, 399
Phonophoresis, for MPS, 133
Phosphokinase A, 64
Phosphokinase C, 64
Physical dependence, 352
Physical therapy
  compression neuropathies, 98
  FMS, 161
  spinal pain, 196–198
Piriformis muscle, 141
Piriformis syndrome, 217–218
  diagnosis, 140–142
  imaging studies, 140
  manual muscle test, 141
  neurologic examination, 142
  pathophysiology, 142
  physical examination, 141
  physical therapy, 142–143
  treatment, 142–143
Plasmapheresis and intravenous gamma
    globulin, combination therapy, 20
Podiatrist evaluation, 20
Polyneuropathies, 95
Polypharmacy, 10
Popliteal artery entrapment, 87
Posterior interosseous nerve syndrome, 91
Postherpetic neuralgia (PHN), 401
  definition, 30
  diagnosis, 31–32
  laboratory tests, 32
  pain, 31
  pathophysiology, 32–33
  prevention strategies, 30
  risk factors, 33
  sensitization, 32
  signs, 31

symptoms, 31
treatment
  acupuncture, 44
  clinical, 36–41
  combination therapy, 41
  invasive interventional strategies, 42–43
  NMDA antagonists, 41
  prevention strategies, 34–36
  topical, 41
  transcutaneous electrical nerve
    stimulation (TENS) therapy, 44
Post-polio syndrome, 87, 94
Posttraumatic piriformis syndrome, 142
Potassium citrate (Urocit K), 255
Pregabalin, 9, 18, 402–403
  PHN, 35–36, 38
  spinal pain, 194
Primary MTRP, 125
Pronator syndrome, 90
Propionibacterium acnes, 249–250
Propionic acids, 330
Propoxyphene, 346
Prosaptide, 19
Prostate cancer, 245
Prostatodynia. *See* Chronic prostatitis (CP)
Protease inhibitors, 16
Protein kinase C (PKC) inhibitors, 338
Prozac, 131
Pruritis, 292
Pruritus, 31
Pseudoaddiction, 352
Pudendal neuropathy, 94
Pyrazolone, 330
Pyrroleacetic acid, 330

QTc interval, 289
Quantitative sensory testing (QST), 104–105
Quantitative sympathetic sudomotor testing,
    106

Radial nerve entrapment syndromes, 91–92
Radiculopathies, 95
Radiofrequency (RF) neurotomy, 199
Radiotherapy, 280
Referred pain, 218
Reflex sympathetic dystrophy, 105
Relaxation, for MPS, 134
Repetitive supination motion injury, 91
Residual limb pain (RLP), 52–53
Respiratory depression, 292
Restless legs syndrome, 159–160

Rheumatoid arthritis, 85, 146
Roxicodone, 351

Sacral neuromodulation, 236
S-adenosylmethionine, 159
Salicylic acids, 330
Samarium-153, 280
Sarcoidosis, 85
Sarcolemma, 122
Satellite MTRP, 125
Sciatica, 92. *See also* Spinal pain
    definition, 182
Sciatic neuropathy, 92
Secretion of antidiuretic hormone (SIADH), 8
Selective norepinephrine and serotonin
    reuptake inhibitors (SNRI), 157–158
Selective serotonin reuptake inhibitors (SSRI)
    antidepressants, 131, 392–395
    FMS, 157
    low back pain, neuropathic, 220
    PHN, 39
    spinal pain, 195
Selective tissue conductance (STC)
    technology, 106–111
Semmes-Weinstein monofilament, 2
Sensations related to amputation, 50
Sensory abnormalities, 104
Sensory dermatomes, 103
Serotonergic system, 328
Serotonin 5-HT3 receptor antagonists, 277
Serotonin norepinephrine reuptake inhibitors
    (SNRIs), 8
Serotonin syndrome, 346
Silastic sweat imprint method, 106
Sjögren's syndrome, 146
Skin biopsy, 17
Skin discoloration, in PHN, 31
Small-fiber neuropathies, 85
Smoking cessation, 10
Sodium channel blockers, 9
Soft-tissue treatment (STT), for MPS,
    133–134
Sorbitol accumulation, 3
Spatial selectivity, 107
Sphenopalatine blocks, 159
Spinal canal stenosis, 216
Spinal cord, 214
Spinal cord stimulation (SCS) treatment, 5,
    201
    of PHN, 43
Spinal nociceptive model, 190

Spinal pain, 181–182
    diagnostic strategies, 187–189
    interviewing a patient with, 184
    mechanical *vs* nonmechanical, 183
    pathophysiology, 189–191
    physical examination, 185–187
    spinal lesion, 183–184
    treatment
        algorithm for management of low back
            pain and sciatica, 188
        bed rest, 192
        facet joint injections, 198–199
        intradiscal electrothermal therapy
            (IDET), 201
        lumbar epidural spinal injections
            (LESIs), 199–201
        oral pharmacology, 193–195
        physical therapy, 196–198
        spinal cord stimulation (SCS), 201
        therapeutic spinal interventional
            techniques, 198
Spondylolisthesis, 216–217
Spondylolysis, 217
Spontaneous electrical activity (SEA),
    123
Stimulus-evoked pain, in PHN, 31
Stimulus-independent pain, in PHN, 31
Strengthening, for MPS, 134
Stretching, for MPS, 133
Stretch injury, 315
Strontium-89, 280
Sudomotor dysfunctions, 106
Sudomotor function tests, 64
Sudomotor pathways, 106
Suprascapular nerve entrapment, 88–89
Sural nerve entrapment, 93
Surgery
    chronic prostatitis (CP), 252–253
    CPP, 268
    diabetic peripheral neuropathy (DPN), 11
    interstitial cystitis (IC), 235–237
    neurogenic thoracic outlet syndrome
        (N-TOS), 316–317
    PHN, 43
    piriformis syndrome, 142–143
    posterior interosseous nerve syndrome, 92
SYDNEY 2 (Symptomatic Diabetic
    Neuropathy 2) trial, 7
Sympathetic nerve blocks, treatment, 42
Syphilis, 16
Systemic lupus erythematosus, 146

Tarlov's cysts, 216
Tarsal tunnel syndrome, 93
Taurin, 4
Taut band, 122
TCA medication, 131
Temporal selectivity, 107
Tender point index (TPI), 147
FMS, 144, 146
Tennis-related injuries, 87
Tetrazepam, 194
Therapeutic injections, 198
Thermal burn injury, 303–304
Thermal pain, 105
Thermal sensation, pure thresholds of, 105
Thermography, 96
Thermoregulatory sweat test, 106
Thoracic outlet syndrome (TOS), 86
Thrombocytopenia, 280
Tiagabine, 278
Tinnel sign, 11, 81, 92
Tizanidine, 131, 194, 334
Tolerance, 352
Topical preparations, of local anesthetics, 336
Topiramate, 195, 278, 400
Tramadol, 9, 19, 220, 327, 335–336, 346
   FMS, 155
   PHN, 40
Transcranial magnetic stimulation (TMS), 5
Transcutaneous electrical nerve stimulation
      (TENS), 5, 26, 44, 134
Transitional cell cancer, 245
Transitional (STC stage T) results, 108
Transurethral resection of the prostate
      (TURP), 252
Transurethral resections (TURs), 236–237
Tricyclic antidepressants (TCAs), 7–8, 18,
      131–132, 195
   adverse effects of, 391
   CPP, 267
   FMS, 156–157
   LFCN, 84

pain relief, 391
phantom limb pain (PLP), 55
PHN, 38–39
topiramate, 84
Trimethoprim–sulfamethoxazole, 251–252
Triple-phase bone scan technique, 64
TRPVI (vanilloid) receptors, 338
Tumor necrosis factor-α, 125

Ulcers, 1
Ulnar nerve entrapment at the wrist, 91
Ulnar nerve entrapment syndromes, 91
Ulnar neuropathy, 85
   at the elbow, 91
Ultracet, 346
Ultram, 350
Unmyelinated fiber abnormalities, 4
Urinary diversion technique, 237
Uterine leiomyoma, 264

Valacyclovir, 35
Valproic acid, 399
Vanilloid receptor (TRPV1), 40
Varicella vaccination, 34
Venlafaxine, 131, 157, 195, 220, 394
Venlafaxine ER, 8
Vibration testing, 2
Vicodin, 350
Videourodynamic evaluation, for CP, 247–248
Vincristine, 41
Vistaril, 335
Visual Analog Scale, 20, 103
Vitamin antioxidants, 308
Voiding diary, 255

"Walking man," 103
Weight loss, 31

Zoloft, 131
"Zone of reference," 124
Zonisamide, 278